AESTHETIC RHINOPLASTY

AESTHETIC RHINOPLASTY

Jack H. Sheen, M.D.

Assistant Clinical Professor,
Department of Surgery, Division of Plastic Surgery,
U.C.L.A. School of Medicine,
Los Angeles, California

with
Anitra Peebles Sheen

Medical illustrator
Hermene Kavanau

1080 illustrations

The C. V. Mosby Company

Saint Louis 1978

SECOND PRINTING

Printed in the United States of America

The C. V. Mosby Company
11830 Westline Industrial Drive, St. Louis, Missouri 63141

Library of Congress Cataloging in Publication Data

Sheen, Jack H., 1925-
Aesthetic rhinoplasty.

Bibliography: p.
Includes index.
1. Rhinoplasty. I. Title.
RD119.5.N67S48 617'.523 78-27554
ISBN 0-8016-4575-1

GW/S/B 9 8 7 6

Preface

It is not my intention to chronicle, review, analyze, or otherwise evaluate the many known concepts and techniques in rhinoplasty. Nor is it my intention to present a complete and comprehensive treatise on the subject. In short, it is not my goal to write the definitive work on rhinoplasty. My intent is, very simply, to offer my personal approach to aesthetic rhinoplasty.

This approach has evolved by a process of selection from a pool of information provided by both predecessors and contemporaries and from my own countless hours of pondering, experimenting, and delving into the exciting problems of nasal surgery. And it continues to evolve. My purpose here is to explain my technique and its underlying rationale in a practical, useful way in the hope that it will not only contribute to the surgical capability of the practicing surgeon but will also contribute to the evolution of rhinoplasty in general.

To say I have a passion for rhinoplasty is not overstated. This passion sustains my work and is manifest in it. This does not mean my results are always good, only that I always invest great energy toward achieving good results.

Understanding that one person's passion is another person's trivia, rhinoplasty is considered by some to be a frivolous undertaking, unworthy of the physician's training or mission in life. Although that attitude may have some validity, I believe that a cavalier approach to rhinoplasty will certainly prevent the surgeon from accomplishing the best possible results, regardless of technique.

I consider this surgery to be not only a technical challenge, but more important, a challenge to one's aesthetic sensibilities and one's ability to appreciate the consequences of minute or subtle details. This keen consciousness of detail is the key to a great result in rhinoplasty.

A beautiful and natural-appearing nose is but one determinant of the excellent rhinoplastic result. The other determinant, of equal importance, is a nose that functions normally and well. Therefore, any discussion of rhinoplasty technique must involve nasal physiology and functionally related surgical anatomy.

By first discussing practical anatomy and physiology and aesthetic concepts, I wish to lay the foundation for the surgical methods and case analyses that follow. Because each aesthetic rhinoplasty is unique, basic principles and individual case review can guide the surgeon only so far, but my hope is that the clinical orientation of this work will provide light and clarity for what is essentially a very personal surgical journey.

Jack H. Sheen

Contents

AESTHETIC RHINOPLASTY

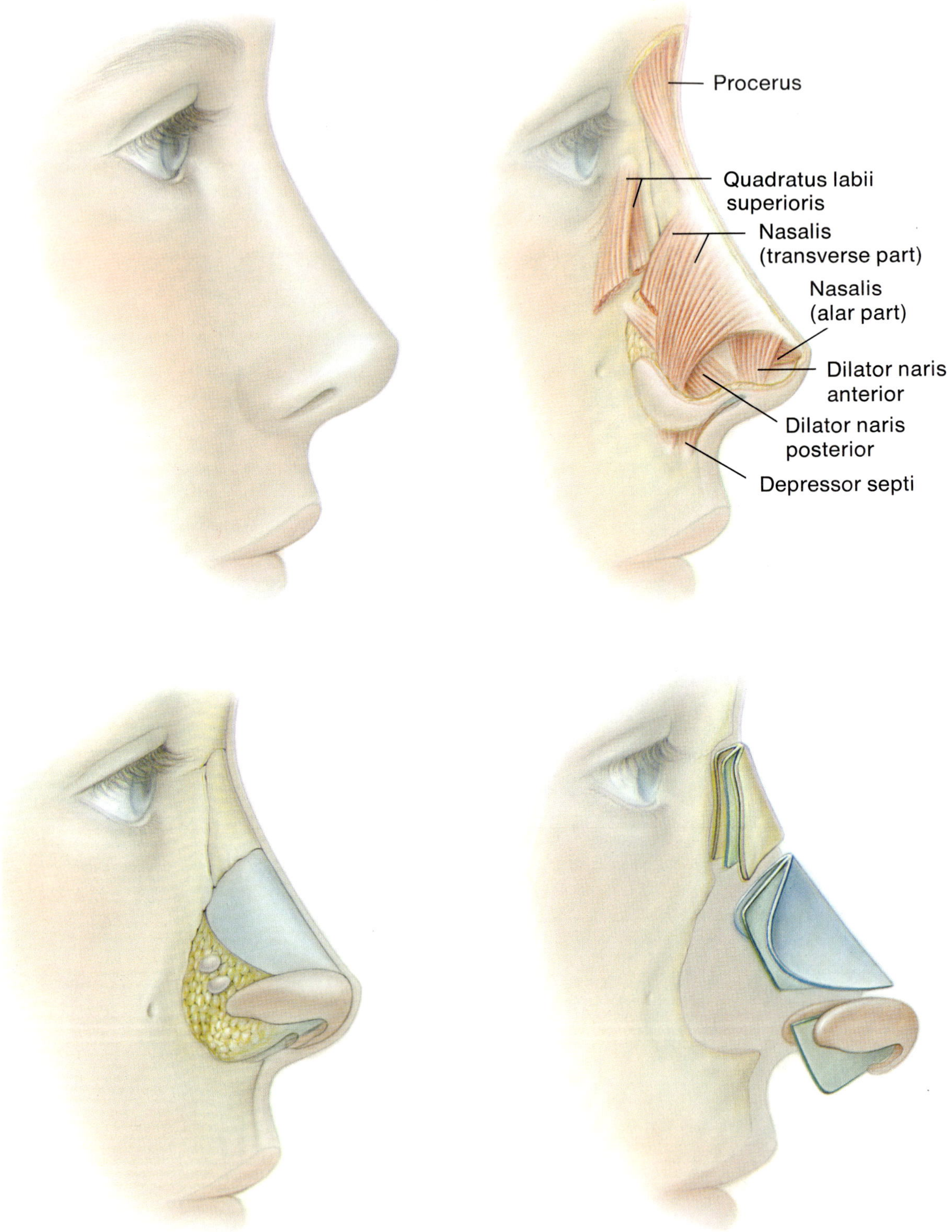
Procerus
Quadratus labii superioris
Nasalis (transverse part)
Nasalis (alar part)
Dilator naris anterior
Dilator naris posterior
Depressor septi

CHAPTER 1

Applied anatomy and physiology

Bony vault
Upper cartilaginous vault
Lower cartilaginous vault
Nasolabial angle
Nasal base
Nasal vestibule
Internal valve
Turbinates

Nasal physiology is too often thought of as an esoteric, kymographic science better suited to medical school laboratories than to the clinician's practice. The idea that nasal physiology is somehow separate from aesthetic rhinoplasty and therefore out of the domain of plastic surgery is frankly wrong. Plastic surgeons routinely change the relationships of nasal parts that are integral to proper nasal function. Because of surgeons' lack of appreciation of these critical relationships, many patients suffer permanent impairment of nasal function—a price too high to pay for a change in nasal contour.

The purpose of this chapter is to present essentials in anatomy and physiology that directly relate to nasal function and that constitute the premise from which all steps in rhinoplasty proceed. The purpose and effect of specific surgical alterations of the various compartments of the nose will be analyzed.

To appreciate the nose as a principal part of respiratory function, it is important to understand how and why it is that breathing through the nose is superior to breathing through the mouth. Superficially, breathing through the mouth would seem to be an easier and more efficient way of getting an optimal amount of air to the lower respiratory tract. But not so. Effortless, effective breathing with its accompanying sense of well-being can be achieved only through nasal respiration, which provides controlled, measured resistance in both the inspiratory and expiratory phases.

On deep inspiration the alar muscles, the alae, and the internal valve work in concert, producing a controlled increase in the resistance to airflow. The physiologic advantages of controlled, variable resistance provided by the nasal structures are as follows:

1. A slower nasal delivery of air against resistance affords a smooth, almost imperceptible change from the inspiratory to expiratory phase.
2. There is an increase in the *negative* intrathoracic pressure directly caused by the work necessary to overcome the resistance in the nose. This has the effect of sucking blood into the pulmonary venous system to aid the right side of the heart by decreasing its work load.

3. When the aperture is narrowed on deep inspiration, the air is spread into a sheet by the internal valve, improving distribution over all of the turbinate tissues for proper conditioning.
4. As the work of the respiratory muscles increases during respiration, the chest expands to a greater dimension (expiration does not occur until the alveoli are dilated), promoting better intercostal muscle tone, and improving the elasticity of the lung tissues, which must expand to the greater thoracic volume.
5. Increased resistance to expiration increases the interalveolar pressure, which improves oxygen absorption. It also extends the time the oxygen is exposed. It is well known that arterial PO_2 is higher during nose breathing than during mouth breathing.

A major disadvantage of mouth breathing is that it causes a bolus of air to be delivered to the alveoli. This bolus of air dilates the alveoli rapidly, triggering the expiratory phase (through the pulmonari vagi) without the slow buildup of pressure necessary to satisfactorily complete the optimum exchange of oxygen and carbon dioxide. Breathing under these circumstances tends to become shallow and jerky. Chronic mouth breathing may produce symptoms of headache, fatigue, and sinus problems. Moreover, many symptoms of the common cold can be attributed to a decrease in respiratory efficiency consequential of mouth breathing.

It is clear then that nasal breathing is physiologically superior to mouth breathing. Thus, it would follow that nasal parts that affect respiration must be treated with particular respect. The nasal components responsible for the control of air delivery to the lower respiratory tract include: the nasolabial angle, the alar muscles, the nostrils, the alar cartilages, the upper lateral cartilages, the internal valve, the turbinates, and the choanae. Of these parts, *only the choanae and turbinates are not affected by a routine aesthetic rhinoplasty.* Therefore, it is incumbent on the surgeon to be meticulous in the exact anatomic reconstruction of the nose during rhinoplasty.

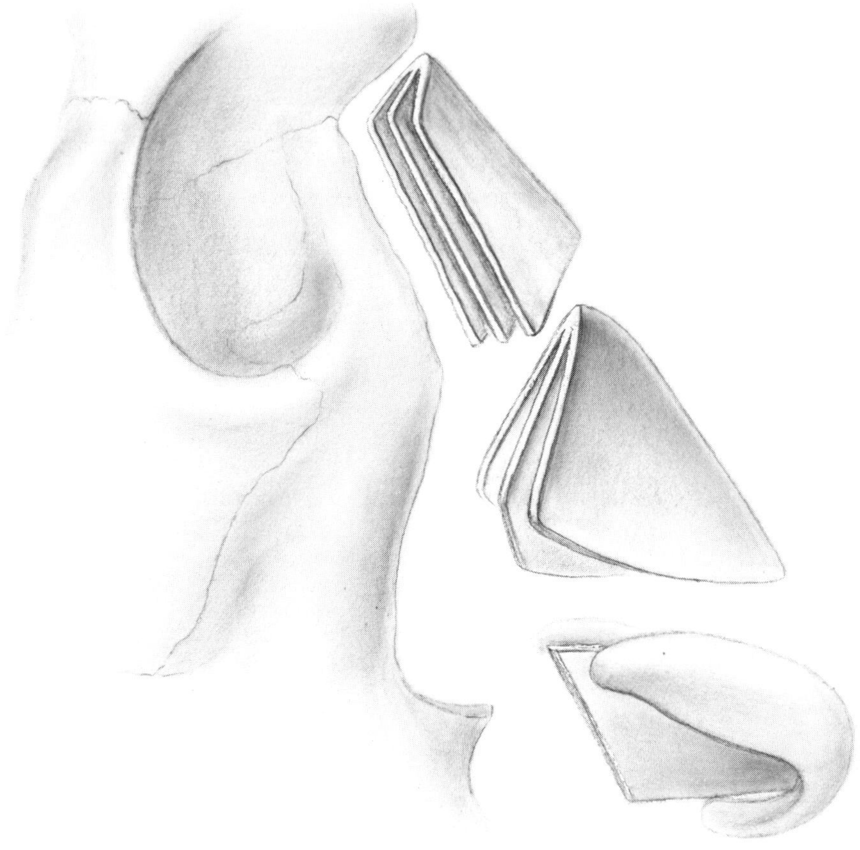

The nose as a functional organ can be divided into three compartments (from *top* to *bottom*): the bony vault, the upper cartilaginous vault, and the lower cartilaginous vault. These have in common a supporting partition, the bony and cartilaginous septum, which in essence creates two separate and complete functioning noses in one.

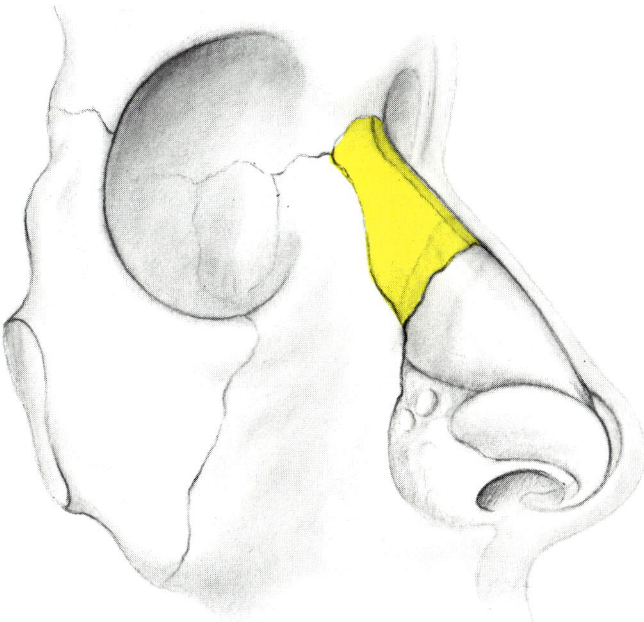

BONY VAULT

The bony vault is a pyramidal bony structure that forms the principal structural base for the nose. It is made up of the upward projections of the frontal process of the maxilla, which articulate with the nasal bones to form an arch with the union of the nasal bones in the midline. The cephalic portion articulates with the frontal bone, and the posterior border is continuous with the maxilla. The caudal arch is a free edge that lies in intimate apposition to the upper cartilaginous vault, joined by a single connective tissue membrane.

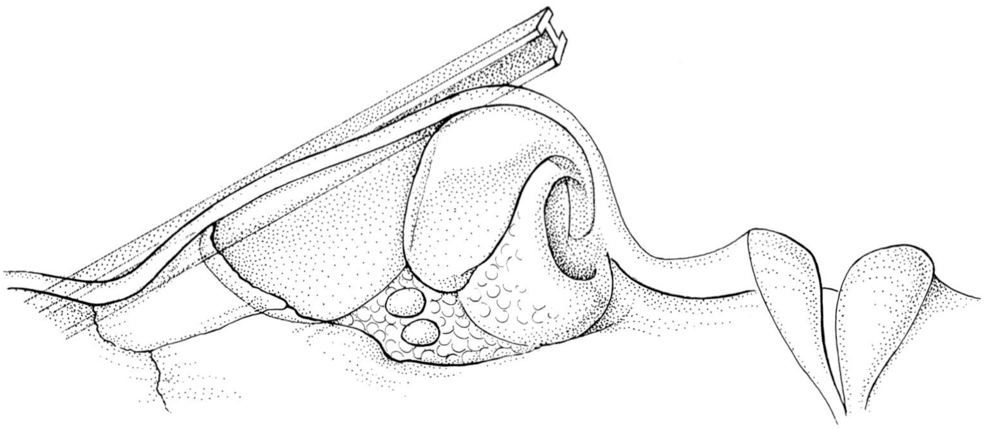

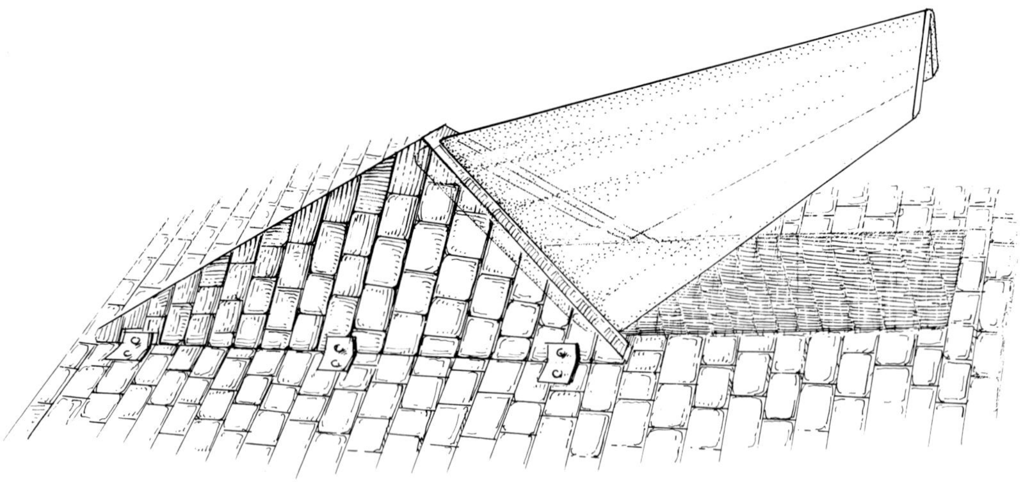

If the nose is thought of as a cantilever, the bony vault forms a stable base, with its protective arch an extension of the skull. The bony vault, with its cantilevered upper cartilaginous vault, fuses with the dorsal border of the septum to form a structural "I beam" extending from the radix to the base. This concept helps one fully appreciate the critical impact of lowering the dorsum during rhinoplasty.

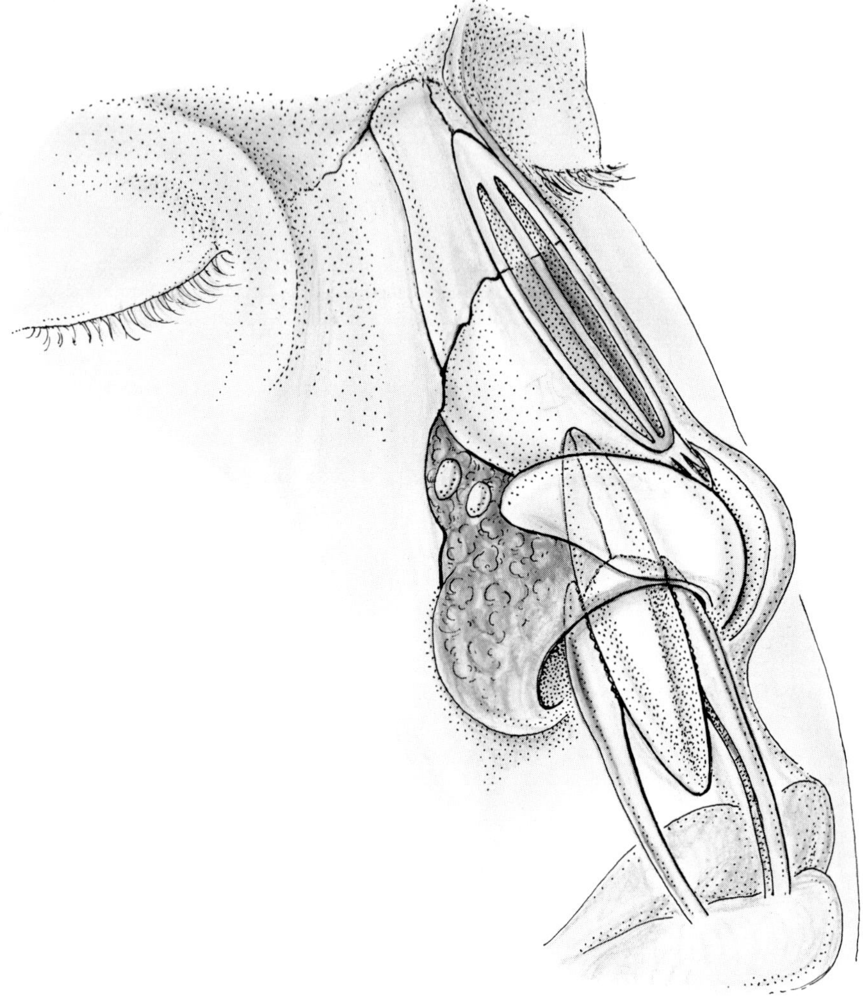

During rhinoplasty the dorsum is resected, removing the I beam of support, separating the bony and cartilaginous vaults from the septal edge, and producing what is commonly known as an "open roof." In addition, to reconstruct the nasal arch it is necessary to detach the nasal pyramid from its footings to allow the nasal bones to move into their new position. Following these maneuvers, the structural integrity of the nose is never quite the same because nasal bones heal by fibrous union, not by callus. Therefore, manipulation of nasal bones should be limited to the particular requirements of each nose, and bony attachments should be preserved whenever possible.

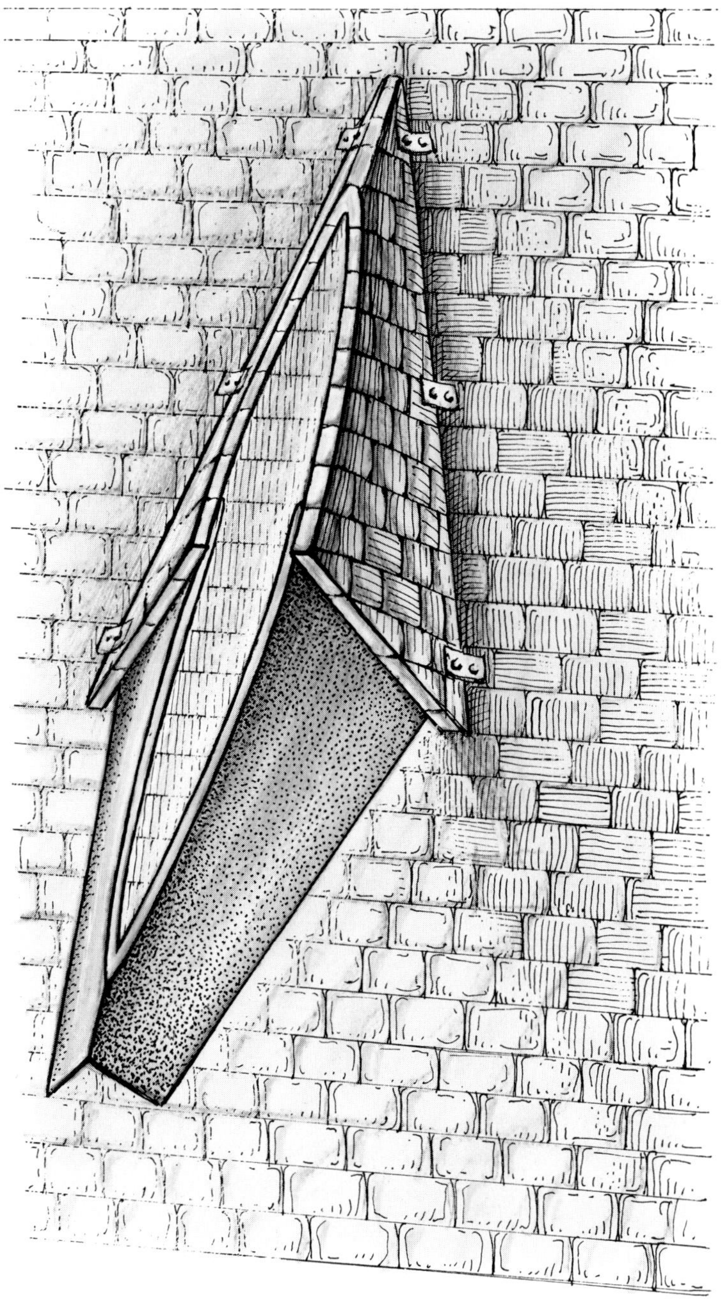

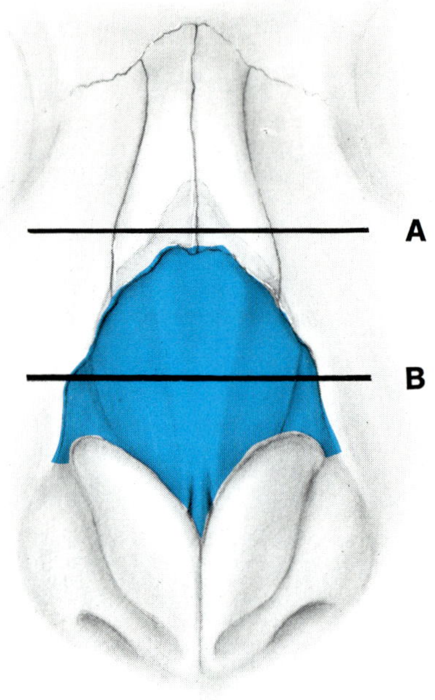

UPPER CARTILAGINOUS VAULT

The upper cartilaginous vault is made up of paired, triangular cartilages that extend from the caudal arch of the bony pyramid as a cantilever. They are attached along the dorsal border of the septum by a dense fibrous union and extend cephalad under the bony arch for a distance of up to 11 mm. The cartilages attach to the undersurface of the lateral walls of the bony vault by side to side apposition. They are joined by a single membrane for a distance of 2 to 4 mm.

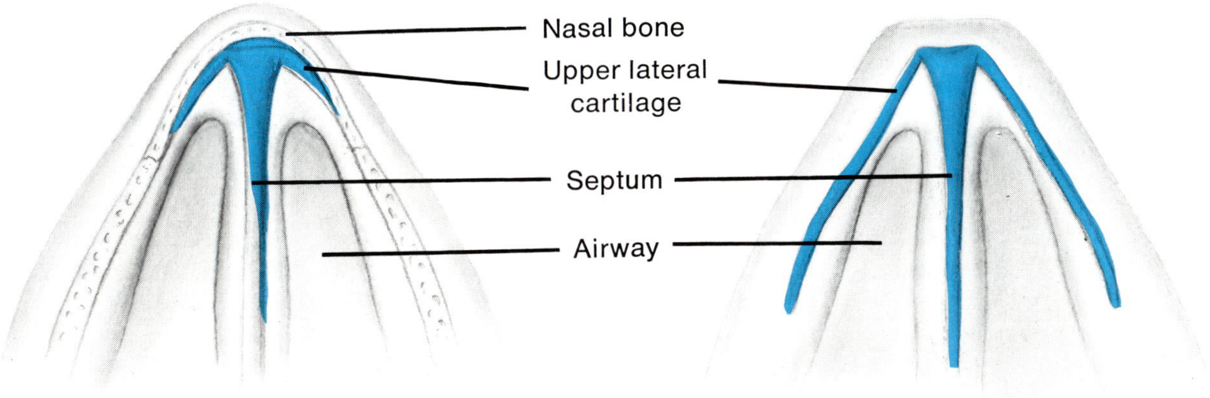

Cross section at A

Cross section at B

The roof, or dorsal segment, of the upper cartilaginous vault has a vital role in the aesthetics and function of the nose. Structurally, the dorsal edge is the bridge that connects the two upper lateral cartilages to give them architectural stability. Also, the dorsal edge acts as a lateral distractor of the upper lateral cartilages, placing them in a favorable relation to the septum so that they can resist the increasing negative pressure that occurs with nasal inspiration to control the influx of air.

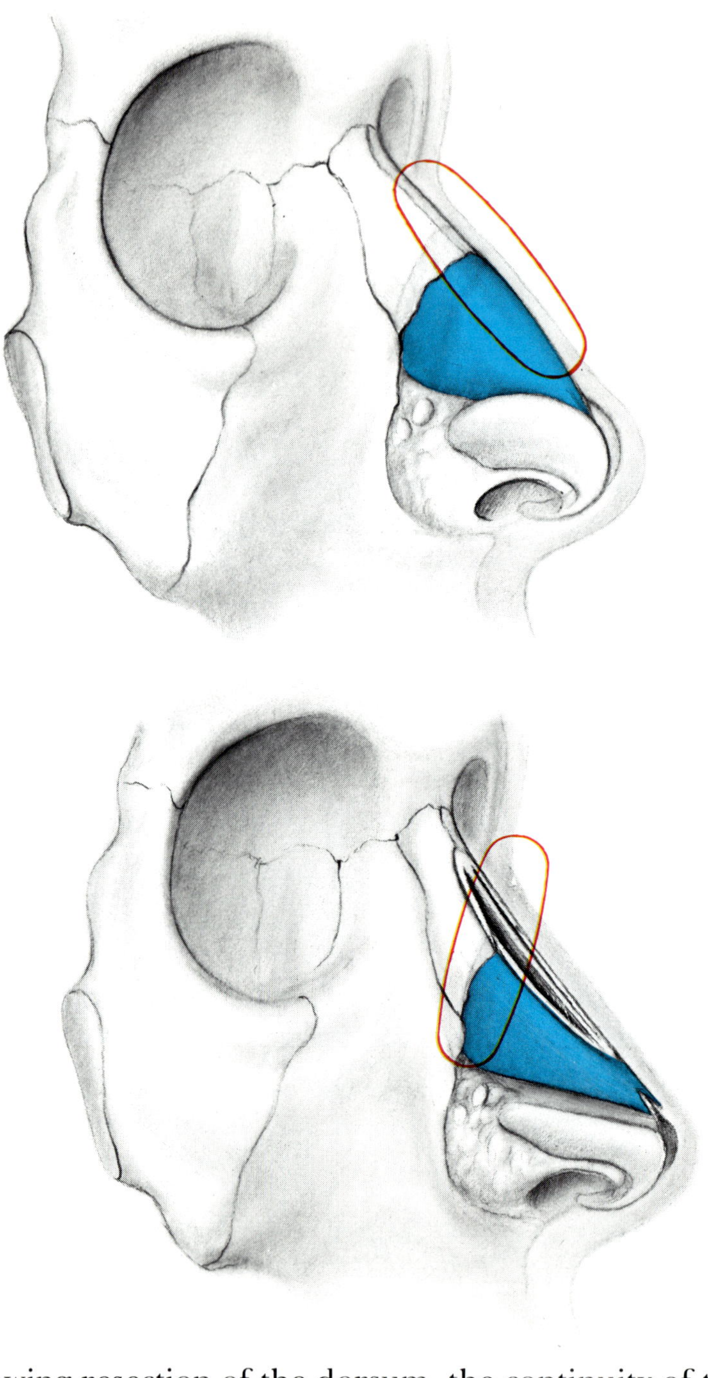

Following resection of the dorsum, the continuity of the upper lateral cartilages with the septum is interrupted, making them independent of each other. Thereafter they must rely on the remaining attachment to the nasal bones for their total support and lateral distraction.

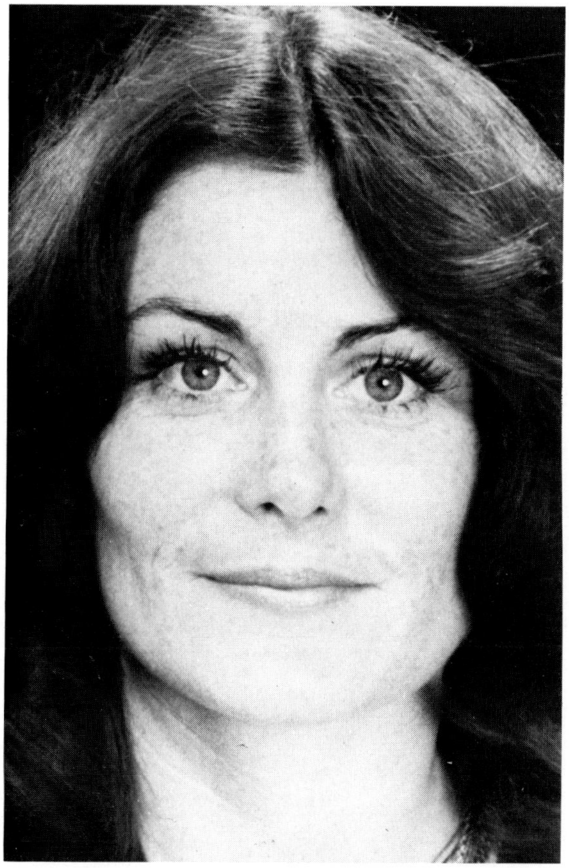

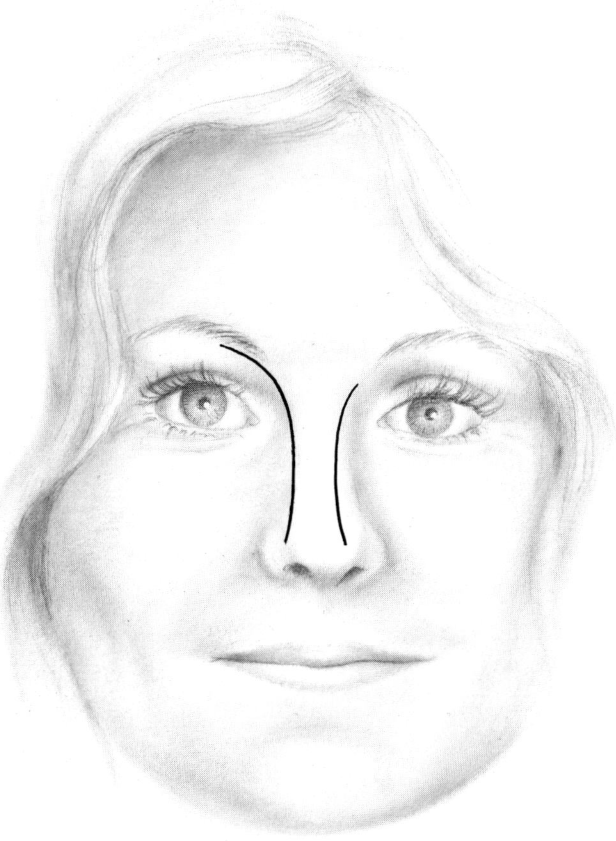

In the normal nose viewed from the front, there is a pair of matching, unbroken lines that are slightly concave extending from the radix to the domes of the lower lateral cartilages.

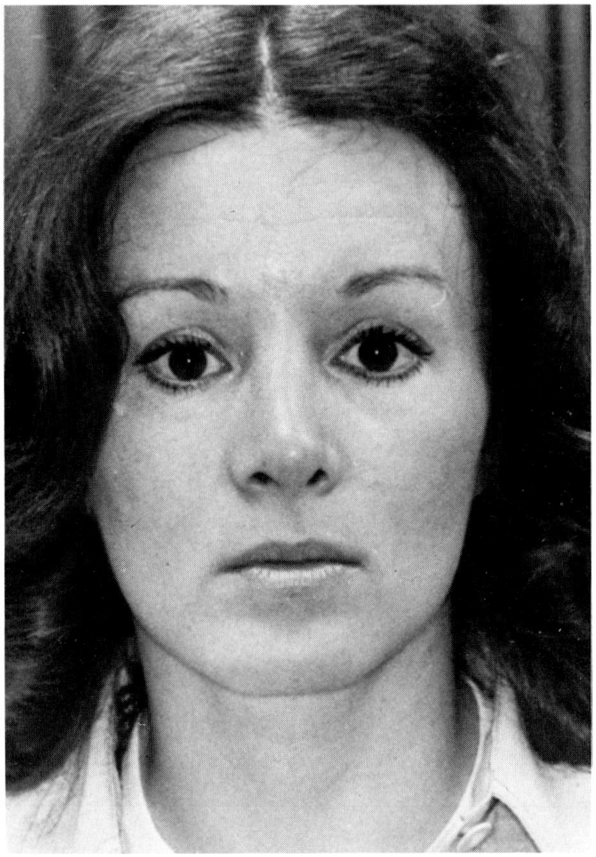

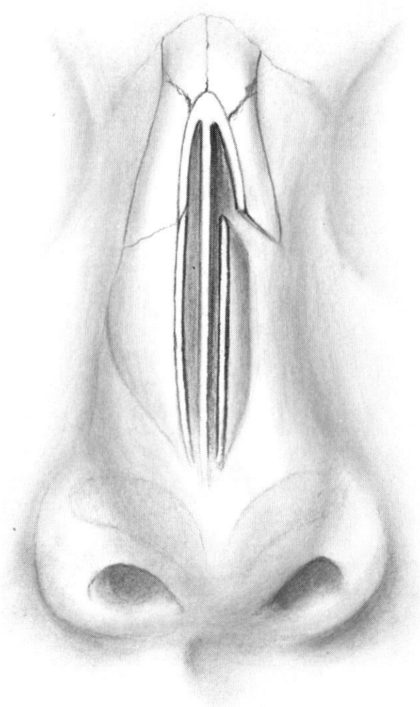

With a unilateral avulsion of the upper lateral cartilage, the patient has a nose that appears crooked by virtue of the resulting concavity on the side of the avulsion. This is more or less noticeable depending on the thickness of the tissues but is usually apparent.

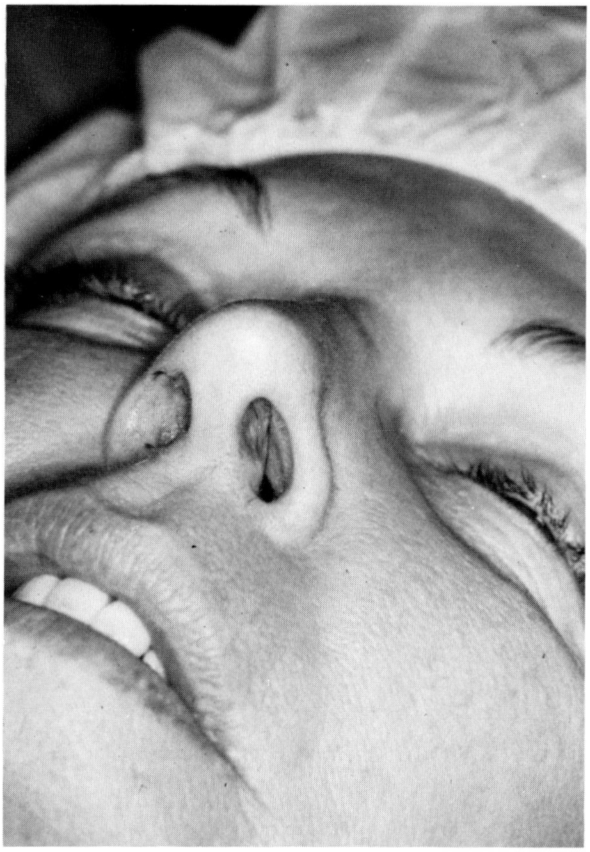

Furthermore, the efficiency of the internal valve can be impaired on the avulsed side because the upper lateral cartilage no longer has support. Without the cephalic support of the nasal bones, a flutter valve action is created; expiration is normal, but on inspiration the unsupported cartilage collapses against the septum.

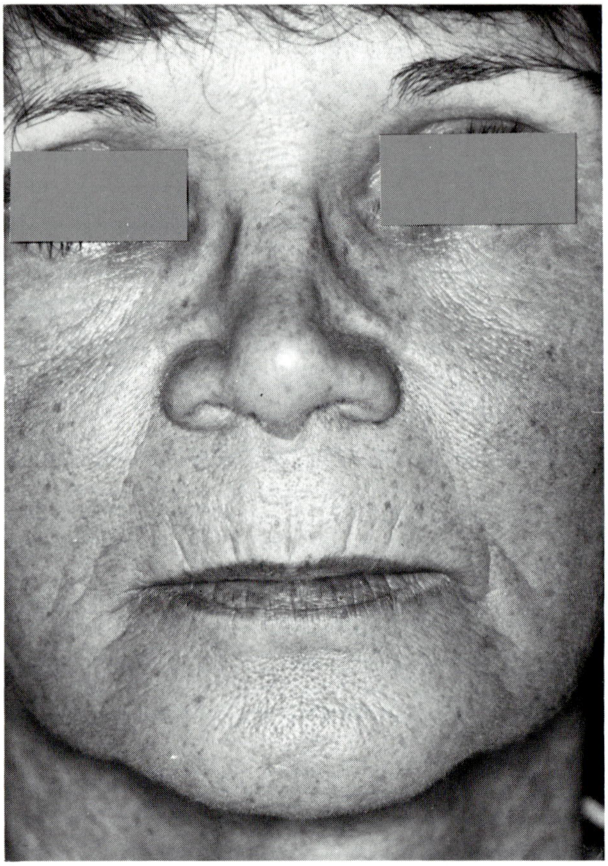

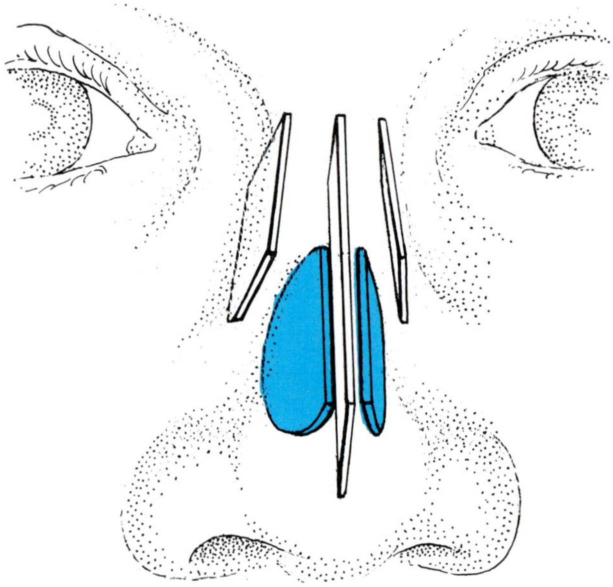

In a bilateral avulsion, the middle third of the nose is compressed, and the nasal bones and upper lateral cartilages are distinctly separated. As a result, the functional capacity of the nose is decreased, and the patient may complain of anosmia because the air currents are directed posteriorly only and not allowed to flow through the upper recesses of the nasal cavity for proper olfaction.

LOWER CARTILAGINOUS VAULT

The lower cartilaginous vault forms the base of the nose. It is made up of all tissues caudal to the free edge of the upper lateral cartilages. These include: paired lower lateral cartilages, medial crura, lateral crura, alae, alar lobules, nares (nostrils), nasal sill, nasal vestibule, columella, and membranous septum.

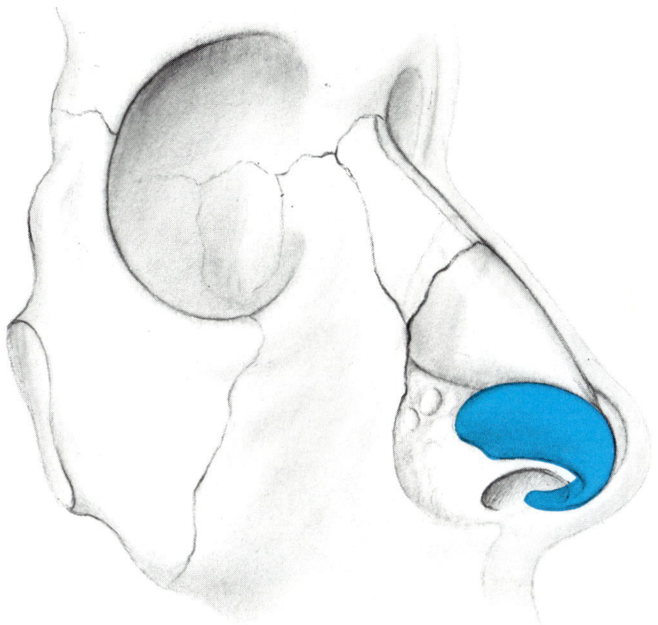

Although the lower vault is relatively independent of the other two vaults, it shares with them the dorsal edge of the septum (septal angle) and the connective tissue attachments to the upper lateral cartilages.

NASOLABIAL ANGLE

Any change in the nasolabial angle changes the direction of air flow into the nasal cavity. Though imaginative studies have been designed to reveal the direction of air flow through the nasal passages, the exact distribution of the air current after it passes the nasal threshold can only be theorized. Not only are the internal nasal structures as variable as fingerprints, but each individual airway changes from moment to moment as it responds to changes in the atmosphere. These variations notwithstanding, there are acknowledged parameters that are important to optimal direction of air flow through the nostril.

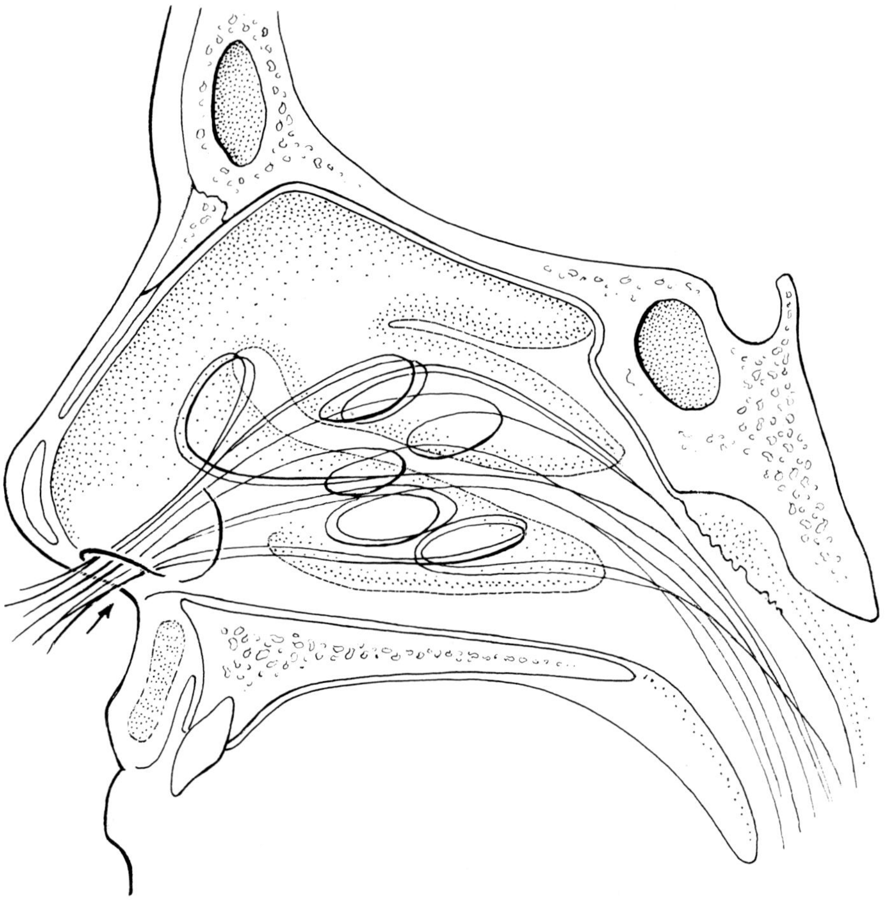

A nasolabial angle functionally and aesthetically should be between 90 to 115 degrees. Within this range, the vestibule is in the best position to effectively deliver columns of air to the internal nasal parts for conditioning. Improperly directed air currents that cause a blast of air against any internal nasal part penetrate the protective mucus blanket, resulting in drying, a loss of ciliary action, and metaplasia.

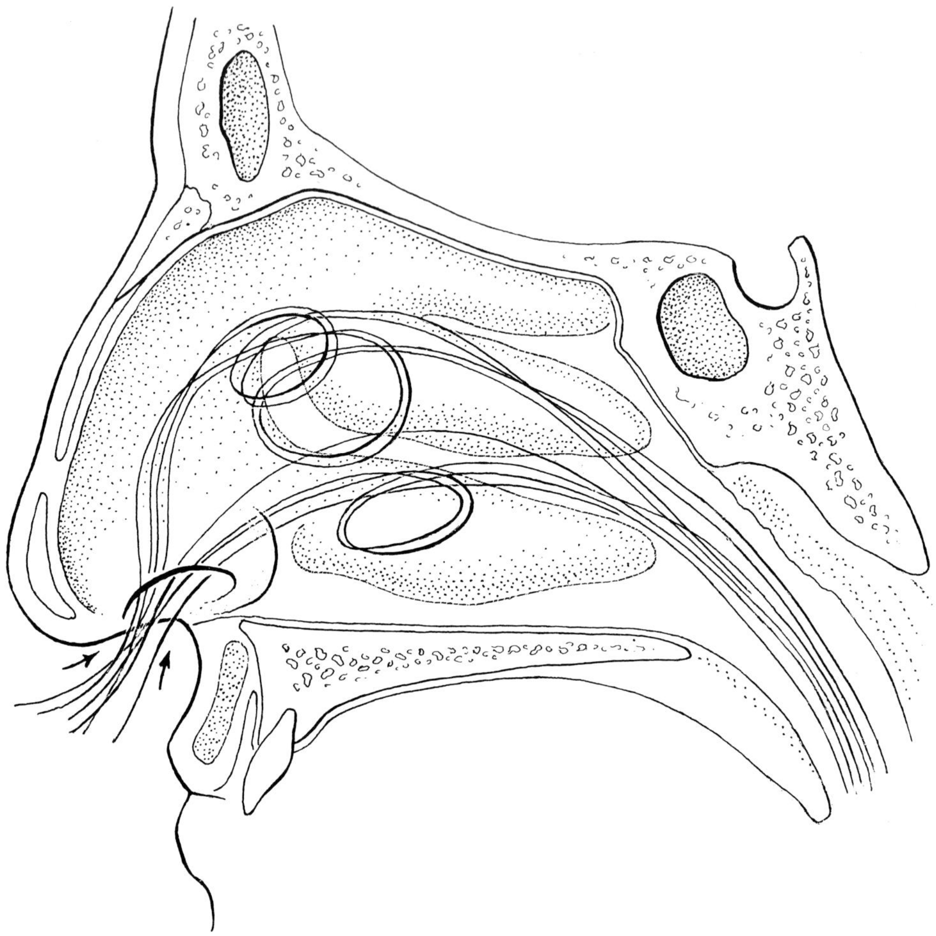

An acute nasolabial angle creates a high thrust of air. This high arch of current creates an excess of eddy currents that increases resistance in the nasal passages, making breathing more work than necessary. The effortless flow of nasal respiration depends on a moderate arch of the air column, curving through the nasal passages down into the larynx.

Areas of metaplasia subsequent to misdirected air currents may be the foci of local infection, foul odors, and recurrent epistaxis. Moreover, symptoms of headache, difficulty in breathing, and sinus pains may have their etiology in poorly directed air currents.

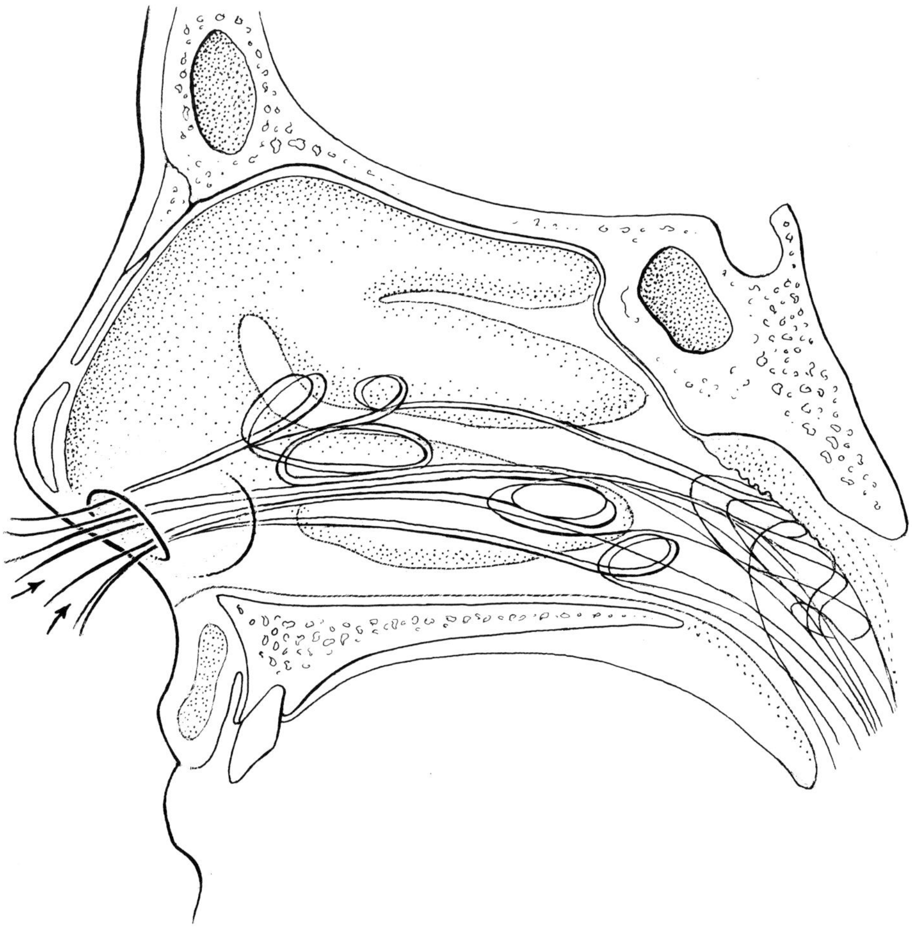

The nasolabial angle that is too wide channels the column of air directly to the posterior pharyngeal wall. There is a decrease in the flow of air through the upper nasal vault, allowing a buildup of nasal secretions. This increase in secretion is paradoxical to the inadequate humidification of air that ultimately produces a feeling of dryness of the throat caused by the blast of air striking the anterior nasal structures and posterior pharynx. A convex air current, distributed over all of the tissues of the turbinates, is mandatory to proper nasal function.

Patients who have adequate airways and a wide nasolabial angle may develop small, atrophic turbinates because of the constant battering of the currents of air on the delicate mucosa. These patients often complain of stuffiness when they appear clinically to have very large nasal airways. Good nasal respiration depends on a certain amount of resistance provided by the turbinates. Without it, excessive drying, improper air conditioning, and the sensation of stuffiness can occur.

NASAL BASE

The shape of the base of the nose is dependent on its supporting structures: the dorsal edge of the septum, the lower lateral cartilages, and the soft tissues. Each is important in determining the contour of the nasal base, but the dorsum is by far the most important support structure. When the dorsum is lowered, tip support is reduced, which causes a decrease in tip projection. As the tip loses projection, the nostrils broaden and change position from vertical to horizontal.

It is helpful to think of the nasal tip as being supported by the I beam that extends from the radix. If the dorsal I beam is lowered, it is apparent that changes in the basal perimeter can occur. In fact, the nasal base can broaden only by reduction of the dorsal edge of the septum, specifically the angle of the septum. A high percentage of alar wedge resections may indicate excessive dorsal resection. Alar wedges should be part of the preoperative plan. If alar resection becomes an unexpected final step in rhinoplasty, it is likely that the dorsum has been overreduced. When support is lost, the tip is pulled down by the tissues, and the base broadens, making alar wedges necessary to bring the nose into proportion. When this occurs, the efficacy of the nostril as an external valve can be compromised.

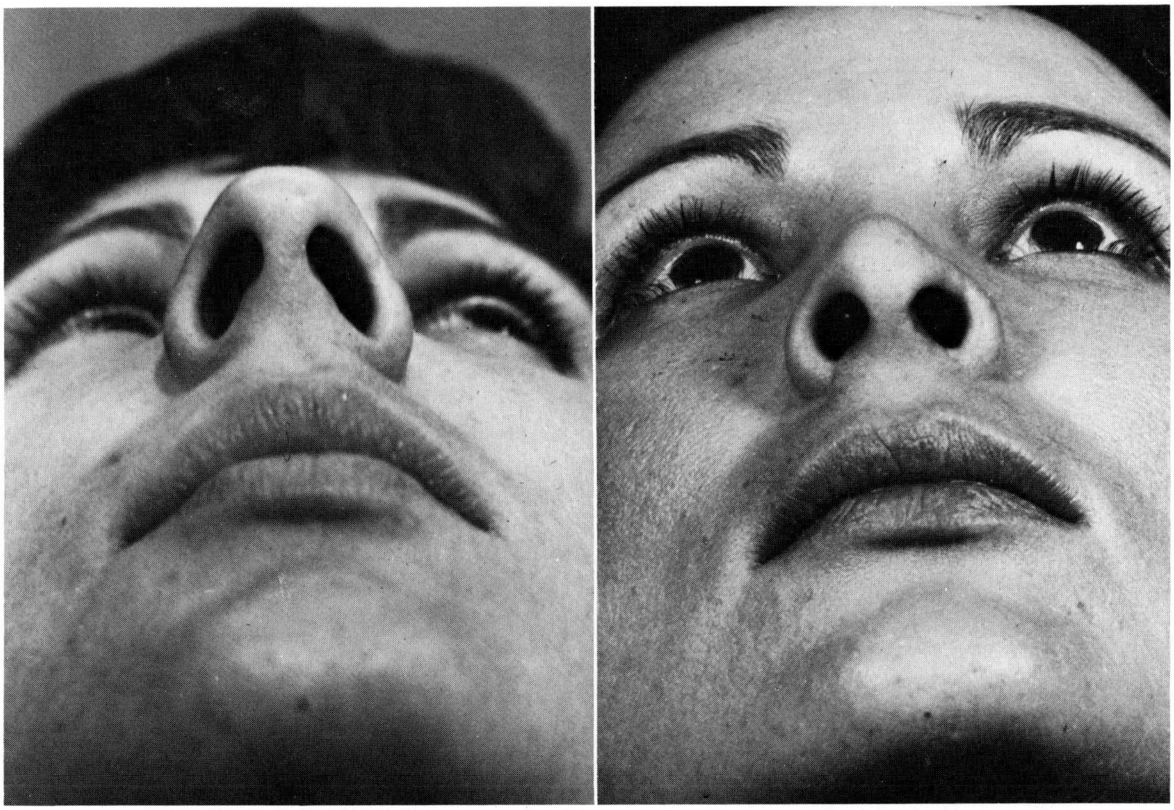

These are basal views of the same patient before and following rhinoplasty. The preoperative view illustrates a well-supported basal configuration that is projecting and triangular, with good relationships of all parts. The nostrils are ideally shaped to deliver air to the internal valve for distribution to the internal nasal compartment. The postoperative view illustrates the change in the basal perimeter. The nostrils are poorly functioning inlets that direct high-velocity columns of air against the septum, which may be the cause of the patient's chronic septal crusting and bleeding.

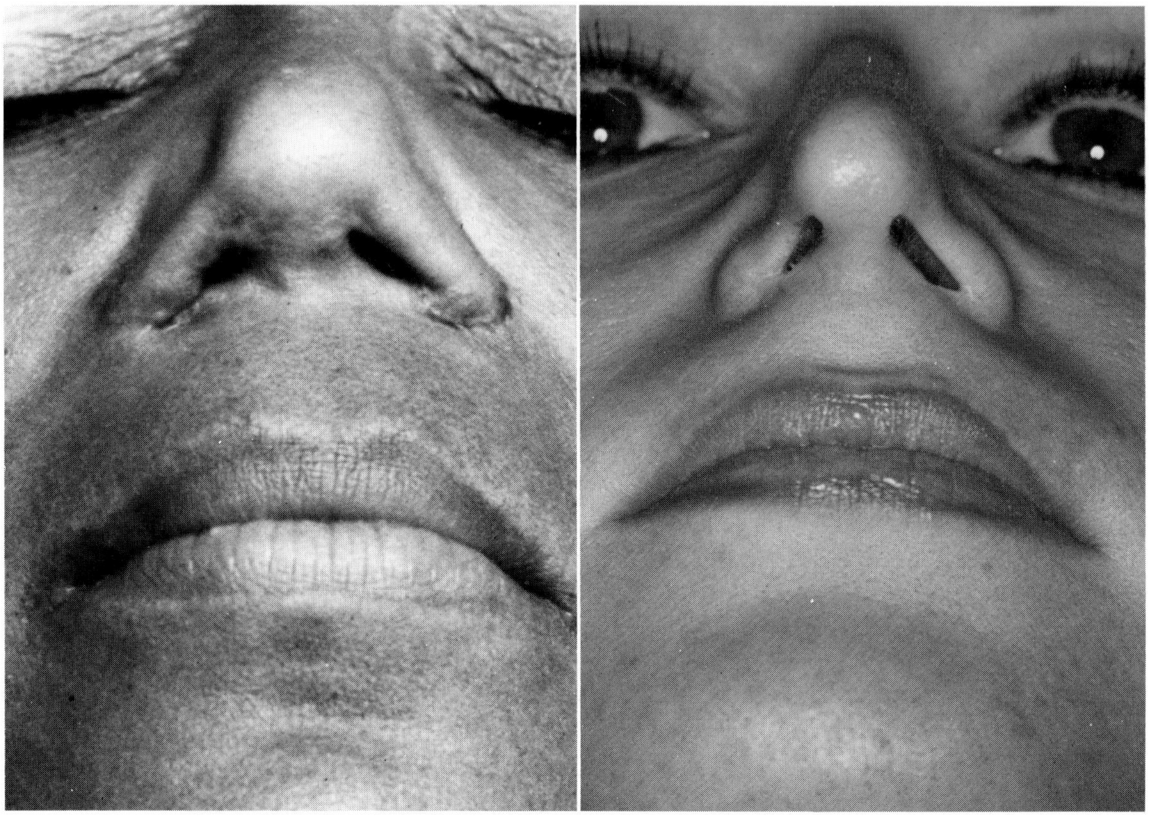

Severe and irreversible aesthetic and physiologic impairment can result from poorly planned alar wedge resections. There is no known way to duplicate the specialized and beautiful contour of the normal nostril.

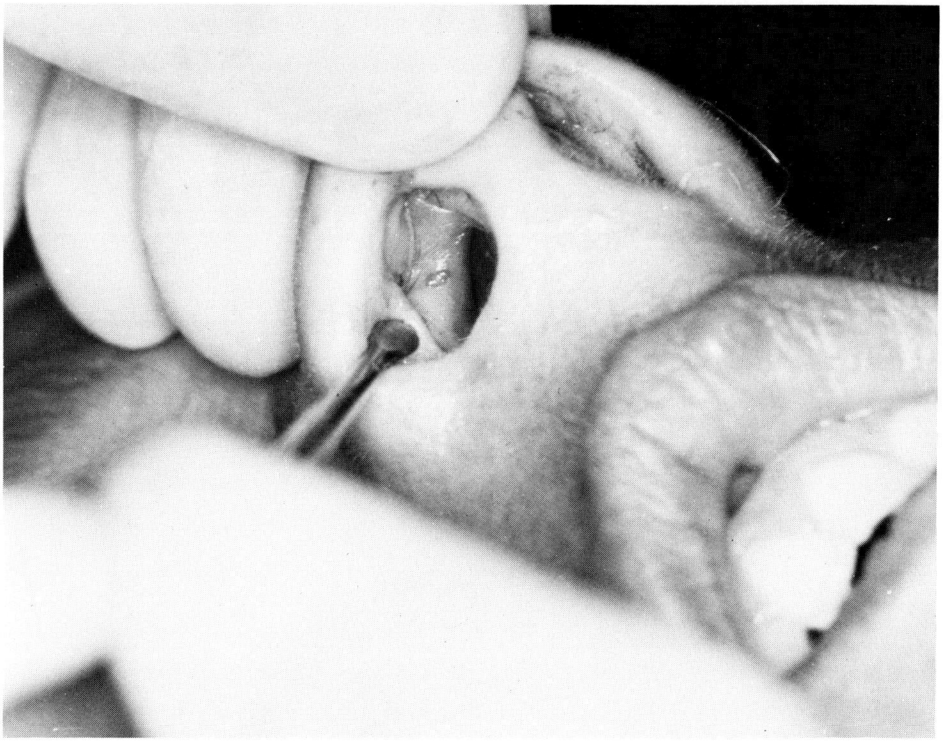

NASAL VESTIBULE

The nasal vestibule is the compartment caudal to the internal valve. The above patient illustrates the appearance of the normal unoperated vestibule. The internal valve can be seen as the caudal reflection of the upper lateral cartilage, its inferior edge arching posteriorly from the angle of the septum, creating a high apex to the vestibule.

Vestibular atresia

The most common evidence of prior rhinoplasty is a reduction of the perimeter of the vestibule by synechiae at the apex. I would estimate conservatively that 75% to 85% of postrhinoplasty patients have some reduction of the nasal vestibule caused by synechiae. These synechial webs are pathognomonic of overresection of mucosa, specifically over the caudal edge of the upper lateral cartilages or over the cephalic edge of the lower lateral cartilages.

The loss of mucosa in this area usually occurs during a routine step in rhinoplasty—the resection of the caudal edge of the upper lateral cartilage with a pair of right-angle scissors (commonly referred to as "upper lateral scissors"), the use of which I hope to discourage.

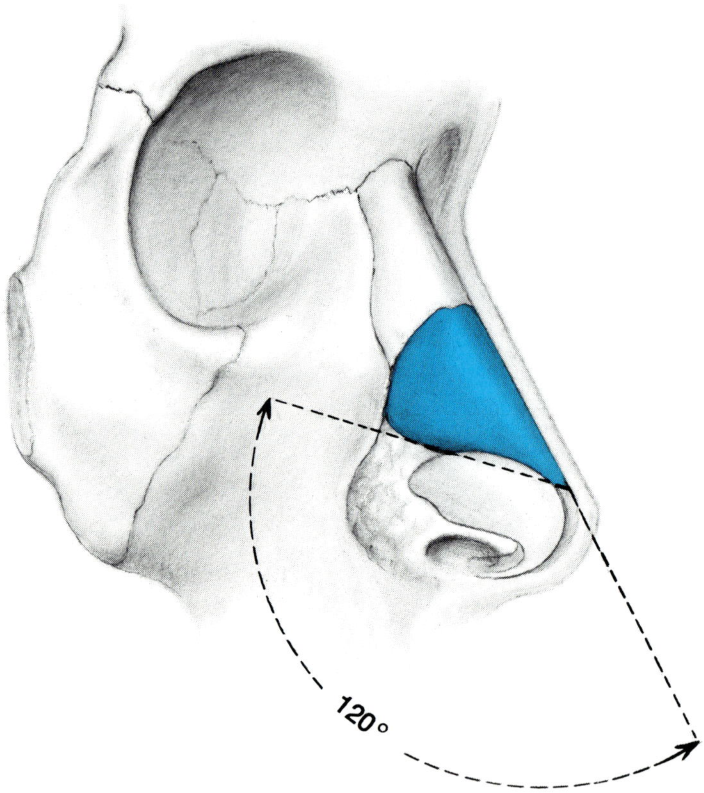

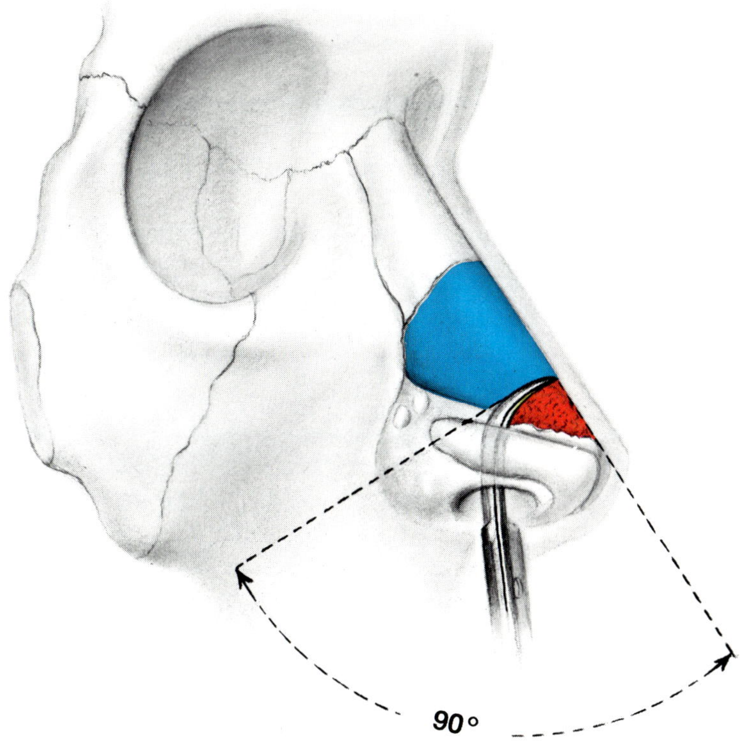

If one examines the relationship of the caudal edge of the upper lateral cartilage to the dorsal edge of the septum, it is usually found to be about 120 degrees, not 90 degrees. The upper lateral cartilages are triangular, not quadrangular. The illustration demonstrates this relationship before surgery and following resection of the caudal edge of the upper lateral cartilage using right-angle scissors. The area in red indicates the predictable loss of mucosal lining using this technique.

This raw area in the vestibule is potentially increased following tip modification, which reduces the width of the lateral crura, allowing the mucosa to retract. Separation of mucosal edges as a result of heedless packing of the vestibule can also cause postoperative vestibular atresia.

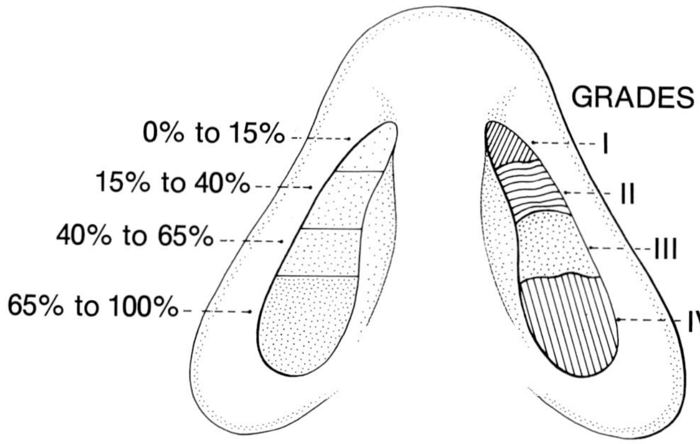

Reduction of the perimeter of the vestibule can be conveniently categorized in degrees of atresia ranging from grade I to grade IV, as shown.

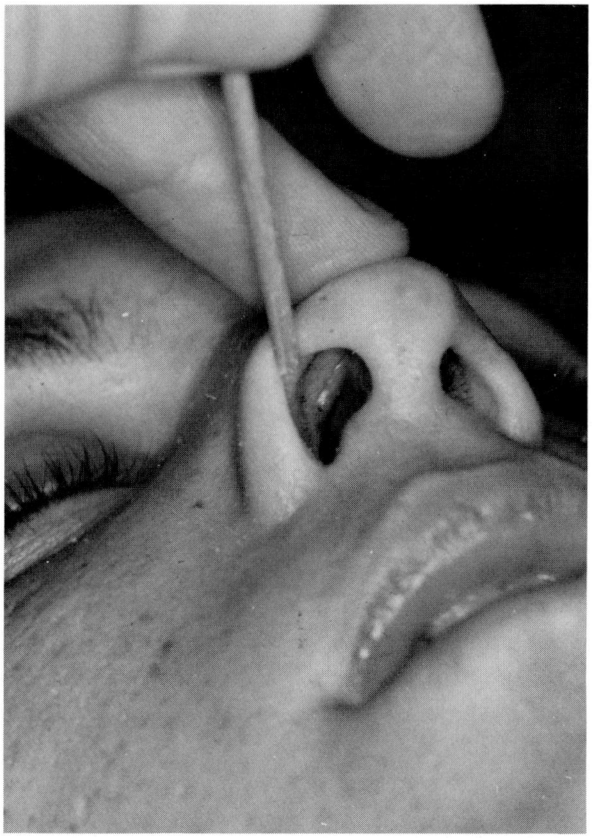

This patient illustrates the correct appearance of the vestibule 8 days following aesthetic rhinoplasty. There is an almost perfect re-creation of the normal anatomy. The internal valve has been reconstructed by preserving mucosa and resecting only the caudal part of the upper lateral cartilage, maintaining 120 degrees to the dorsal edge. The caudal edge of the upper lateral cartilage is close to the angle of the septum and allows for a high apex of the vestibule at the interval valve.

GRADE I ATRESIA

These postrhinoplasty patients illustrate grade I atresia. Patients with grade I atresias usually are not bothered functionally and may not even be aware that there has been a loss of vestibular volume. Occasionally a patient will complain of some difficulty cleaning the nose if there is anterior webbing, since crusts can accumulate in a blind pouch behind the web. Ingrown hair resulting from the tangle of vestibular hairbearing skin and scar can be a recurrent problem also. Treatment is rarely necessary.

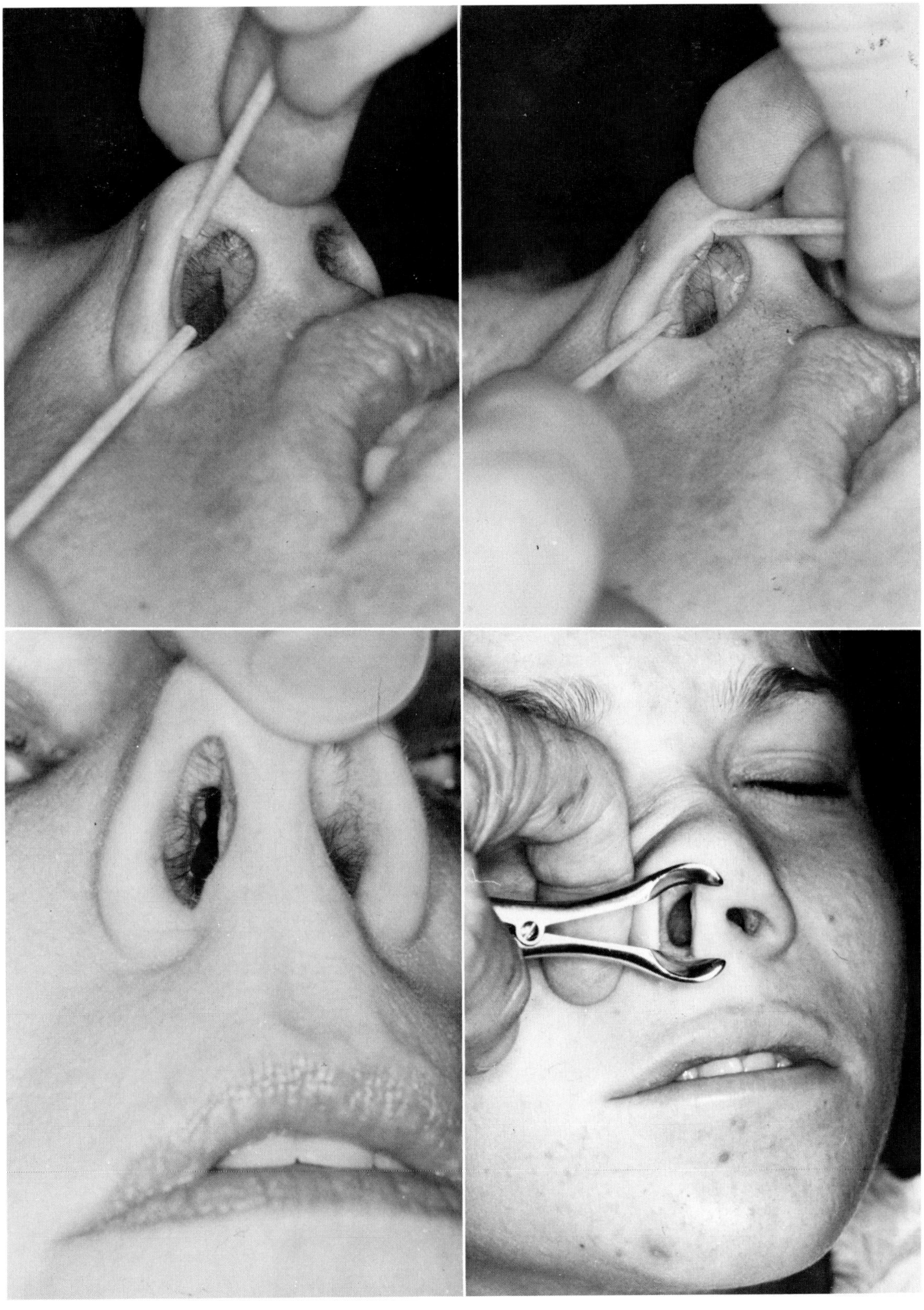

GRADE II ATRESIA

These patients illustrate grade II atresia. Patients with grade II atresias have a reduction in vestibular volume that is more than 15% but less than 40%, which usually impedes respiratory function. As a result, areas of metaplasia on the turbinate or the septal wall, with crusting and intermittent epistaxis, can occur. Treatment is beneficial.

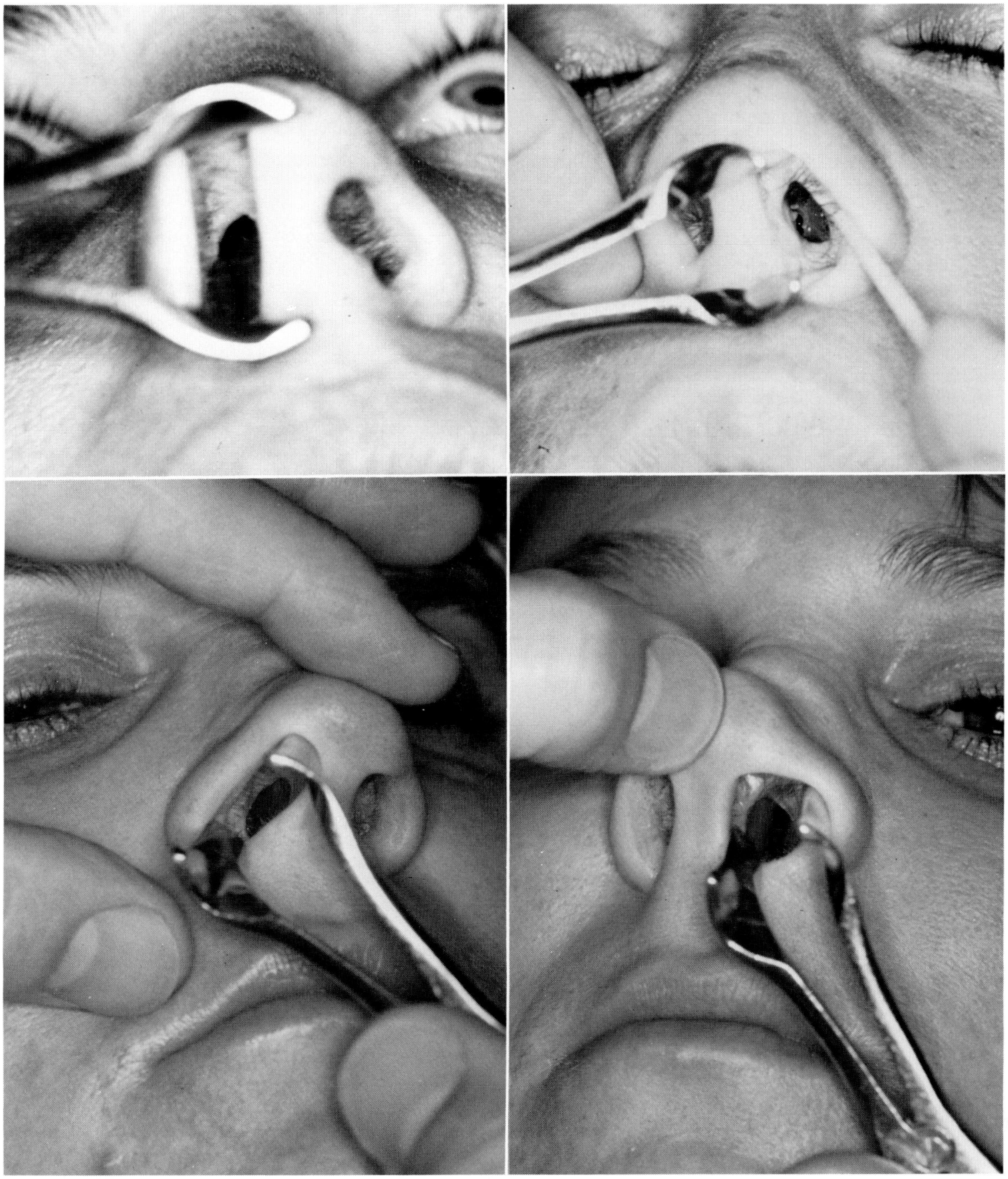

GRADE III ATRESIA

These patients illustrate grade III atresia. Patients with grade III atresias have a reduced vestibular volume of more than 40% and less than 75%. Patients are aware of their impeded airway, and they must resort to mouth breathing when the need for air is increased only slightly. Metaplasia, increase in nasal secretions, and symptoms attributable to partially obstructed airways can be found in these patients. Improved function can be gained only through surgical repair.

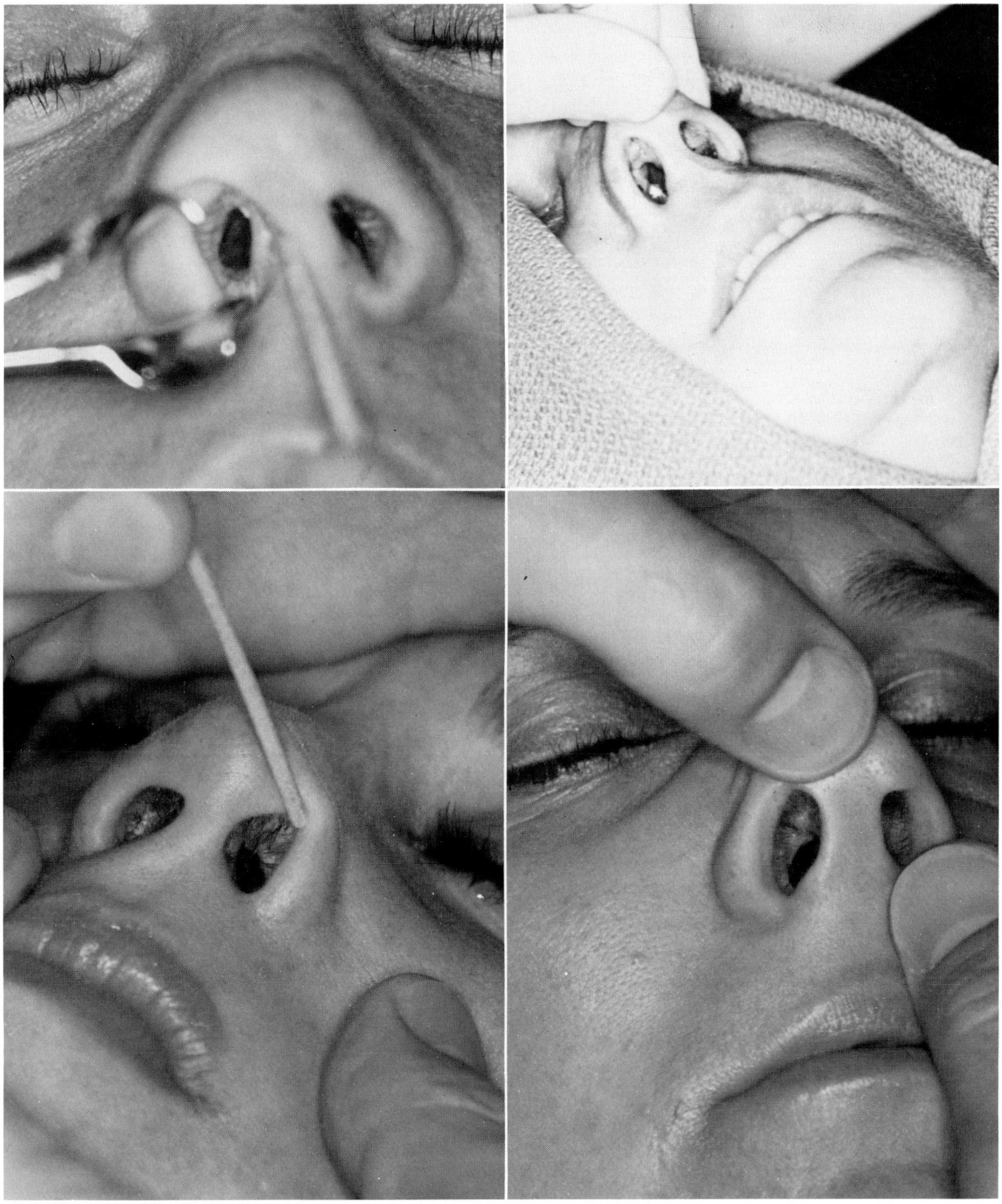

GRADE IV ATRESIA

These patients illustrate grade IV atresia. Patients with grade IV atresias have a vestibular volume that has been decreased by more than 75%. These deformities are not common, but when they do occur, they are devastating to both patient and surgeon. The patient becomes a virtual respiratory cripple. Many develop great anxiety about their breathing and are subject to chronic clinical problems associated with mouth breathing. Surgical repair is mandatory.

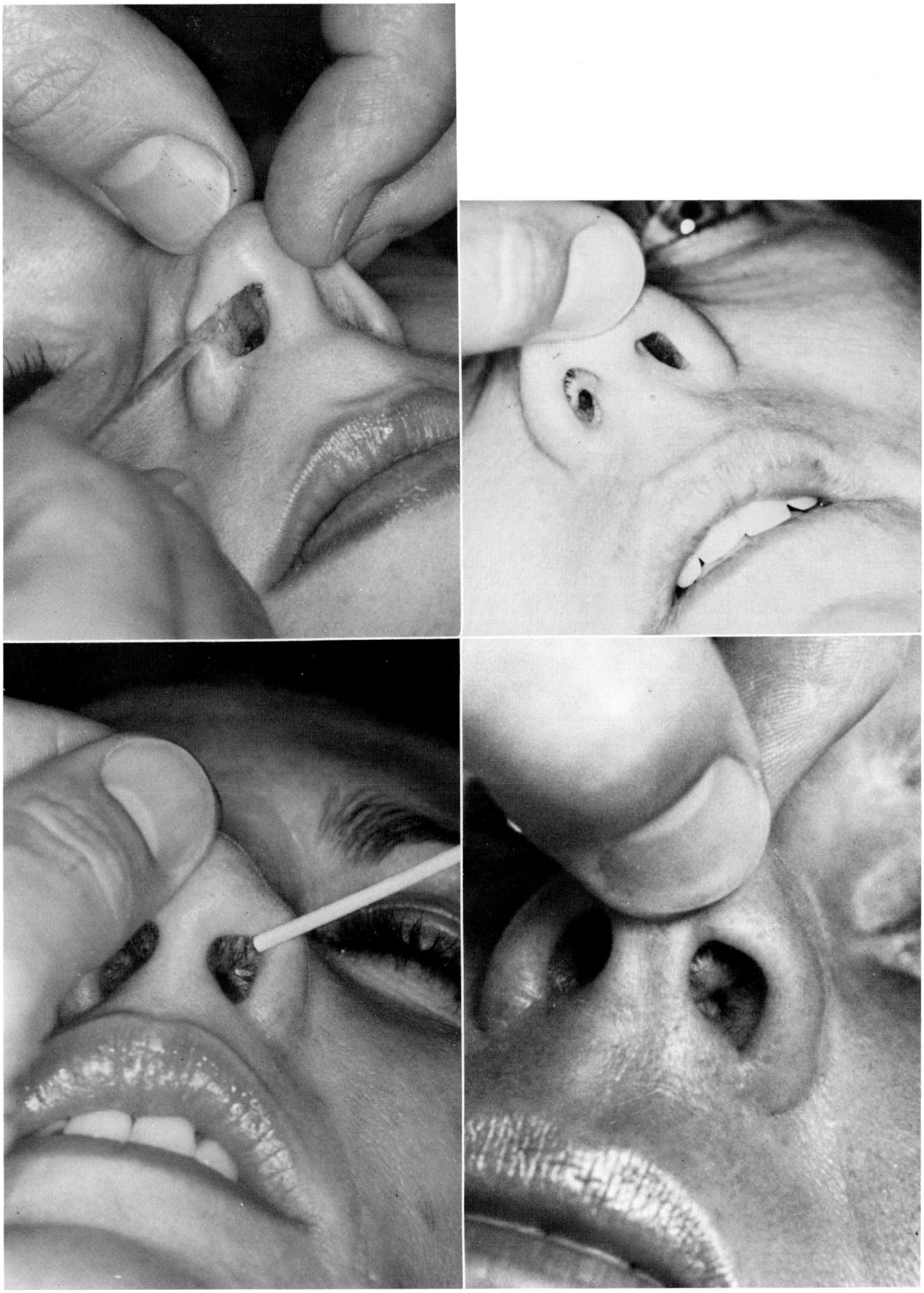

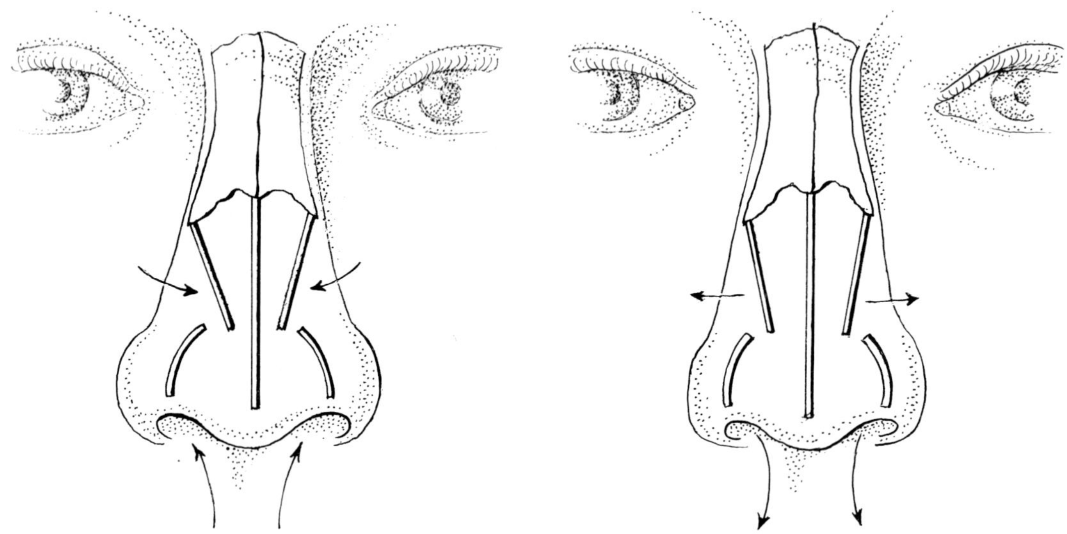

INTERNAL VALVE

The internal valve can be described as an isosceles triangle formed by the caudal free edge of the upper lateral cartilage, the septum, and the nasal floor. It is paradoxical in its action, narrowing on inspiration and widening on expiration.

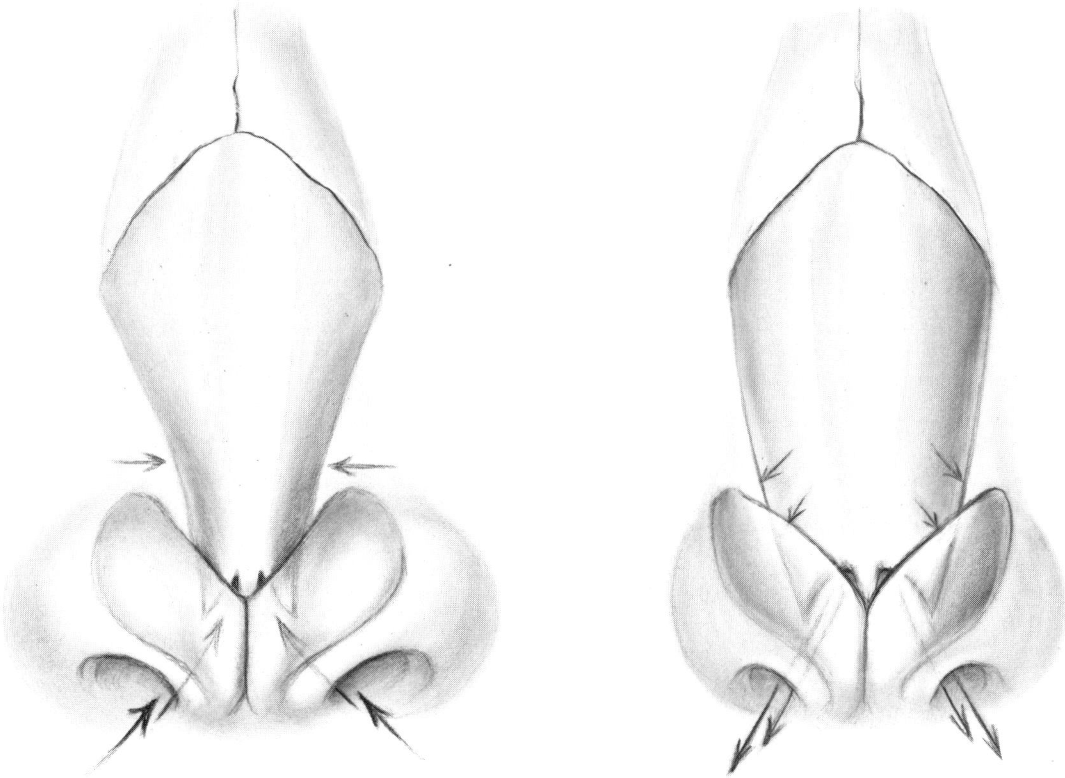

On deep inspiration, the secondary muscles of respiration are brought into play, forcibly expanding the chest wall and sharply increasing the negative pressure of the entire upper respiratory tract. In the lower cartilaginous vault, the nostrils flare, increasing the diameter of the external valve. The internal valve is narrowed by the increase in negative pressure and the action of the flaring nostril, which causes the cephalic border of the lateral crus to fold medially as the caudal border flares laterally. This reciprocal action changes the contour of the internal valve to increase resistance and modify the currents of air entering the nasal cavity.

On expiration, there is a shift from negative to positive intranasal pressure. This forces the upper lateral cartilages away from the septum, thereby widening the internal valves and allowing air to escape easily. The nostrils relax to their normal position, which shifts the upper edges laterally and the lower edges medially.

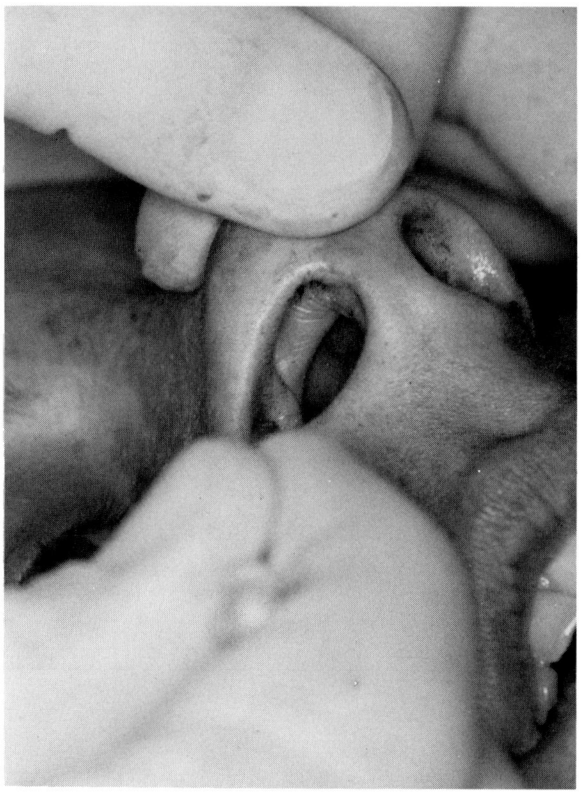

In this photograph of an unoperated nose, the tip is distracted in a cephalad direction, exposing the internal valve. The caudal edge of the upper lateral cartilage begins close to the angle of the septum (an important consideration in reconstruction of this part during rhinoplasty) and arches posteriorly and superiorly toward the lateral inferior corner of the pyriform aperture.

The angle formed by the attachment of the upper lateral cartilage to the septum must be 10 to 15 degrees. If this angle is less than 10 degrees, it is likely that the patient will have difficulty on inspiration because of a flutter-valve action of the internal valve. An important preoperative check is the determination of the position of the upper lateral cartilages to the septal wall. If the posterior portion is close to the septum (or if the angle is less than 10 degrees), it is a warning that osteotomy could completely defeat the action of the internal valve by further narrowing. Therefore, no fracture should be done, and reconstruction of the roof of the upper cartilaginous vault should maintain mucosal continuity. Placement of Solvang (spreader) grafts is recommended.

TURBINATES

Anatomy and physiology of the nose would not be complete without mention of the principal air-conditioning structures of the nose—the turbinates.

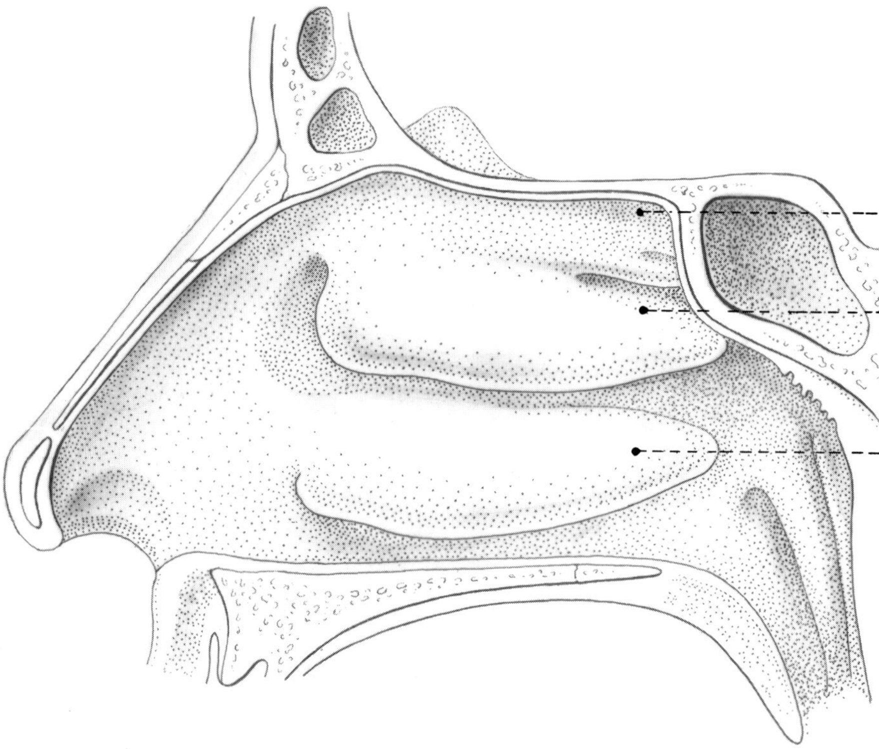

There are three pairs of turbinates: superior, middle, and inferior. Occasionally there is a fourth—the supreme. The superior turbinate is ethmoidal in origin and is covered by pseudostratified ciliated columnar epithelium. It has very few mucous glands and no venous lakes or pools. It is located just below the cribriform plate, although it is often rudimentary or absent. Because of their size and location, the superior and supreme turbinates are not involved with nasal obstruction.

The middle turbinate is a downward projection of the ethmoid bone with its lateral wall adjacent to the osteum of the maxillary sinus. It is covered by ciliated epithelium and has few venous pools. Mechanically, the middle turbinate has little or no control of airflow through the nose. Its principal function is the secretion of mucus. Chronic or recurring sinusitis and the "turbinate headache" are most often associated with hypertrophy or malposition of the middle turbinate.

The inferior turbinate is covered by ciliated epithelium and has many venous lakes. Because of its erectile capacity, it can change its mass quickly, functioning as a valve to control the air volume delivered to the lungs. It thereby plays a major role in maintaining proper intranasal resistance.

The inferior turbinate is a sensitive and responsive organ that is exposed to a wide range of stimulants, such as alcohol, smoke, excessive carbohydrates, air pollution, and rapid temperature changes through artificial air-conditioning and emotional excesses. All of these irritants are of special interest in light of the fact that turbinate tissue responds to stimulation of any kind, by hypertrophy. When the turbinate becomes obstructing, it ceases to function normally, which leads to chronic hypertrophy. Chronic hypertrophy leads to hyperplasia, and chronic hyperplasia leads to polypoid degeneration. This cycle of events can be aborted by the judicious resection of turbinates when indicated.

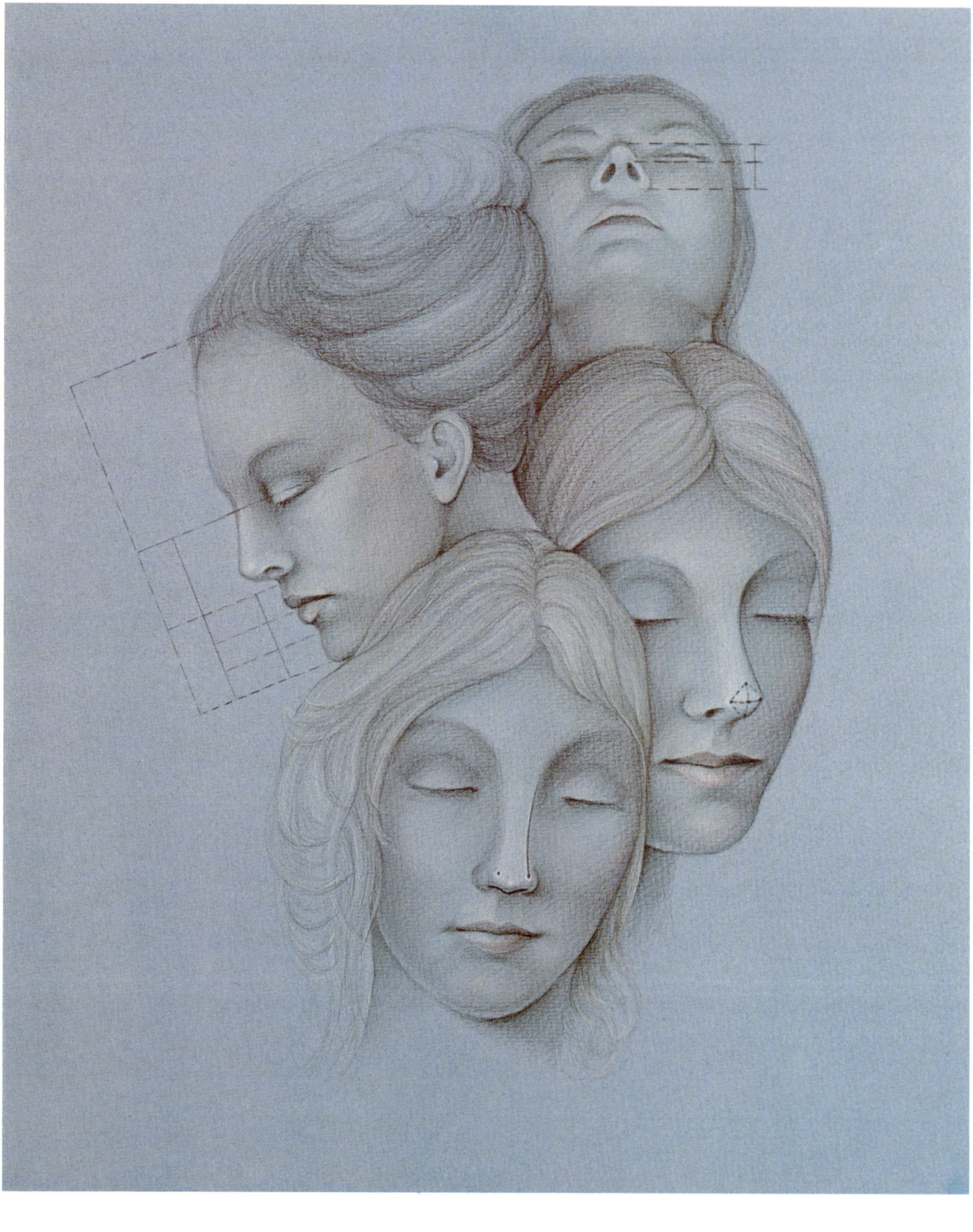

CHAPTER 2

Aesthetics

It is neither possible nor desirable to impose a preconceived "ideal" nose on every face. Nor can one acquire good aesthetic judgment by utilizing a table of average measurements or an instrument with six joints and a set of screws. However, certain ideal nasofacial and intranasal relationships are essential for an optimal aesthetic result. For this reason, well-defined nasal relationships should form the basis for the preoperative evaluation and the postoperative goals.

The purpose of this chapter is to present some basic concepts pertaining to the relationship and character of nasal parts, concepts that are central to the formation of a successful operative plan.

RADIX

The nose should have no discernible beginning but should be a continuation of lines that are graceful extensions of other facial parts. The root of the nose, or radix, should be part of an unbroken curve that begins in the superior orbital ridge and continues along the lateral nasal wall.

The width of the radix is in good alignment with the supraorbital curve in most patients. With few exceptions, the use of surgical procedures designed to narrow the radix is unnecessary and contradicts a basic aesthetic premise, that is, that lines should flow uninterrupted.

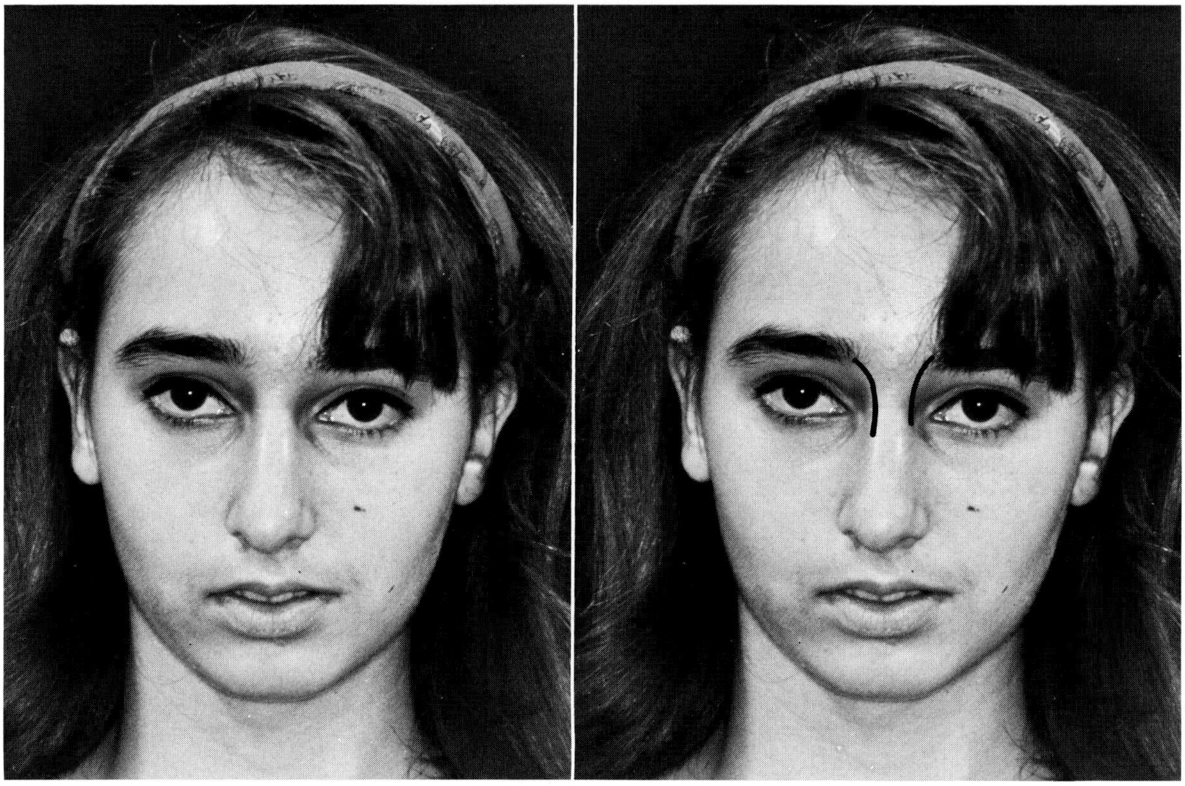

Normally there is an uninterrupted curve from the orbit to the lateral nasal wall. This patient illustrates the normal conjunction of the superciliary ridge to the lateral nasal wall, which must be preserved during rhinoplasty. Wedge resection of bone at the radix or comminution and overmobilization of nasal bones result in a nose that is too narrow and that is incongruent with the natural facial curves.

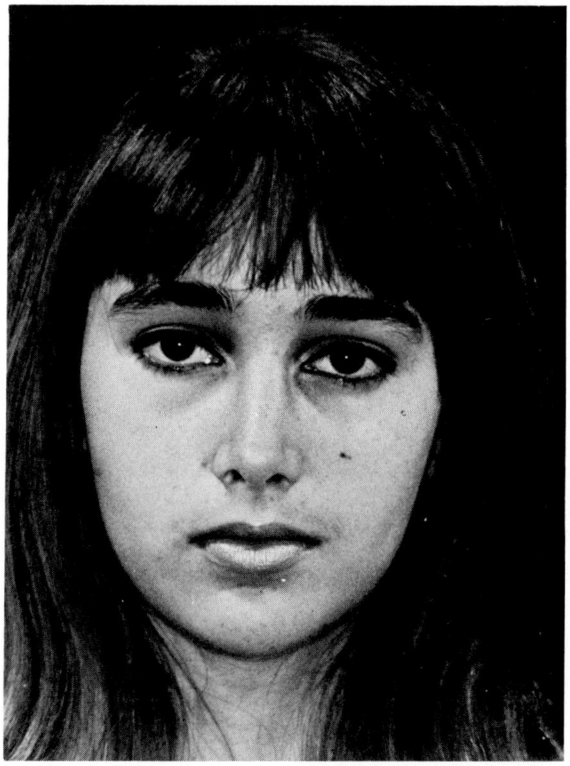

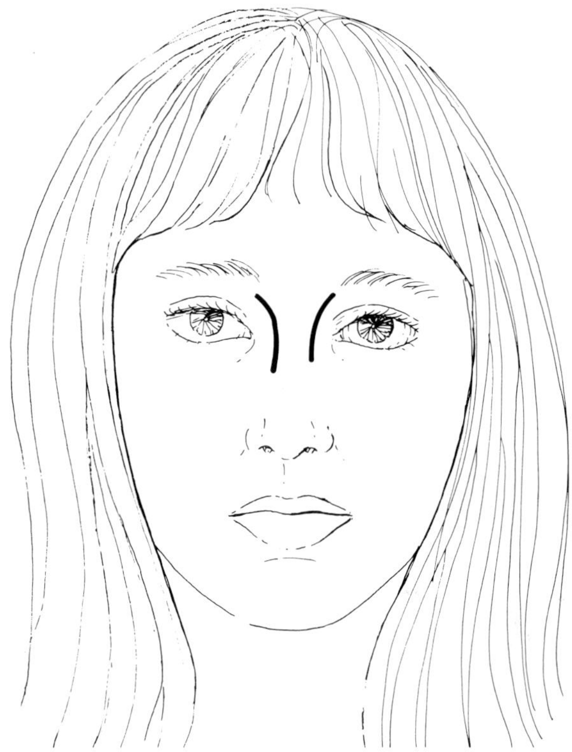

The postoperative view illustrates the preservation of the continuity from the superciliary ridges to the lateral nasal walls. The radix remains as wide as it was preoperatively, which retains this patient's characteristic relationship of radix to orbit.

DORSUM

Dorsum on front view

Viewed from the front, the dorsum connects the radix with the lateral projections of the crura of the lower lateral cartilages by two divergent concave lines that are unbroken extensions of the superciliary ridges.

Though the dorsum is generally considered to be of greatest importance in profile, the impact of the frontal view of the dorsum on the appearance of the midface must be appreciated. The dorsum on front view should be of sufficient height to provide the appearance of an anatomic part separating the eyes. Overreduction of the dorsum causes a change in the characteristic orbital-nasal relationship of each individual.

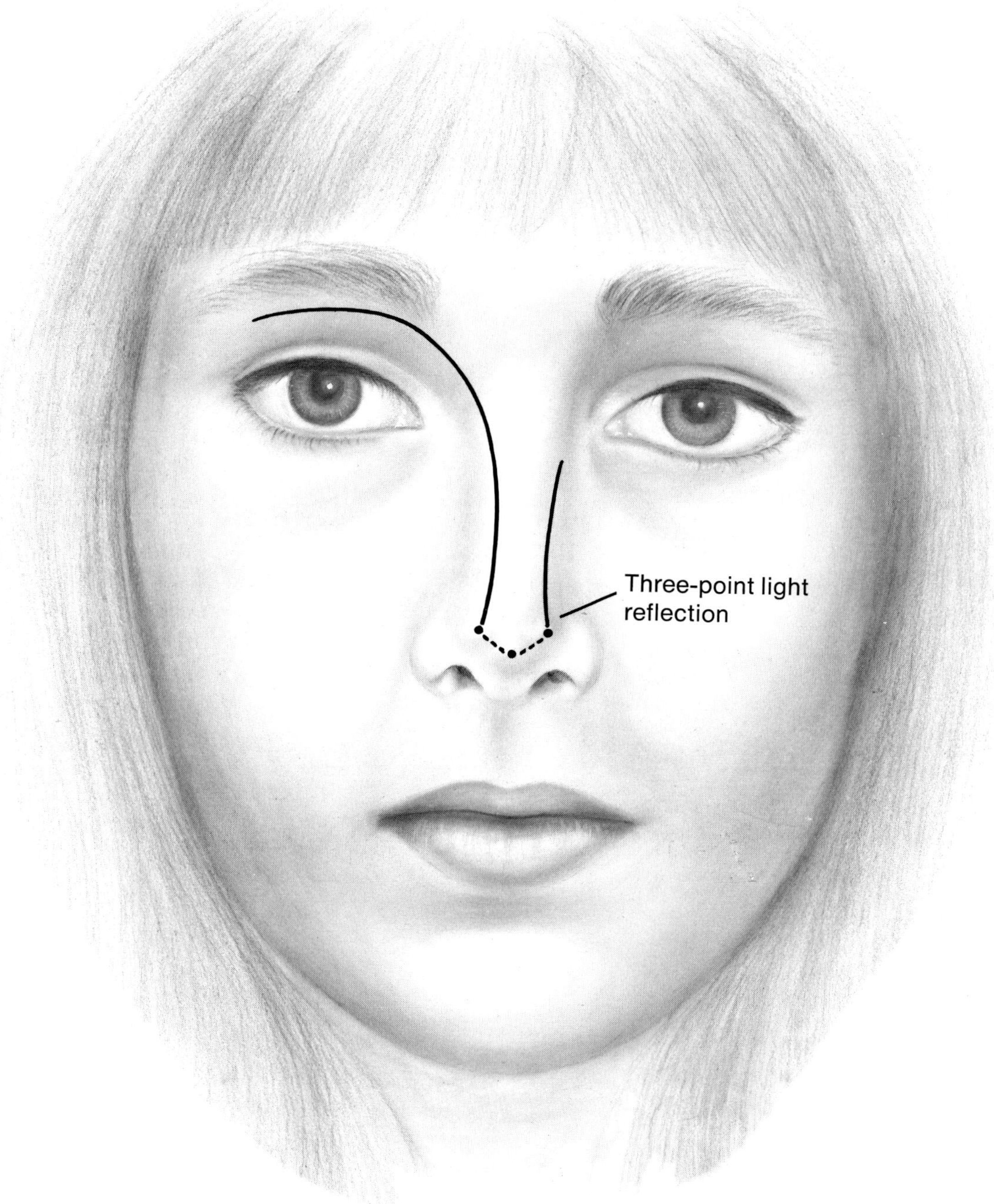
Three-point light
reflection

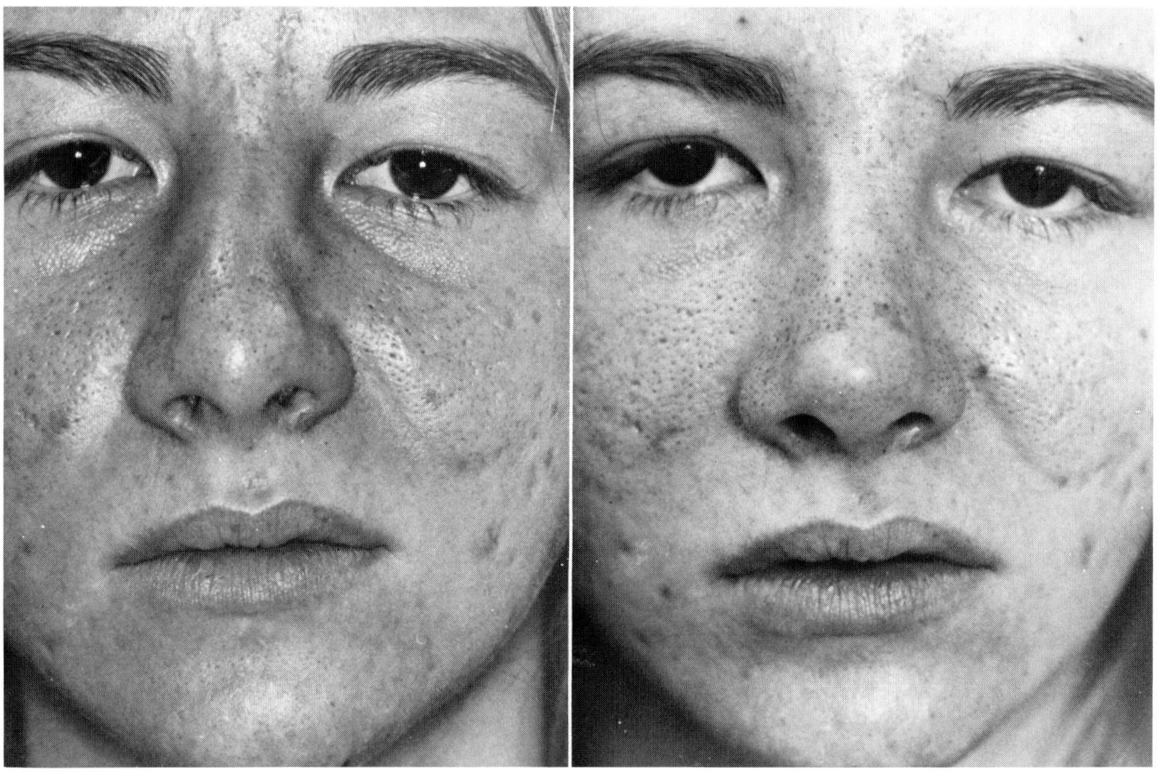

Whenever there is a disruption of the smooth line of flow from the orbit to the lateral walls to the tip, there is immediate focus of attention on the area of discrepancy. This patient had bilateral avulsion of the upper lateral cartilages from the bony pyramid following rhinoplasty, resulting in irregularities of the lateral nasal lines.

An aesthetic improvement was obtained by augmentive cartilage grafts over the depressed upper cartilaginous vault and lateral osteotomies to narrow the bony pyramid.

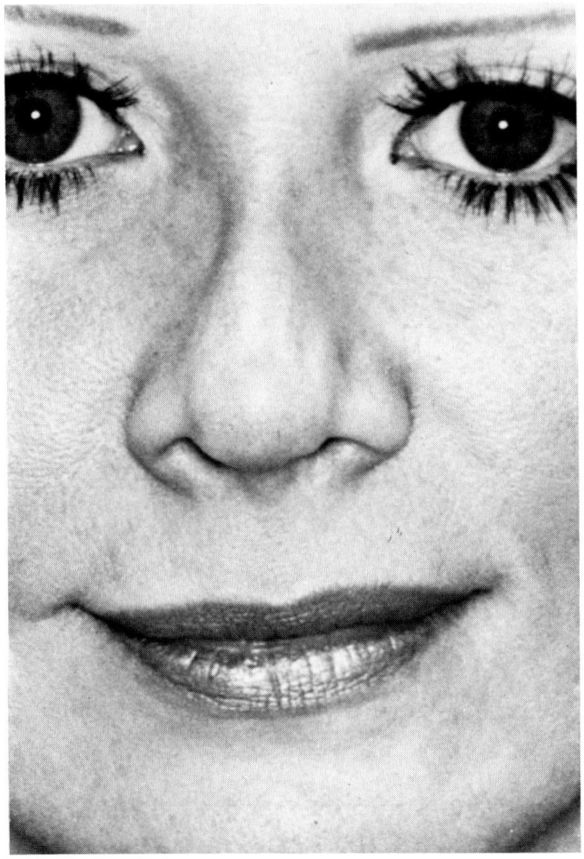

This patient illustrates the result of a surgical attempt to narrow the root of the nose. The consequence is a loss of continuity of the lines from the orbit to the lateral nasal walls and a radix that remains unchanged. The overly narrowed nasal pyramid is incongruent with both the root and the base of the nose.

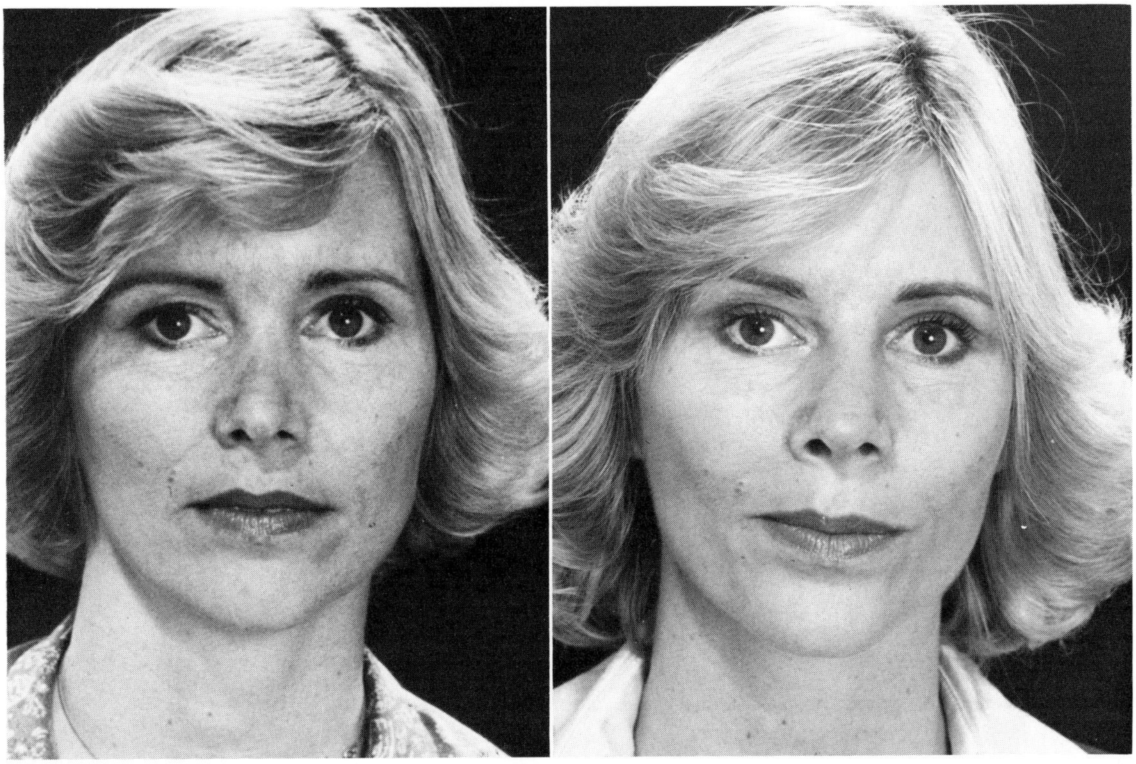

Patients who have had an overreduction of the dorsum, as this patient has, frequently complain that "something funny has happened to my eyes." The lack of height of the dorsum produces a flatness across the midface, which patients often translate as an unfavorable change in the appearance of their eyes.

The patient received a 3-mm cartilage augmentation of the dorsum. With this slight dorsal augmentation, the change in the appearance of the midface has restored the normal look that the patient had lost following her first surgery. There is also a restoration of the proper nasal-orbital relationship, as evidenced by the smooth lines from the superciliary arches to the lateral nasal walls.

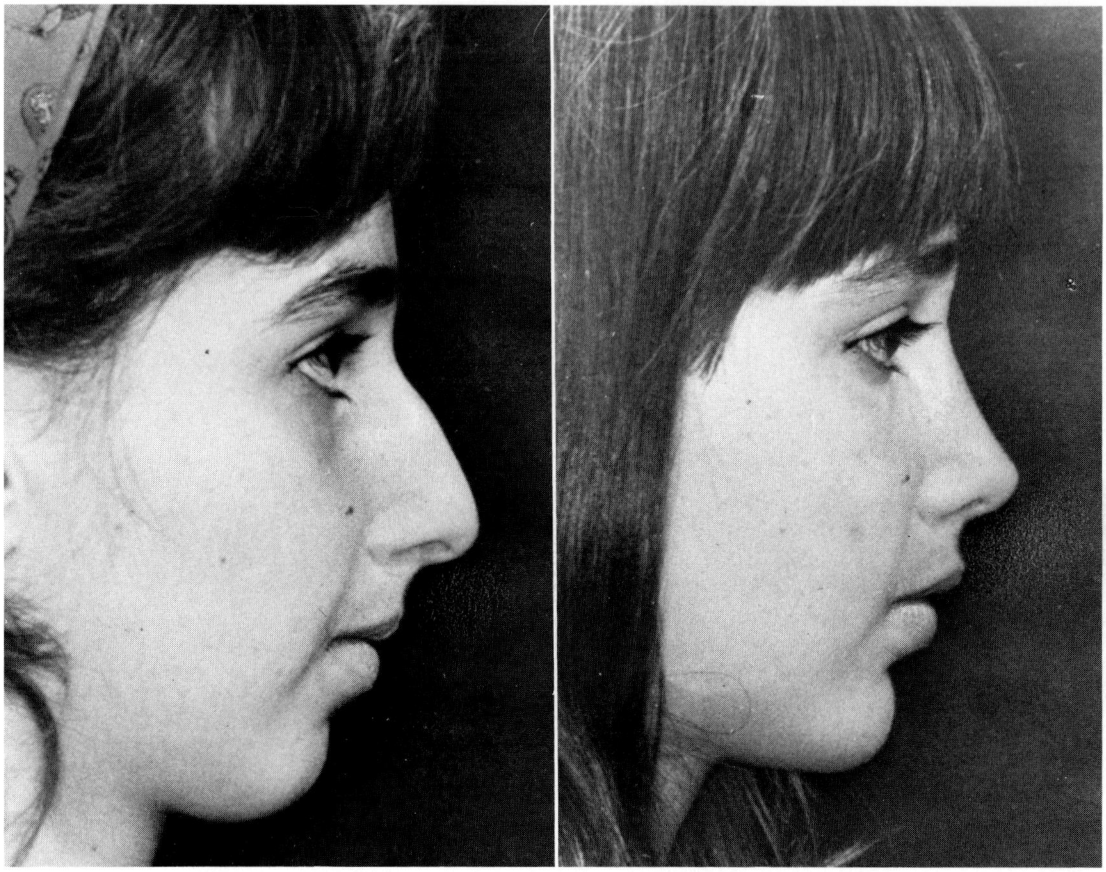

Dorsum on lateral view

The relationship of the dorsum to the tip has a strong influence on the apparent attitude of the tip. This patient's nose preoperatively has the appearance of a downward tilt in spite of an open nasolabial angle.

The middle third of the face is overwhelmed by the nasal convexity and prominent nasal spine, which are in turn emphasized by a retrusive chin.

Postoperatively, the dorsal line begins at the radix and descends in a relatively straight line to the tip, which has become the highest point in the nasal profile. This change in the relationship of dorsum to tip changes the apparent inclination of the nasal tip from a downward to an upward slant.

The imbalance of the middle third of the patient's face has been improved by partial resection of the projecting nasal spine and conservative augmentation of her chin.

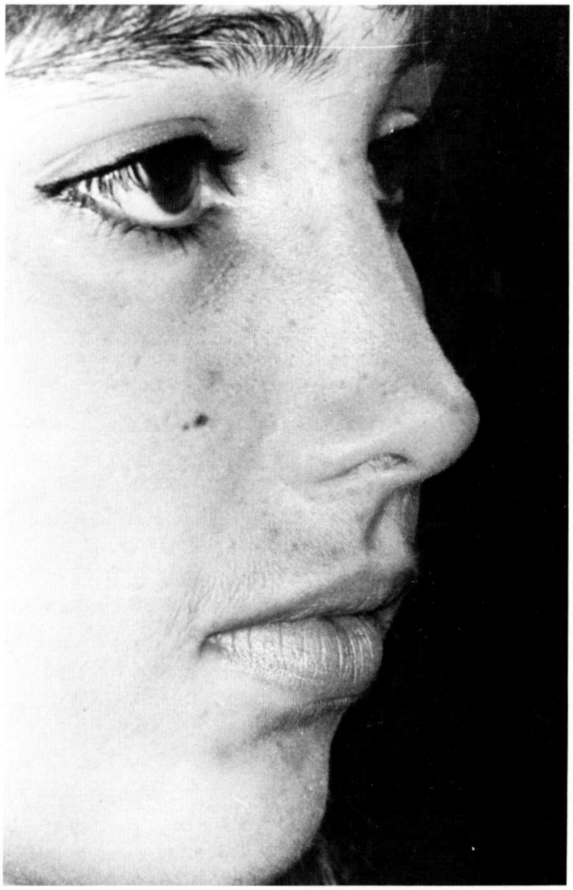

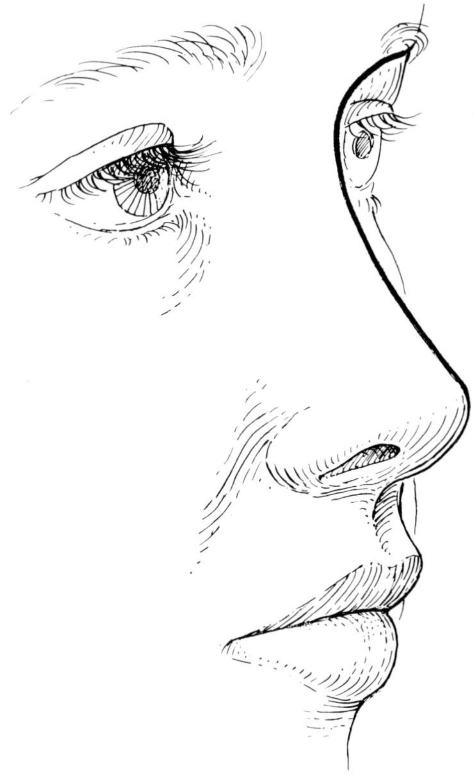

Dorsum on oblique view

On oblique view, there should be an unbroken line that extends from the supraorbital ridge to the radix and along the dorsal line to the dome of the lower lateral cartilage.

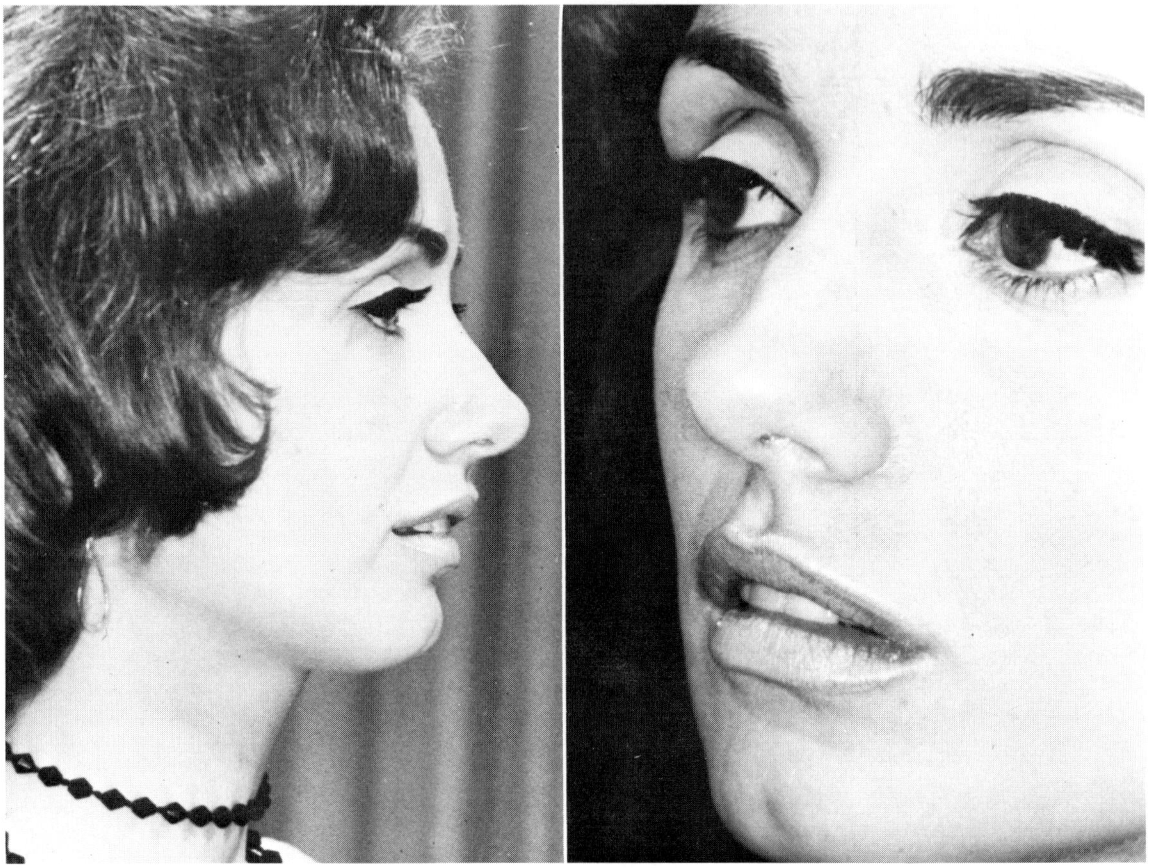

Too often the oblique view of the dorsum is omitted in the evaluation of the nose. This preoperative lateral photograph shows a straight dorsal line; however, on oblique view there is marked irregularity caused by the disparity between the caudal edge of the bony vault and the upper cartilaginous vault. This irregular line on oblique view occurs with short nasal bones or with patients who have extremely thin skin and cartilage.

Differing oblique views reflect the relative positions of the lateral nasal walls to the dorsum. In the posttraumatic nose with a concavity on the left, the dorsum on the right oblique view appears to be concave. The normal or laterally displaced right side appears to have a dorsal hump on left oblique view (see p. 355).

NASAL TIP

There is no greater challenge in rhinoplasty than the predictable construction of a nasal tip that is elegant and distinct. And there is no other problem in rhinoplasty that involves so many variables. The dorsal edge of the septum, the caudal septum, the nasal spine, the size, position, and substance of the lower lateral cartilages, the position of the domes of the lower lateral cartilages, the character of the skin, and the relationships and size of the nostrils all play a role in determining tip configuration. A thorough understanding of the influence of these various factors on the tip and a well-defined conception of the surface anatomy serve to guide the surgeon in the assessment and management of the nasal tip.

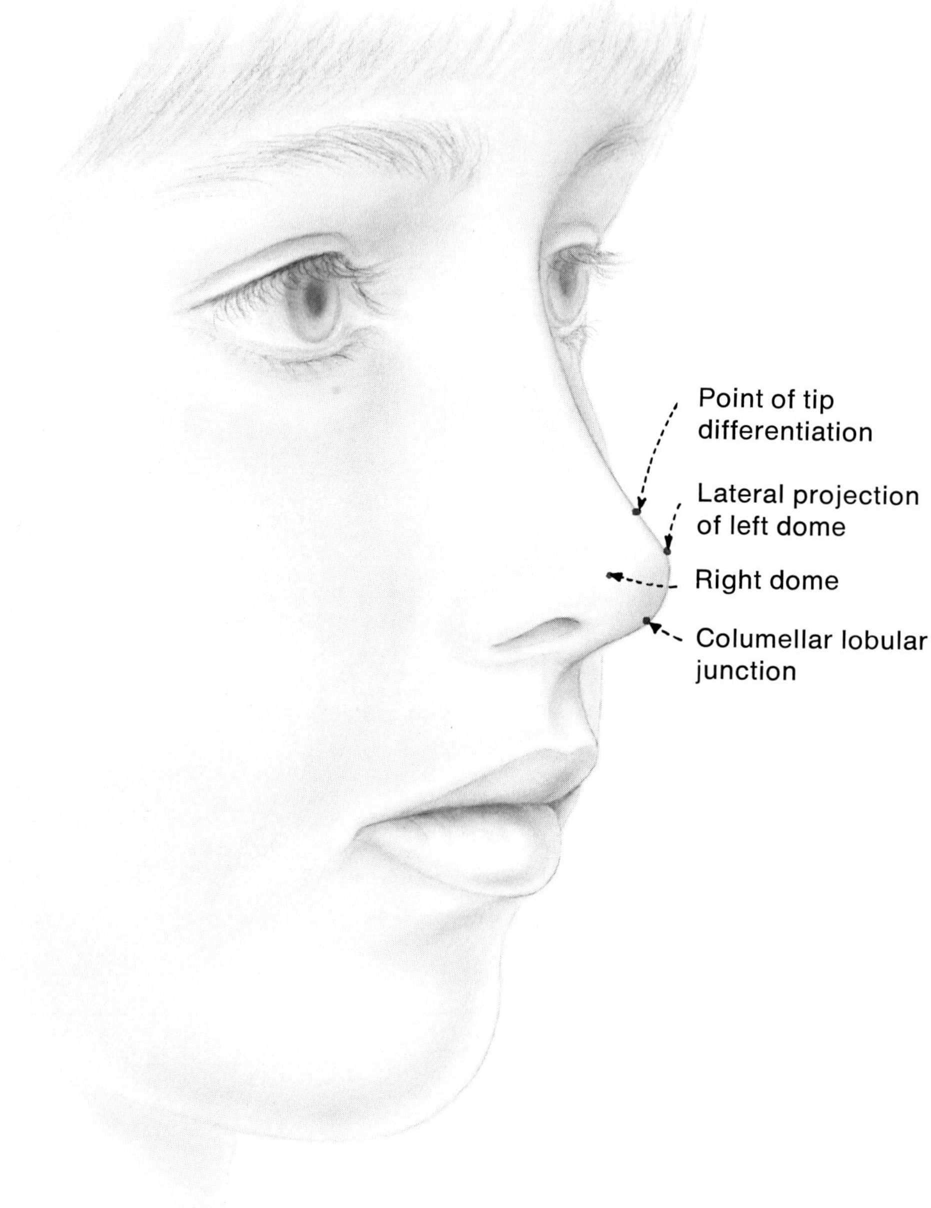

The refined tip is characterized by four essential landmarks:

1. Lateral projection of the left dome
2. Lateral projection of the right dome
3. Point of tip differentiation from the dorsum
4. Columellar lobular junction

These four reference points are seen on any view of the nose and are manifest by either light reflexes or projections.

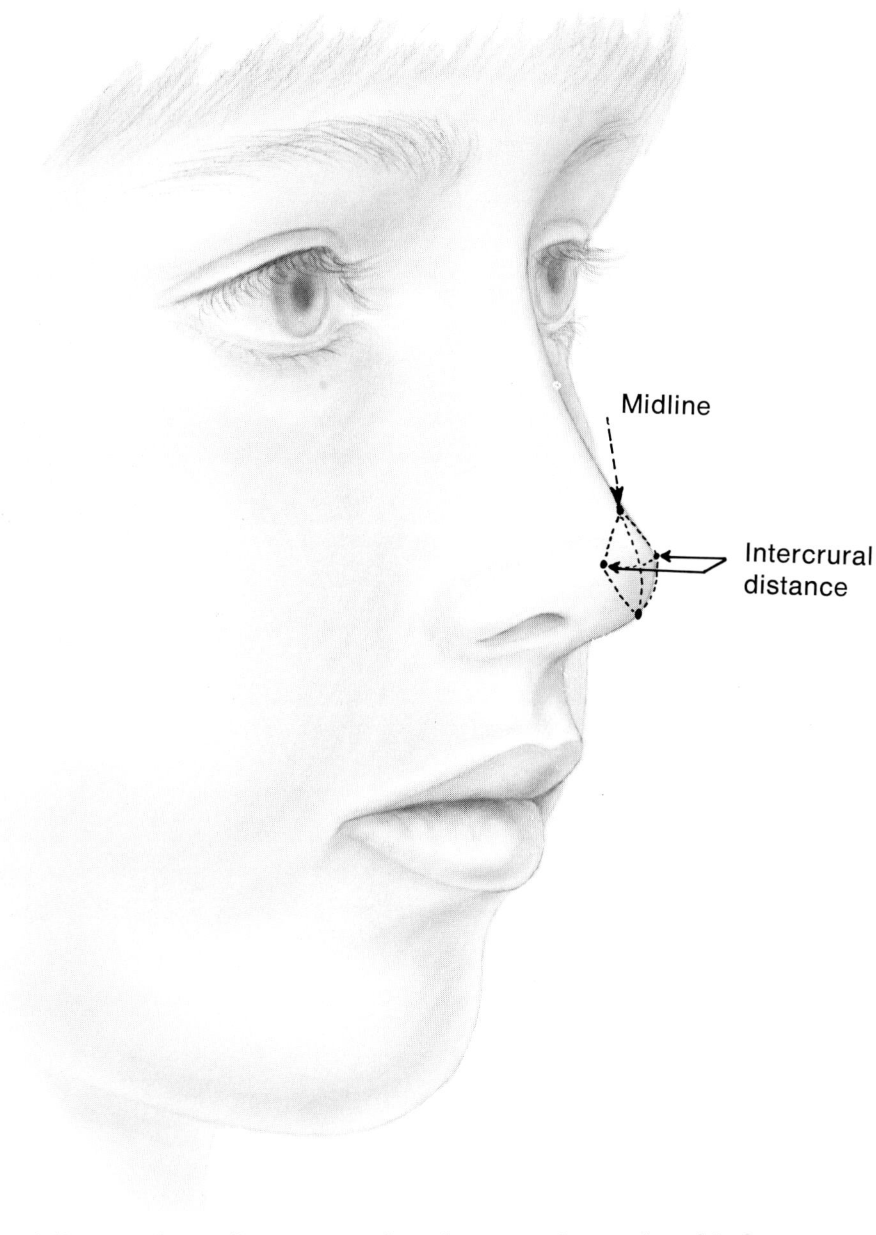

On oblique view, for example, these points should form two equilateral geodesic triangles with a common base, the length of which I refer to as the intercrural distance, or ICD. The apex of the superior triangle is the point of tip differentiation from the dorsum. The apex of the inferior triangle is the point of the columellar lobular junction. The apogee of the curved line that connects the two domes of the lower lateral cartilages should be the highest projecting part of the nose from whatever angle the nose is viewed.

Nasal tip on front view

On front view the nasal tip must appear as a continuation of the lateral nasal walls. The end points of the diverging lines appear as light reflexes. The normal anatomy of a nasal tip produces a light reflex from three areas—the two lateral domes of the lower lateral cartilages and the central arch of the line that joins them. These reflections are ideal aesthetically if they follow the equilateral tip triangle that I have described.

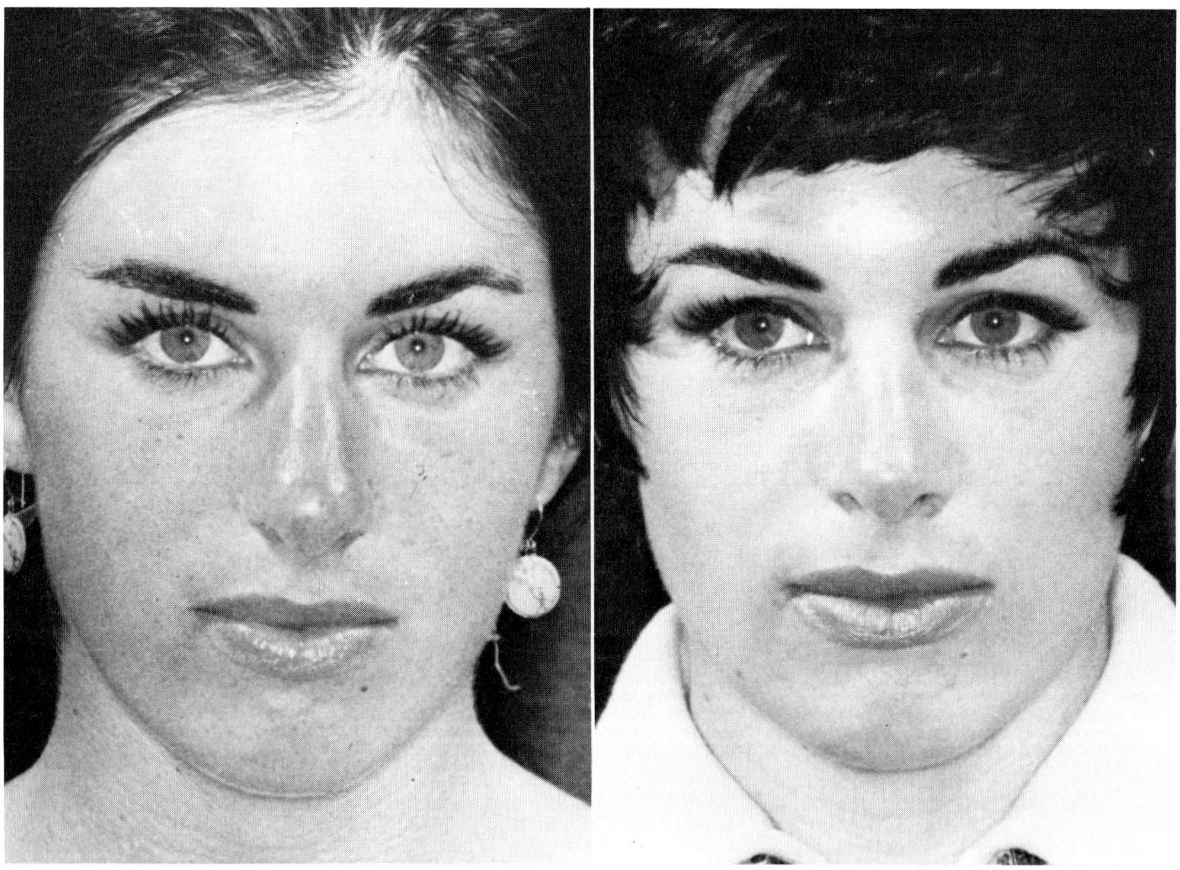

The preoperative photograph of this patient illustrates a three-point reflex that is broad. Clinically the tip was bulbous. Following surgery, the exact placement of the alar domes is confirmed by a corresponding three-point reflex.

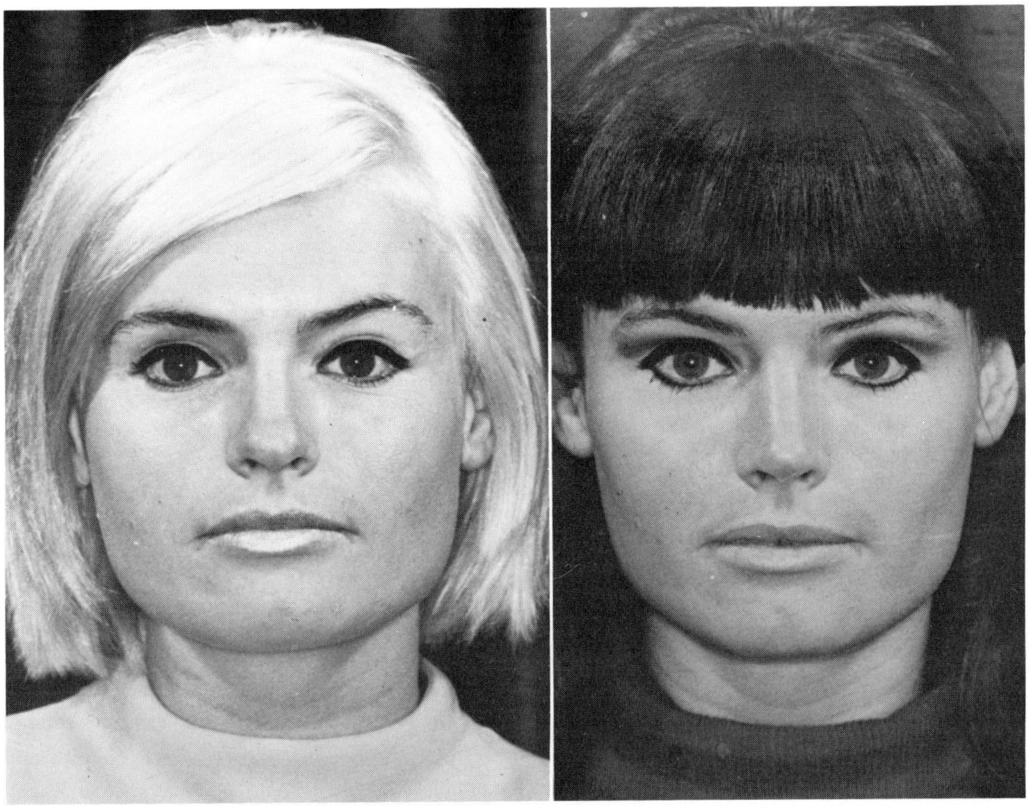

In this preoperative photograph the patient's tip cartilages are broad (long ICD), producing a ball-like tip. An illusion of shortening results because of the high position of the cephalic edges of the lower lateral cartilages. The light reflecting from the tip confirms a long intercrural distance.

Postoperatively, the nose appears longer even though it is actually shorter. The lines from the lateral nasal walls flow into the tip and end at the point of the lateral projection of the lower lateral cartilaginous domes. This produces a three-point light reflex that gives the tip a delicacy that can be obtained only with proper position of the domes of the lower lateral cartilages.

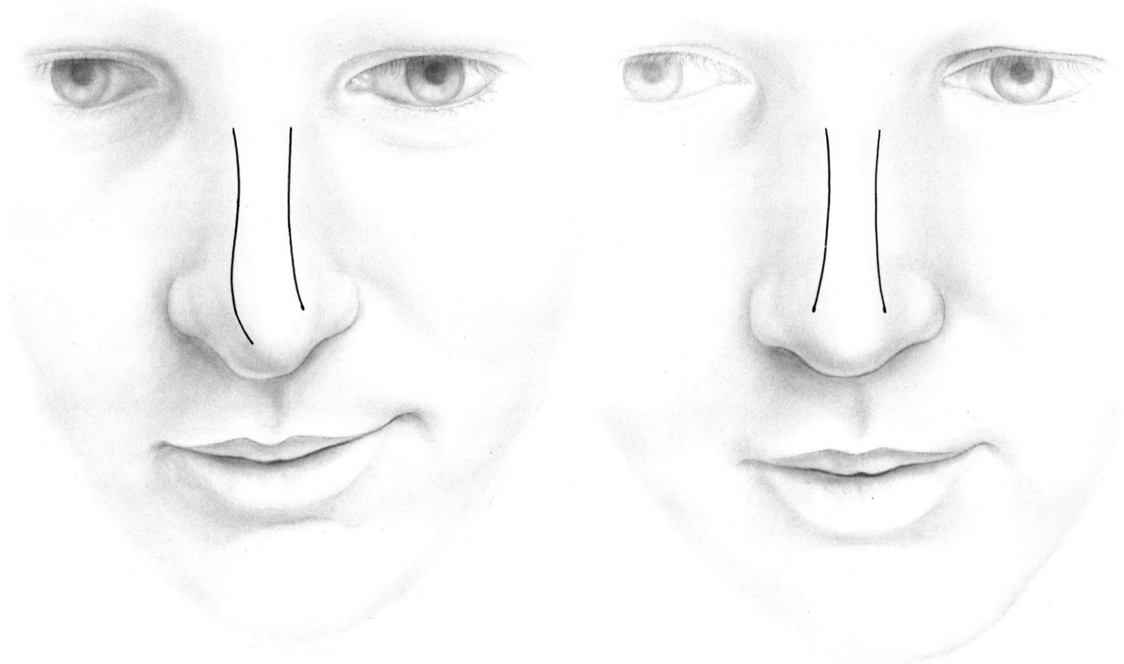

The ICD must be consistent with the rest of the nasal tip—not too wide or too narrow. The significance of the placement of the domes equidistant from the midline becomes immediately apparent when shown schematically. Any change or loss of one or both of these important landmarks results in a tip that appears asymmetrical or distorted.

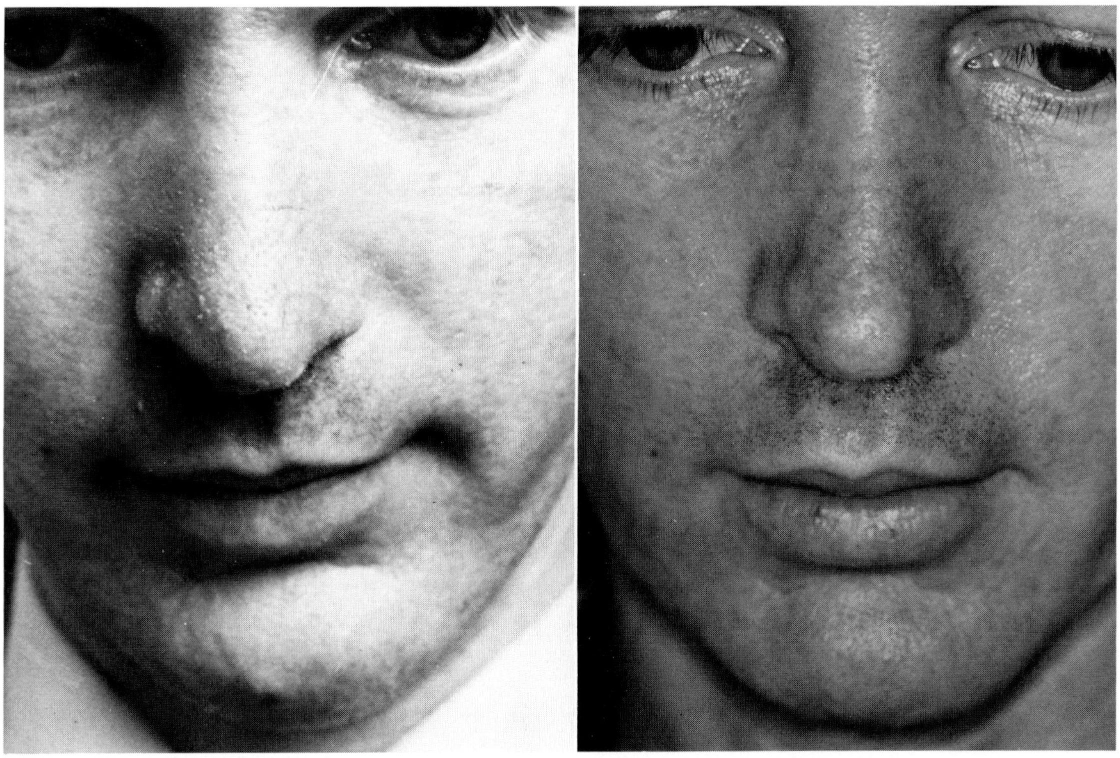

Preoperatively, the right alar dome lacks projection. This is manifest by a flatness to the right side of the nose. Postoperatively, the projection of the right dome was created by use of a cartilaginous tip graft, resulting in a more symmetrical nasal tip.

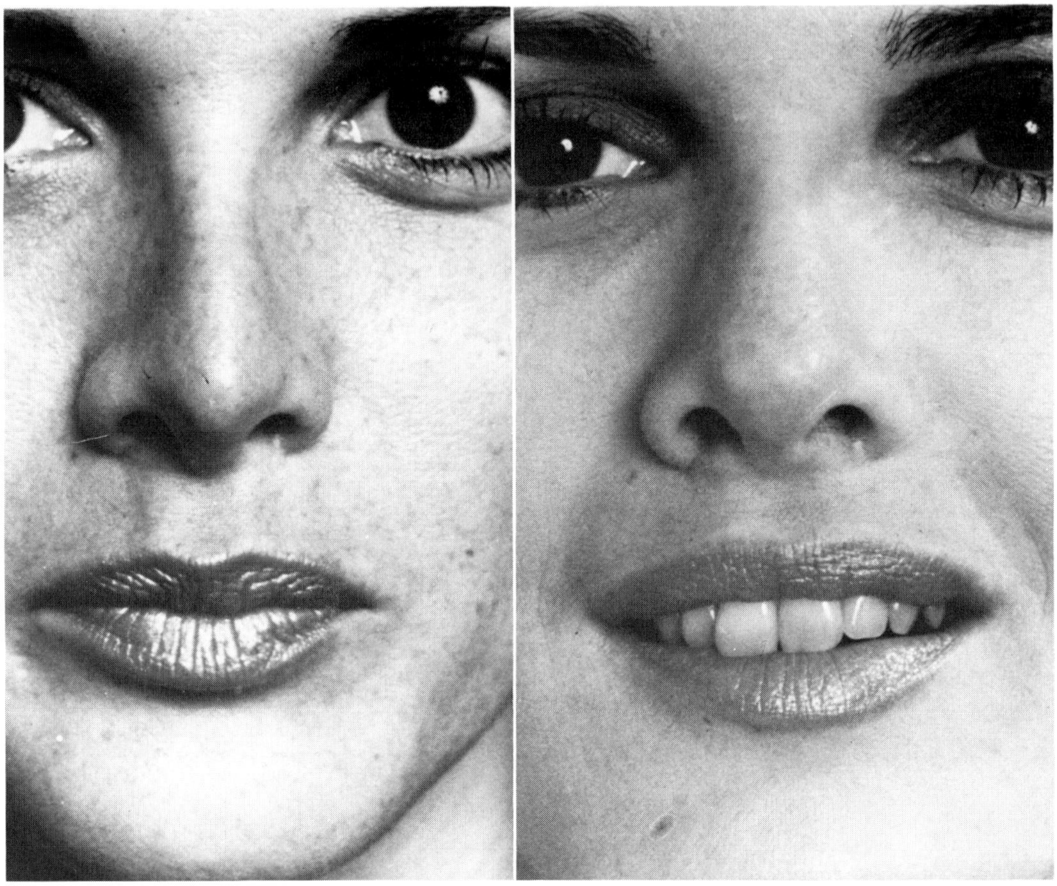

This patient has had a primary rhinoplasty. There is a single light reflex in the middle of her nasal tip, indicating a short or imperceptible ICD. This can occur with resection of the domes of the lower lateral cartilages by suturing the medial crura together or by using central struts. The lines from the lateral nasal walls converge on this point, giving the tip a pinched appearance. Moreover, the nasal tip appears disproportionately small for this nose.

The patient underwent tip reconstruction to re-create the lateral projections of the alar domes. The lines from the lateral nasal walls diverge, and the nasal tip configuration is consistent with the rest of the nose.

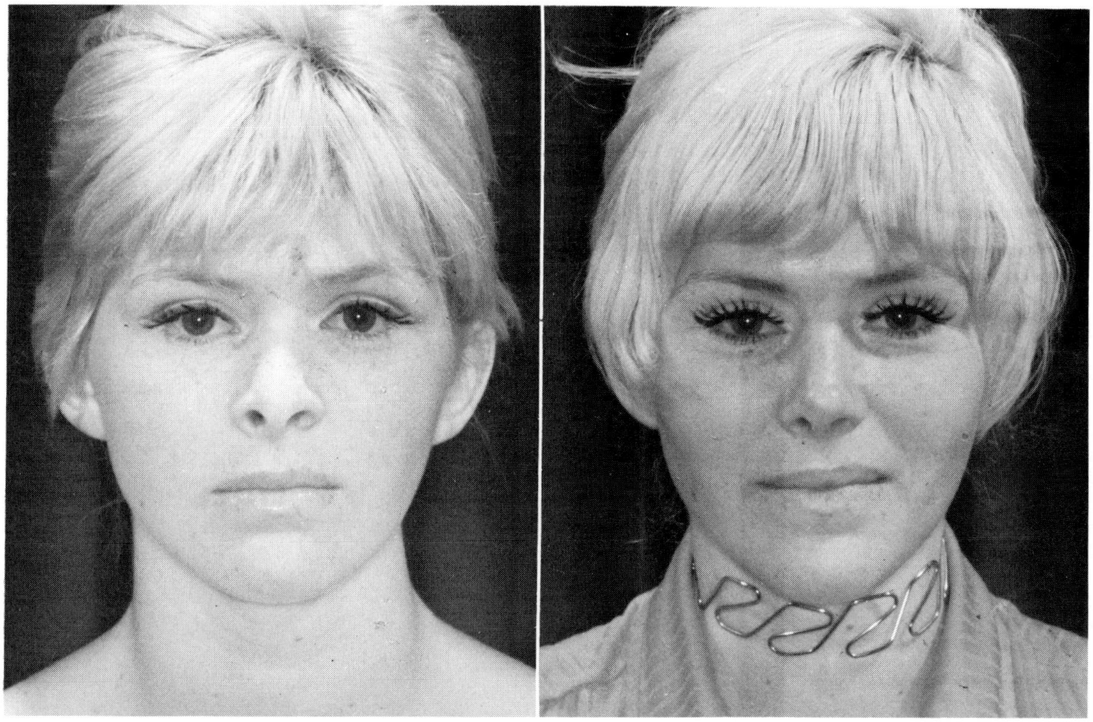

Following primary rhinoplasty, this patient has a rounded nasal tip with no appearance of the lower lateral cartilages. There are no landmarks or projections—in short, no definition. This front view illustrates the lack of definition as light reflects across the tip. The low bridge again illustrates a flat look in the midface.

After revision, the nasal contour flows smoothly from the superciliary ridges, diverging to two lateral points that have been constructed to duplicate the normal domes of the lower lateral cartilages. The aesthetic restoration of the nasal tip is made evident by the symmetrical three-point light reflex. Elevation of the dorsum with a graft has reestablished the normal separation of the eyes.

Nasal tip on oblique view

The oblique view places the dome of the opposite lower lateral cartilage as the highest projecting part in the nasal silhouette. The alar dome should be the terminal point of the smooth line that descends from the radix. This lateral projection of the dome must be of sufficient distance from the midline to cause this visible projection. In the event that one dome has been surgically ablated, there is a striking difference in the appearance of the nose from one oblique view to the other.

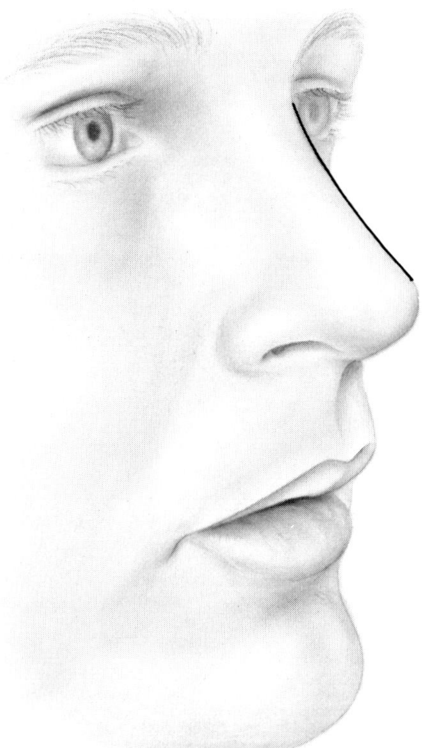

A right oblique view illustrates the position of the dome of the left lower lateral cartilage in the nasal silhouette.

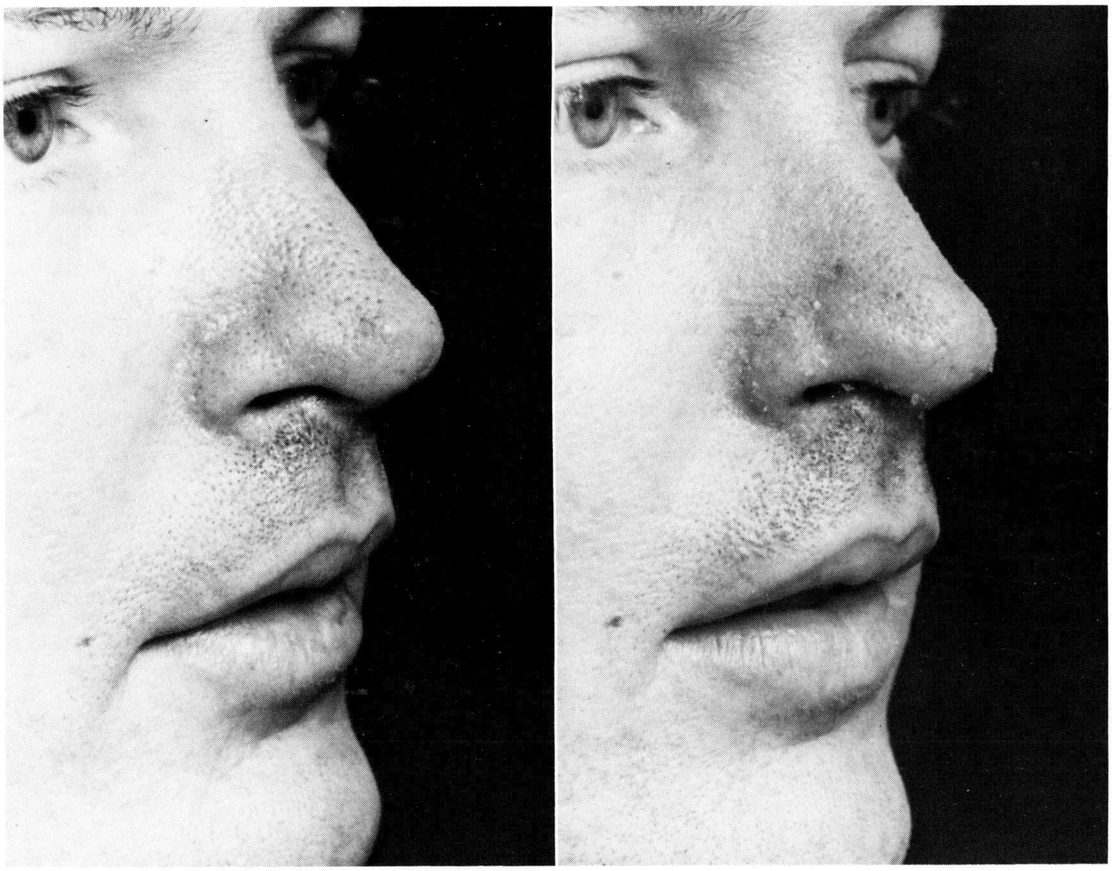

These photographs of the right oblique view illustrate the projection of the dome of the left lower lateral cartilage, which appears as the highest point in the nasal profile. Examining the pictures closely reveals a light reflex in the postoperative photograph *(right)* that corresponds to the lateral projection of the right lower lateral cartilage.

The intercrural distance must be sufficient to provide lateral tip projection on oblique view. An insufficient ICD places the dome of the alar cartilage in poor position relative to the rest of the nasal base, causing a flatness to the nasal tip on oblique view.

The preoperative left oblique view illustrates the amputated appearance of a nasal tip with the dome of the right lower lateral cartilage absent or too near the midline.

The postoperative photograph demonstrates the reconstructed dome. All of the important landmarks are visible: adequate ICD, two equilateral geodesic triangles, and projection of the dome of the right lower lateral cartilage, which provides an end point for the regular line from the root to the base.

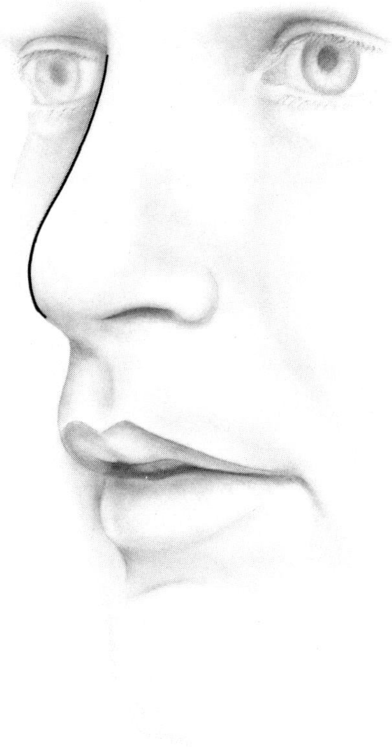

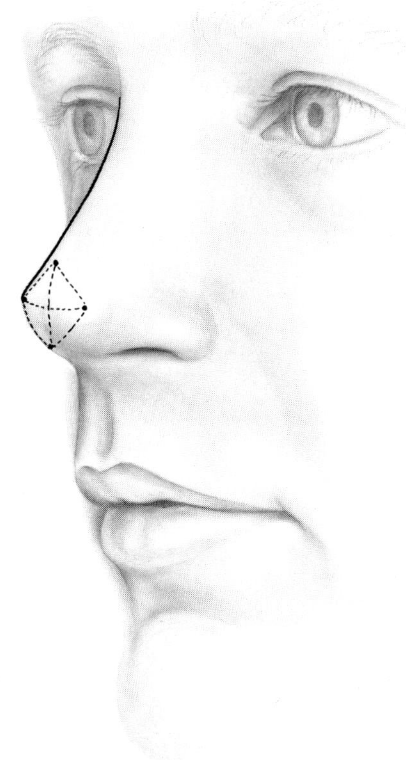

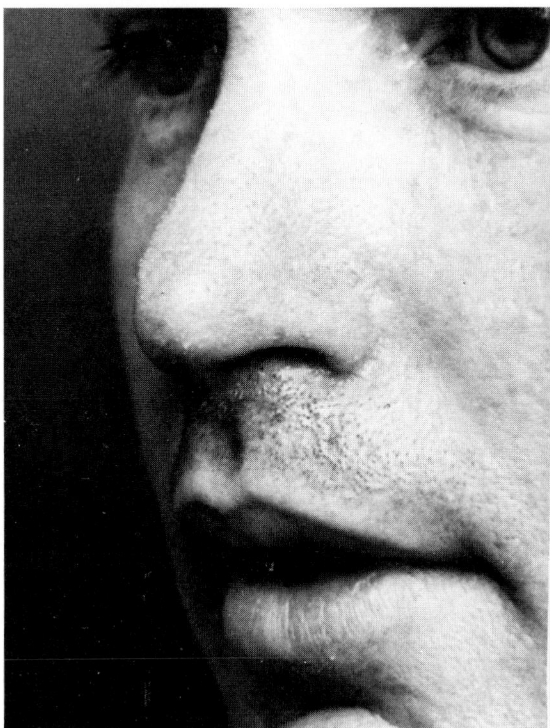

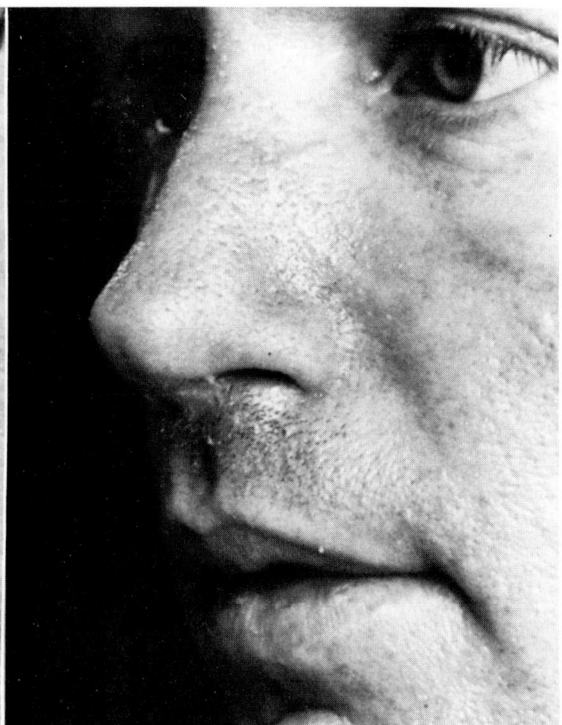

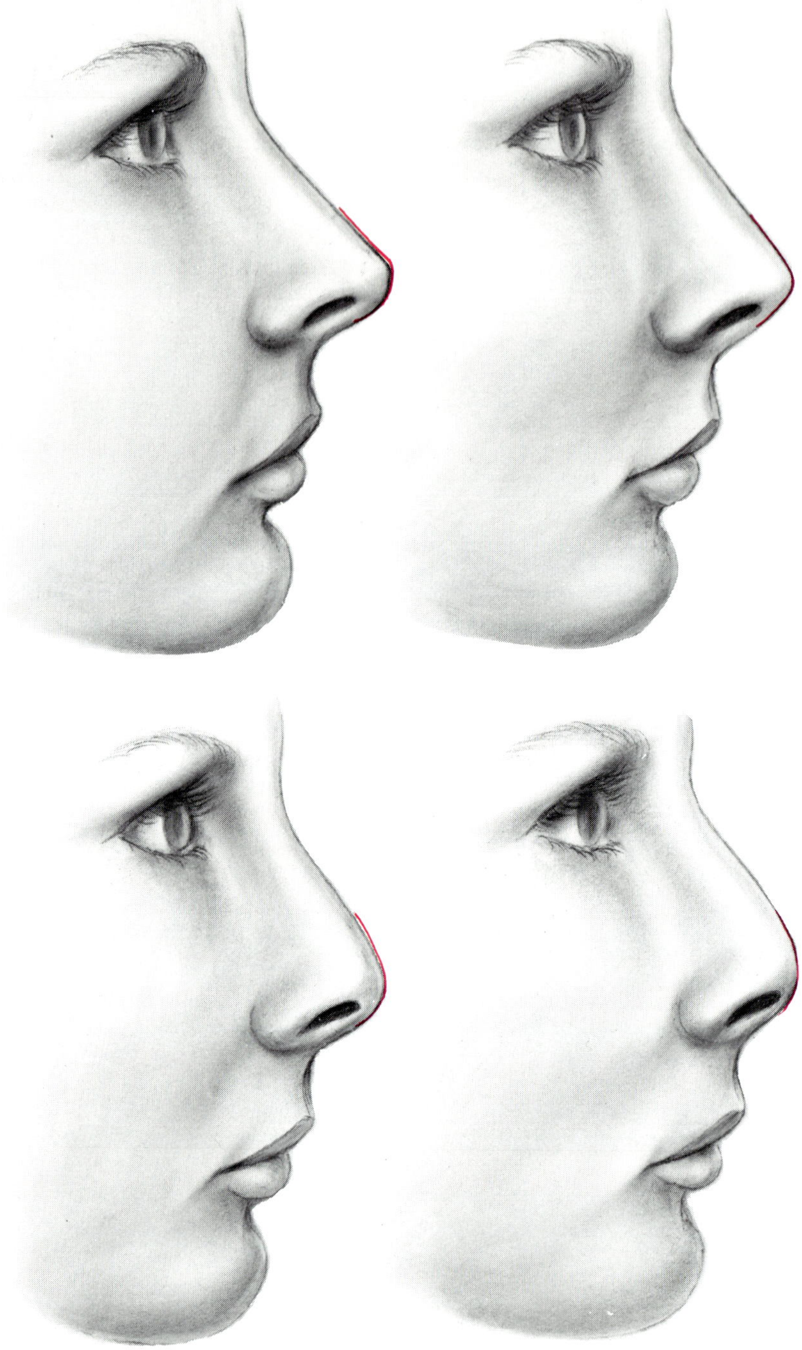

Nasal tip on lateral view

The character of the nose—its delicacy, inclination, length, and width—is influenced by the contour of the nasal tip. These four lateral views are identical except for the tip configuration (in red). The dramatic changes that are illustrated underline the importance of the structure of the nasal tip to facial aesthetics. The influence of the nasal tip on the apparent length of the nose cannot be overstressed.

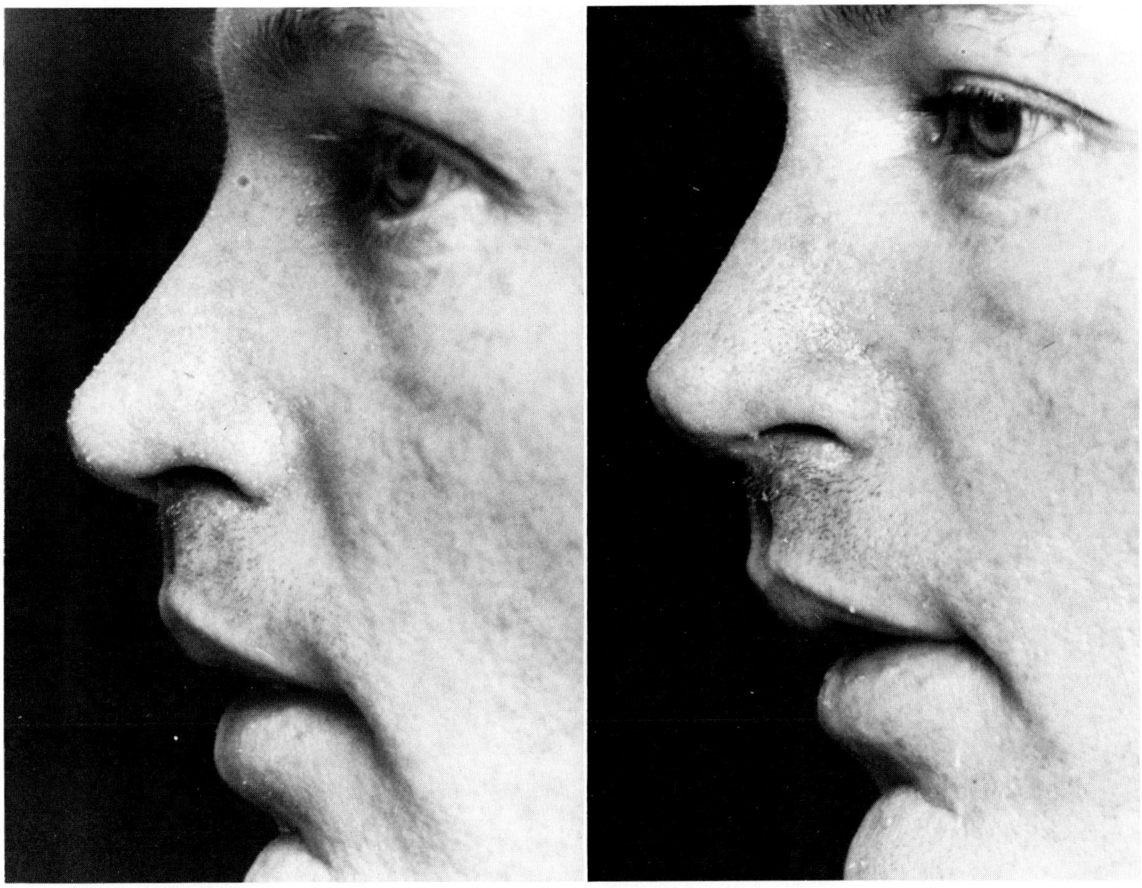

On left lateral view, the preoperative nasal relationships are satisfactory, but there is less delineation of the tip than is desirable. In the postoperative view, the projection of the right dome, with slight rotation of the tip cephalad, has sharply improved the profile.

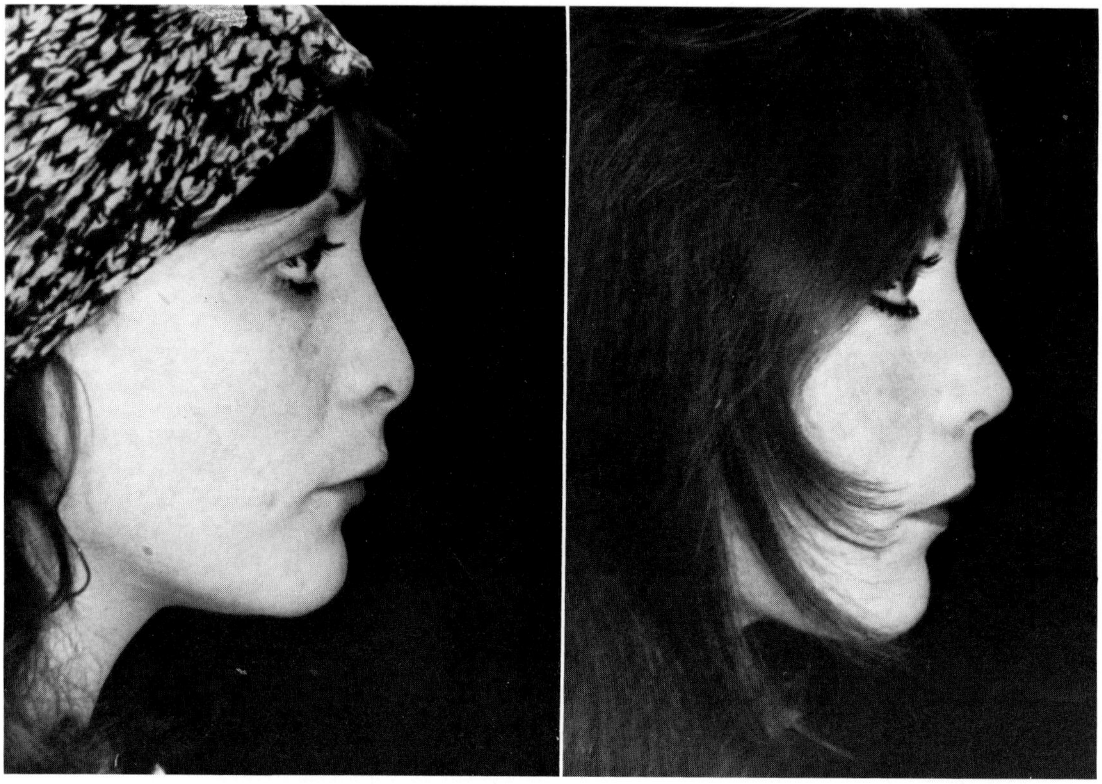

Following reduction rhinoplasty, the lowering of the dorsal line and overresection of the domes of the lower lateral cartilages can result in this classic postoperative look with no definite end points to the nasal profile.

After revision, restoration of good nasofacial and intranasal relationships has been accomplished by dorsal augmentation and tip reconstruction.

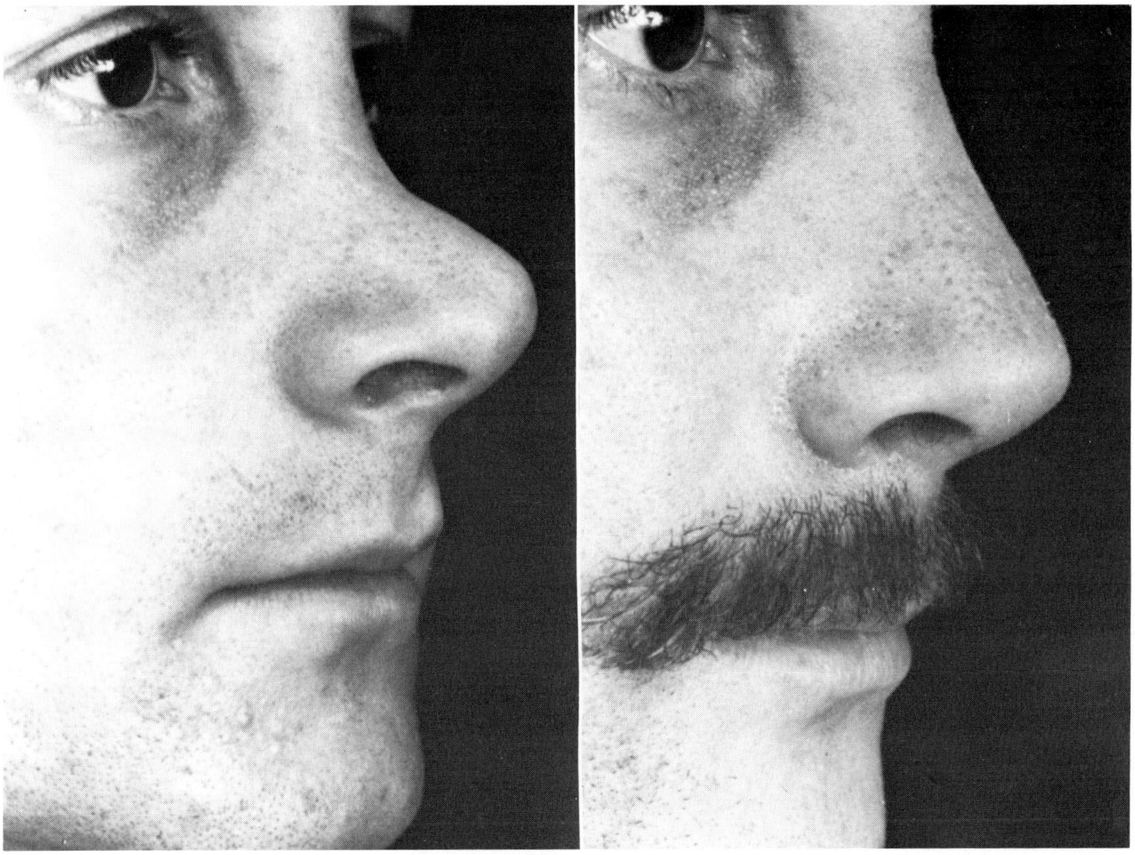

Overprojection of the nasal tip in relation to the rest of the nasal parts produces a result that may be totally inconsonant with the face and the nasal configuration. This patient has an overreduced dorsum and unreduced projection of the angle of the septum with transection (not resection) of the domes of the lower lateral cartilages.

Postoperatively, augmentation of the dorsum superiorly and reduction of it inferiorly have brought the parts into appropriate alignment. Modification of the caudal septum and nasal spine and tip reconstruction were also done.

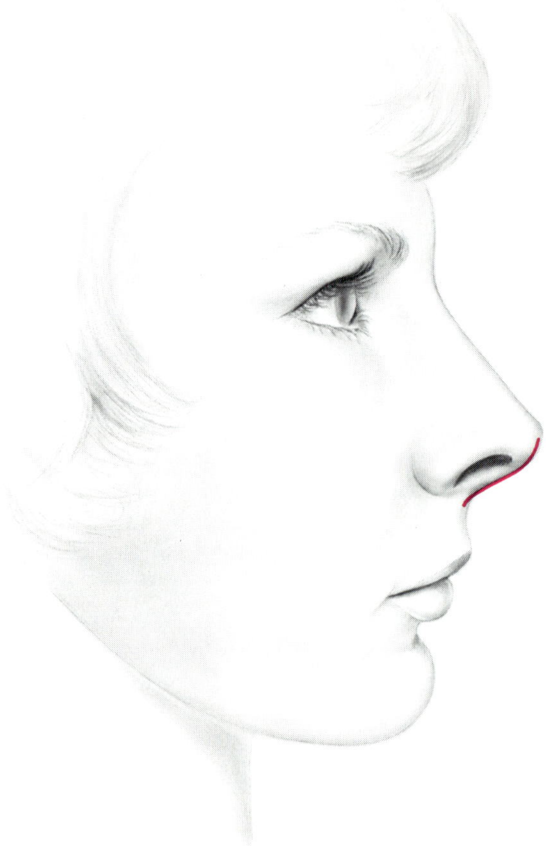

COLUMELLAR ALAR COMPLEX

The line that extends from the tip to the base of the columella is broken at the area of the columellar lobular junction. This break occurs at the apex of the inferior triangle of the nasal tip and on lateral view becomes a subtle but necessary part of the ideal nasal tip.

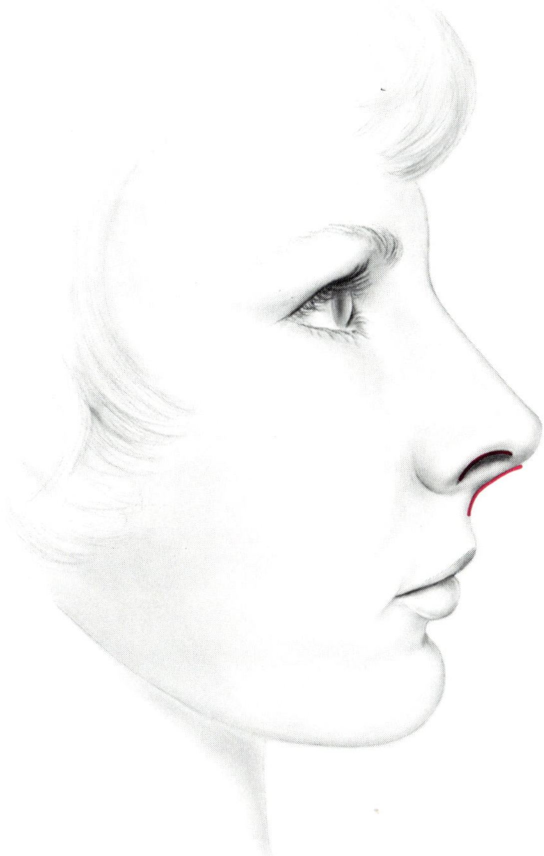

The columella must be of sufficient length to provide the necessary projection of the nasal tip above the dorsal line. It should form an obtuse angle with the lip and should be 2 to 3 mm lower than and parallel to the alar rims.

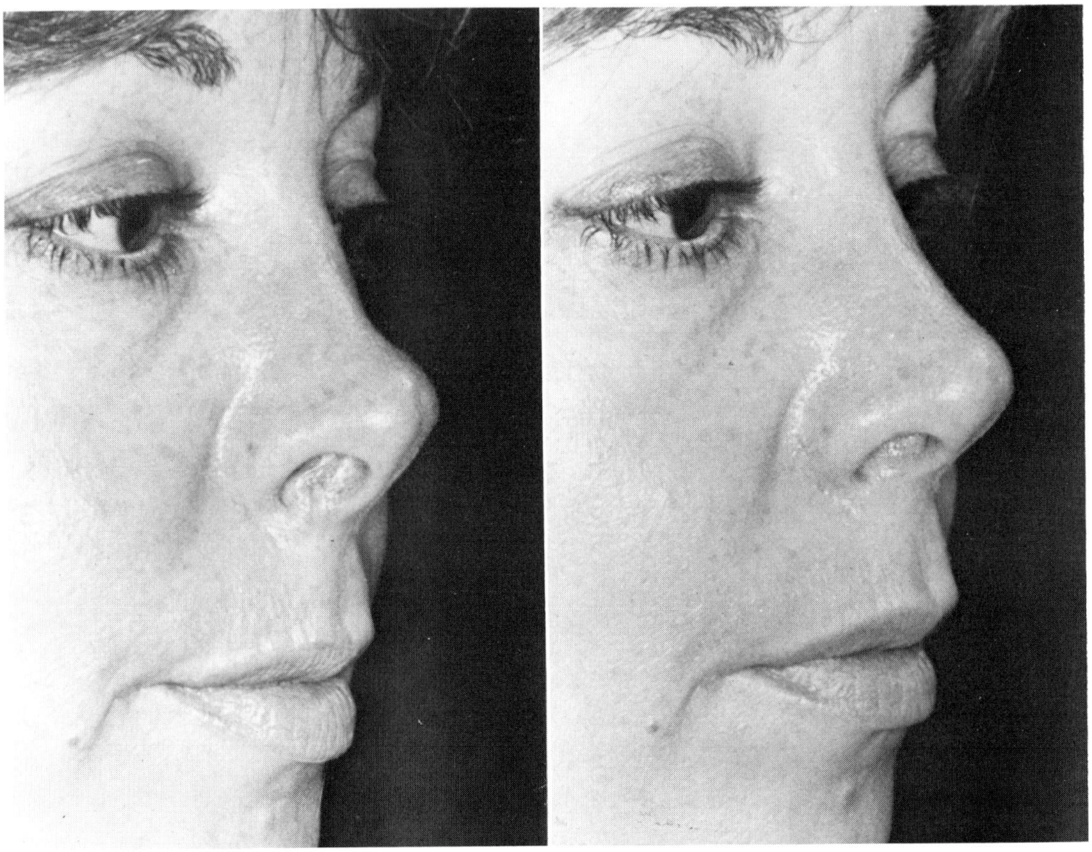

The poor alar-columellar relationship most often involves the caudal septum and nasal spine. This patient illustrates the effect of a low columella (6 to 7 mm below the alar rims). There is unattractive exposure of the membranous septum and vibrissae. The upward tilt of the nasal tip seems extreme because the overly full subnasion causes a nasolabial angle that is too shallow and too wide.

After revision, resection of the membranous septum with conservative reduction of the nasal spine and dorsal augmentation have brought the nasal base into better alignment.

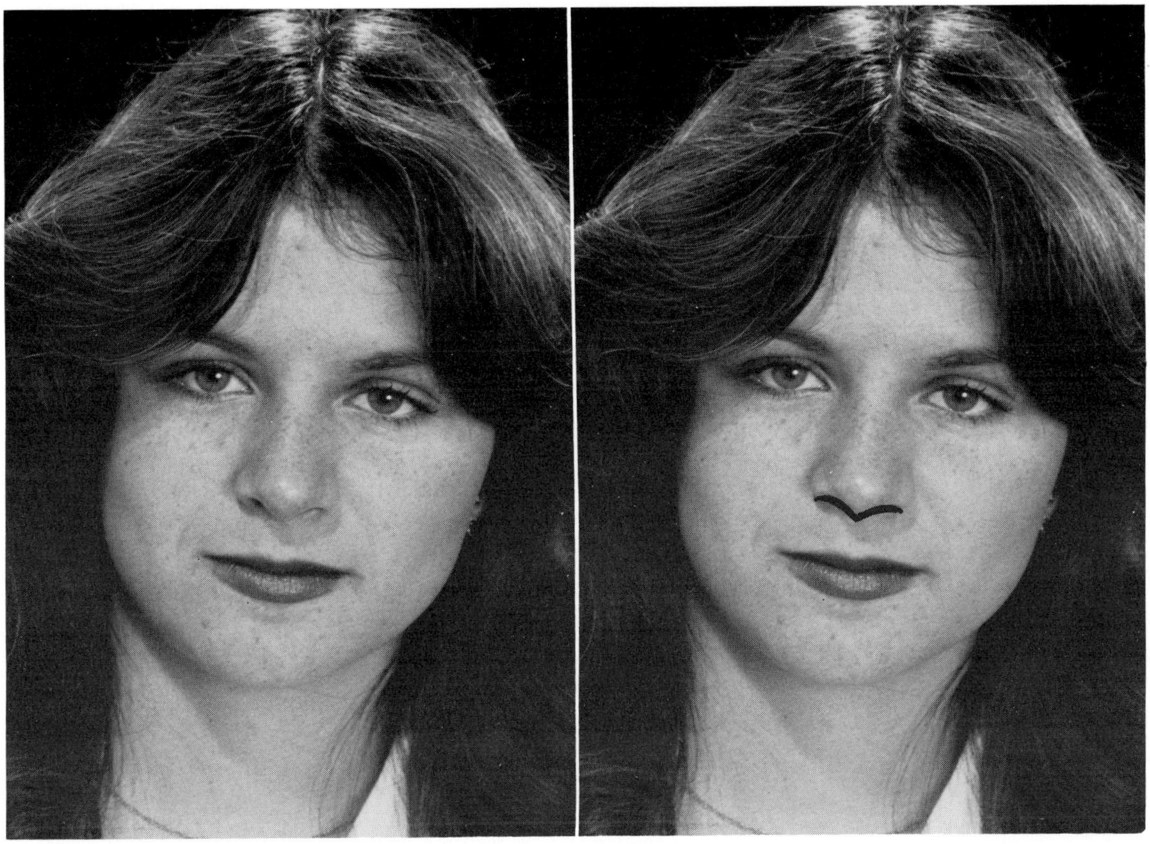

Columella on front view

On front view, there is a gull-in-flight contour to the base of the nose (the columella forming the body and the alar rims the wings). Aesthetically, the columella must be slightly lower than and parallel to the alae when viewed from any direction.

The position of the columella is governed by the cartilage of the caudal septum. Shortening the nose without appropriate caudal resection can produce a columella that hangs too far below the alar rims, whereas overresecting the caudal septum may cause retraction of the columella.

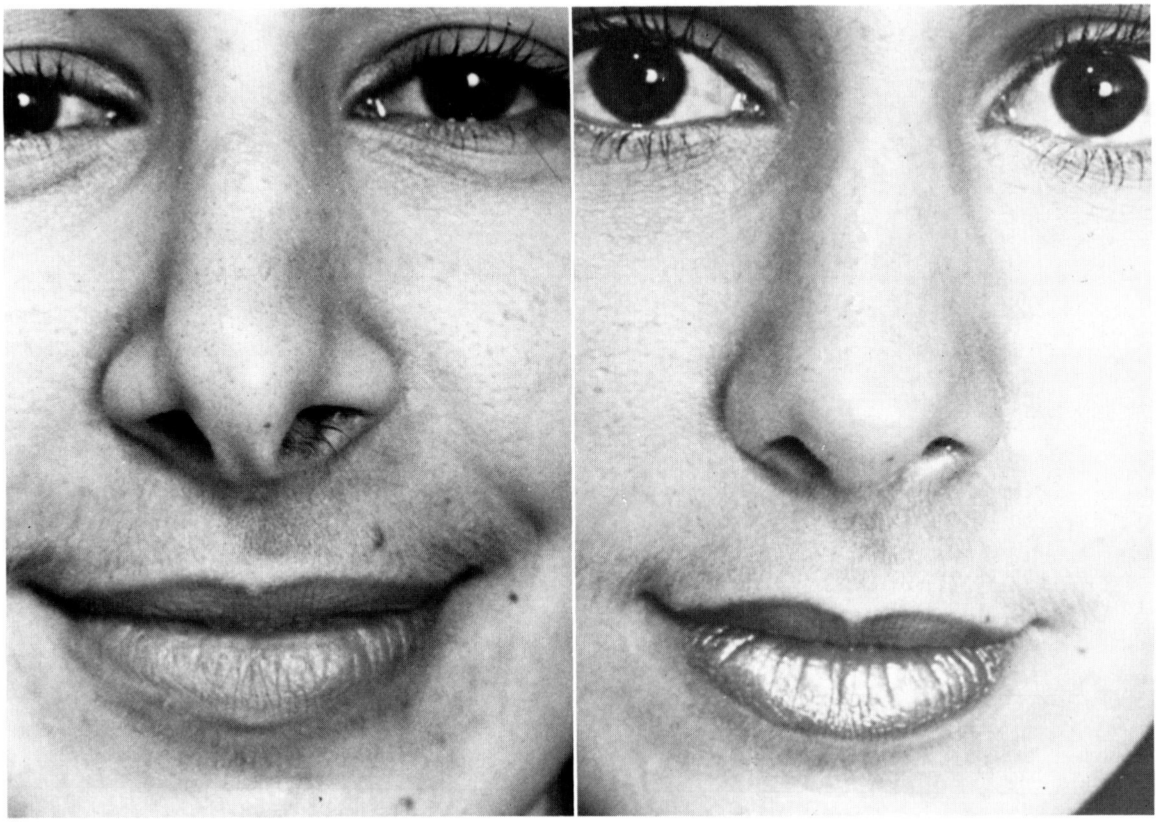

When the columella is too low in relation to the nostrils on front view, there is an unnatural prominence to the columella. Furthermore, there is an unattractive show of nasal vestibule and vibrissae.

Conservative resection of the caudal septum, tip grafting, and alar wedges have brought the base of this nose into better balance.

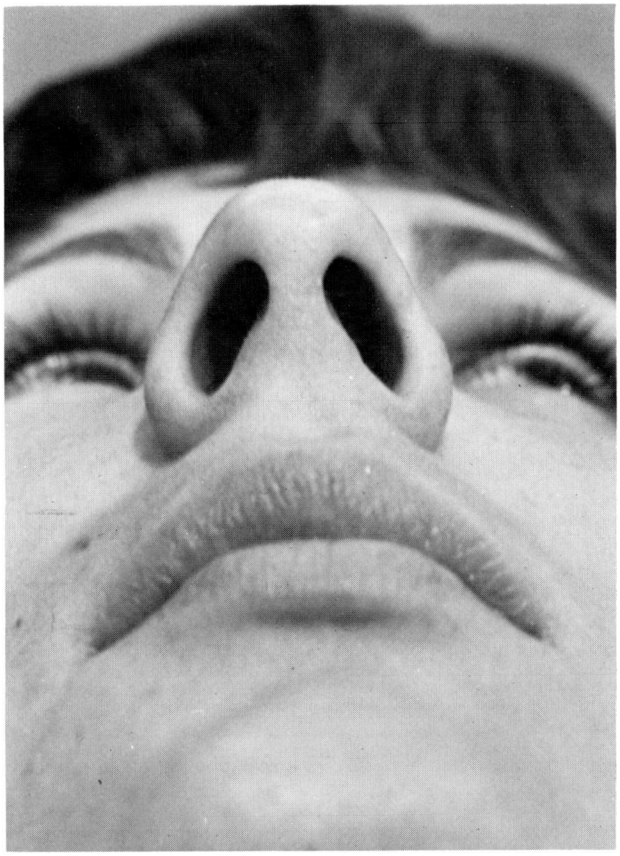

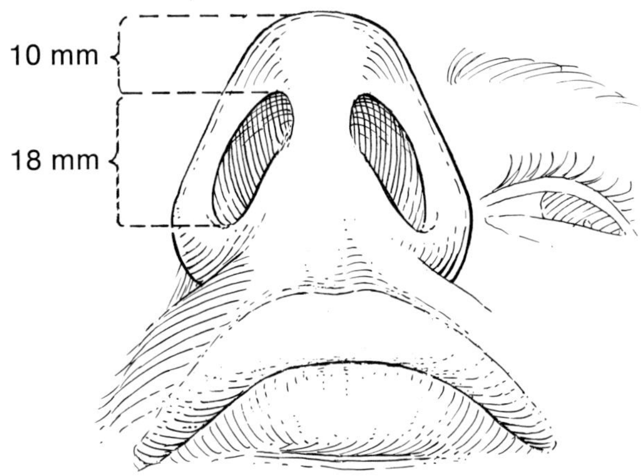

NOSTRILS

Irregularities of the nostrils can best be evaluated from the basal view. Ideally, nostrils should be elliptical to pear shaped, with the greater diameter near the nasal sill. They should incline toward the apex of a trianguloid that is formed by the basal perimeter.

Although nostrils may have a variety of contours, in order to obtain congruence with the rest of the nasal base, the greatest diameter of the nostril should not be less than the height of the lobule or greater than two times its height. Note the upper limit of the nostril size in relation to the tip.

Patients with a nostril-lobular disparity must be considered problem cases requiring special treatment. This patient illustrates the aesthetic impact of a nostril that is less than one-half the height of the tip lobule. The nose appears tip-heavy. The small nostrils and short columella are red flags that warn that the tip does not have the structural potential to project above the dorsal line following hump removal (see pp. 370-396). Patients with this configuration should be advised of the unalterable heaviness of the nasal tip and the problems relating to inadequate tip projection.

To obtain the necessary tip projection it was necessary to add length to the tip lobule, further increasing the nostril-lobular disproportion. The dilemma of improving one relationship at the expense of another is not always easily resolved, but the decision is usually in favor of overall rather than specific effect.

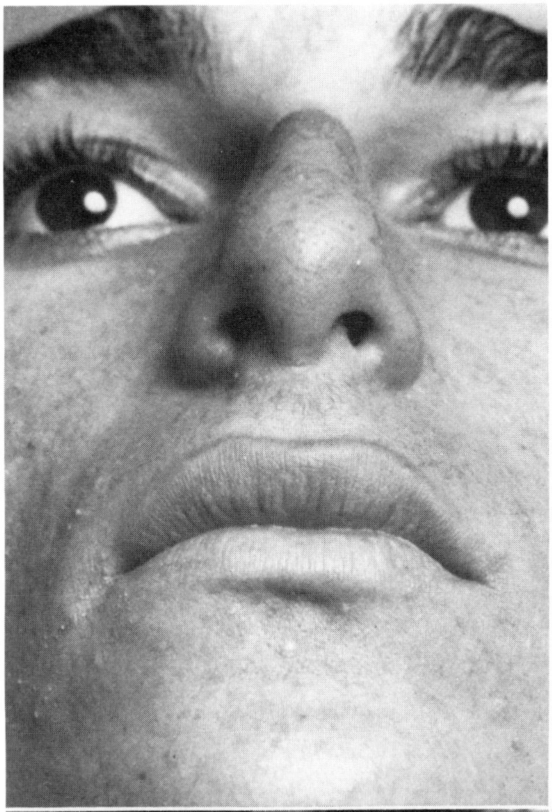

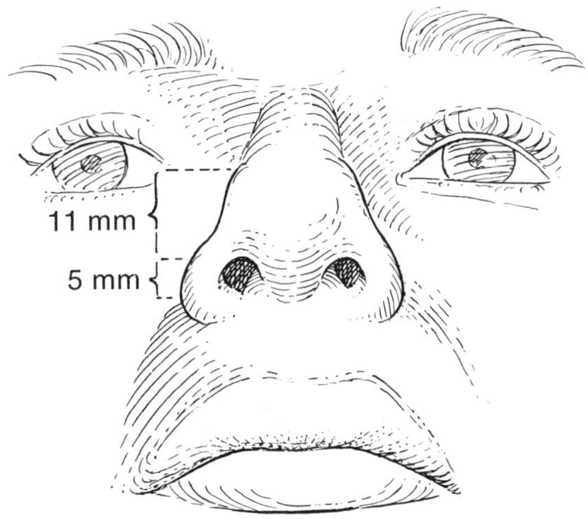
11 mm
5 mm

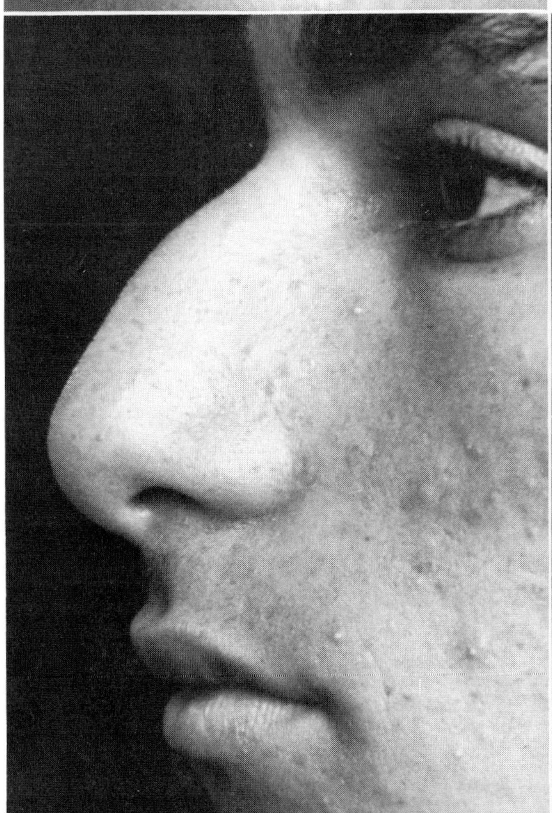

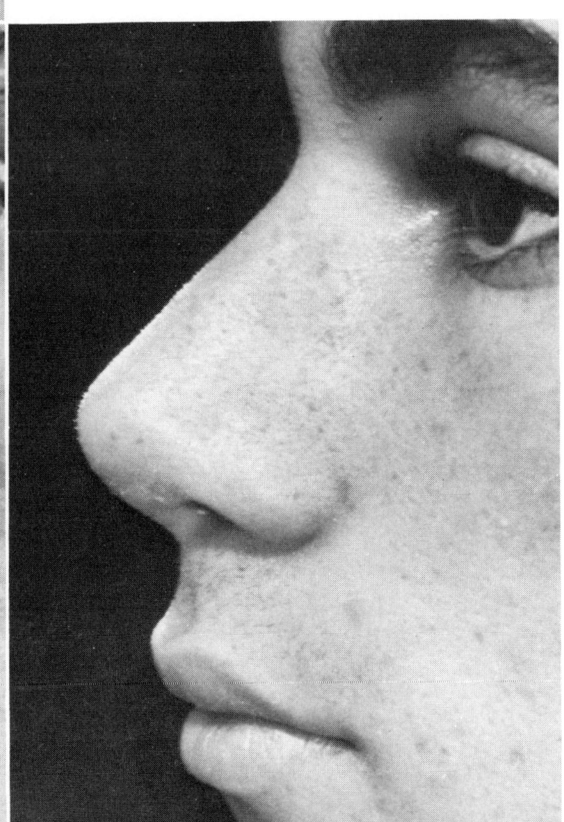

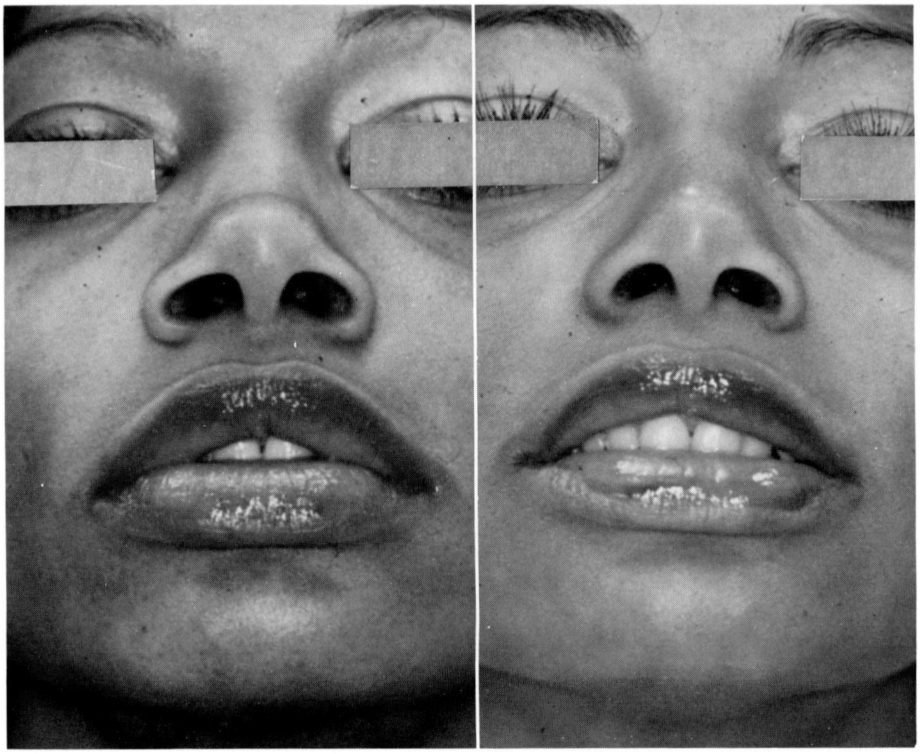

The black nostril is a special problem in rhinoplasty because of its horizontal position and the importance of maintaining ethnic character. The nostril-lobular ratio is still important in making judgments concerning alar resection in blacks.

In this patient, the measurement of the nostril in its longest axis is about equal to the height of the tip lobule. This would indicate that the further reduction of the nostril by alar wedges would disrupt the ratio, making the patient's nose tip-heavy.

Resection of the alae with narrowing of the nostril produced a greater discrepancy between the nostril and the lobule, but this discrepancy was felt to be a fair exchange for obtaining an improved position of the nostrils. The remaining width of the nasal base is aesthetically consistent with her racial features.

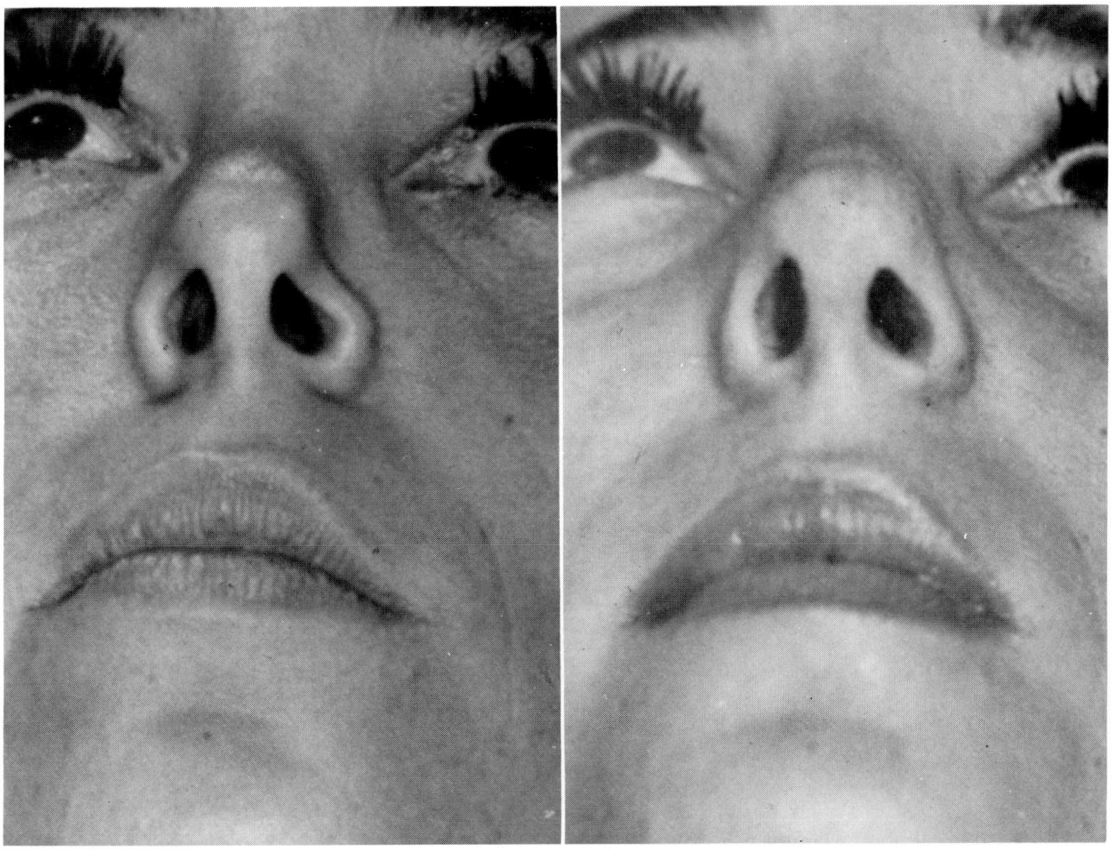

Reshaping nostrils

Notching of the nostril, caused by scar contracture or overresection of the lateral crus of the lower lateral cartilage, can be improved by composite grafts or full-thickness grafts with implantation of a spicule of perpendicular plate. The latter technique was used for this patient.

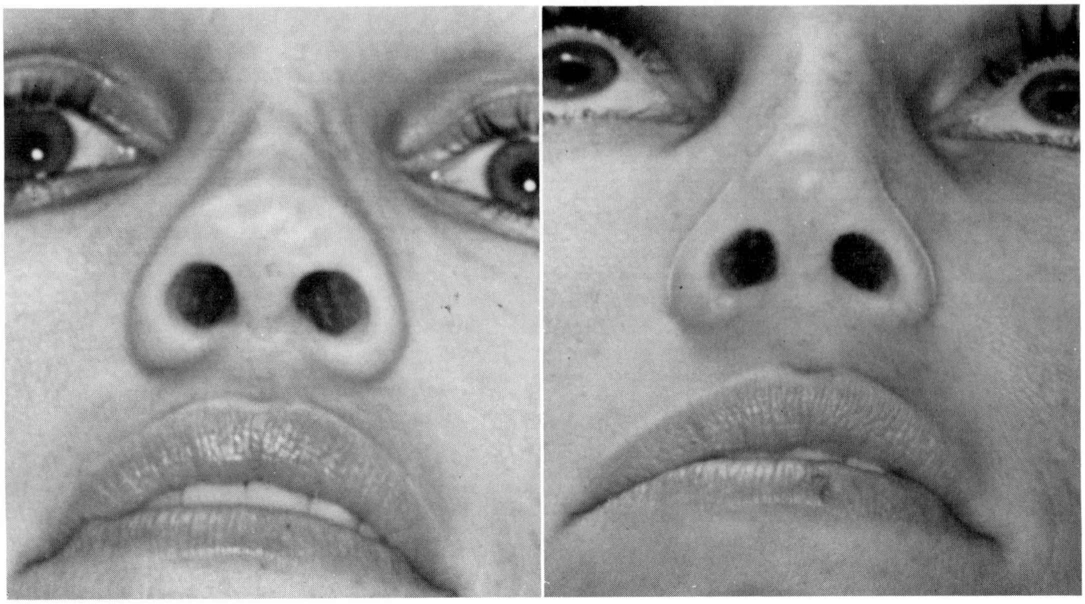

It is not enough for nostrils to be symmetrical; they should also have an elliptical contour. Round nostrils often reflect an over-reduced dorsum. Therefore, elevation of the dorsum is a constructive way to rectify nostril distortion. The nostrils of the patient above were improved by a dorsal graft, tip graft, and conservative alar wedge resections.

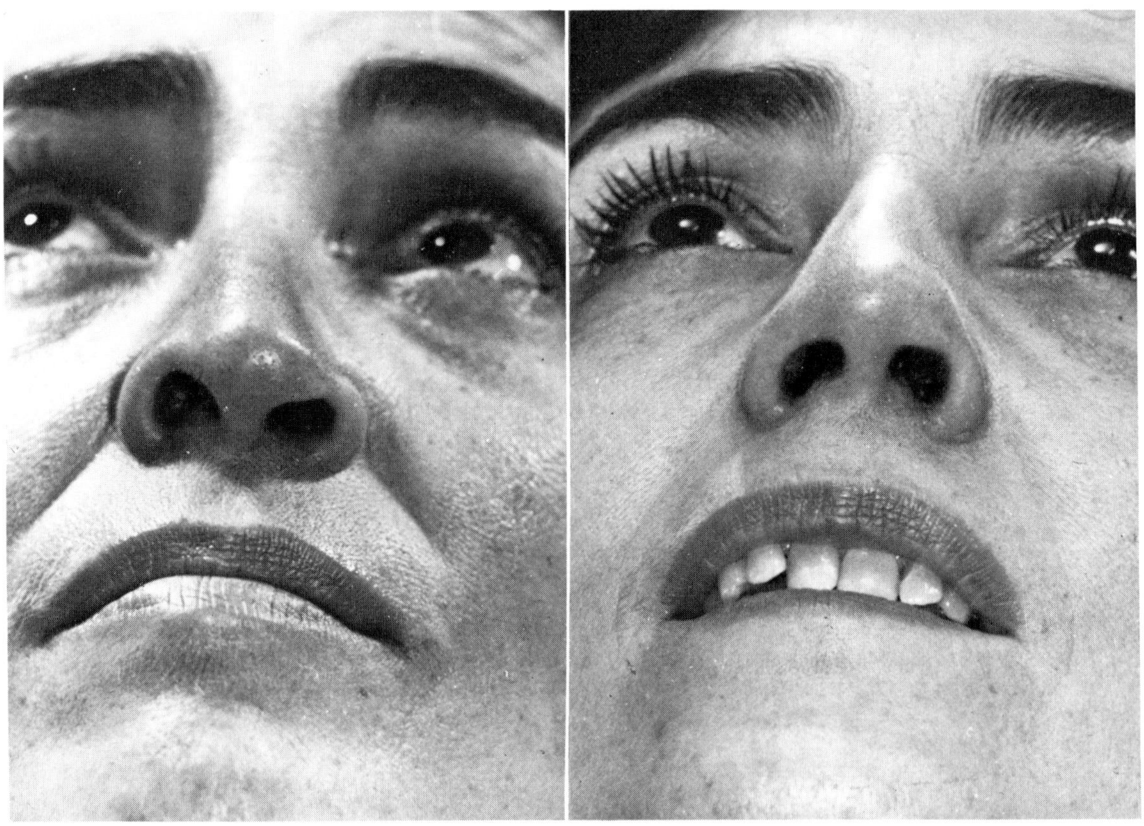

Occasionally all parts of the nose are involved in the correction of nostril distortion. This patient required dorsal augmentation, a tip graft, a skin graft to the right vestibule, bone implantation into the right nostril, and alar wedges to reshape her nostrils.

EPILOGUE

As a beginner I was impressed by the quasi-magical aura that surrounded rhinoplasty. In texts there was some talk of aesthetic surgical objectives and of facial planes and angles, but in the operating room the surgeon's eyes were fixed on some distant spot while his hands were busy with stereotypic movements. Something vague and mystical seemed to be happening under those hands within the unlighted, unseen recesses of the nose. From time to time the surgeon would look down at the results of his handiwork but in a nonspecific way. If in the end the nose was smaller, the job was done. There seemed to be no relation between those textbook aesthetic standards and the practical reality of performing a rhinoplasty. It was as if there were no clear-cut aesthetic criteria that could be applied clinically. It was as if the surgeon had neither the conception nor the control to effect specific, precise changes. For lack of applicable theory, the surgeon resorted to instinct and feel.

In my discussion of nasal aesthetics I have tried to dispel the mystique of the rhinoplastic result. By identifying specific factors that constitute a beautiful nose and by demonstrating how these factors can be manipulated surgically, I have attempted to convey an aesthetic construct that is both comprehensible and usable.

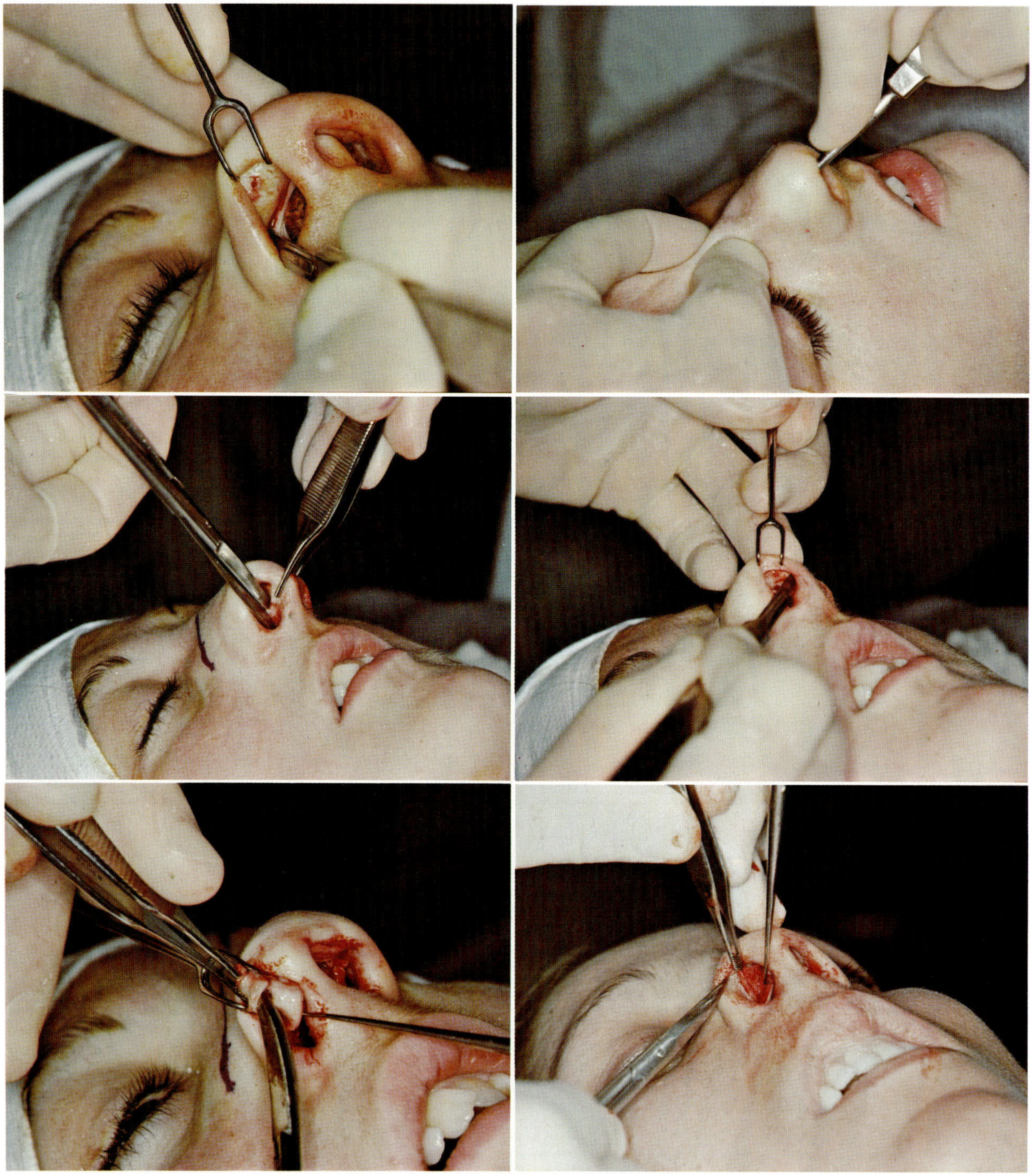

CHAPTER 3

Basic technique

Success in rhinoplasty comes from a deep respect for the procedure, honest and continuing intellectual assessment, and perpetual dissatisfaction. A masterfully performed rhinoplasty appears deceptively simple and has the rhythm and development of an art form.

There is a logical sequence of operative stages in any surgical procedure. However, I feel that rigid adherence to *steps* in rhinoplasty prevents the surgeon from responding to the special problems and opportunities that arise during the course of the procedure.

Because rhinoplasty is performed with an ideal in mind, the anatomic part that deviates most from the ideal should be changed first. One must be free to modify this distracting part out of prescribed order to be able to make accurate judgments about the management of other parts.

Rhinoplasty is like a game of chess being played between the surgeon and the nasal anatomy. To win, the surgeon must think ahead several moves, modifying the surgical plan according to the response of the tissues. For example, following cephalic rotation of the tip, it may be found that the new position has improved the relationship of the dorsum to the tip, making less dorsal resection a part of the revised strategy. Each move the surgeon makes elicits a response on the part of the patient's anatomy that should direct the surgeon in making a logical following step.

Listed below are the stages necessary for performing a rhinoplasty. To encourage flexibility in surgical planning, they are not numbered.

- Anesthesia
- Separation of soft tissues from the skeleton
- Preliminary modification of skeletal parts
  - Bony
  - Cartilaginous
- Preliminary modification of tip cartilages
  - Osteotomy
  - Final contouring of all parts
  - Fixation of soft tissues
  - Reconstruction of internal valve
  - Dressing

ANESTHESIA

Usually general anesthesia is unnecessary because most patients tolerate local anesthesia without untoward effects. The placement of an endotracheal tube during general anesthesia distorts the patient's mouth, limits free handling of the patient's head, and visually obstructs parts of the face. However, when emotional or physical factors dictate, general anesthesia may be elected. In these patients, the addition of the usual local infiltration is recommended to ensure proper hemostasis.

Rhinoplasty performed with local anesthesia is pleasant and uncomplicated under the following conditions:

1. The patient must be relaxed, quiet, and cooperative during the procedure.
2. The entire nose, including mucosa, must be well anesthetized, and the amount of bleeding must be minimal.

Relaxed, quiet, cooperative patient

Preoperative medication not only relieves the patient's anxiety but is a valuable indicator of the response to medication. This response serves as a guide to the administration of intravenous medications in the operating room. Morphine is preferred because of its proven clinical safety and the feeling of euphoria it produces in the majority of patients. In addition, the incidence of nausea is low. For the patient who weighs between 55 to 80 kg, 15 mg of morphine is given 1 hour before surgery, and 10 mg is given to the patient who weighs between 45 to 55 kg. With these dosages of medication the average patient enters the operating room tranquil but responsive.

After the patient is placed on the operating table and the cardiac monitor is attached, an intravenous infusion is begun using 500 ml of Ringer's lactate solution. An initial dose of diazepam (Valium), not exceeding 2.5 mg, is given over a 1-minute period of time. The patient is then observed for 2 minutes for any untoward response to the medication. During this time casual conversation serves to distract the patient and indicates his or her response to the medicine. In the absence of any adverse response, an additional 5 to 20 mg of Valium is given over a 5 to 10-minute period of time.

As the patient becomes tranquil, 100 mg meperidine (Demerol) is added to the intravenous solution, and it is allowed to drip at approximately 60 drops per minute (1 mg/minute). During this time the anesthetic solution is prepared by the surgeon in preparation for infiltration. Fifty ml of plain 1% lidocaine (Xylocaine) is placed in a sterile glass with 1 ml of unautoclaved 1:1,000 adrenalin added to it. This combination makes a solution of 1:50,000 Xylocaine with epinephrine.

As the patient becomes somnolent, there may be a verbal response, but most often the patient will not remember the injections of local anesthetic. A 10-ml three-ring syringe with a 27-gauge 1¼-inch needle is used for infiltration. The total amount of anesthetic material injected usually does not exceed 8 ml, and as little as 5 ml can suffice if there is a need to limit the amount of epinephrine. Following infiltration the intravenous drip is slowed and is titrated as needed during the procedure.

Although this titration method of medication is relatively slow (20 to 30 minutes), it has real advantages. It is relatively safe, affords the best chance for a bloodless field, and provides excellent contact with the patient who frequently is in need of reassurance from the operating surgeon during the immediate preoperative period.

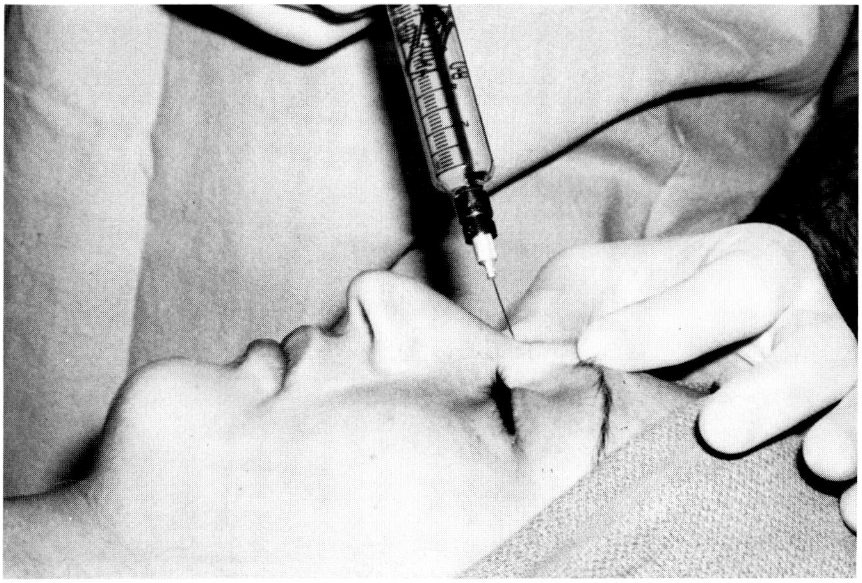

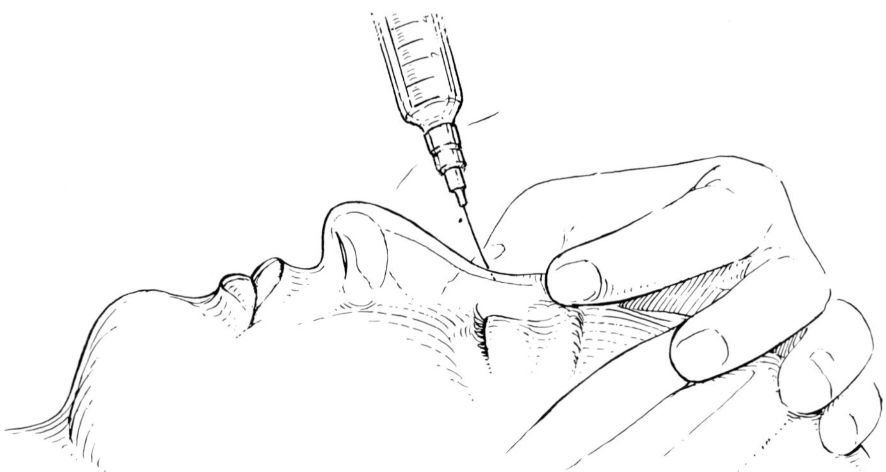

Well-anesthetized nose and minimal bleeding

Anesthesia begins at the radix where approximately 0.5 ml of the anesthetic solution is injected into the soft tissues.

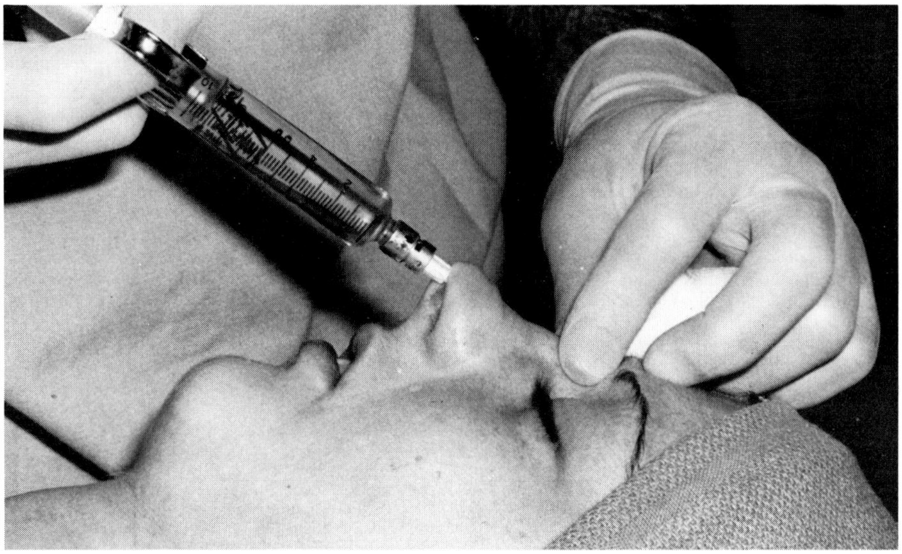

The needle is placed at the angle of the septum and inserted to the radix.

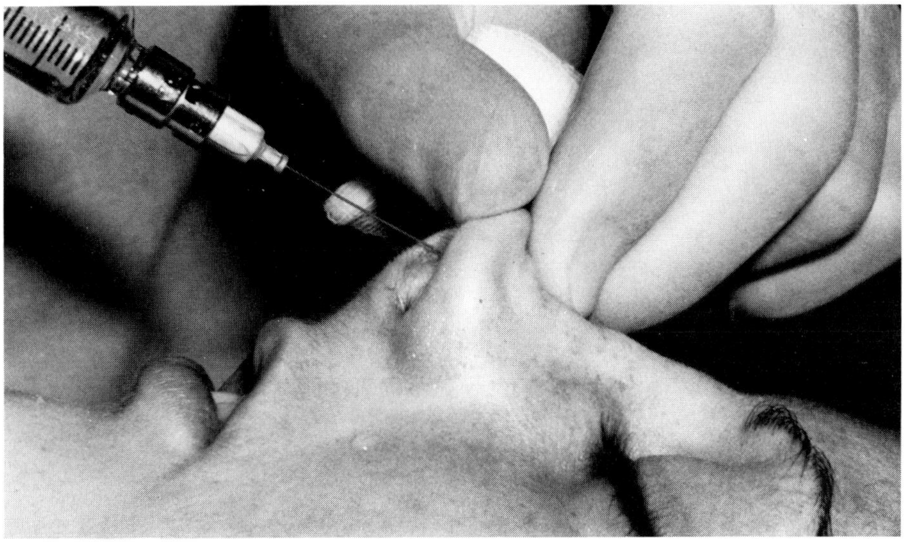

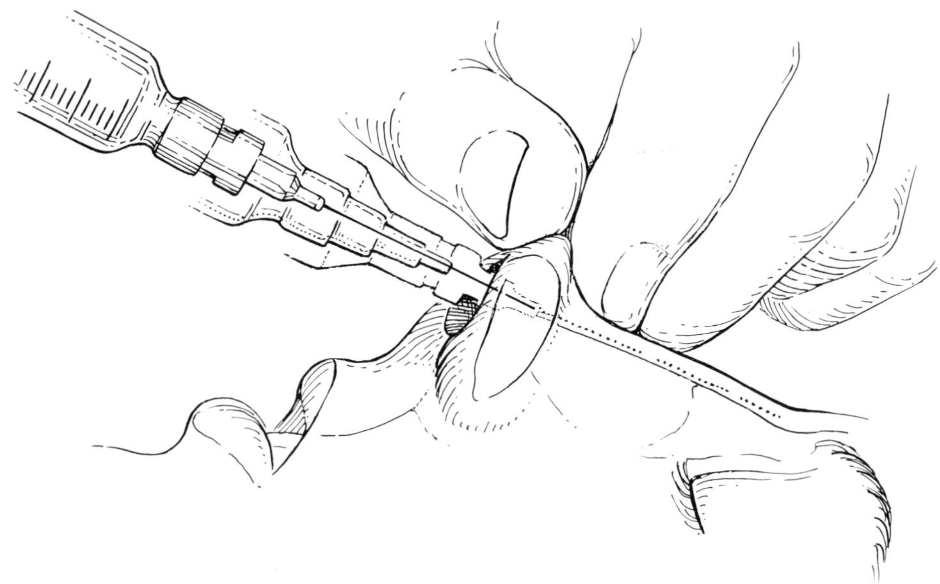

It is slowly withdrawn, placing approximately 1 ml of anesthetic solution just over the dorsal edge of the bony and cartilaginous vaults.

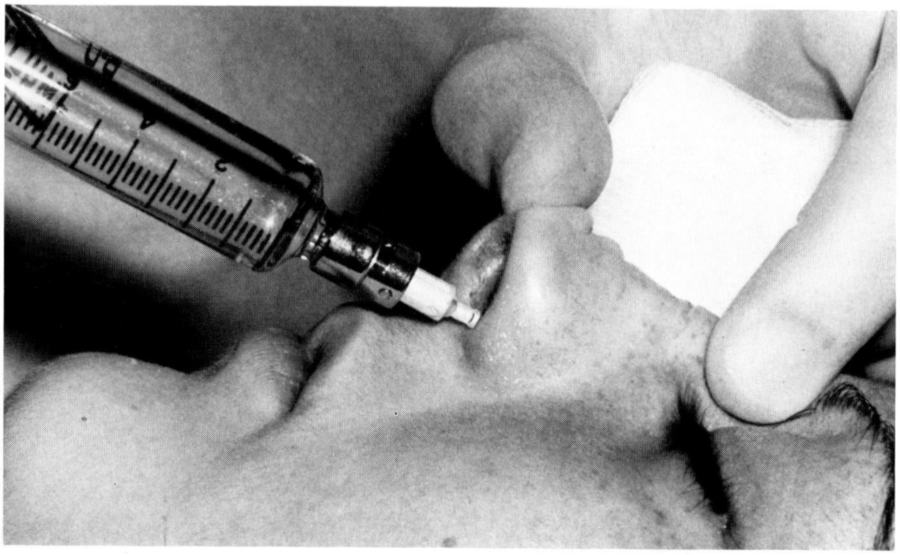

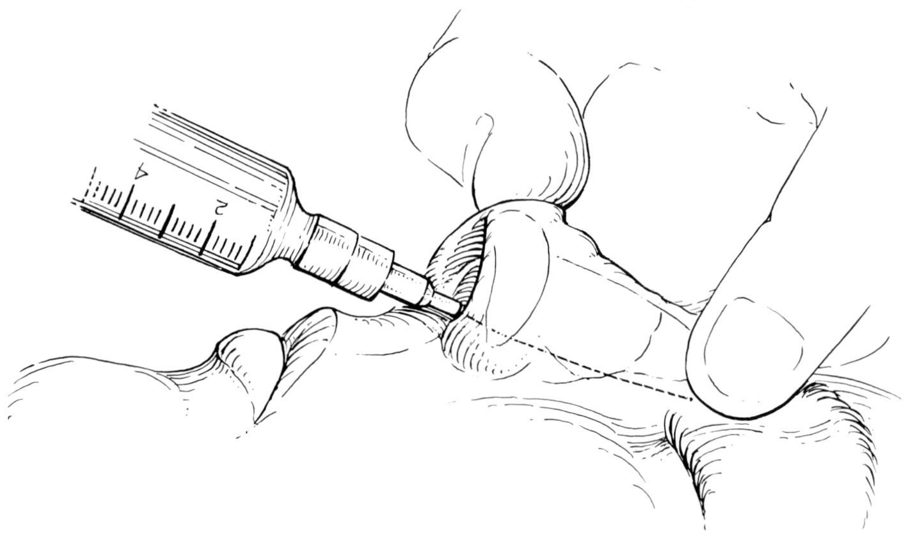

The needle is introduced just over the site of the incision for osteotomy and goes cephalad, close to the maxillary bone toward the radix.

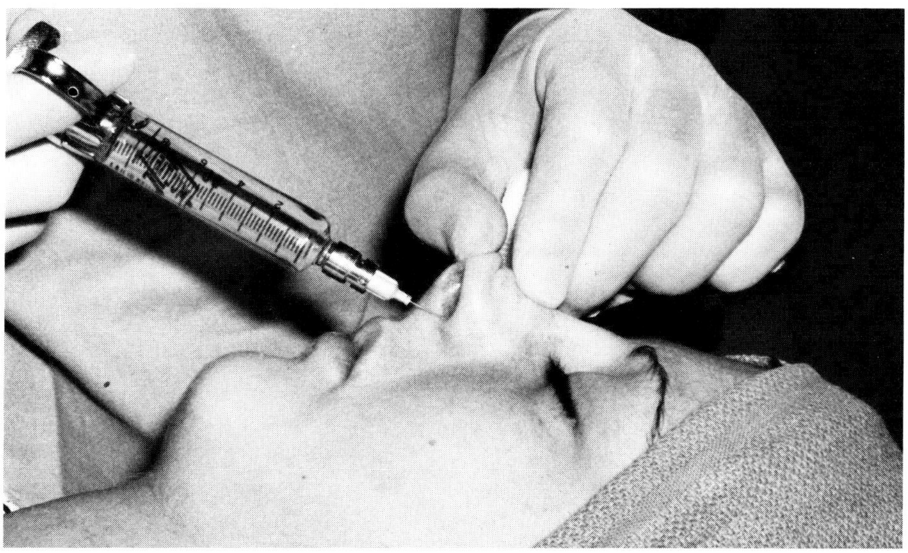

It is then slowly withdrawn, injecting approximately 1 ml of anesthetic solution. This is repeated on the opposite side.

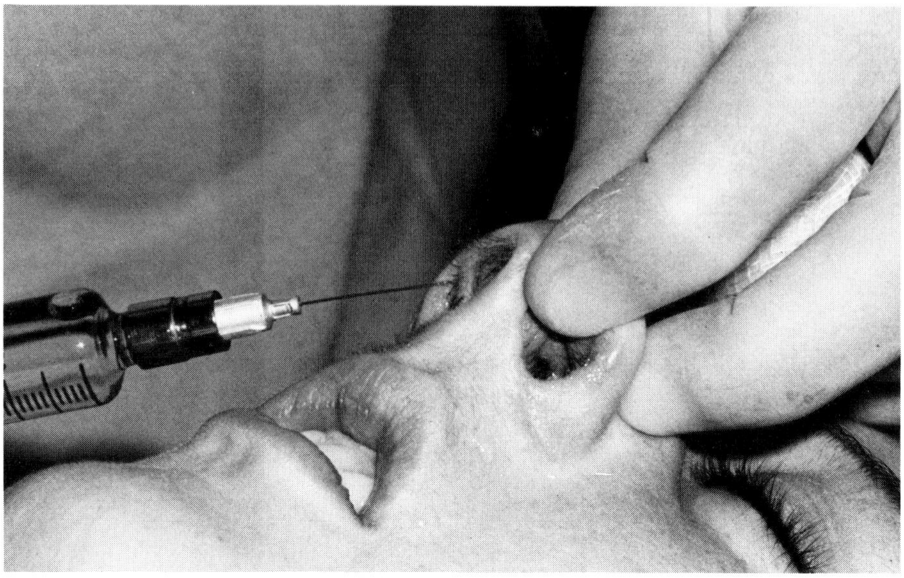

Anesthesia and hemostasis of the tip are best obtained by direct infiltration. It begins at the base of the caudal reflection of the lateral crus with the needle inserted anterior to the cartilage.

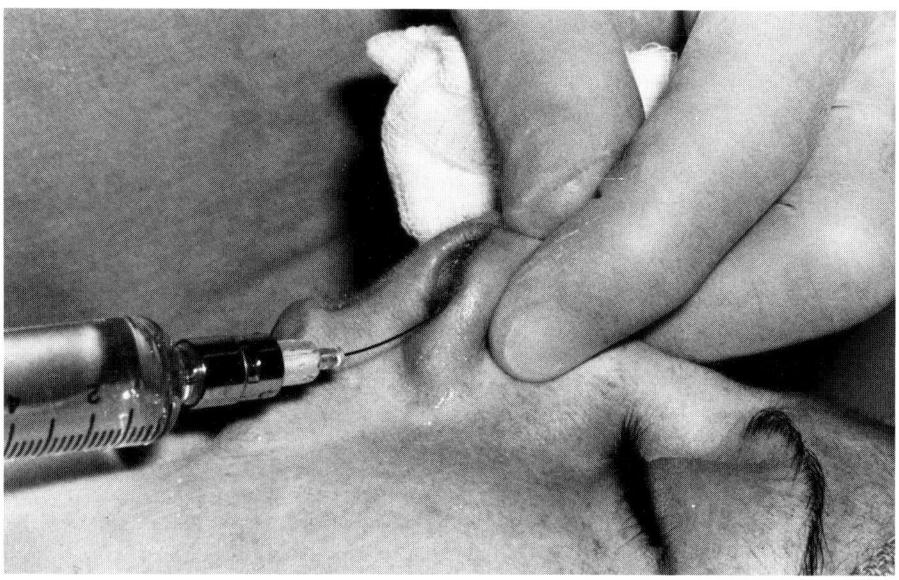

The needle is then advanced to the area of the dome. Less than 0.5 ml is sufficient to obtain excellent hemostasis. This is repeated on the opposite side.

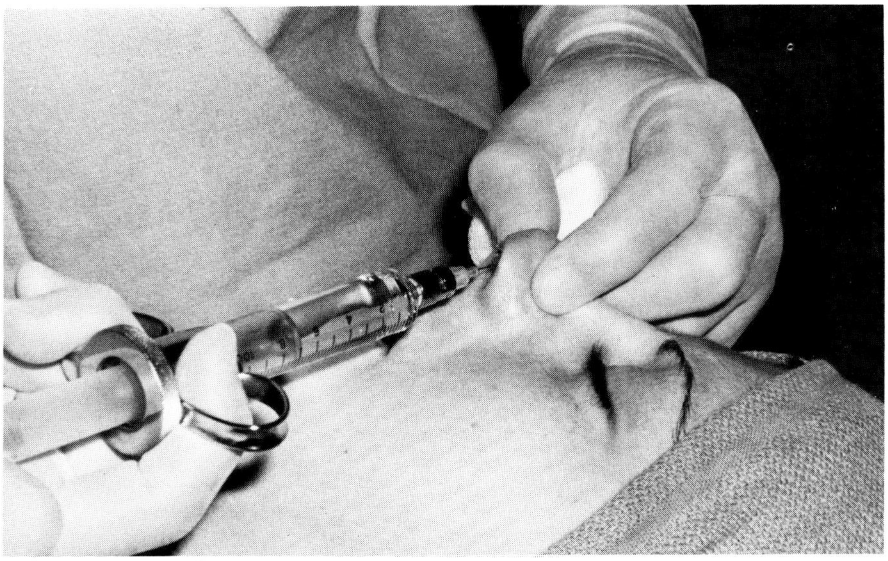

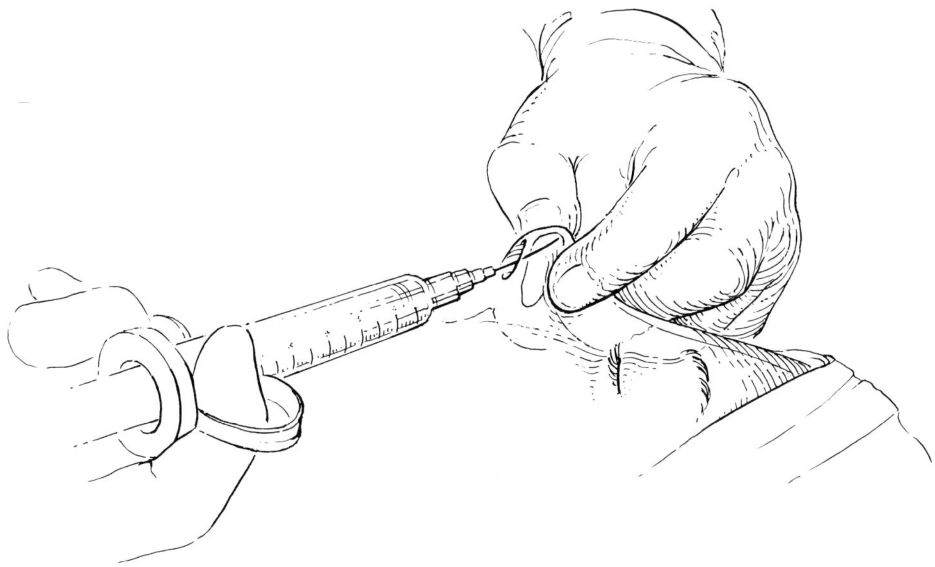

Direct injection of the anesthetic solution is critical to proper anesthesia and hemostasis. Regional blocks do not afford the necessary hemostasis for critical modeling of the cartilages when the rim technique is used.

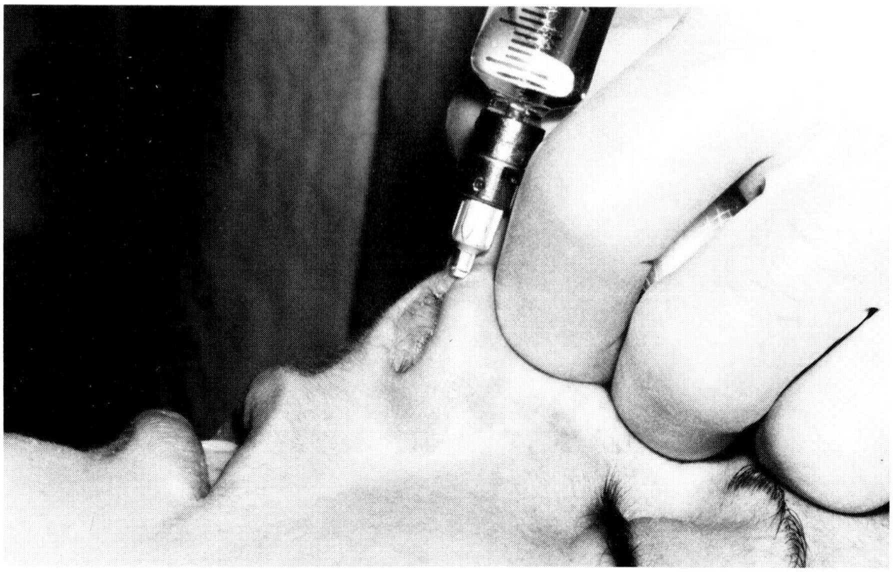

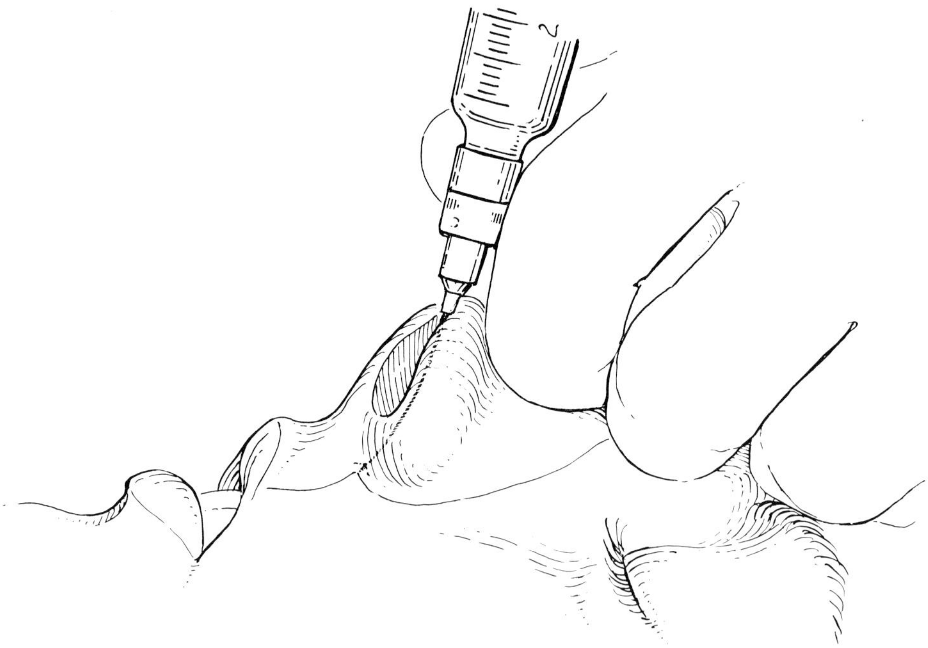

The needle is placed at the angle of the septum and caudal to it and then inserted along the membranous septum to the spine. As the needle is withdrawn, 1 ml of anesthetic solution is injected.

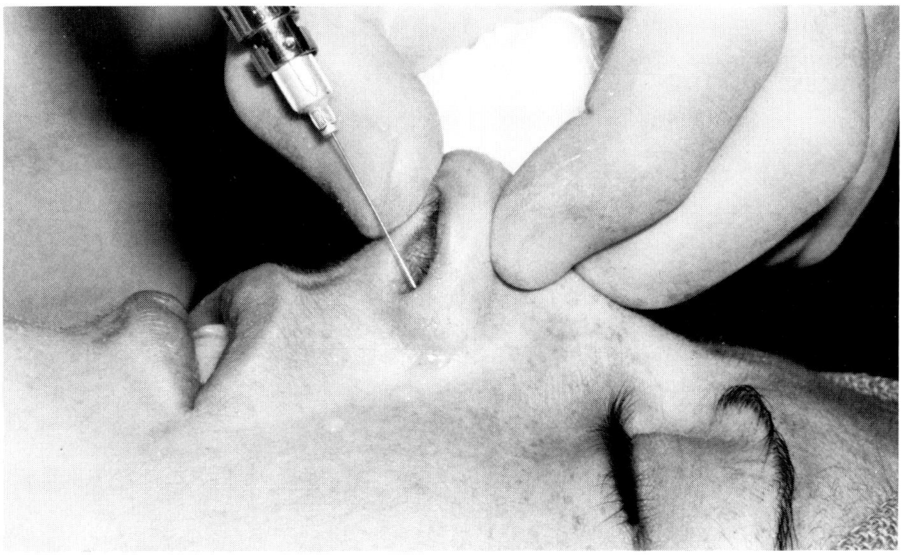

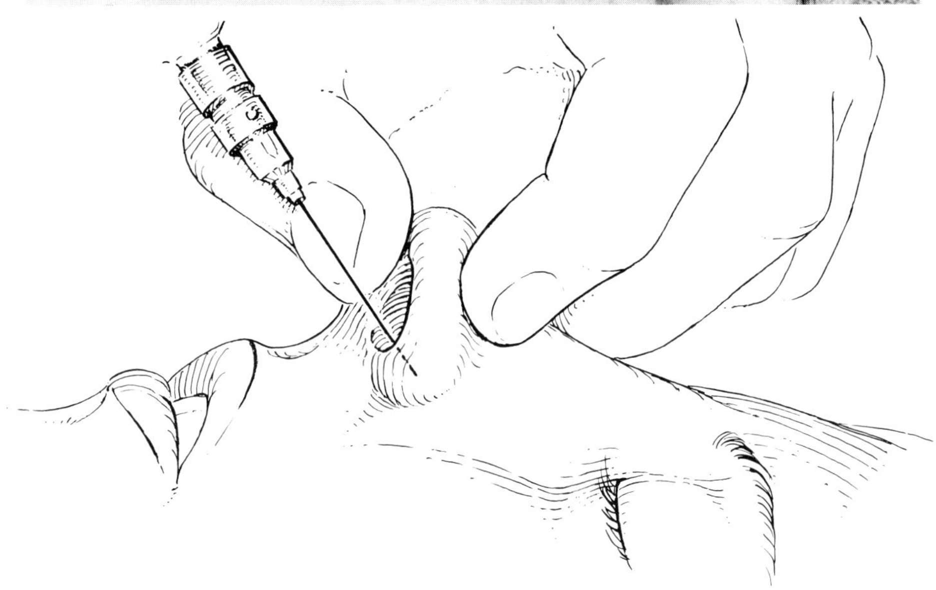

If alar wedge resections are planned, 0.25 ml of anesthetic is injected directly into the alar lobules.

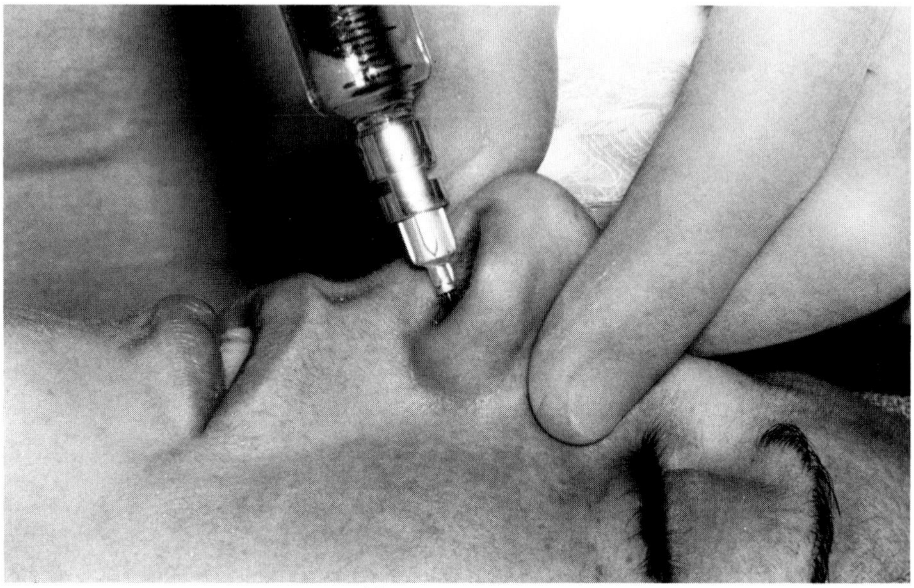

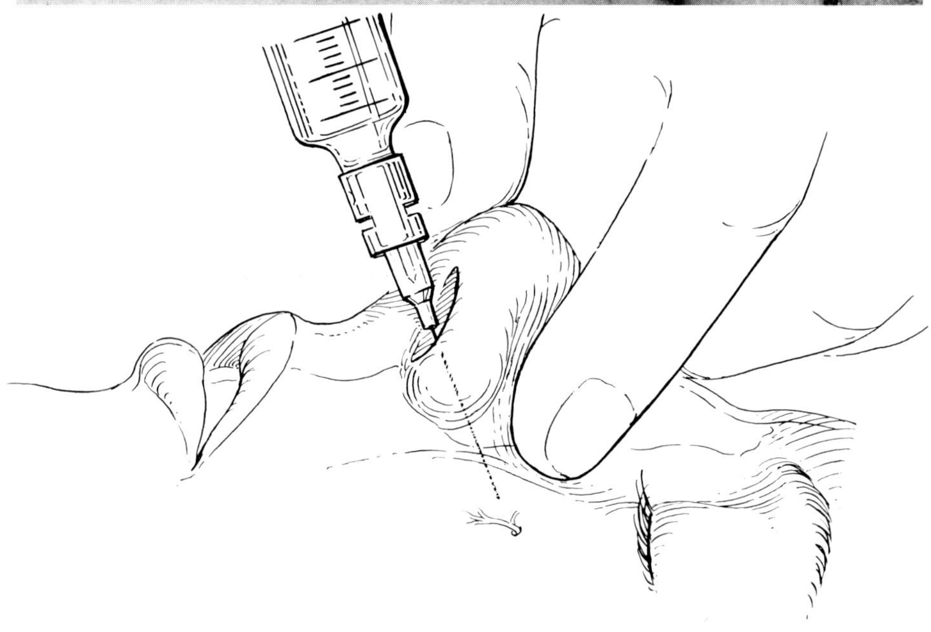

The final injection is placed near the infraorbital foramen with approximately 0.5 ml injected on each side.

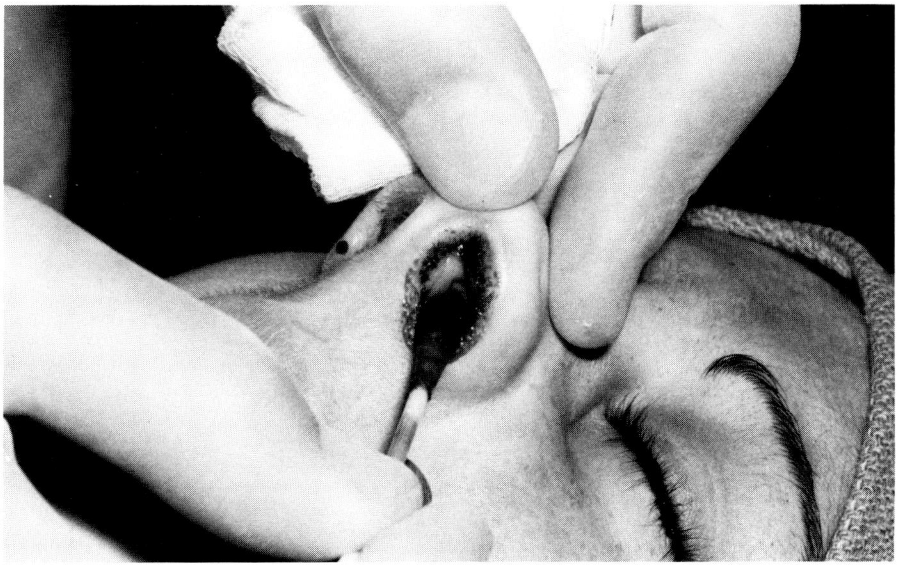

The vestibules are meticulously cleaned with a solution of povidone-iodine (Betadine), with special attention to the apices. The cleansing procedure extends to the area of the internal valve.

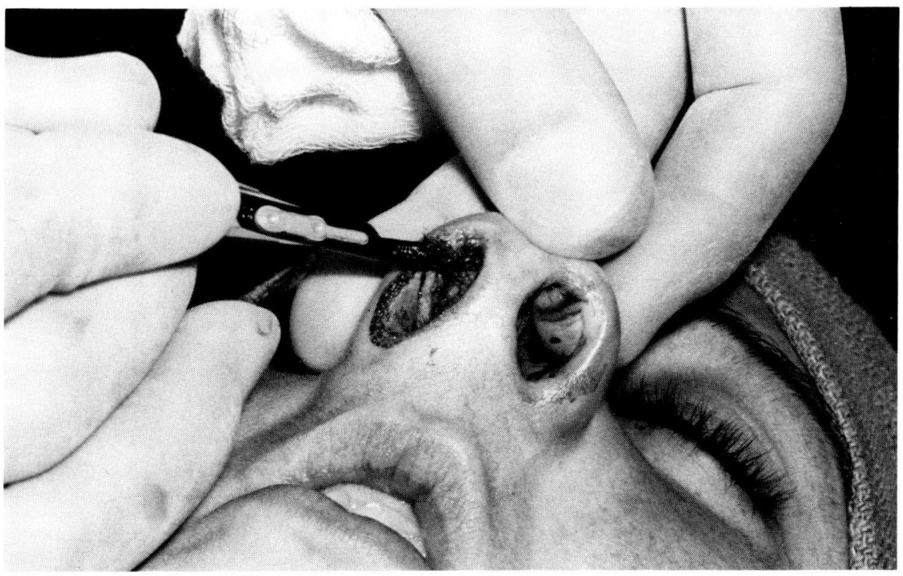

Following the initial cleansing, the vibrissae are shaved close to the vestibular skin with a No. 15 blade. This is followed by a second cleansing with Betadine solution.

Sterile technique is followed for the placement of packing. Sterile cotton and 4 ml of a 5% solution of lightly colored cocaine (200 mg of cocaine hydrochloride) is placed in a sterile medicine glass. No adrenalin is added.

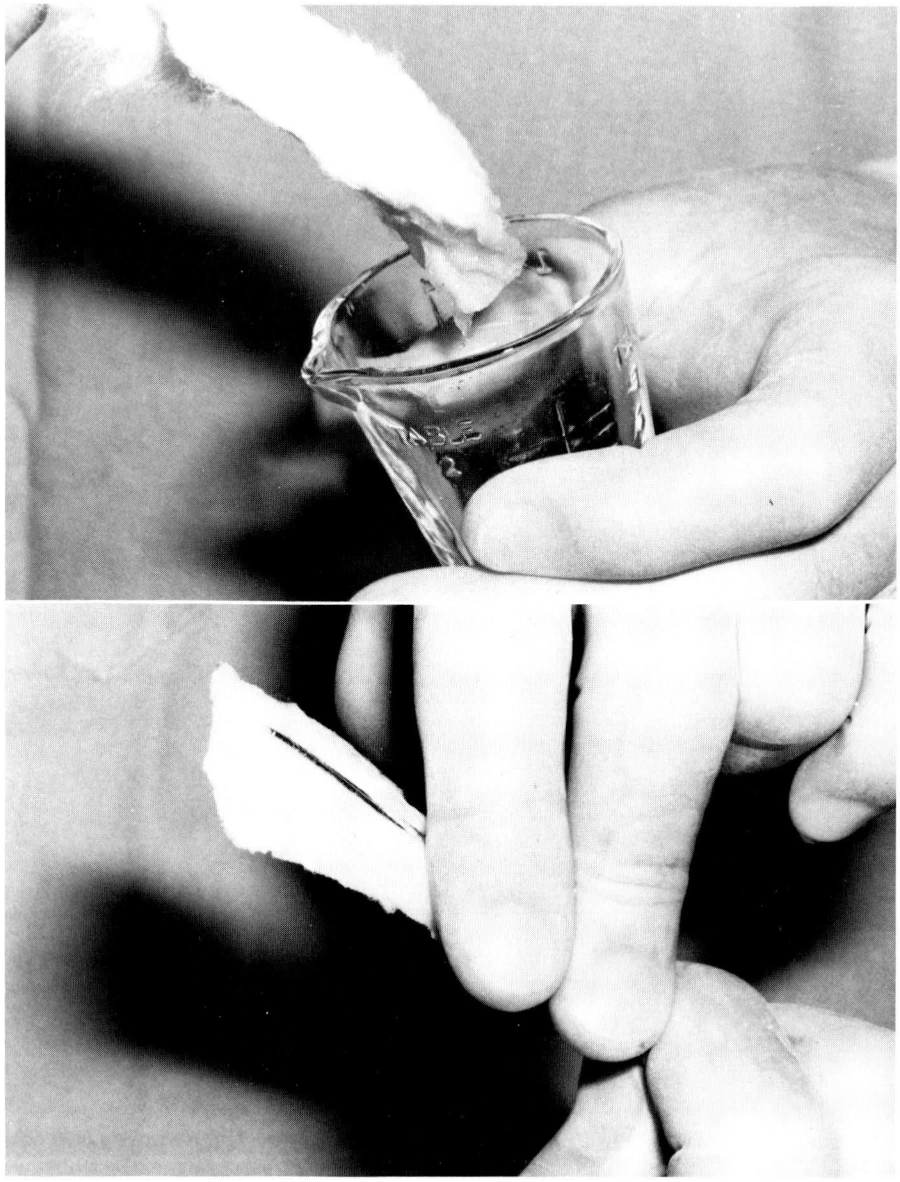

The cotton is dipped into the cocaine, which is then stripped down the cotton.

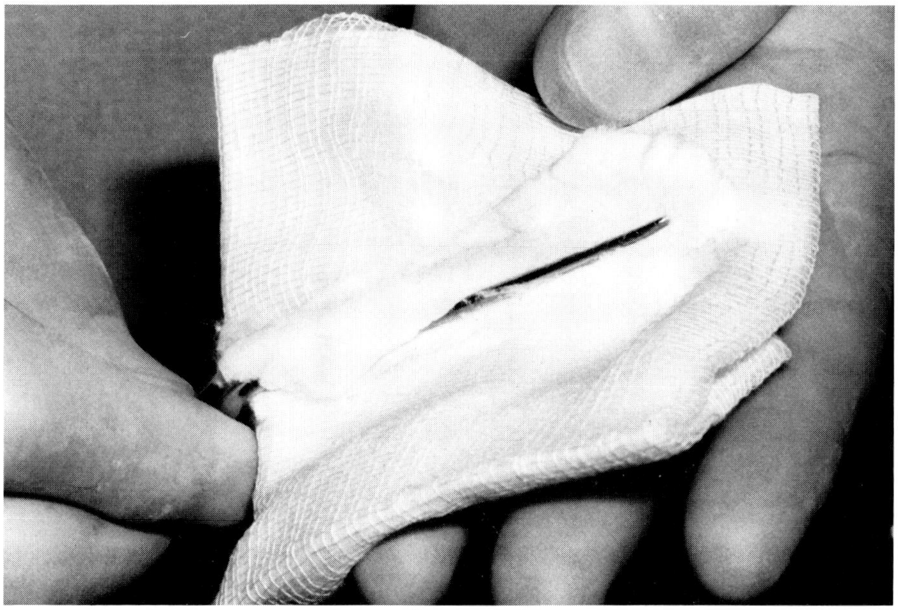

The saturated cotton is pressed between a dry sterile 4 × 4 inch gauze.

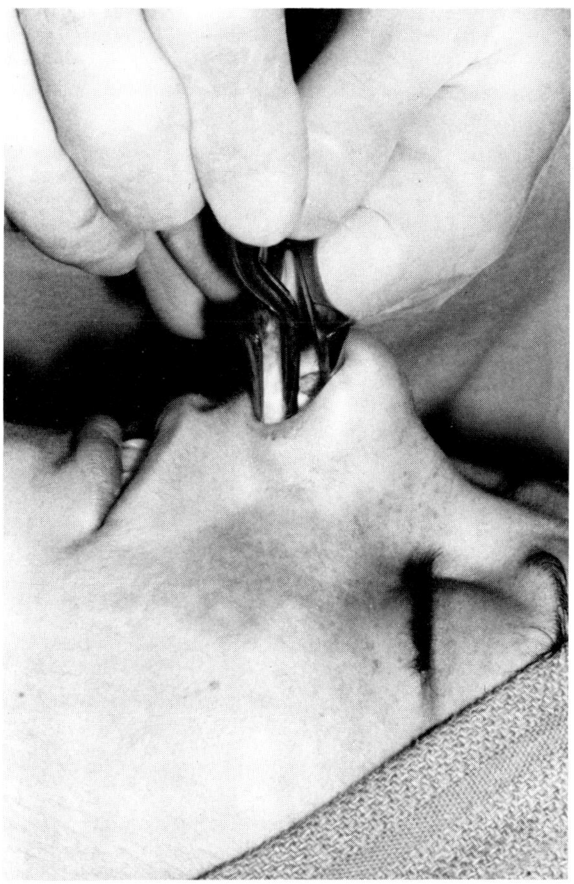

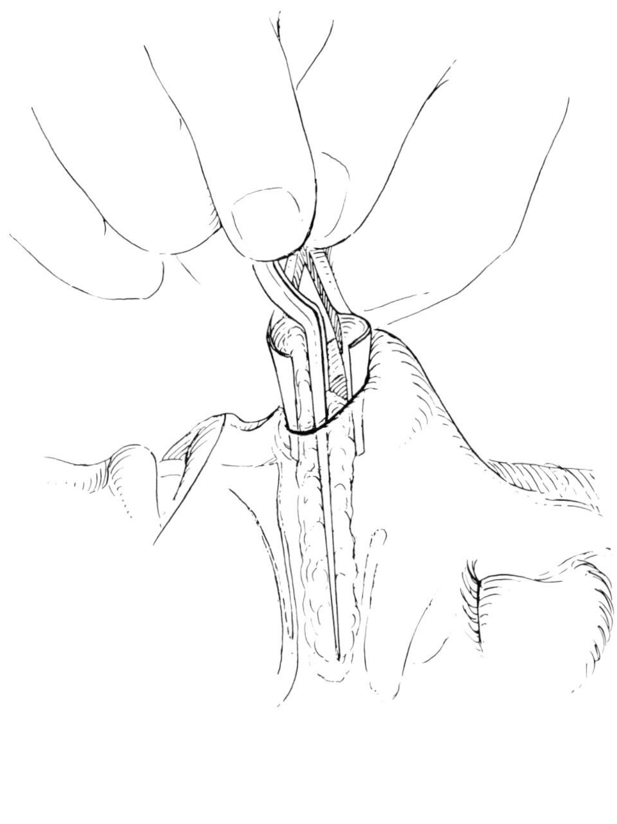

The first and larger pack is placed along the nasal floor between the septum and the inferior turbinate.

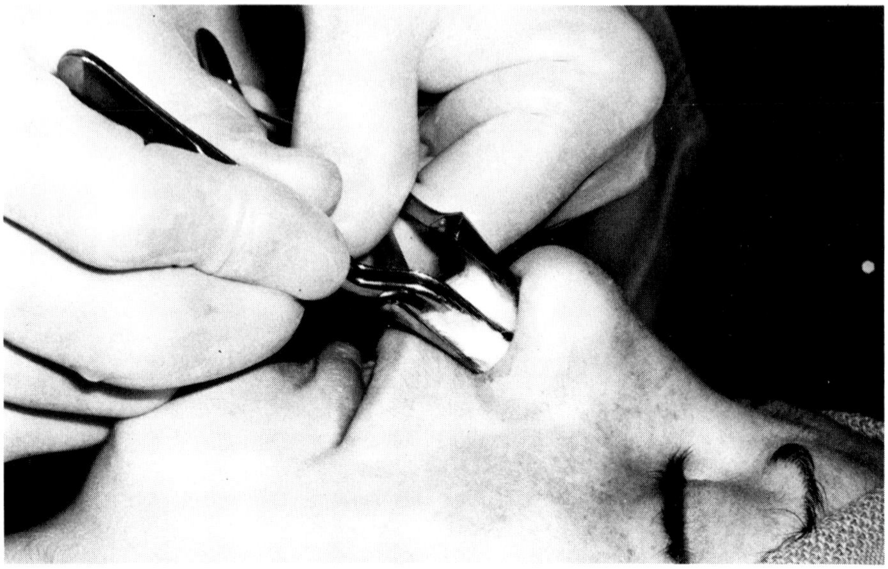

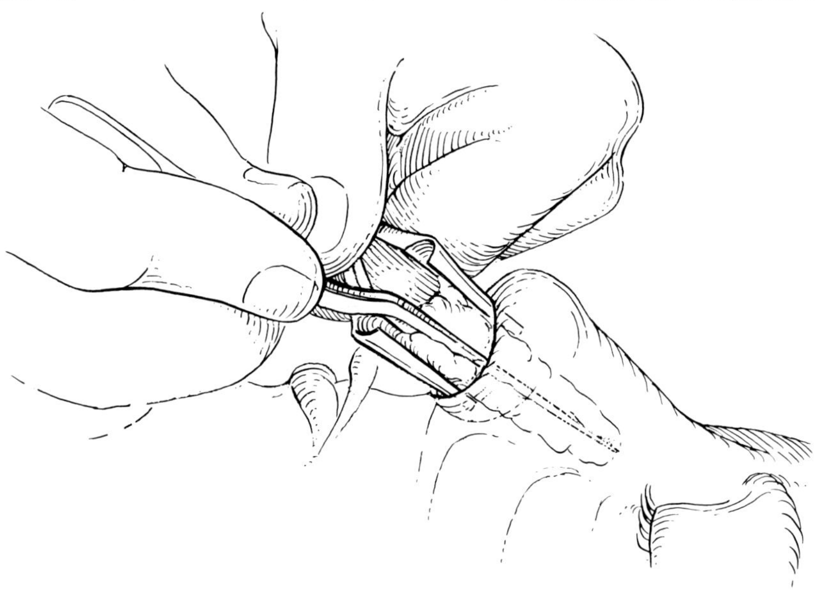

The second and smaller pack is placed along the roof of the nasal cavity to anesthetize the mucosa overlying the area of dorsal resection and lateral osteotomy.

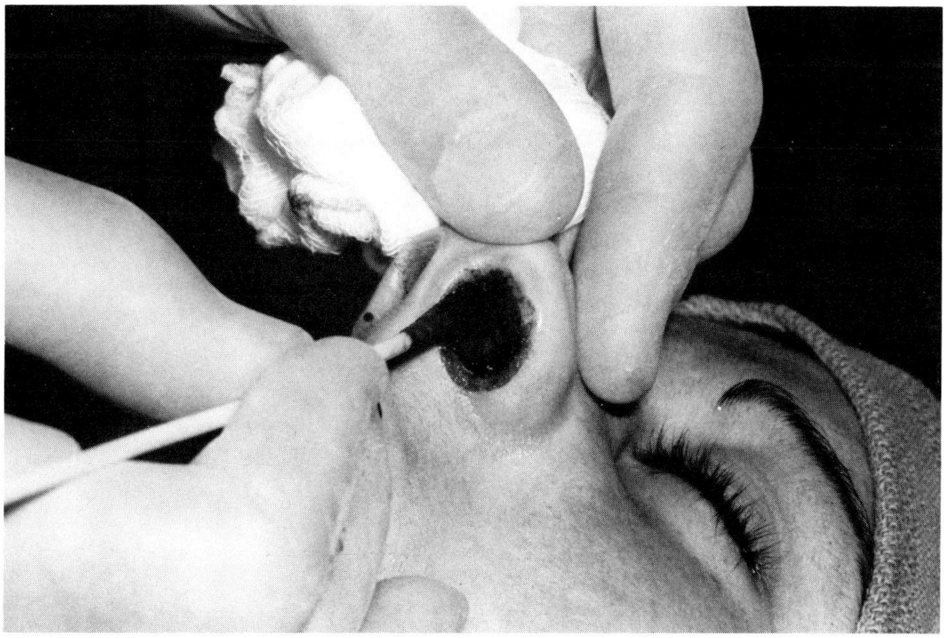

A final cleansing of the base of the nose and vestibules prepares the patient for the usual prep and drape. The surgeon cannot depend on, or expect, the regular operating room staff to sufficiently prepare the vestibule of the nose. This should be considered an important part of the operative procedure.

SEPARATION OF SOFT TISSUES FROM THE SKELETON

The purpose of skeletonization is twofold: (1) to gain access to the skeletal structure and (2) to allow the tissues to redrape over the newly formed framework. The degree of skeletonization varies from patient to patient. It is much less for the thin-skinned patient with a good nasolabial angle than it is for a middle-aged person with thick tissues and an acute nasolabial angle. The former needs only access for structural modification, whereas the latter requires greater mobility of the skin sleeve to facilitate the movement of soft tissue in a cephalic direction.

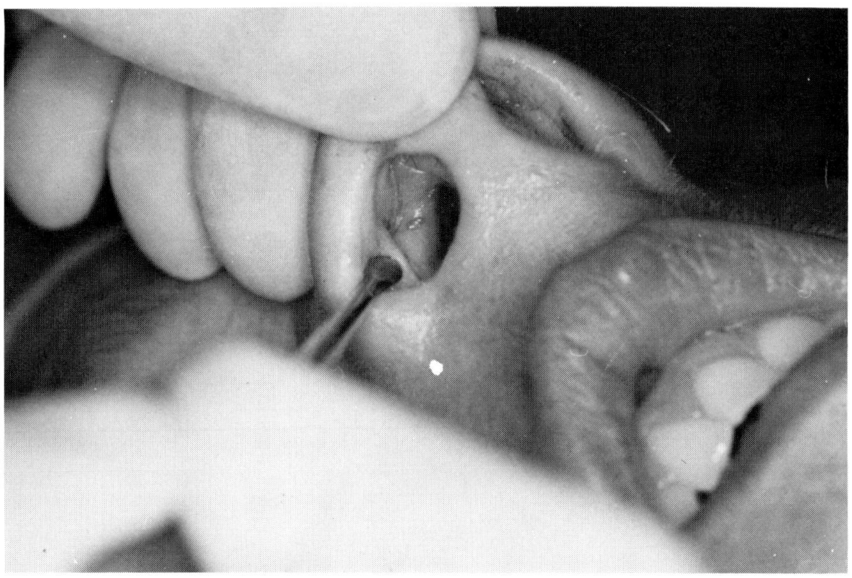

The initial incision for freeing the soft tissues from the skeleton begins just above the reflection of mucosa over the caudal edge of the upper lateral cartilage. It is important to note the relationship of the caudal edge of the upper lateral cartilage to the angle of the septum because this relationship is to be re-created in the final stages of the procedure.

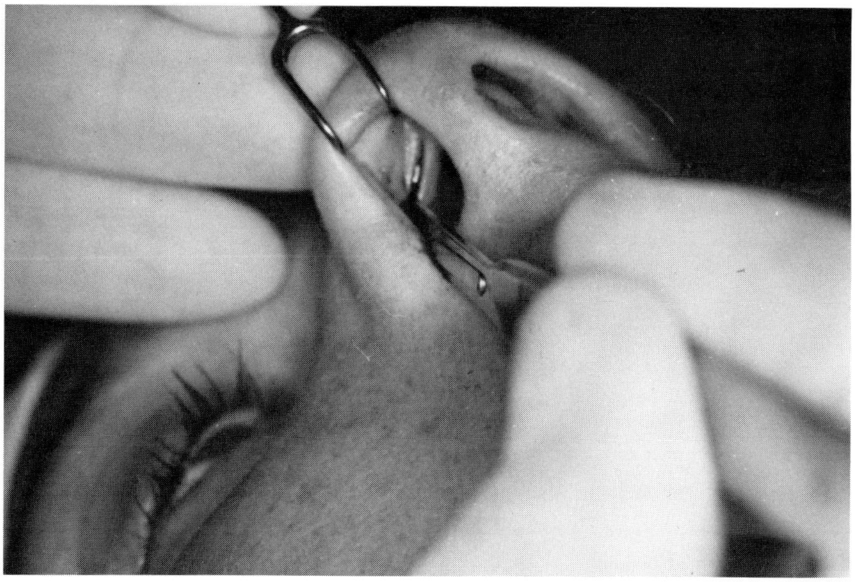

The nostril is retracted with a double hook. With the finger of the left hand checking the position of the No. 15 blade, an incision is made just over the caudal reflection of the upper lateral cartilage.

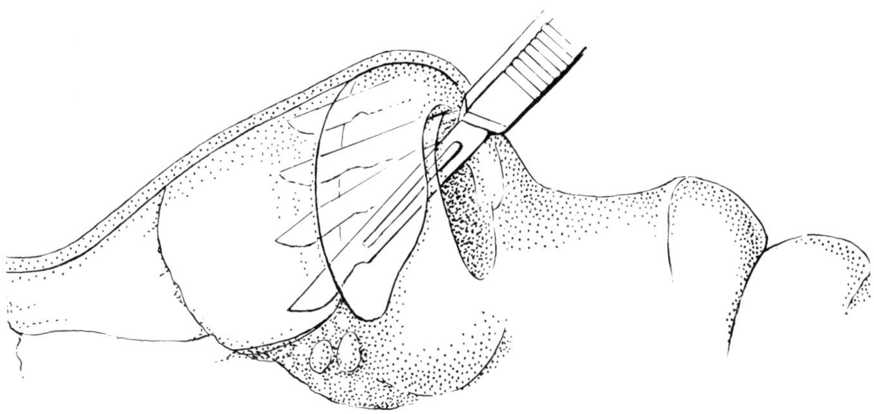

The extent of skeletonization over the upper lateral cartilage is decided preoperatively. If much rotation of the tip is necessary to achieve a satisfactory nasolabial angle, skeletonization is extensive; if little or no rotation of the tip is necessary, it is minimal. The knife sweeps along the caudal edge of the upper lateral cartilage close to the base of the pyriform aperture.

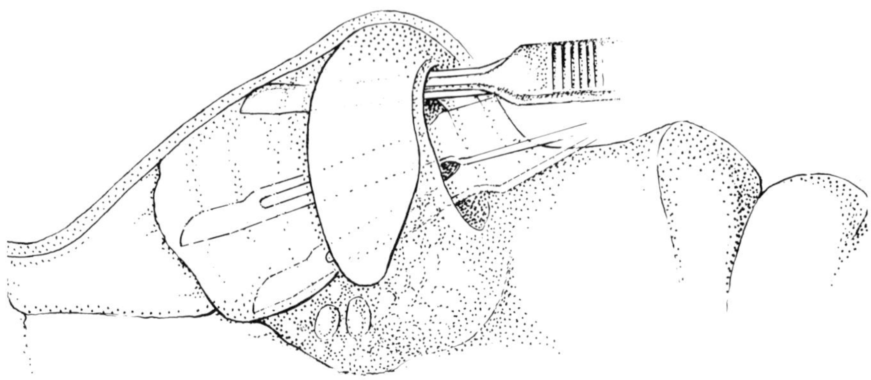

The blade is turned over, and the dissection is carried over the entire upper lateral cartilage, extending over the dorsum.

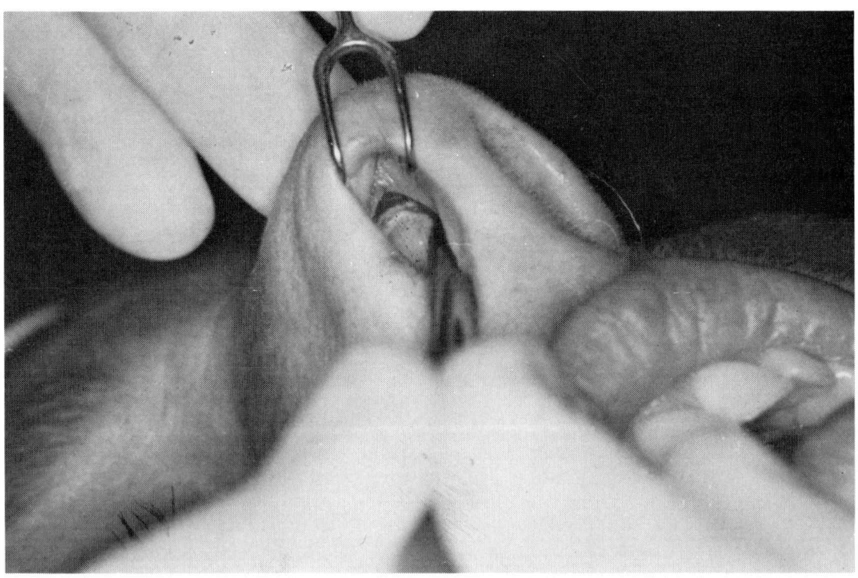

The incision ends past the angle of the septum. The same procedure is carried out on the opposite side.

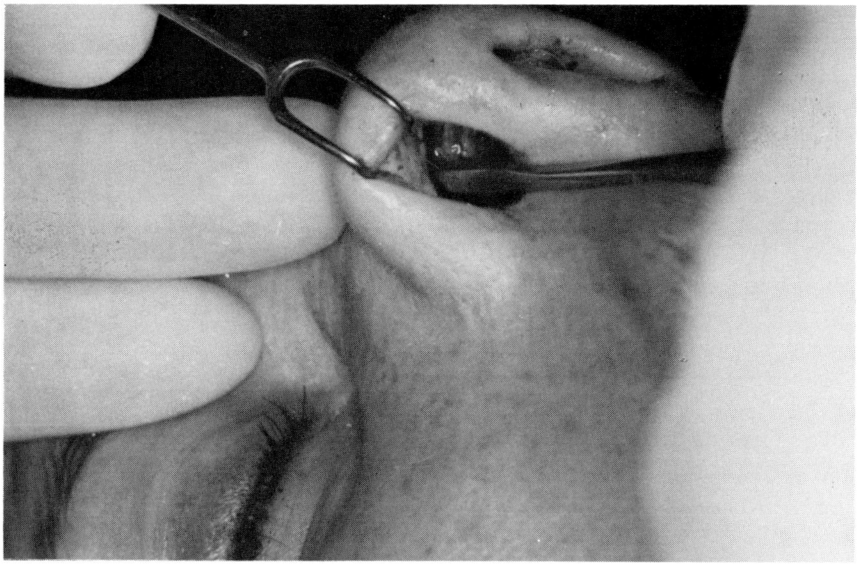

A Joseph periosteal elevator is inserted over the upper lateral cartilage and placed at a point caudal on the bony pyramid that is the lateral limit of the dissection.

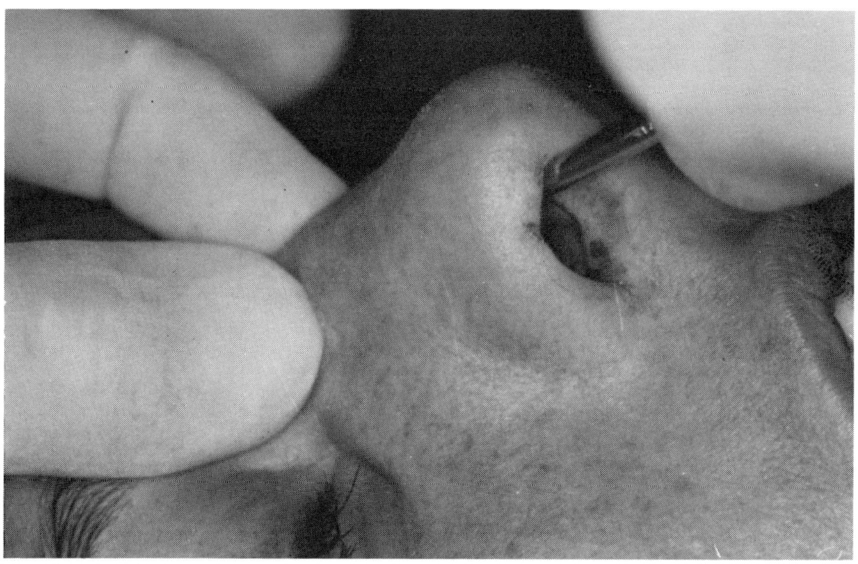

Assisted by external pressure from the thumb, the Joseph periosteal elevator slips under the periosteum with a gentle rocking motion and moderate pressure on the point of the instrument against the nasal bone.

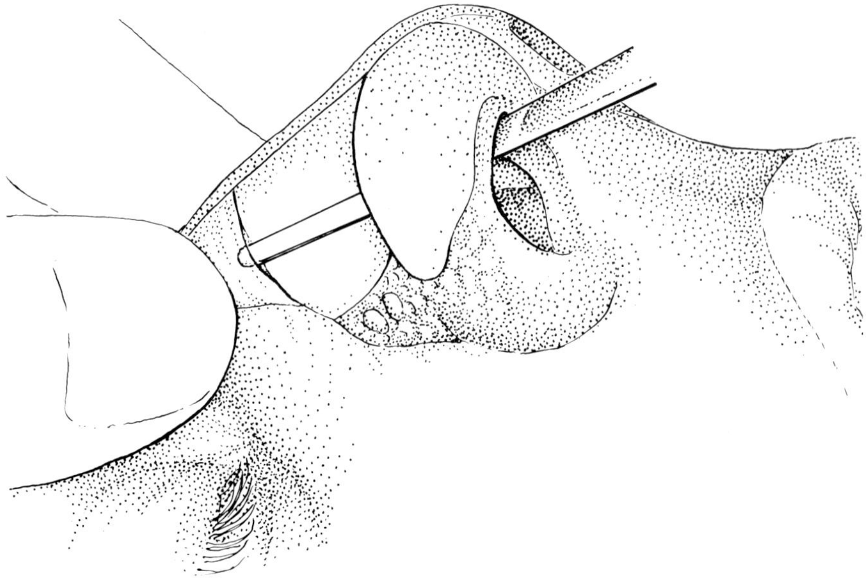

Once under the periosteum, the elevator is advanced to the area of the radix. Care is taken that the lateral limit of the dissection is kept to a minimum. This ensures the necessary support of the nasal bones by the overlying skin.

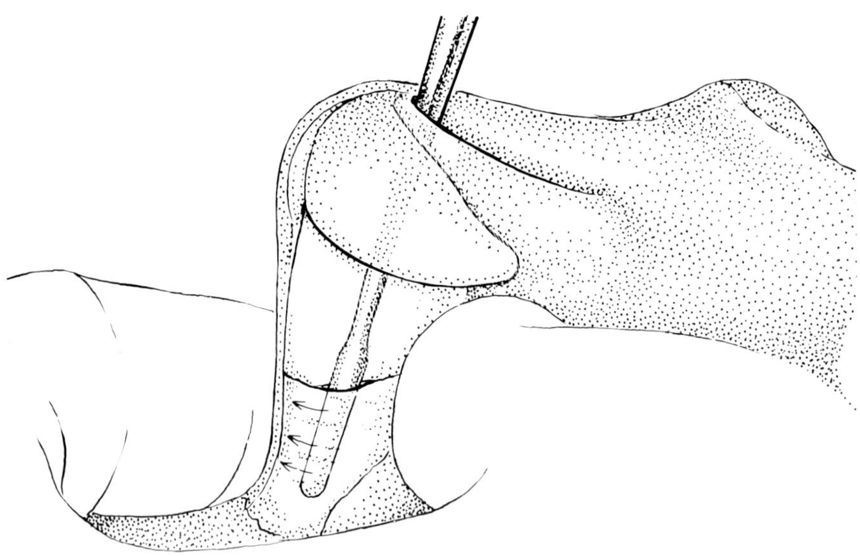

The extent of the dissection of periosteum away from the dorsal edge of the bony pyramid varies but is usually just enough to accommodate reduction of the dorsum.

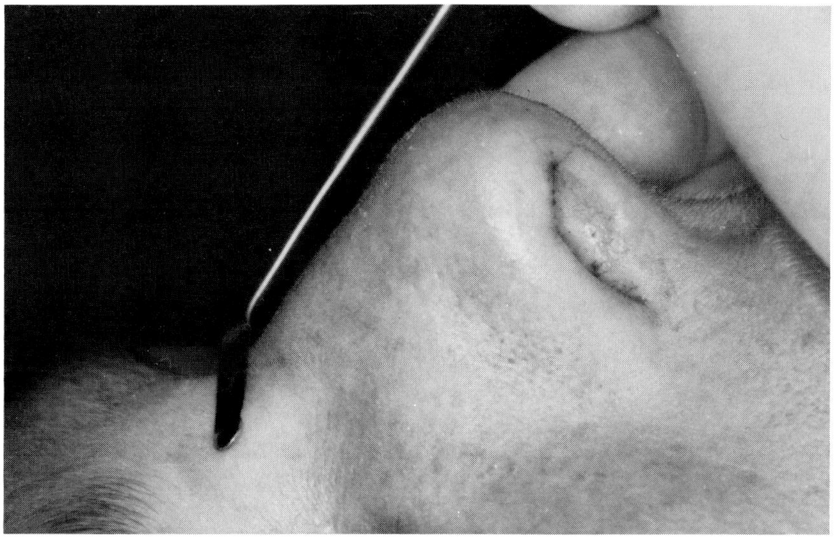

Following skeletonization, a right-angle knife is placed across the radix.

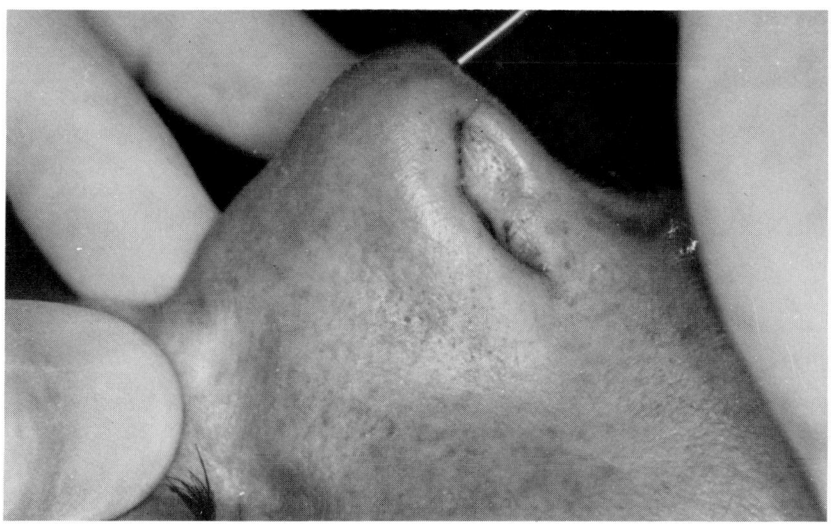

With a downward pull, the cutting edge is angled toward the skeleton with the handle of the instrument held lower than the dorsal line. This ensures that no tissue is unnecessarily resected from the overlying skin.

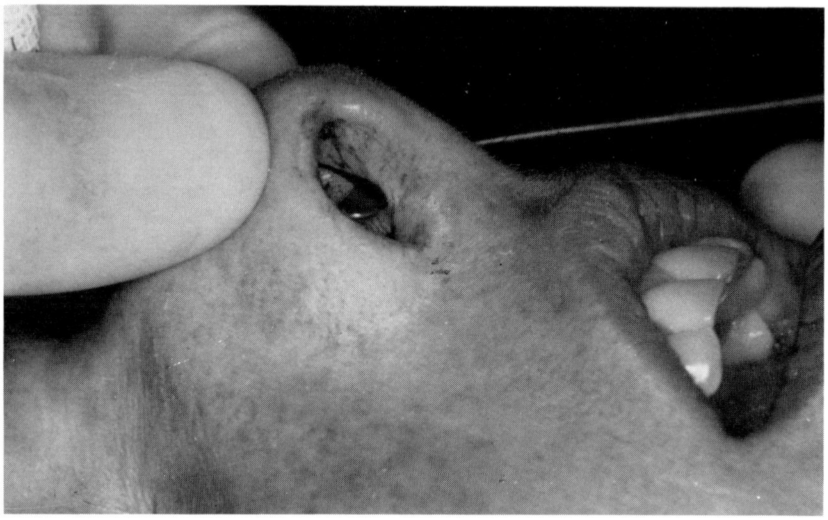

The transection is completed as the knife is drawn across the angle of the septum, completely separating the soft tissues of the nose from the skeletal parts.

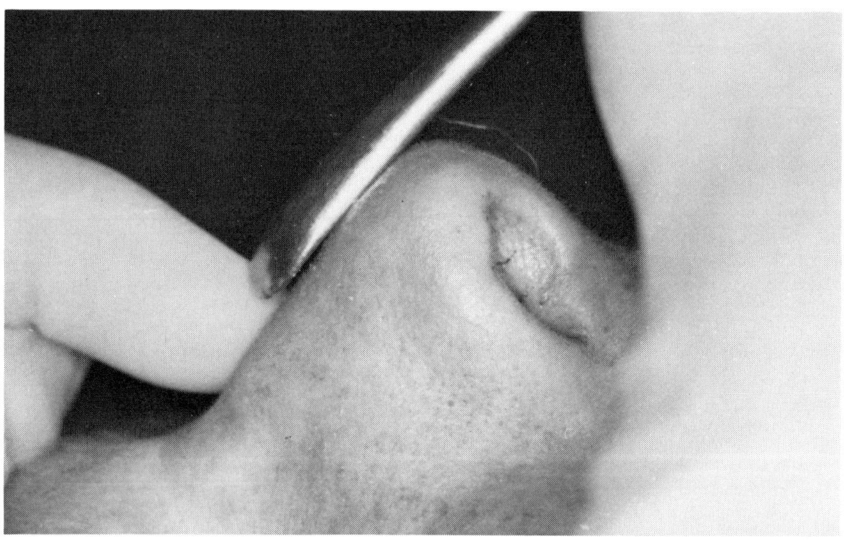

A Cottle periosteal elevator is used to clear off any residual soft tissue from the bony vault. Its broad dissecting edge makes it ideal for this purpose.

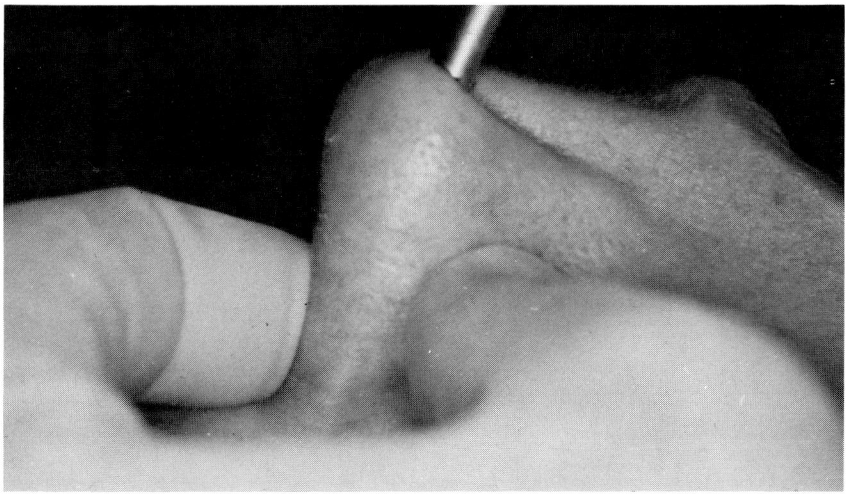

The elevator is placed over the dorsum, and all of the remaining soft tissue and periosteum is scraped from the dorsal edge of the bony pyramid.

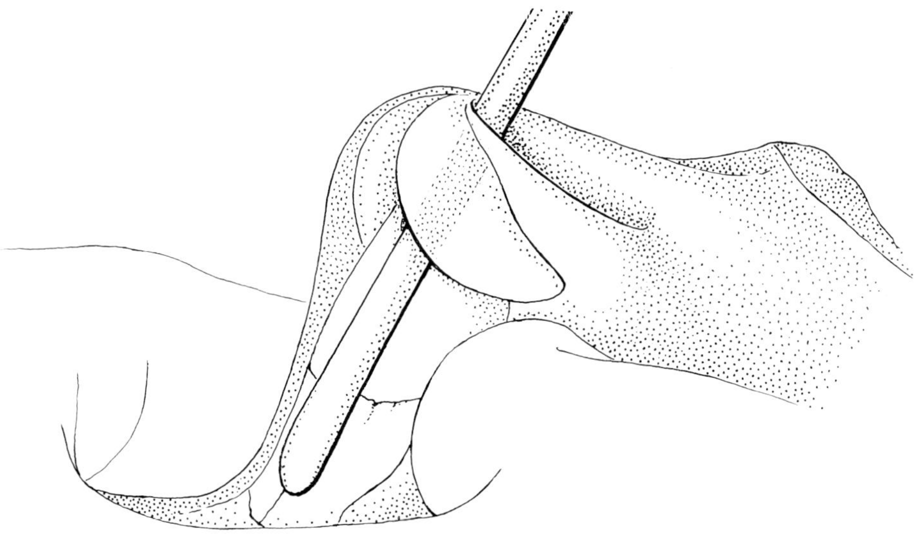

The stripping of soft tissue prepares the bony pyramid for rasping.

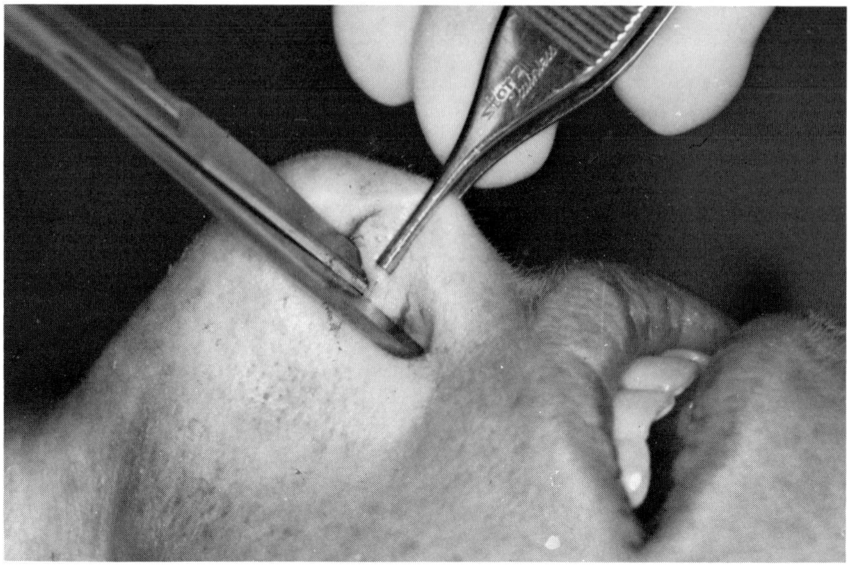

Transfixion of the membranous septum can be done most simply and symmetrically by grasping the columella with a pair of Brown Adson forceps and then using straight Mayo scissors to make a single cut to the nasal spine. The decision to transfix the membranous septum is made preoperatively and should be done only if there is a need to alter the nasolabial angle or if modification of the nasal spine is planned.

MODIFICATION OF BONY SKELETAL PARTS

Nasal spine

The nasal spine is a small, triangular projection of bone arising from the maxilla on the inferior border of the pyriform aperture. It is the saddle for the caudal edge of the septum. The aesthetic importance of this small triangle of bone is rarely discussed, yet its presence or absence plays an important role in facial aesthetics. Because its influence is limited to the area of the subnasion and the lip and not the nasal contour itself, it is usually the first bony part to be reduced following skeletonization. The decision to modify the nasal spine should be made preoperatively.

The prominent nasal spine with its accompanying caudal septum can affect the appearance of the lip by shortening it or causing excessive protrusion. An overly protruding nasal spine creates disharmony of the columella with the alar rims, and it frequently causes a look of webbing in the area of subnasion. Although the features mentioned are undesirable, retrusion of the nasal spine is equally undesirable.

When reduction of the nasal spine is indicated, conservative resection is mandatory to preserve the soft curve of the subnasion and a suitable position of the lip.

Conservative and well-planned resection of the nasal spine can improve the appearance of the mouth by adding length to the lip and by deepening the nasolabial angle.

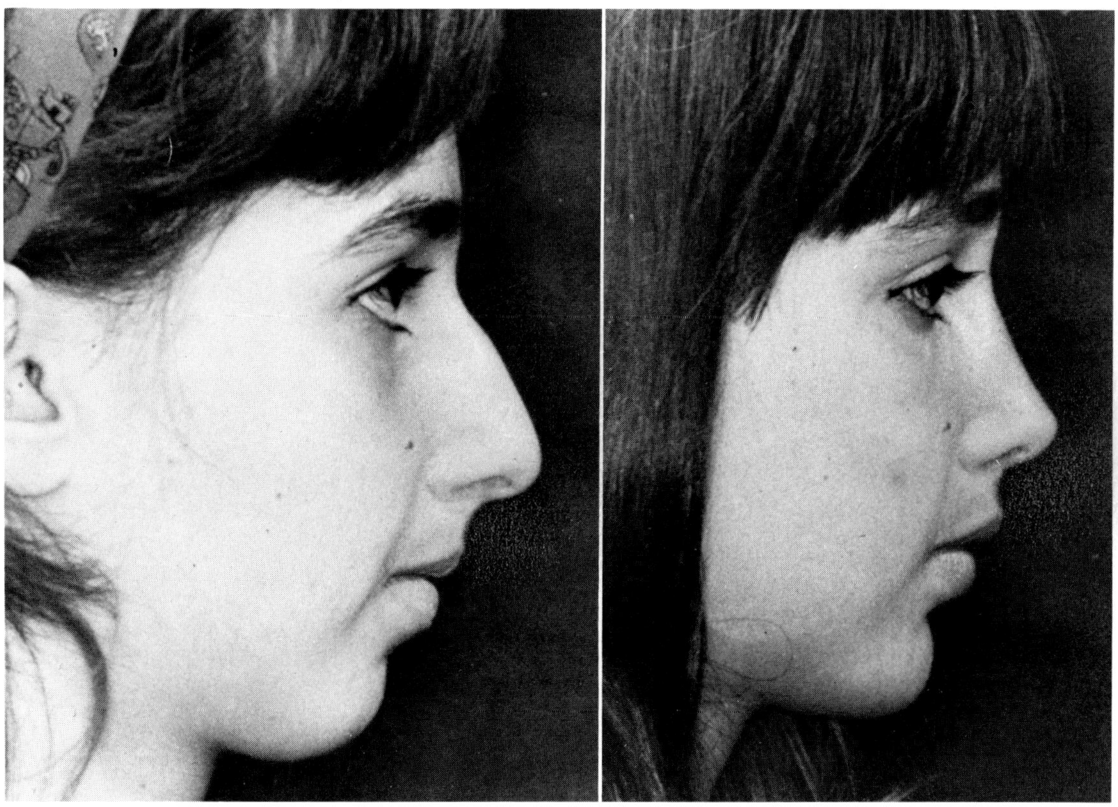

This patient illustrates the effect of appropriate reduction of the spine. There is a deepening of the nasolabial angle, but the soft curve over the subnasion is retained. The vertical line of the lip is parallel to the facial plane.

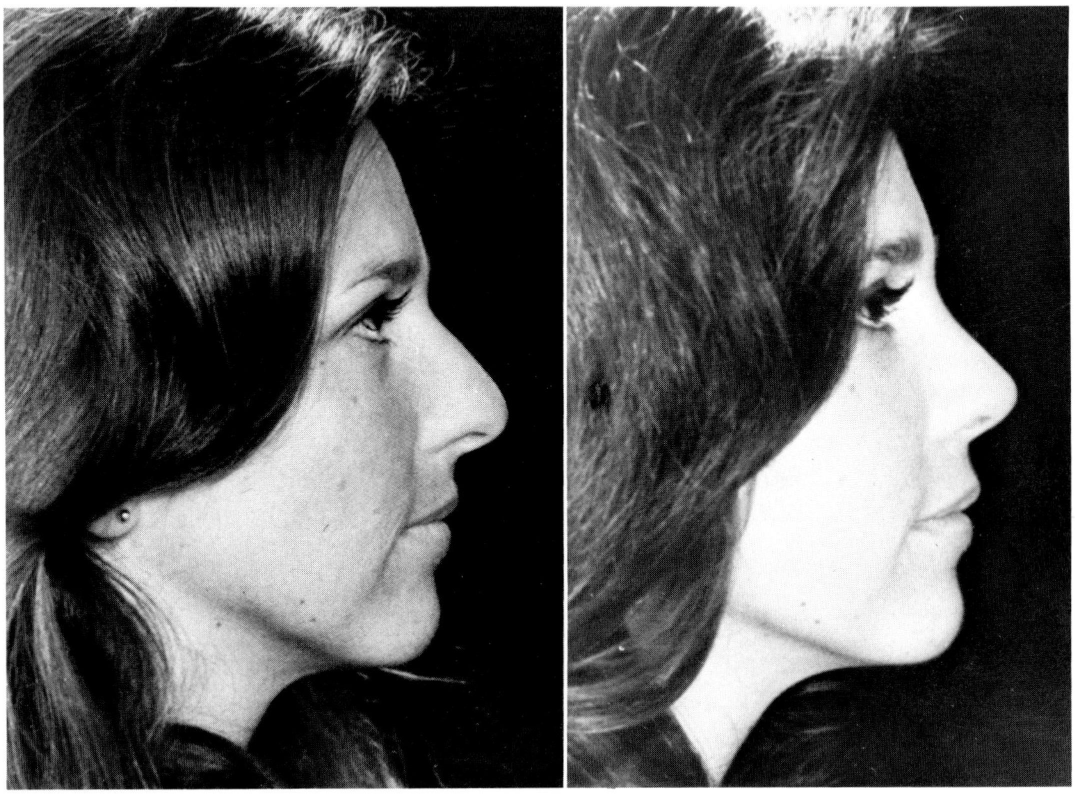

Although this patient has a satisfactory result, she exhibits the effects of slight overresection of the nasal spine. The soft curve over the subnasion has been altered to a sharp angle and has been made slightly retrusive. The vertical line of the lip has been moved from an anterior to a posterior position relative to the facial plane. The overall effect is a definite, undesirable change in the appearance of her mouth.

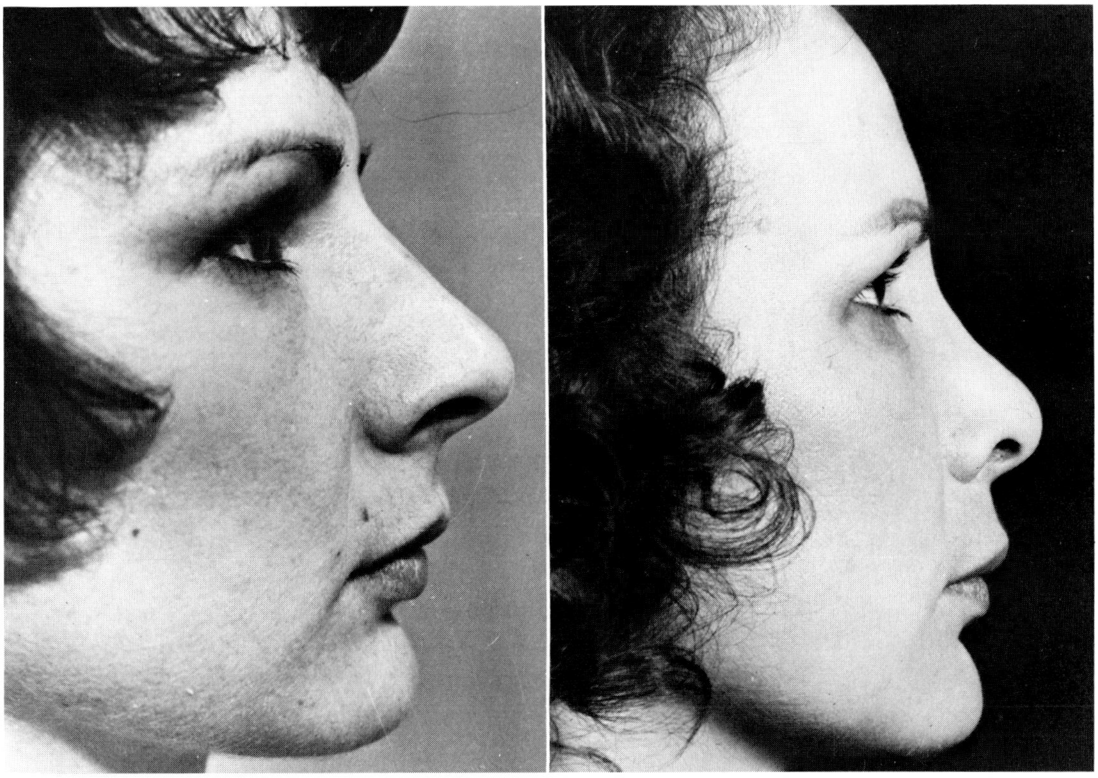

This patient is a dramatic illustration of the effects of overreduction of the nasal spine. The full subnasion has been altered to a sharp retrusive angle. The plane of the lip has been moved posteriorly, giving the lip an unattractive retrusive look.

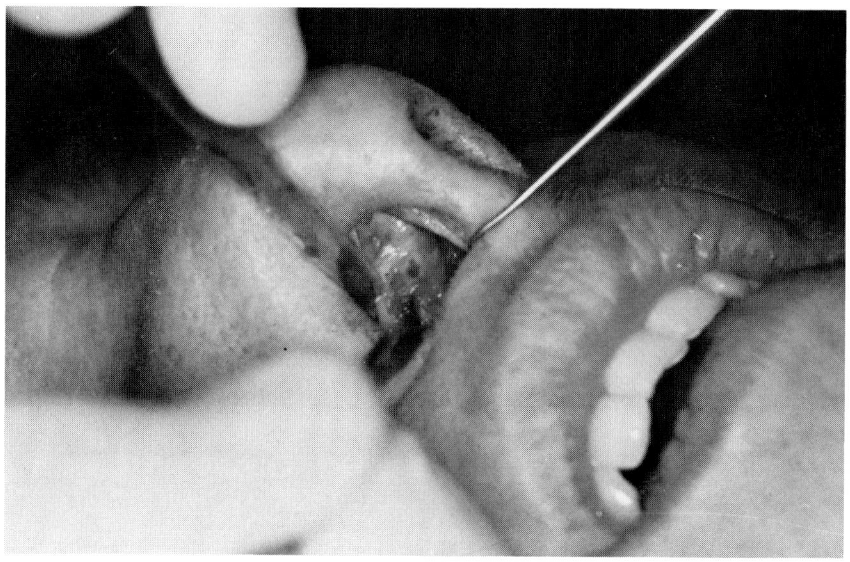

REDUCTION OF NASAL SPINE

Following transection of the membranous septum to the base of the nasal spine, the columella is retracted while the spine is cleared of all soft tissues with a Joseph periosteal elevator.

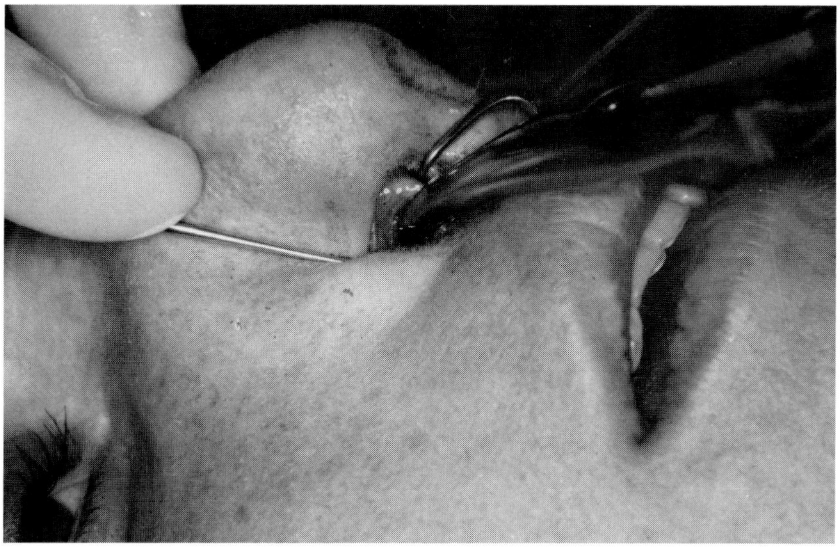

A double-action bone rongeur is used to resect part of the spine and a segment of the caudal septum.

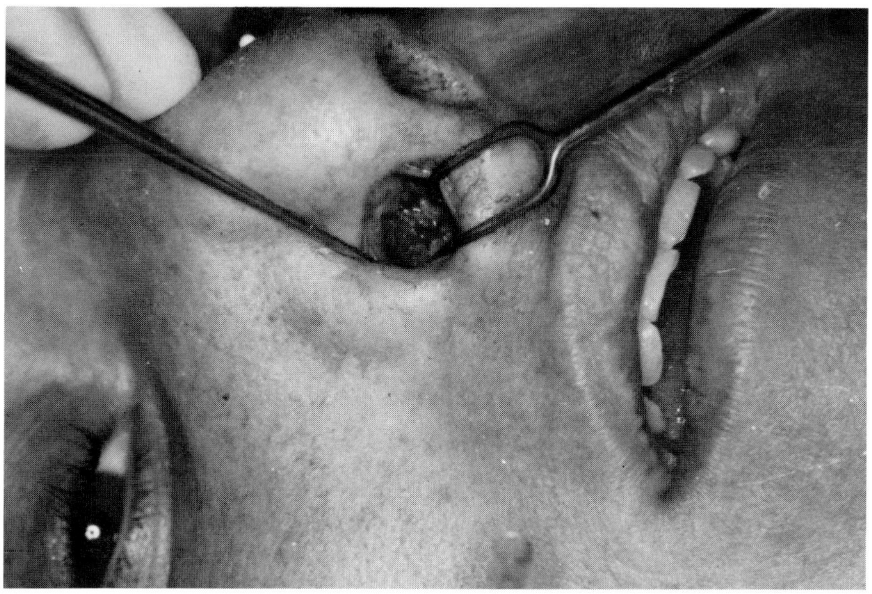

The appearance of the area of the spine following reduction is shown. Bone wax is rarely necessary but may be used if bleeding is excessive.

Bony dorsum

The estimation of the amount of bony dorsum that should be resected is the most common pitfall in rhinoplasty. Most often, the correct amount of resection is deceptively small and frequently less than 3 mm. Because of the small amount of bone that is required to reduce the height of the bony pyramid, the choice of instrument for lowering the dorsum is important for success. There is little chance of obtaining a 3 mm resection of the bony vault using the saw technique unless the saw is used as a rasp.

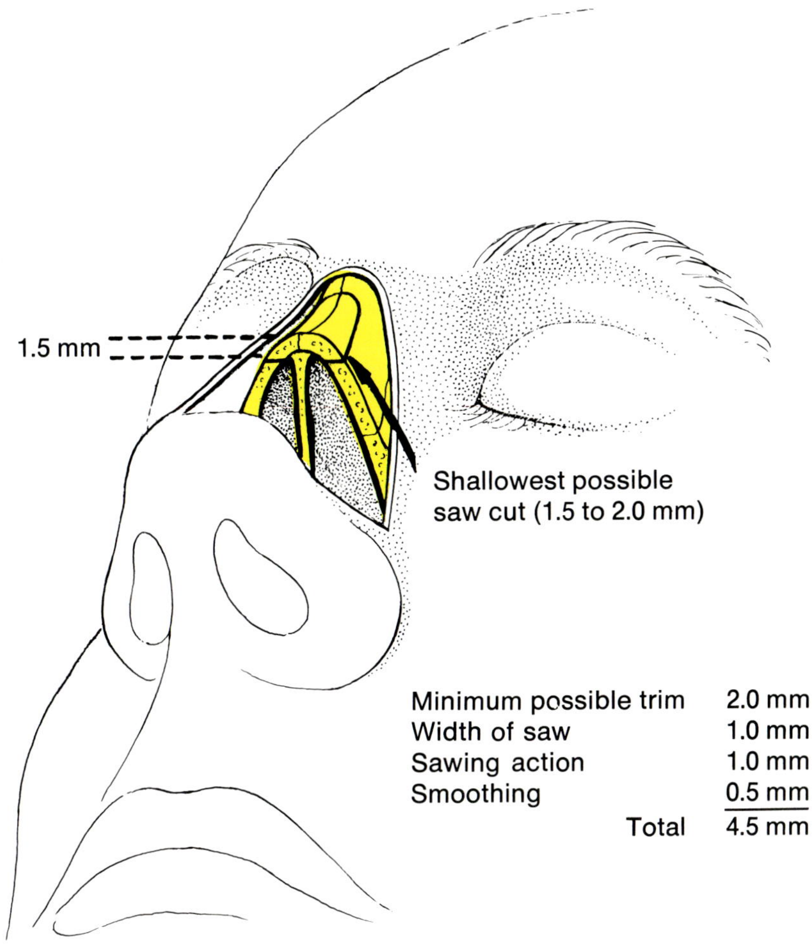

The illustration demonstrates the inevitable bony reduction if a saw is used. To get the necessary purchase of the instrument on the bone, it must be placed below the solid bony arch. This is usually 1 to 2 mm thick. Because it is virtually impossible to get a straight, perfect cut, there is a variation in the cutting stroke of 1 mm or more. Therefore, in order to get the least reduction of dorsum possible using a saw, one is committed to a 4.5-mm reduction, which in many cases would be excessive, setting the stage for a predictable series of errors.

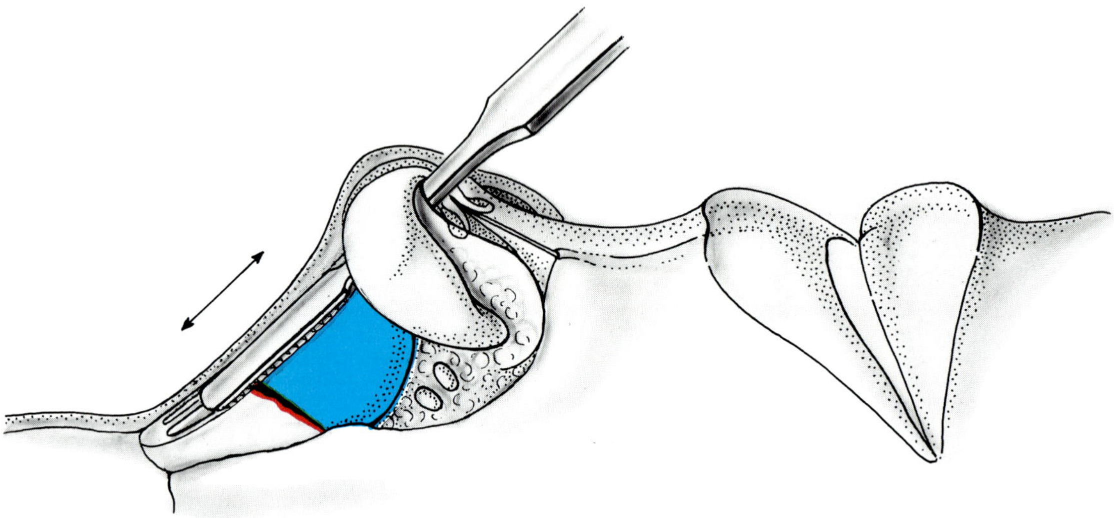

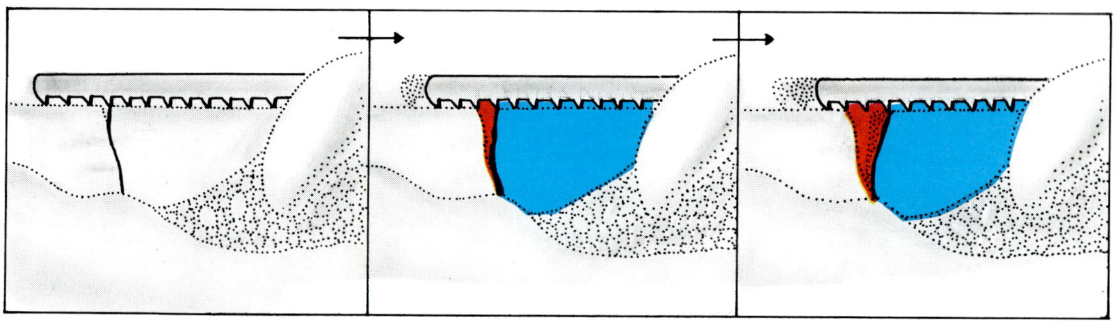

A coarse Foman rasp is recommended because it is effective and easily controlled. The rasp should be sharp enough to cut and fine enough not to avulse the upper lateral cartilages. Deeply ridged rasps should be avoided because of the danger of avulsion.

Since the relationship of the upper lateral cartilages to the bony vault is vital to normal function and to aesthetic symmetry, special care is given to reduction of the dorsum at the osteochondral junction. Separation of this articulation may occur if the direction of pull is in line with the dorsum, placing the greatest pulling force on the area of conjunction.

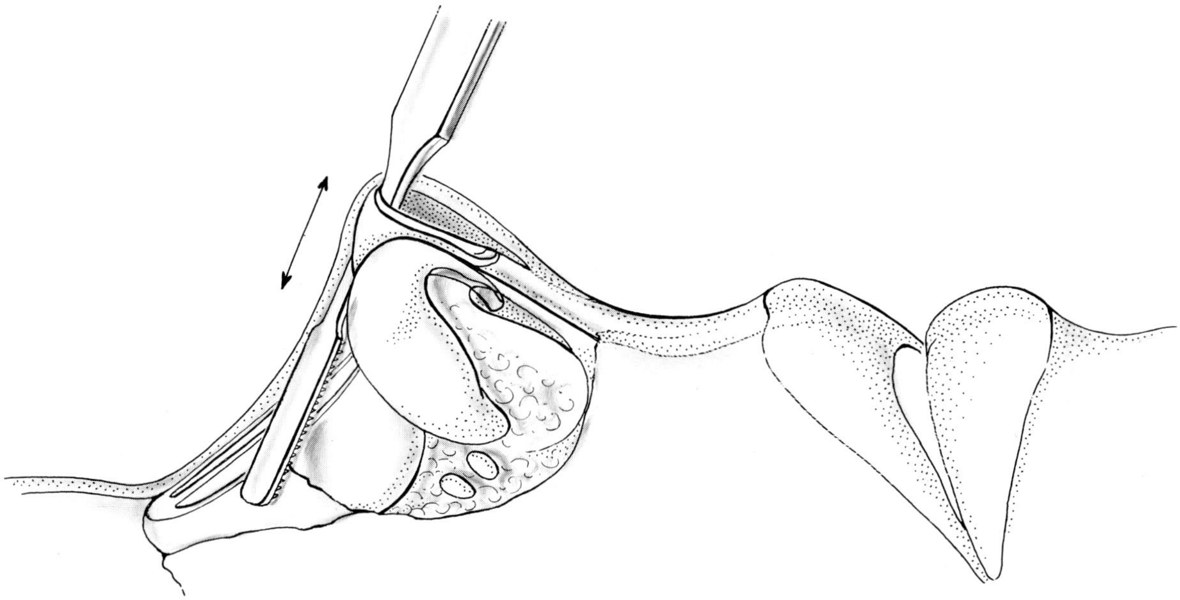

The chance of avulsion can be decreased by gently rasping on the bias to place as little pull as possible on the attachments of cartilage to bone.

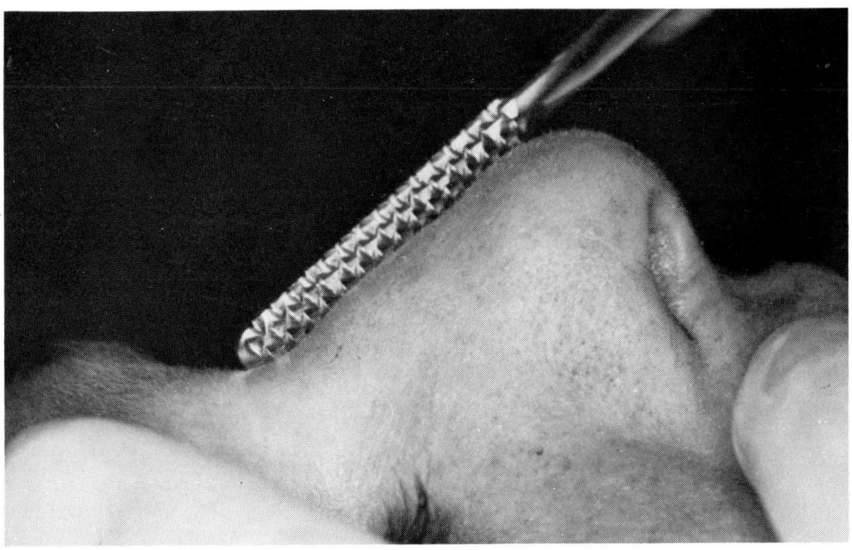

The cutting edge of the Foman rasp is shown next to the dorsal edge to be lowered. It is estimated that approximately 2 mm of the bony dorsum is to be reduced.

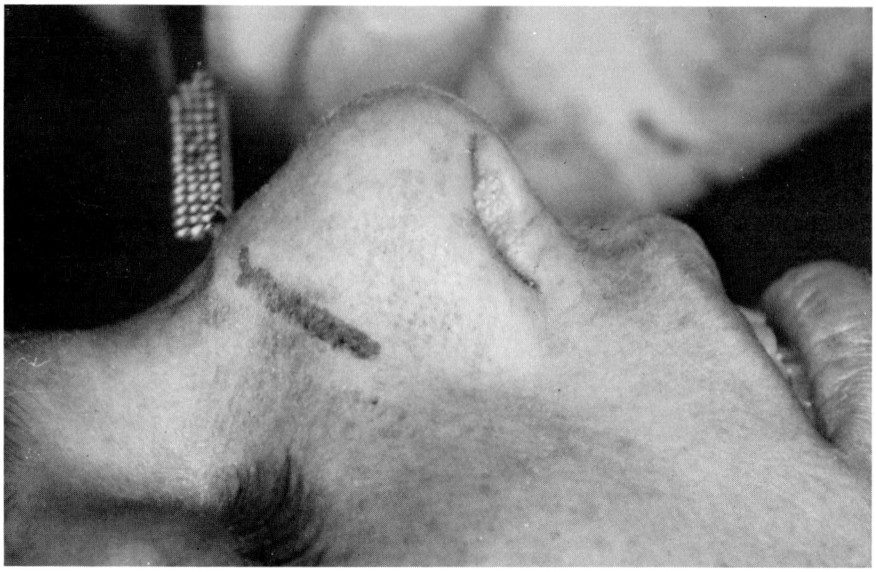

The bony vault has been marked with gentian violet. The rasp is shown following the reduction of the dome of the bony vault, which has produced an "open roof" caudal to the solid arch of bone at the radix.

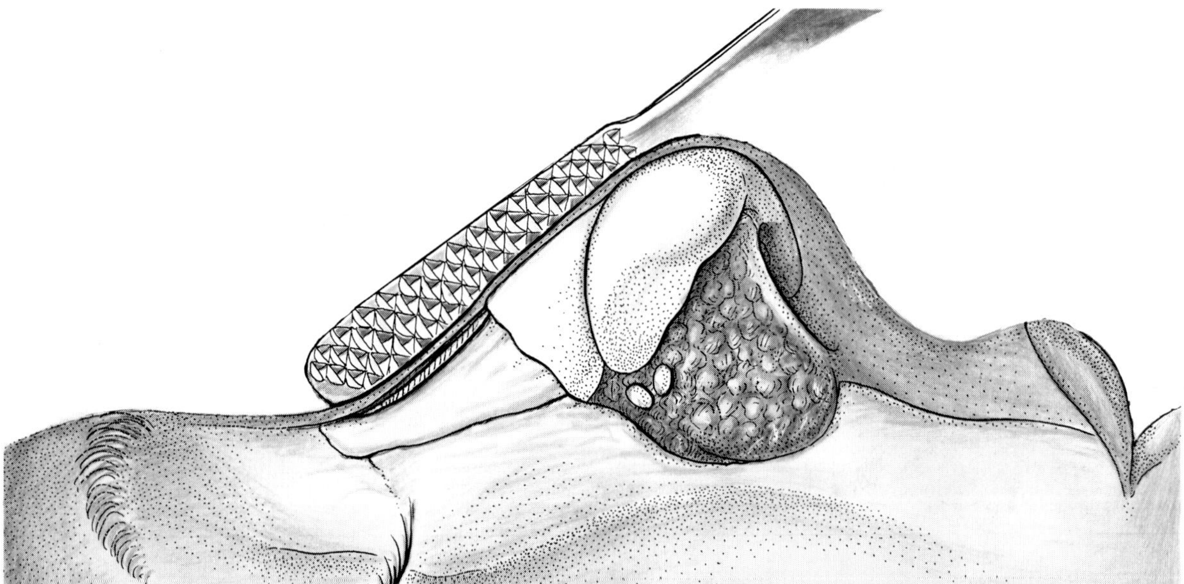

The reduction has uncovered the roof of the bony vault, but has left the cartilaginous portion of the dorsum untouched. Cartilaginous parts should then be modified by sharp dissection for greatest control and least trauma.

MODIFICATION OF CARTILAGINOUS SKELETAL PARTS

The upper lateral cartilages in conjunction with the septum form double arches, or the letter m, as seen in cross section. The m configuration is manifest when the cartilages of the middle vault are integrated into a functional unit. When the domes of the arches are resected or split, the domes may become sharp angles, which if reduced to less than 10 degrees, impair the function of the internal valve. Therefore, any technique of lowering the cartilaginous dorsum should maintain the m configuration by preserving mucosal continuity whenever possible.

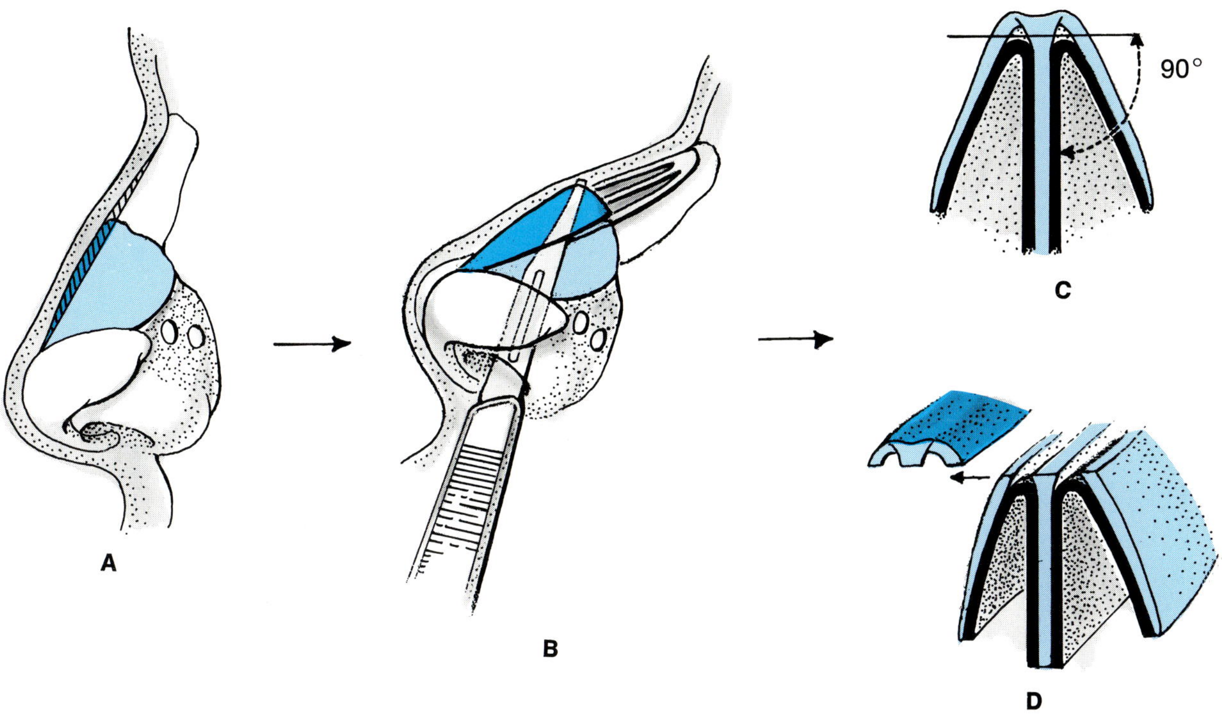

When the roof of the upper cartilaginous vault is resected, symmetry is assured by maintaining a 90-degree angle between the knife and the septum. The illustration shows the following:

A. The area to be reduced (shaded)
B. The bony hump removed and the knife in position to resect cartilaginous roof
C. The position of the cutting edge in cross section
D. Roof removed and the intact mucosa

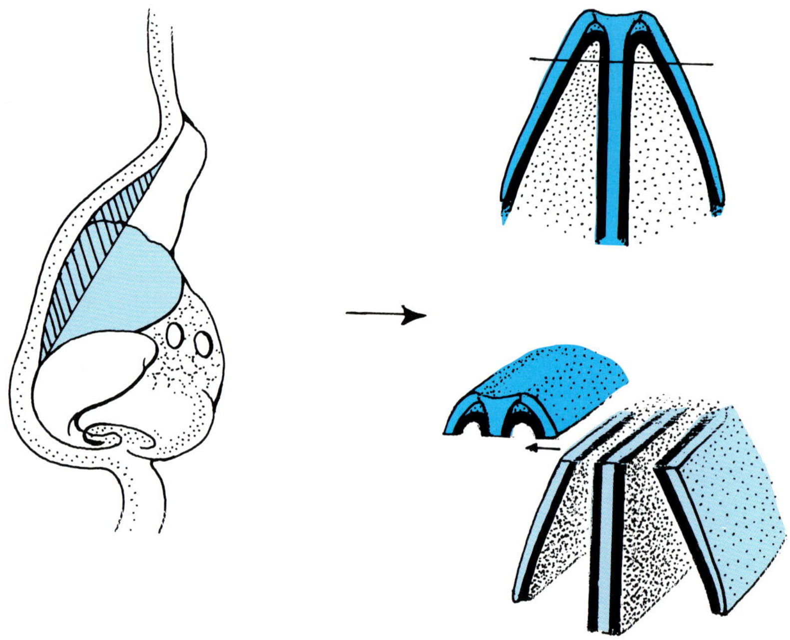

In cases where the dorsum is excessively high, the cut is made as shown. The loss of mucosal continuity increases the potential of excessive narrowing of the middle vault, with subsequent impairment of the internal valve. Mucosal continuity can be maintained in this circumstance only by submucous dissection before resection of the roof.

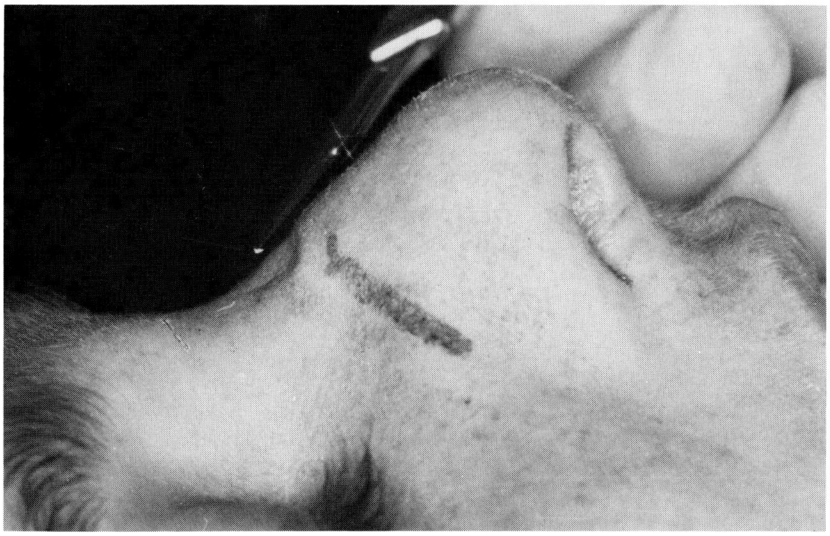

A No. 11 blade is used for dorsal resection because of its long straight cutting edge. Because of the danger of perforation, the tip is broken off by placing it between the handles of a Mayo scissors. Note the 90-degree relationship of the cutting edge to the roof.

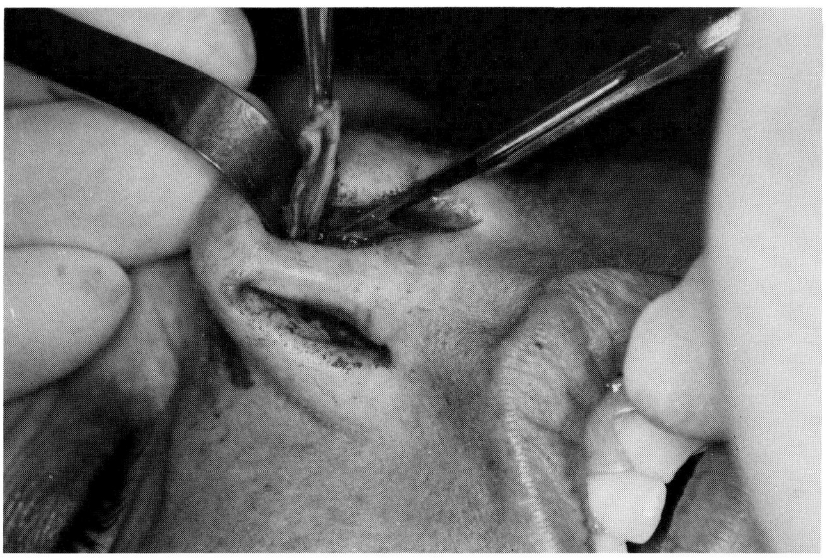

The cut is made under direct vision, and the assistant removes the resected dorsum with a pair of Brown Adson forceps.

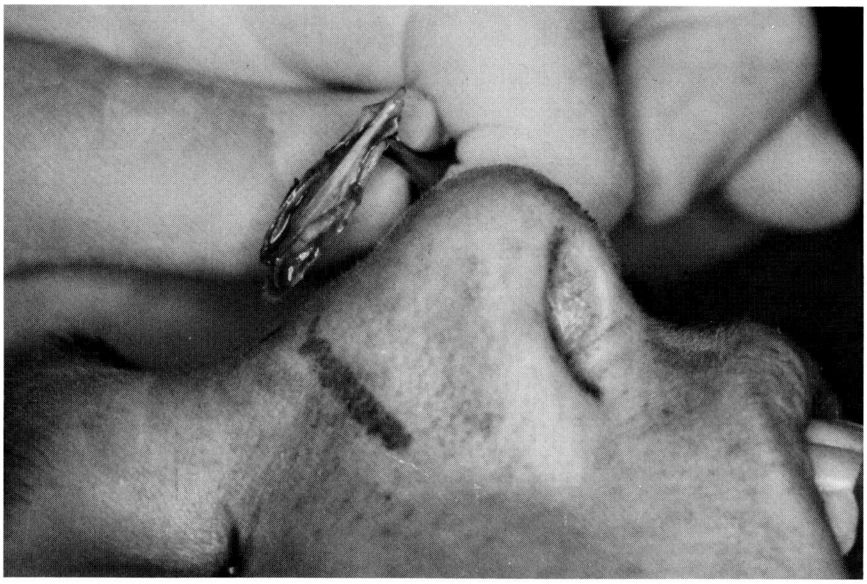

The specimen is shown from the posterior surface where the central septal cartilaginous part, with its lateral extensions to the upper lateral cartilages, can be seen. The cephalic bulge of the lower lateral cartilages is made more evident by the lowering of the dorsal line.

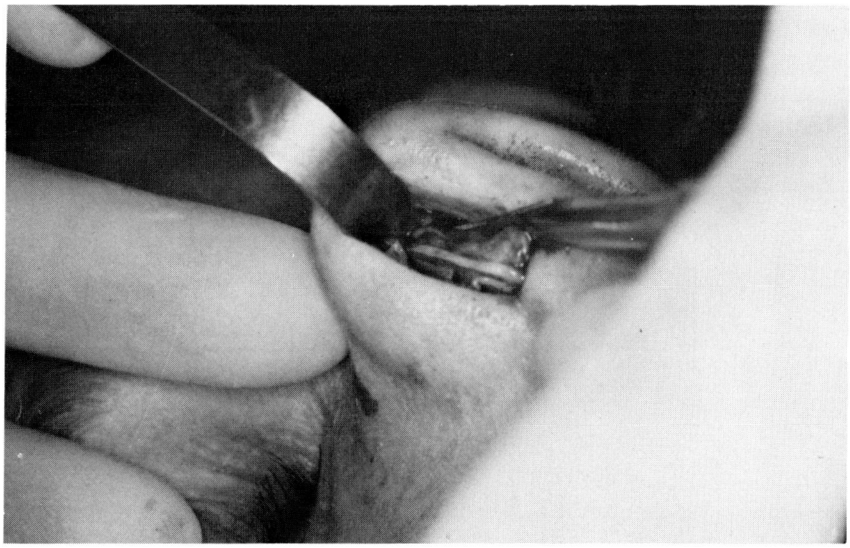

Since the remaining dorsal edge of the septum becomes the new skeletal support for the soft tissues, its contour from radix to the angle of the septum must be absolutely smooth and straight. It is neither anatomically correct nor necessary to overcorrect (over-resect) the dorsum to avoid supratip fullness. If the new dorsal line has been correctly estimated according to the desired contour and the limitations of the patient's tissues, it should retain its contour postoperatively.

Nasal tip

The accomplishment of a well-defined, beautifully contoured nasal tip is a challenge to the surgeon's finesse in judgment and skill. Because of the delicacy of the structures involved, any plan for changing the architecture of the nasal tip must be precise in conception and execution.

In most cases, I feel that the rim incision with delivery of the cartilage is the procedure of choice because it provides direct view of the cartilage, thereby affording the surgeon full control of the amount and manner of resection, especially in the area of the dome. In my experience, this technique produces a predictable and nonsurgical-appearing nasal tip. In approximately 5% of cases, when only slight refinement of the tip is required, the retrograde or cartilage-splitting technique can be used.

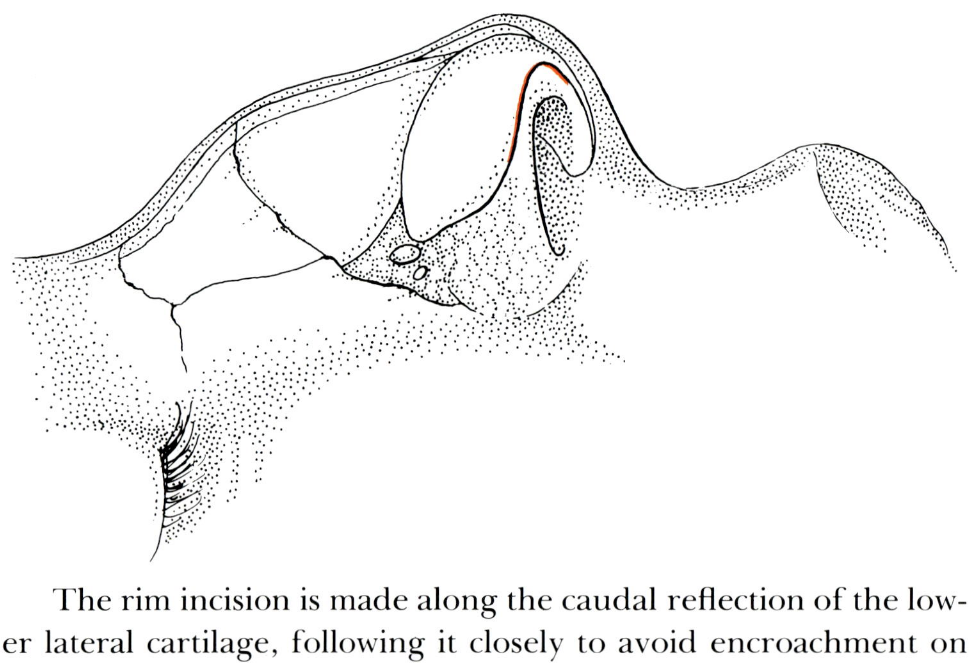

The rim incision is made along the caudal reflection of the lower lateral cartilage, following it closely to avoid encroachment on the soft triangle. The cephalic portion of the rim incision is made with the initial incision for rhinoplasty—the intercartilaginous incision.

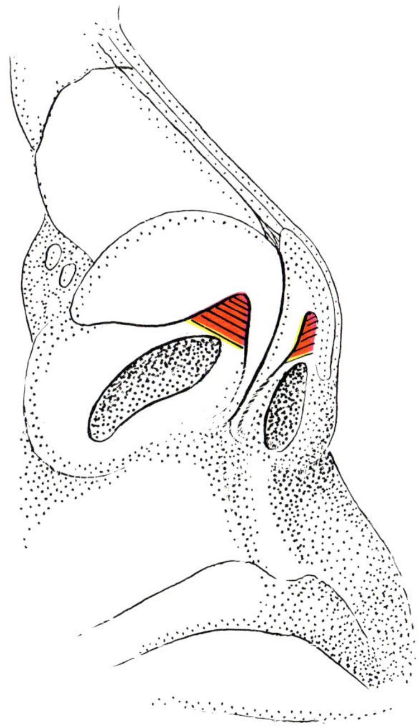

The soft triangle, as described in Converse's *Reconstructive Plastic Surgery,* is that area just caudal to the dome of the lower lateral cartilage where skin is juxtaposed to skin, forming one of the facets important to tip aesthetics. Any incisions in the soft triangle may cause deformity of the tip.

A double-hook retractor everts the nostril, making the caudal reflection of the lateral crus visible. The incision begins approximately 15 mm lateral to the dome and closely follows the caudal reflection of the lateral crus.

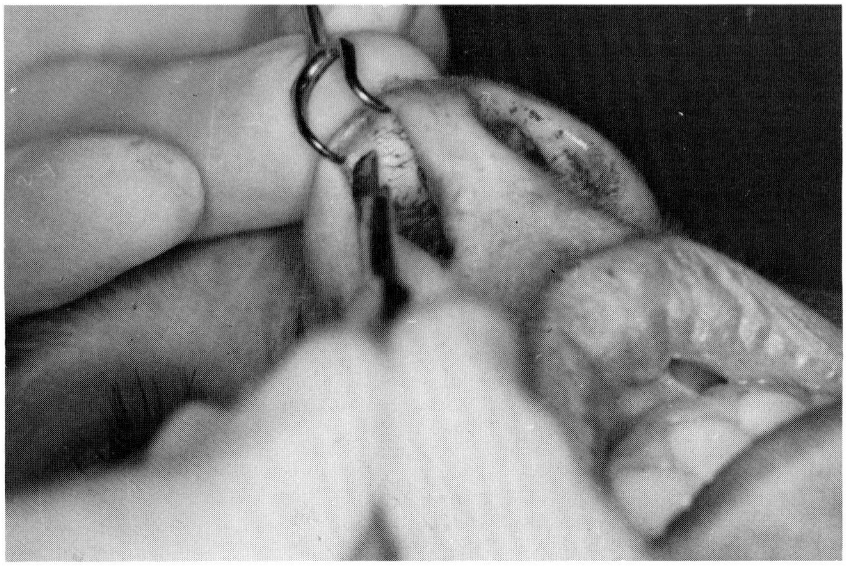

This photograph illustrates the method of reflecting the area of the soft triangle. The scalpel has completed the incision of the lateral crus and is just entering the area of the dome. The soft triangle is between the hook and the scalpel.

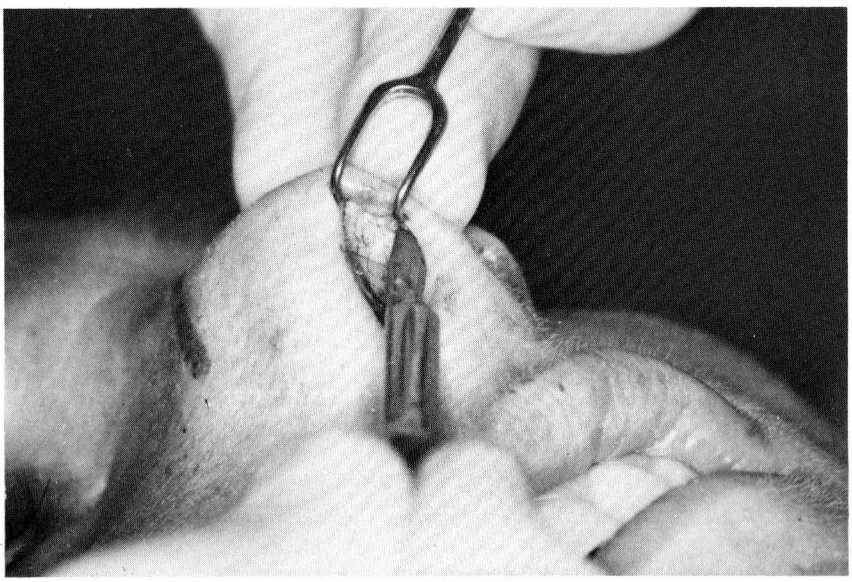

The incision continues from the area of the soft triangle along the caudal reflection of the medial crus and ends at the middle third of the columella.

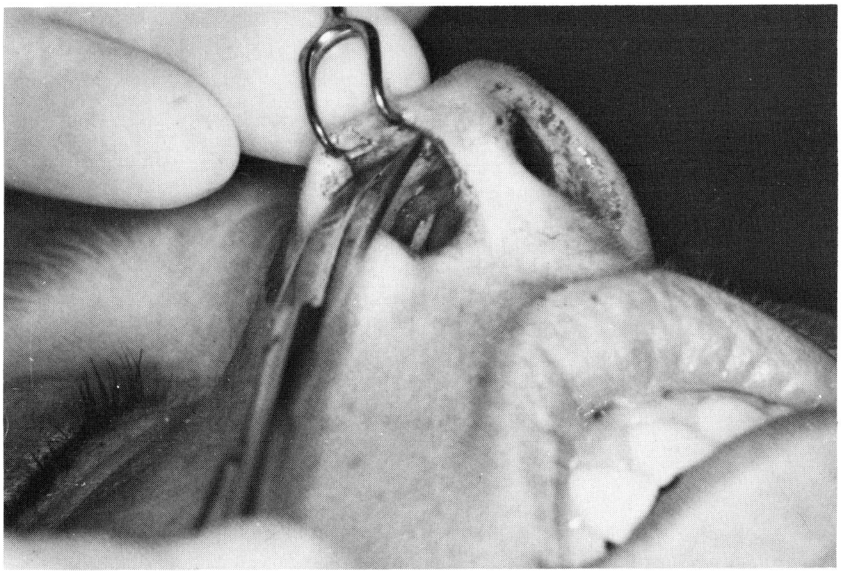

Following the incision, a pair of Joseph scissors is used to dissect the cartilage from the overlying skin. At this point the dissection can be used to trim the fibrofatty tissues overlying the cartilage by developing a plane closer to the surface of the skin. Note the width of undisturbed skin in the area of the soft triangle between the hook and the scissors.

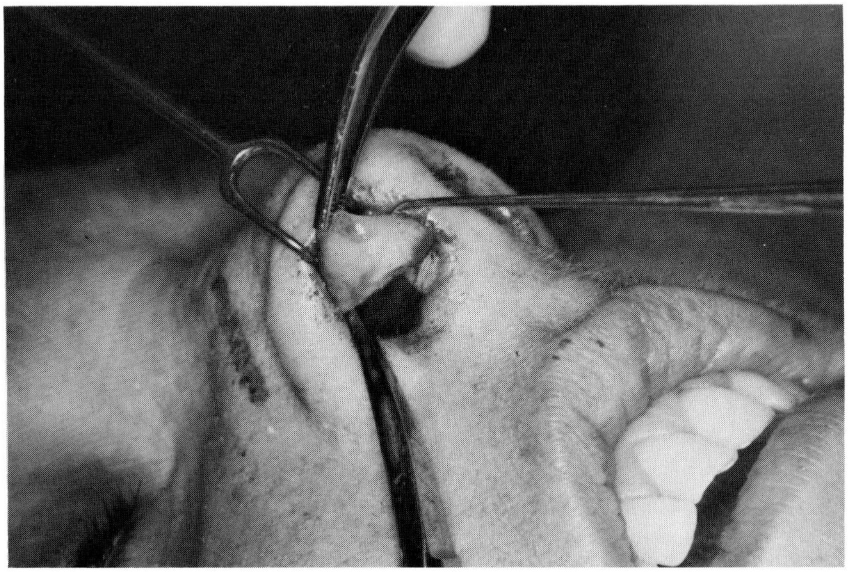

The dissection is kept close to the cartilage, which is delivered as a glistening white structure. Delivery as a bipedical mucochondrial flap allows assessment of the entire cartilage. It should be noted that the cartilage narrows at the area of the dome, contrary to many artists' drawings of this part.

The width of the dome is a major determinant of tip refinement. Ideally it should be 3 to 4 mm wide. Surplus cartilage should be excised; however, if the domes are made narrower than 3 mm, postoperative blanching, or "knuckles," can occur.

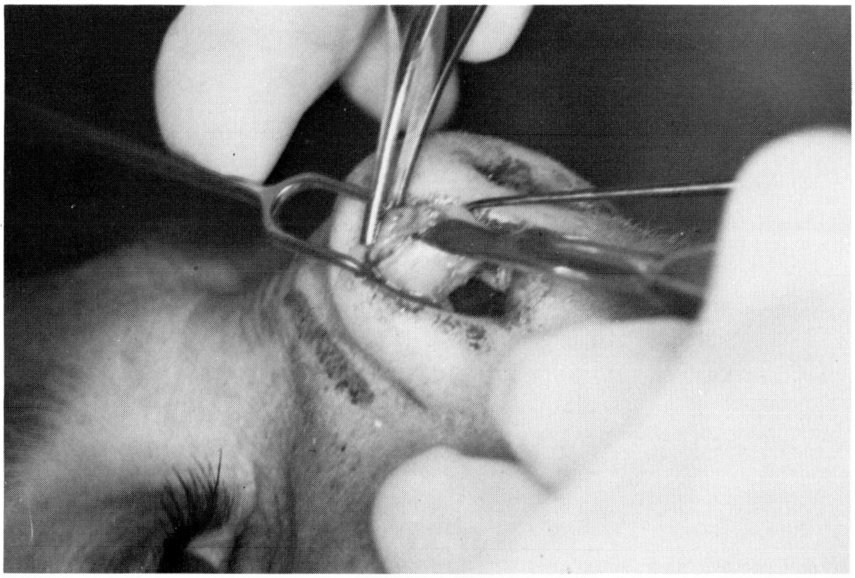

The broad, cephalic part of the lateral crus is trimmed initially. The area of the dome is left untouched. Then, once the cephalic border is resected, the cartilage is returned to its normal position, and the result of the resection is appraised.

Of special importance is the preservation of as much lateral crus as possible consistent with obtaining the desired refinement. Techniques designed to leave only a thin strip of lateral crura, or to totally ablate them, may be successful if the alae are substantial enough to retain their shape without skeletal support. On the other hand, if the alae are thin, they tend to collapse without adequate support, especially on inspiration.

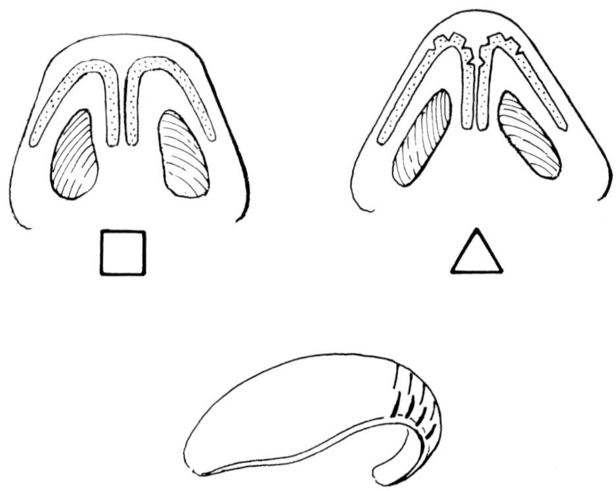

To achieve a narrower, more projecting tip, the cartilage at the dome can be weakened, thereby narrowing the arch and producing a slightly higher and angular dome. Weakening, or attenuation, of the dome is best accomplished by interdigitating partial-depth cuts. This is a champion technique because it changes the contour of the cartilage while preserving its structural integrity. Morselization of the dome is hazardous because it may cause a weakness that is so extreme that loss of contour and projection results.

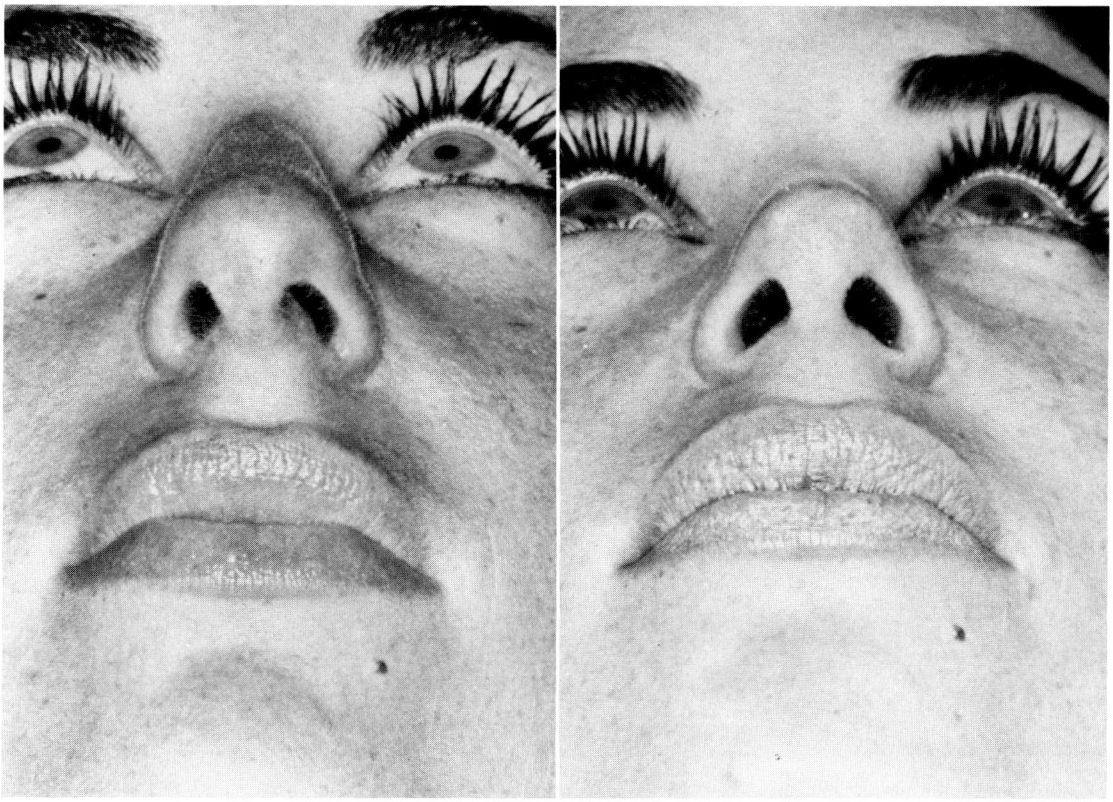

Resection of the cephalic portion of the lower lateral cartilages and attenuation of the domes has changed an almost square basal configuration to a more triangular one.

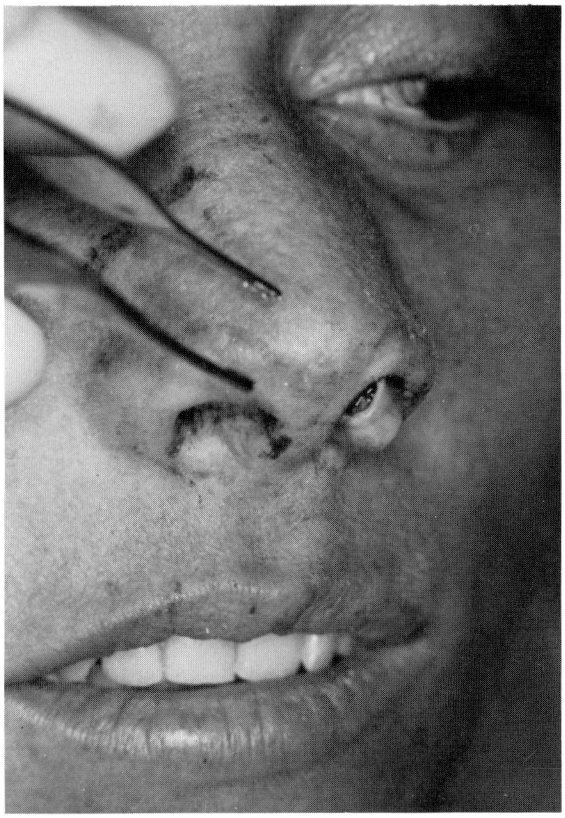

The broad arch of the dome of the lower lateral cartilage is illustrated.

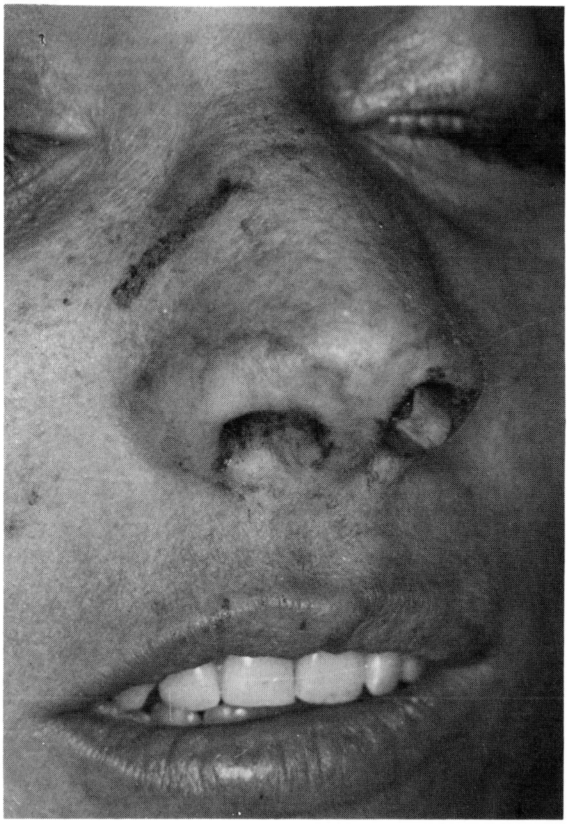

Following attenuation of the dome, a narrower angle and increased projection can be seen. Inasmuch as control of the height and width of the dome is crucial to tip refinement, delivery of the cartilage has an obvious advantage over the blind cartilage-splitting incision.

OSTEOTOMY

Following reduction of the dorsum and preliminary contouring of the lower lateral cartilages, the nasal bones are fractured to re-form the nasal pyramid.

With the use of a series of triangles as a model, an analysis of the changes in the pyramid following fracture can help one understand the mechanics of mobilizing the bony framework and the rationale for the "low to high" osteotomy.

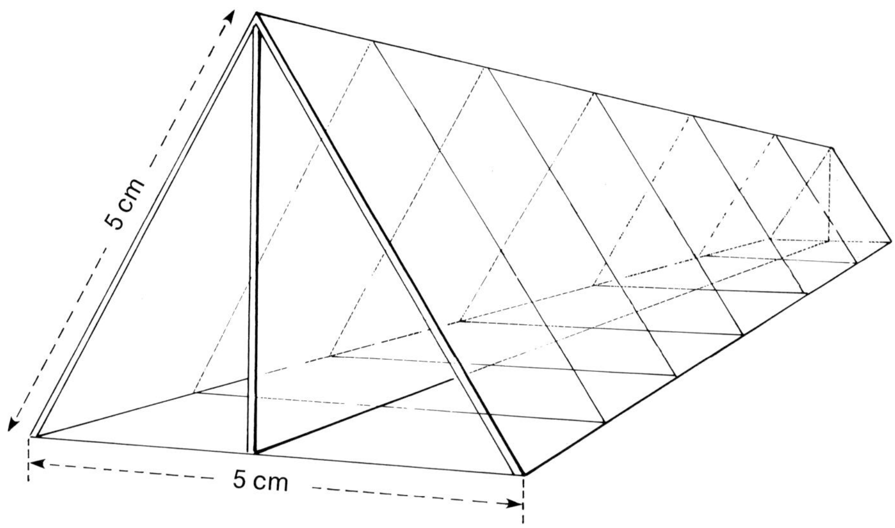

If an imaginary floor were placed at the base of the frontal process of the maxilla on a skull, the nasal pyramid would be seen on cross section to form equilateral triangles of increasing size, going from the smallest at the radix to the largest at the caudal end of the nasal bones.

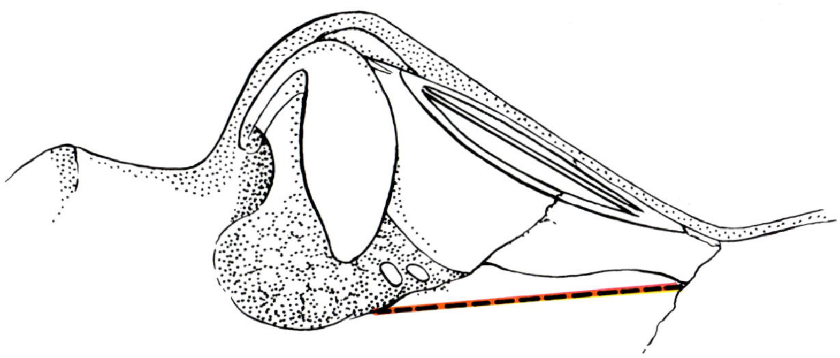

Following dorsal resection, there is loss of the apical part, producing an "open roof." In order to close the open roof and reconstruct a smaller pyramid, the line of osteotomy should converge on the fixed dorsal line following the base of the triangles (in red) as the triangles grow smaller toward the radix. This is referred to as a low to high osteotomy.

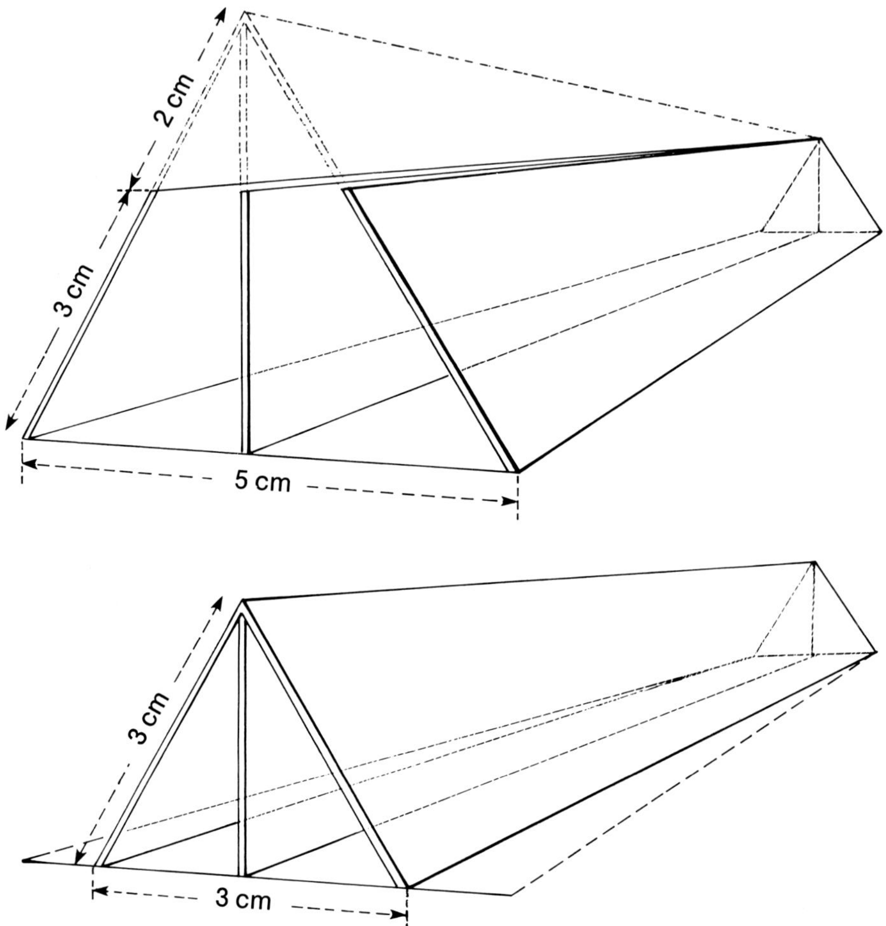

Once the triangles are separated at their bases, the common lateral walls are moved medially, re-forming the pyramid with the greatest medial movement caudally and the least at the radix.

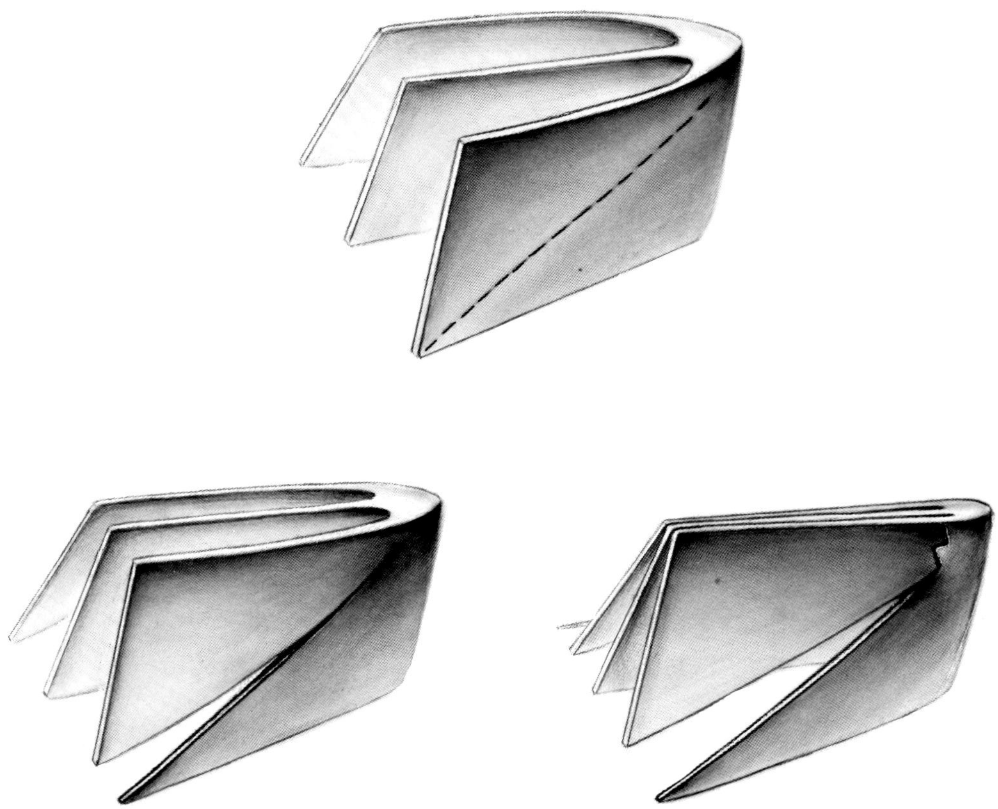

A model representing the bony pyramid following resection of the roof is shown. It demonstrates that a low to high osteotomy produces the proper size and shape of the lateral walls to re-form the normal, tapering nasal pyramid.

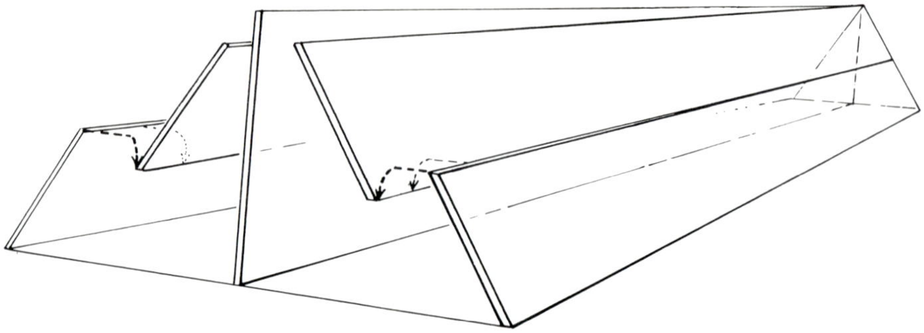

The line of osteotomy must follow along the bases of the equilateral triangles as they decrease in size (low to high osteotomy). If a high to high osteotomy is done, a step deformity with an unsatisfactory re-formation of the pyramid will result. Accordingly, the clinical importance of beginning the osteotomy as low as possible on the pyriform aperture is evident.

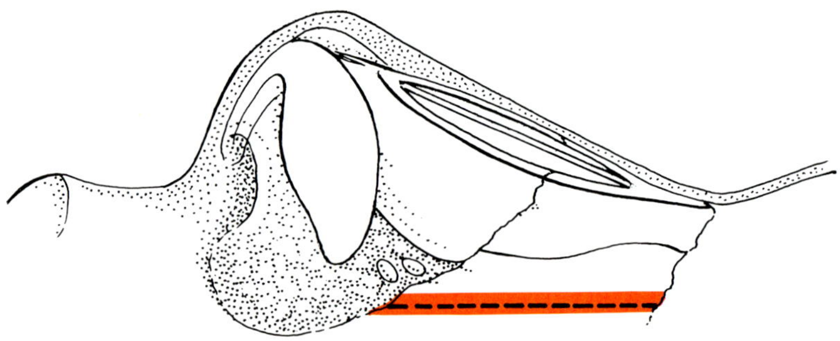

A low to low osteotomy is depicted in many current textbooks. With this type of osteotomy, the caudal position is proper, but the line of fracture almost parallels the dorsal line, producing a very wide cephalic portion of nasal bone. The resulting fragments cannot reconstruct the normal tapering nasal pyramid because of their rectangular shape. In the low to low osteotomy, medial osteotomy and outfracturing become necessary in order to mobilize the bones medially and to obtain a controlled fracture at the radix.

When a low to high osteotomy is performed following reduction of the bony dorsum, the need for medial osteotomy occurs only rarely.

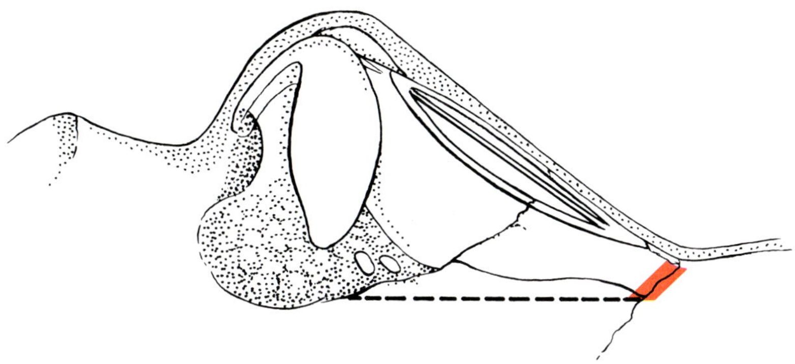

In a properly placed osteotomy that follows along the bases of the equilateral triangles, the unfractured segment extending from the lateral osteotomy to the dorsum is very narrow (in red). This small segment can usually be fractured by slight digital pressure.

Because bony continuity is important for a natural postoperative nasal contour, the best results are obtained when the remaining cephalic segment is broken by a green-stick fracture, whenever possible.

Outfracturing, infracturing, and disarticulating the nasal bones are unnecessary to accomplish the simple task of re-forming the pyramid. The width of the radix is a fixed dimension that is in good continuity with the orbital rims. With few exceptions, attempts to narrow the radix causes postoperative deformity by disrupting the normal alignment of orbital rims to nasal walls.

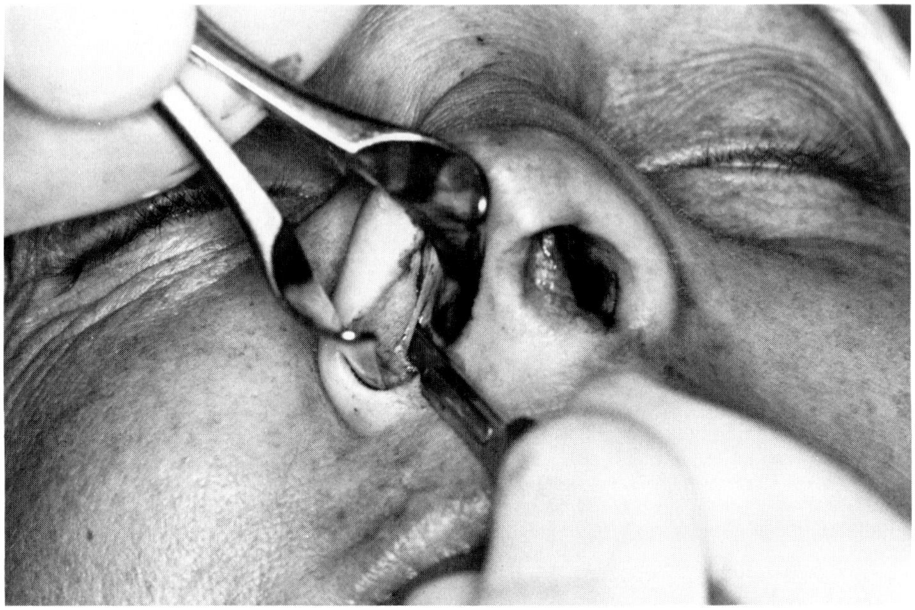

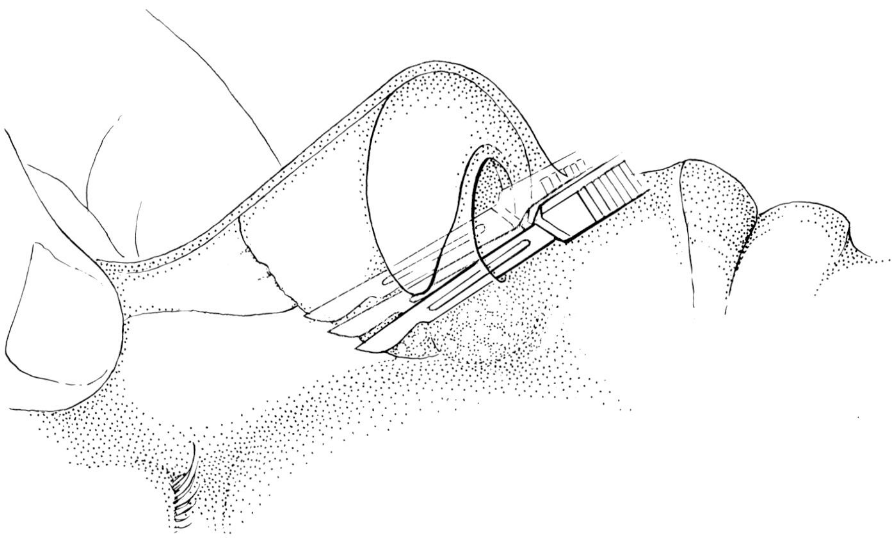

Technique

The incision for the lateral osteotomy is made at the base of the pyriform aperture and extends to the bone.

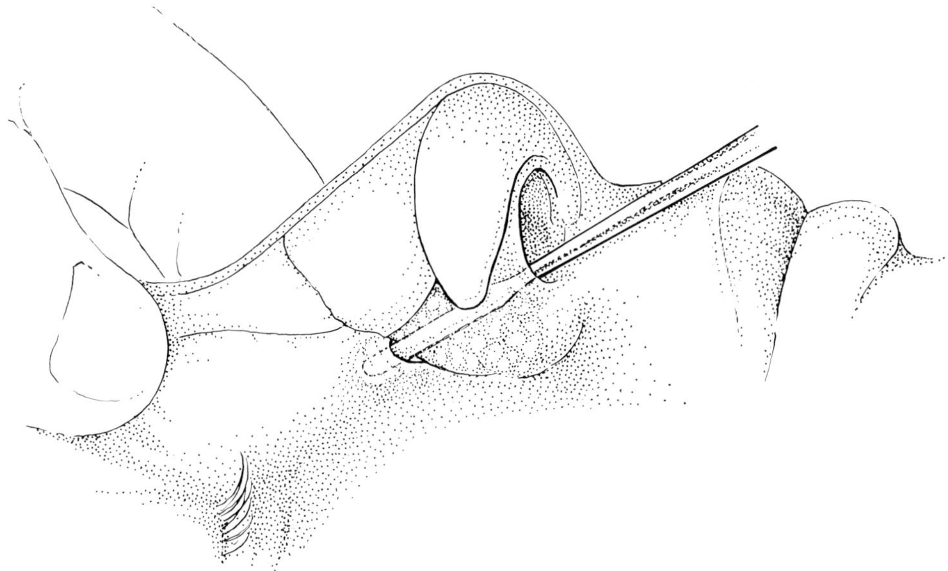

The periosteum is elevated with a Joseph periosteal elevator just enough to place the osteotome in its proper starting position.

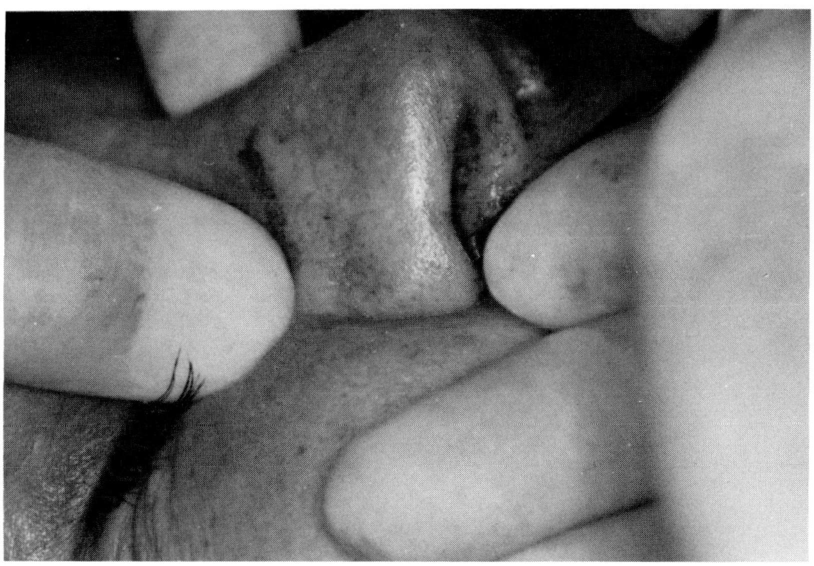

The position of the curved osteotome is checked with the thumb of the left hand to make certain that it is placed at the base of the pyriform aperture.

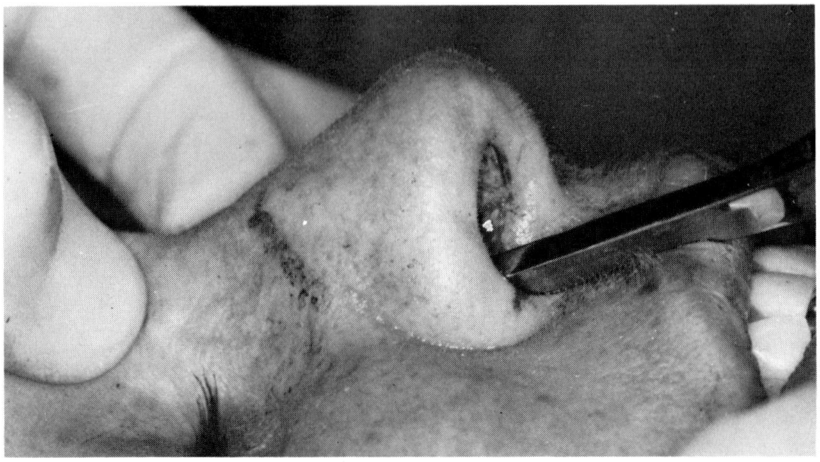

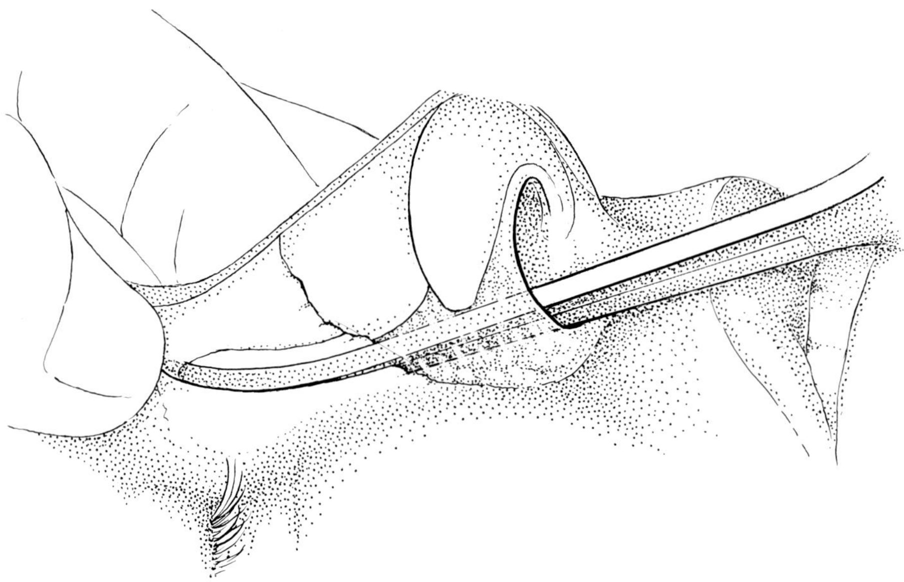

At the completion of the osteotomy, the curved osteotome finishes high at the cephalic end. The assistant stops hammering when the tapping tone changes.

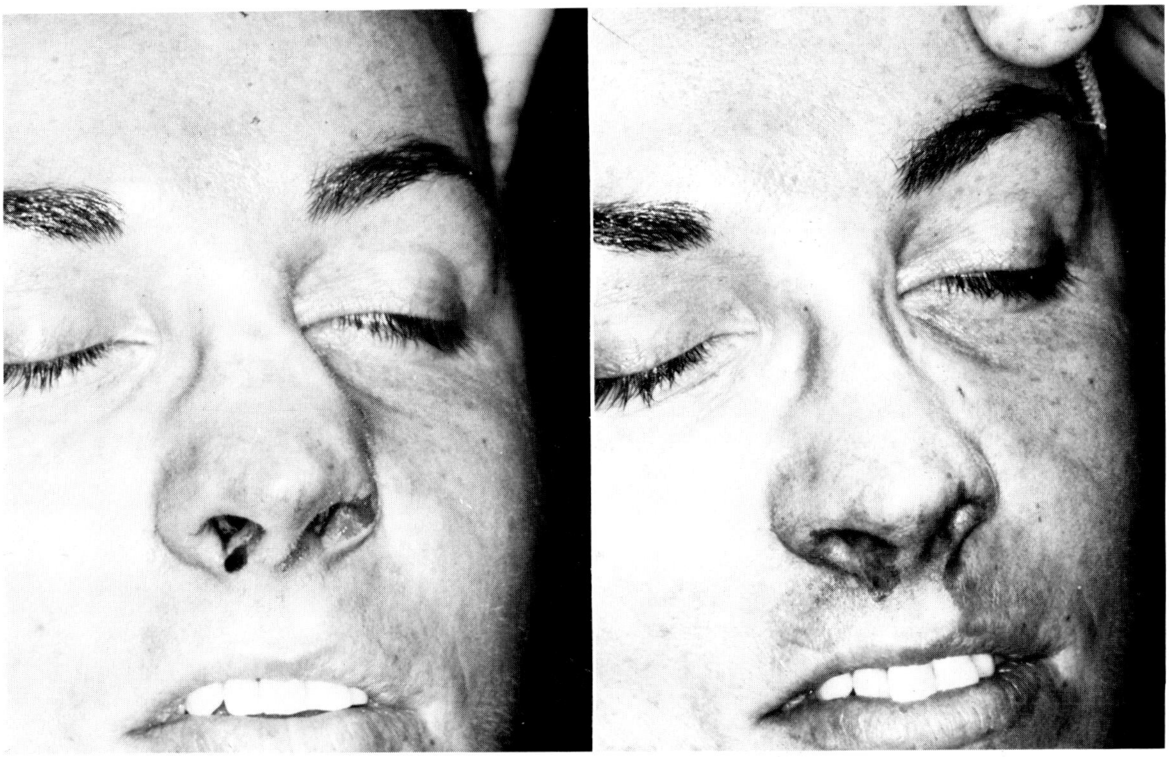

Following resection of the dorsum, there is a flat, broad appearance to the nose, which is caused by the open roof. This is well illustrated by this patient following reduction of the dorsum.

Because this patient had a low to high osteotomy, a medial osteotomy was not necessary. With slight digital pressure, the nasal bones moved medially, fracturing at the cephalic edge to re-form the pyramid.

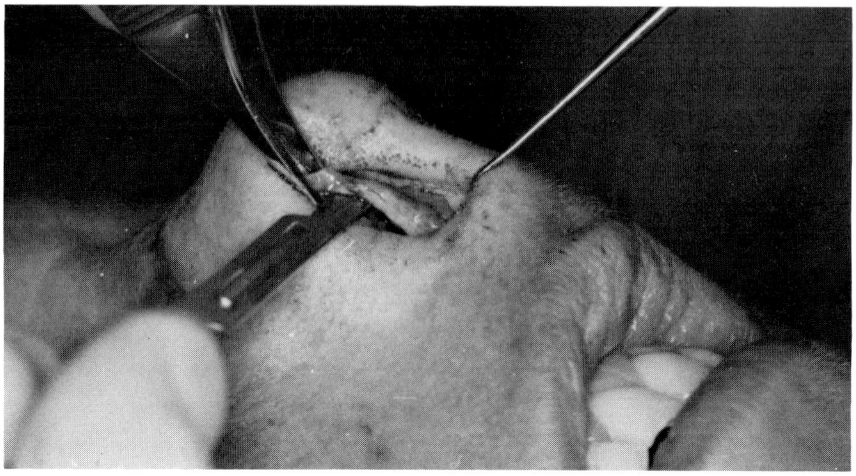

FINAL CONTOURING AND FIXATION

Following reconstruction of the nasal pyramid, the final trim of the caudal septum is carried out to align the columella with the alar rims.

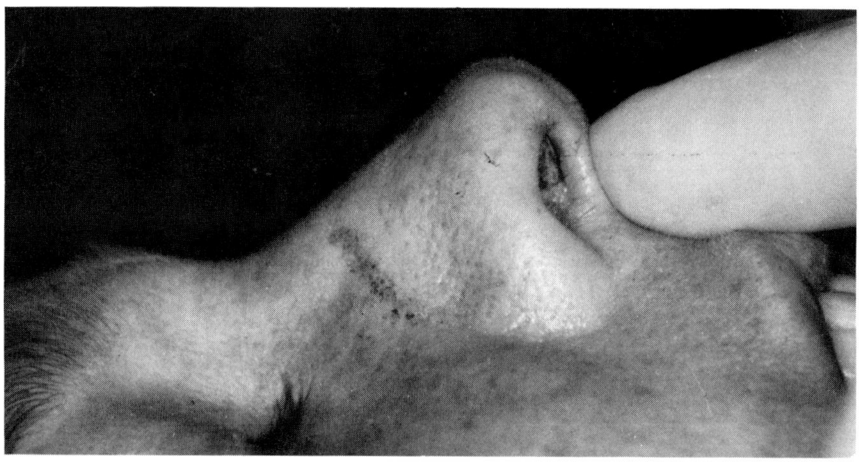

The relation of columella to alar rims can be tested by placing gentle pressure against the columella.

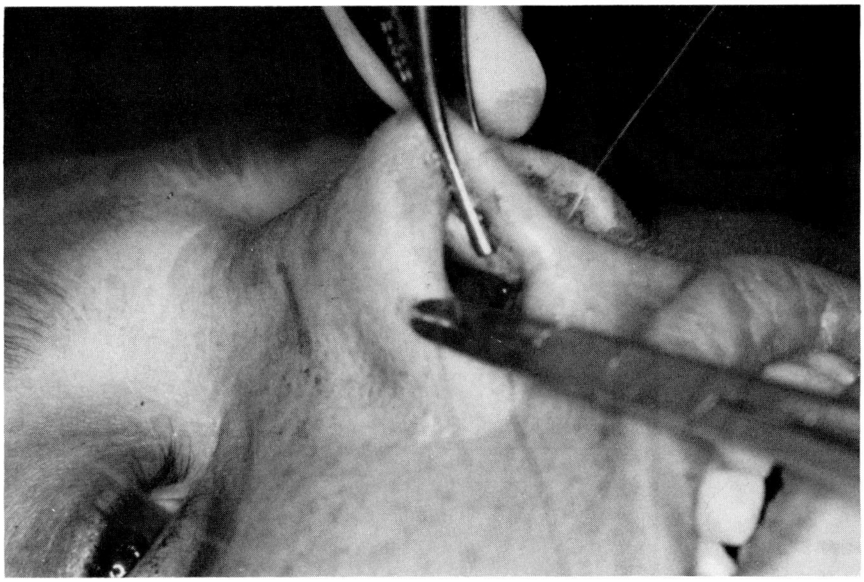

Following the final assessment of all skeletal parts, a transfixing suture is placed to attach the soft tissues of the base of the nose to the caudal septum.

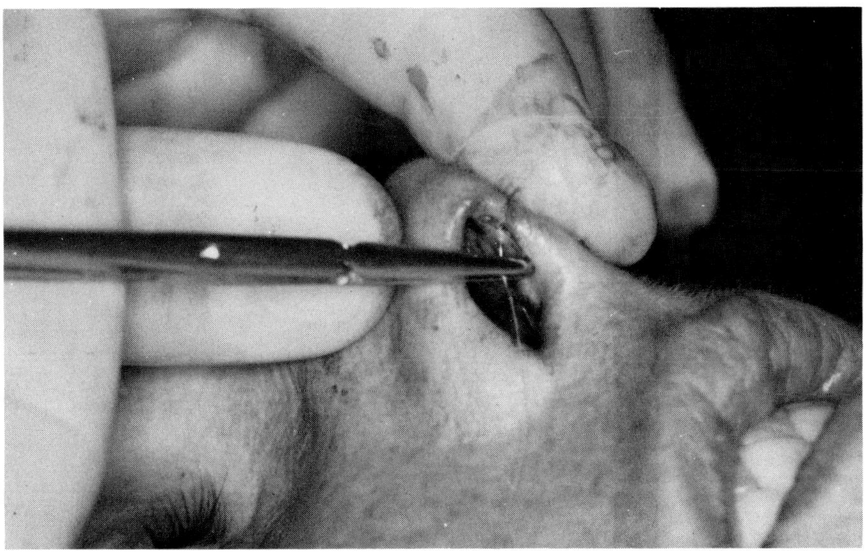

This is followed by suturing the rim incision using interrupted 5-0 catgut.

RECONSTRUCTION OF THE INTERNAL VALVE

Reconstruction of the internal valve by resection of the caudal end of the upper lateral cartilage is the last step of the procedure. It should not be undertaken until final adjustments of the caudal septum have been made and transfixing sutures have been placed. This ensures an accurate judgment of the amount to be resected.

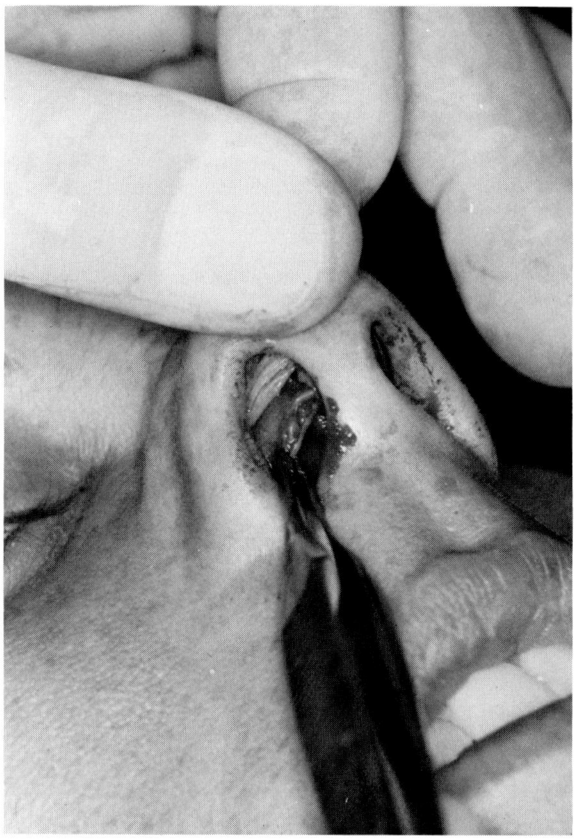

Following fixation of soft tissue, the mucochondrial flap is brought down with a pair of forceps, and the estimated amount of cartilage to be resected is marked mentally.

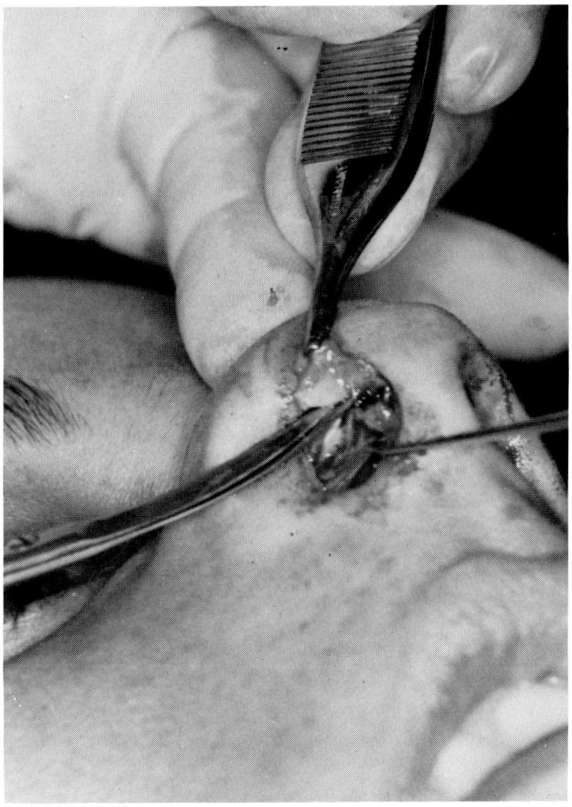

While an assistant holds the mucosa with a single hook, the caudal edge is dissected from the mucosa, and the surplus cartilage is resected. The amount of cartilage should approximate the amount of shortening and cephalic rotation of the tip.

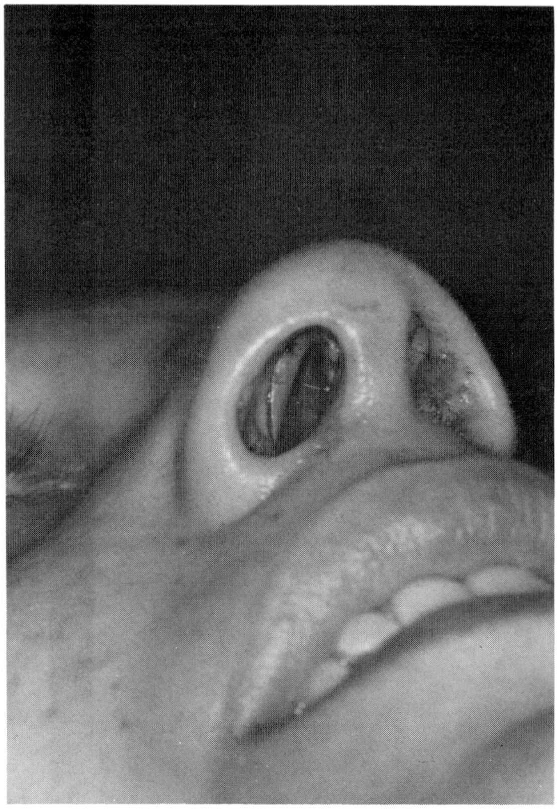

After submucous resection of the caudal part of the upper lateral cartilage is done, special attention is given to the position of the anterior caudal part in relation to the angle of the septum. The mucosal edges should fall together with a slight redundancy of the covering mucosa, which re-creates the functional border of the internal valve. Occasionally, resection of surplus mucosa may be required.

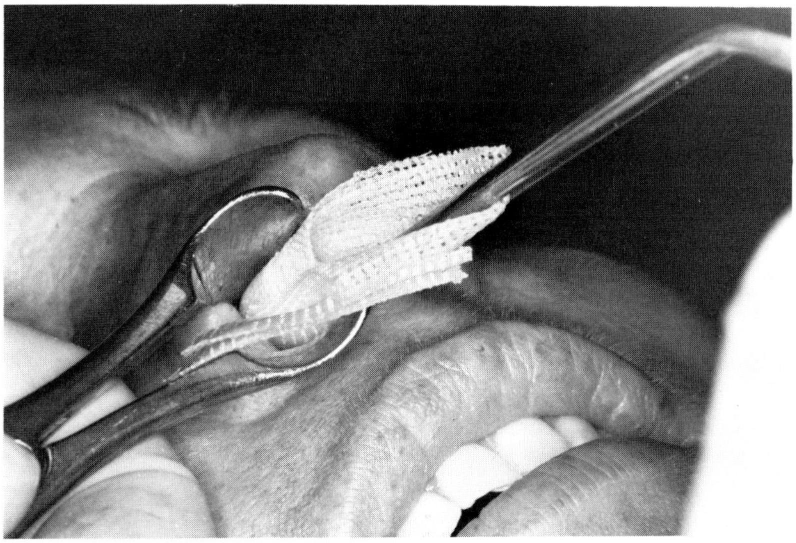

DRESSING

In the absence of septal or turbinate surgery, the packing is kept to a minimum. The purpose of packing the vestibular area is to ensure good tissue approximation in an area where distortion by hematoma or displacement by the splinting could occur. A 3 × 3 inch Adaptic gauze is split diagonally, and a triangle of gauze is placed in each vestibule. The packing should not displace the mucosa over the caudal end of the upper lateral cartilages. In 24 hours the packing is removed.

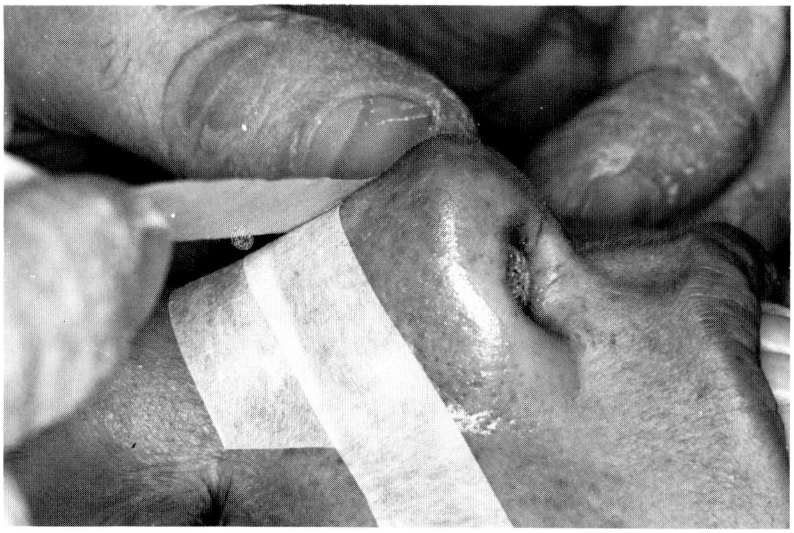

A thin coating of tincture of benzoin is wiped over the nose and malar area with cotton applicators. Patients are asked to close their eyes before application. Because paper tape (Micropore) causes minimal skin reaction, it is used as the skin contact layer. It is placed in overlapping layers to the supratip.

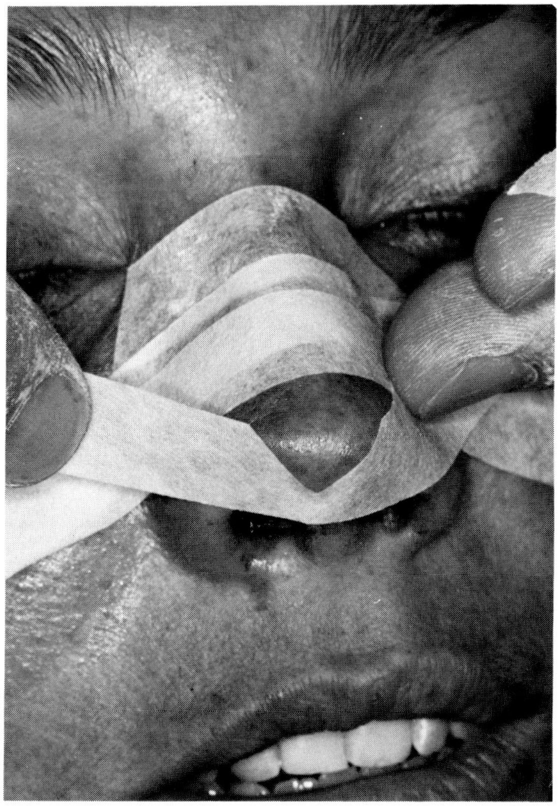

A V notch is cut out of the tape to form a sling for the tip structures.

A second layer of cloth tape is placed over the paper tape. Patients with tape allergy are not affected by this layer as long as there is no direct skin contact. The cloth tape supplies a base for the plaster cast.

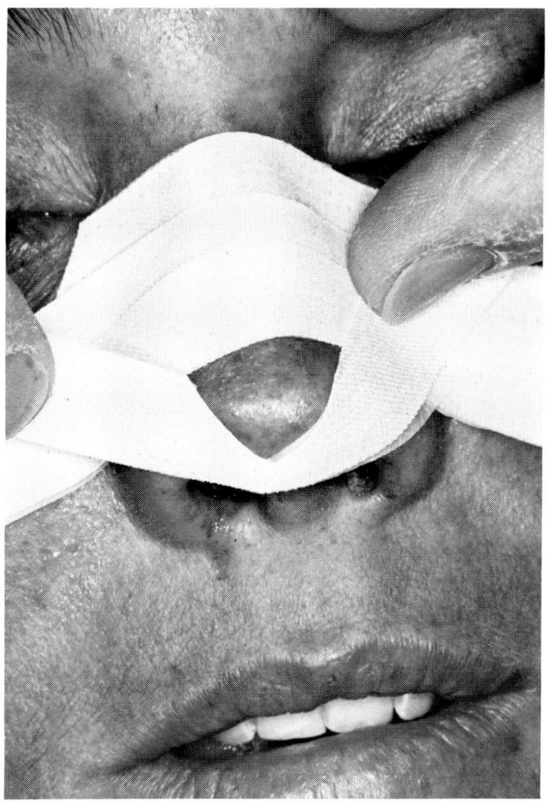

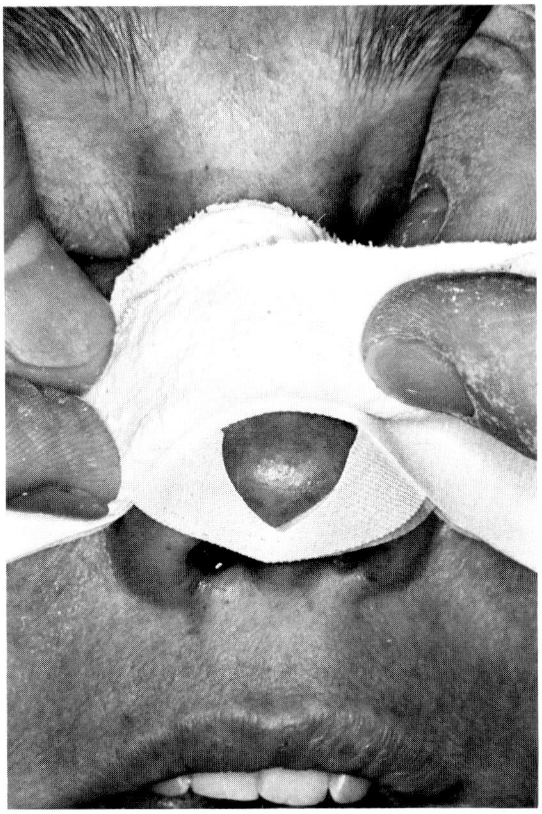

A four-ply triangular piece of plaster is devised, and the apex is cut off to conform to the height of the nasal bones at the radix. It is then dipped in warm water and applied over the dorsum. The caudal end is folded back on itself to provide an eight-ply plaster cast over the central third of the nose. Because of the tight adherence of the plaster to the cloth tape, edema will not displace it.

Two overlapping strips of cloth tape are placed over the plaster extending onto the malar area to further secure its fixation.

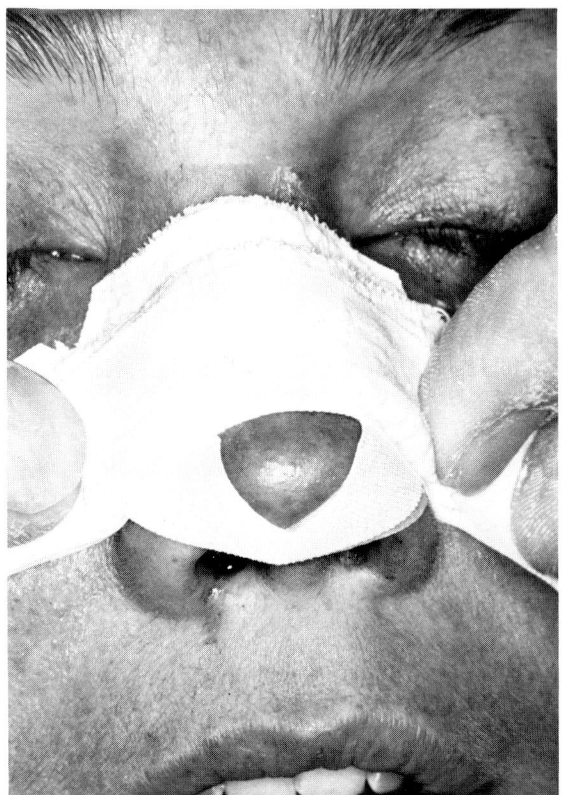

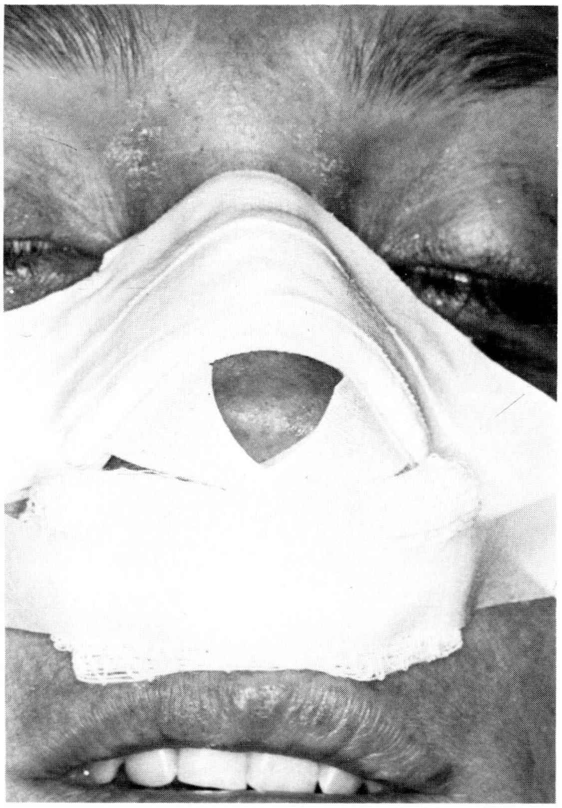

A 2 × 2 inch gauze is applied under the nose and held in place by a ½-inch paper tape sling.

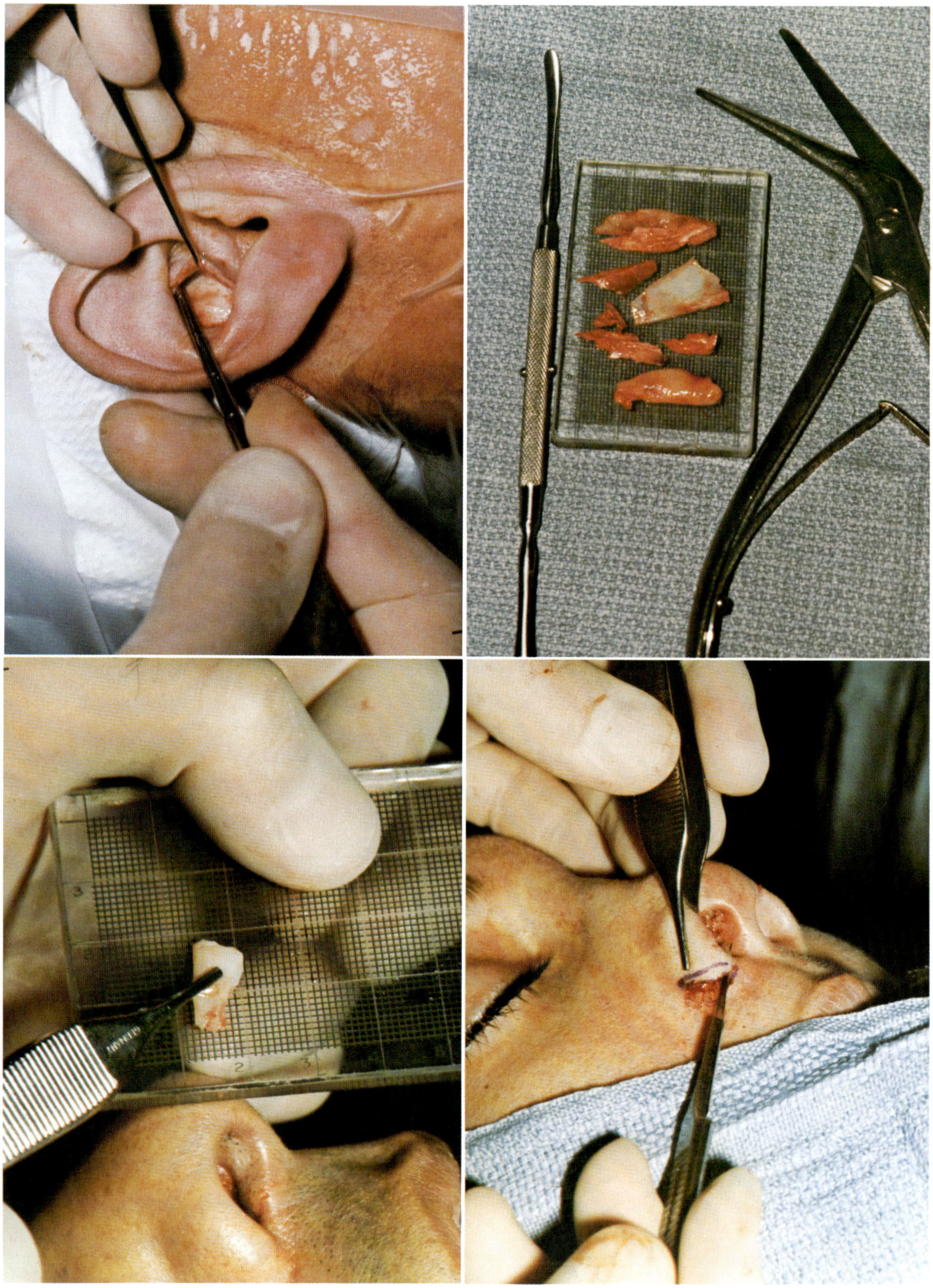

CHAPTER 4

Adjunctive techniques

Septal surgery
Turbinate surgery
Maxillary augmentation
Alar resection
Tip graft
Ear cartilage grafts

SEPTAL SURGERY

Since many rhinoplasties necessarily include correction of airway obstruction or grafting of septal cartilage, or both, proficient septoplasty is an essential part of the plastic surgeon's rhinoplasty repertoire. Septal cartilage is a precious material and should not be wasted. Except for the specific harvesting of material, only distorted or obstructing septal parts should be removed. After these have been extracted, the surplus fragments should be replaced into the septal pocket (crushed if necessary). Then the patient has the double benefit of a rigid septum and the cosmetic effect of the cartilage graft(s).

Whether septal surgery is performed to correct nasal dysfunction or to obtain reconstructive material, a dorsal and caudal segment of at least 1-cm width must be retained for adequate support. Furthermore, at least one mucoperichondrial flap must remain intact to prevent septal perforation.

The following technique provides excellent access to the septum and enables the surgeon to obtain graft material of a usable size.

Surgical procedure

Following preparation of the mucosa by cotton packing saturated with 5% cocaine solution as described in Chapter 3, the packs are removed, and 1% Xylocaine with 1 : 100,000 epinephrine is injected into the septal mucosa using a 22-gauge 3½-inch needle. If the solution is injected subperichondrially, the cartilage will separate from the perichondrium. The infiltration is continued posteriorly past the bony junction. It extends into the entire area of proposed dissection.

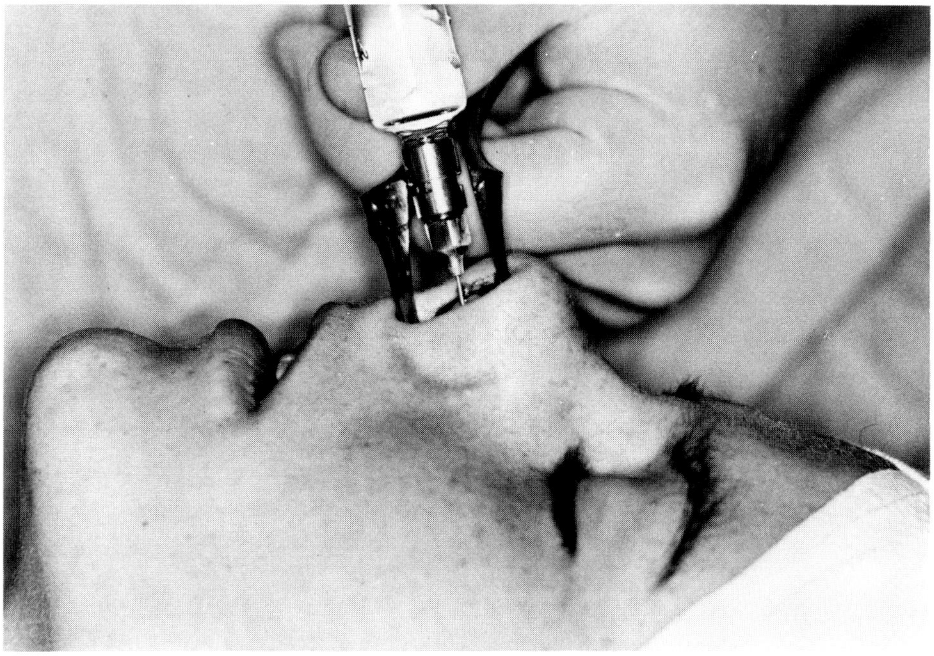

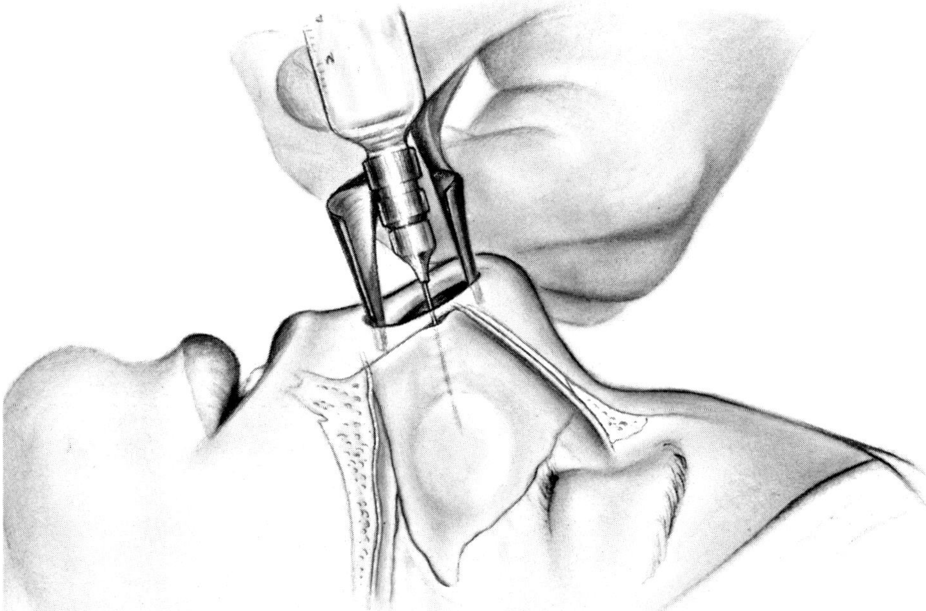

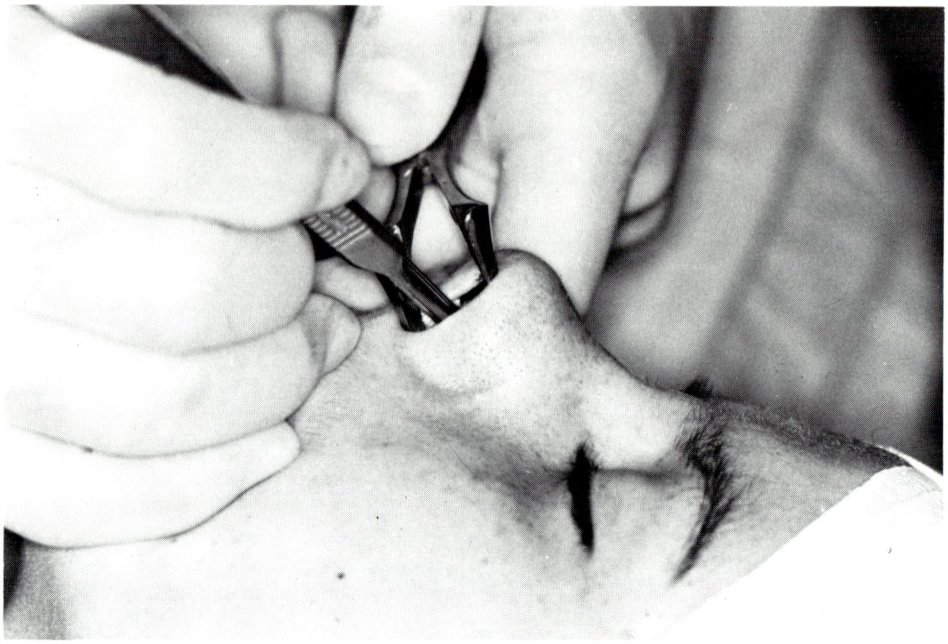

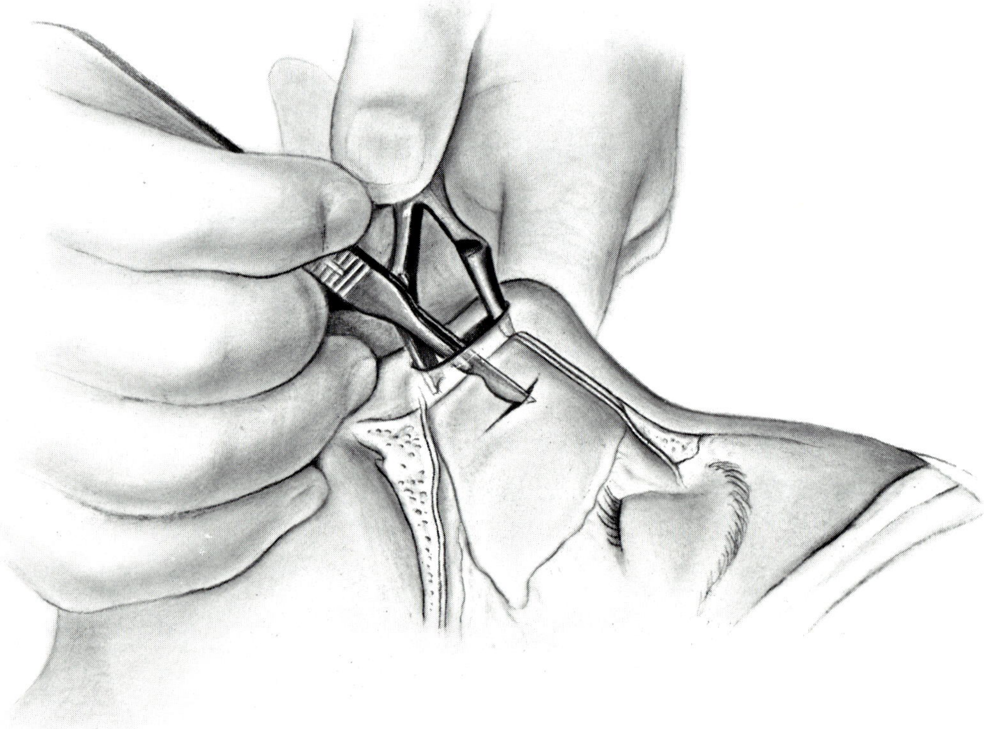

The initial incision is made parallel to the caudal border of the septum and 1.5 cm cephalad to it. When the procedure is done for nasal obstruction, the incision is made just caudal to the deviation. The incision is into but not through the cartilage and extends approximately 2 cm.

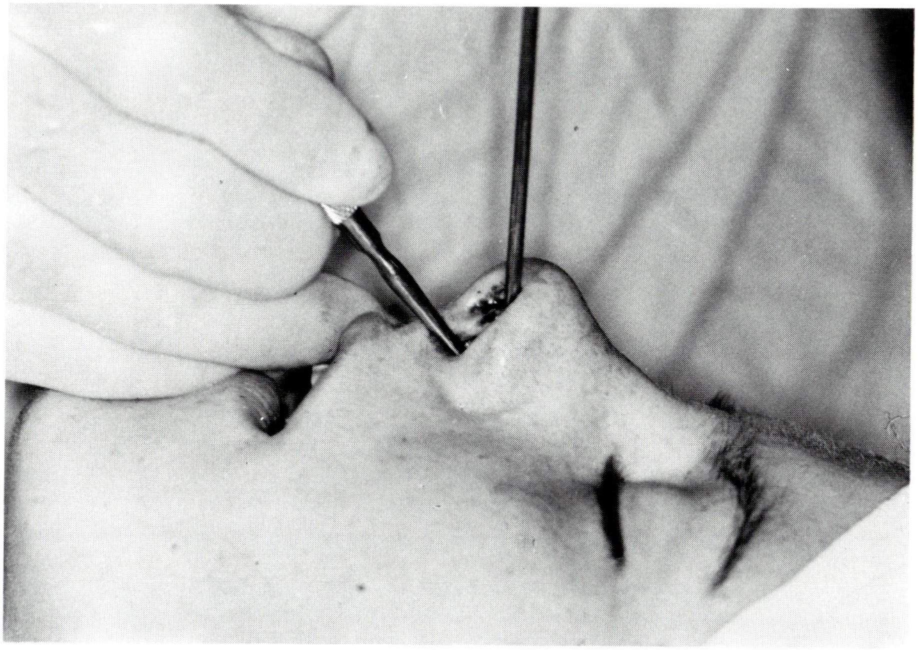

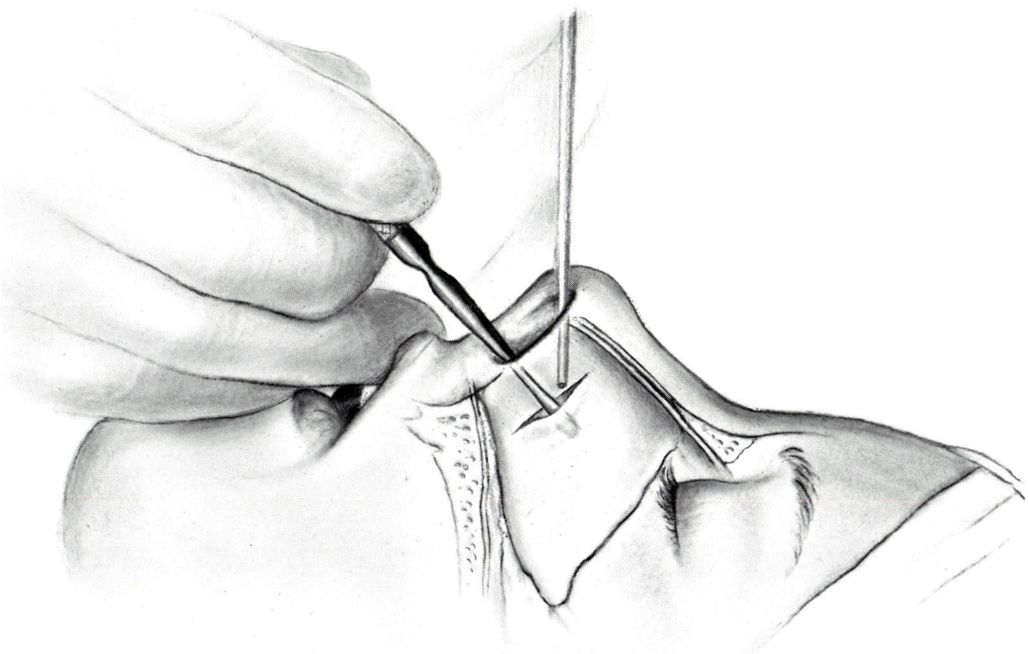

The subperichondrial plane is positively identified using a Frazier suction tube and the sharp end of a Freer elevator. Once the perichondrium is separated from the cartilage, the dissection continues using the blunt end of the Freer elevator and extends 15 to 20 mm past the osteochondral junction.

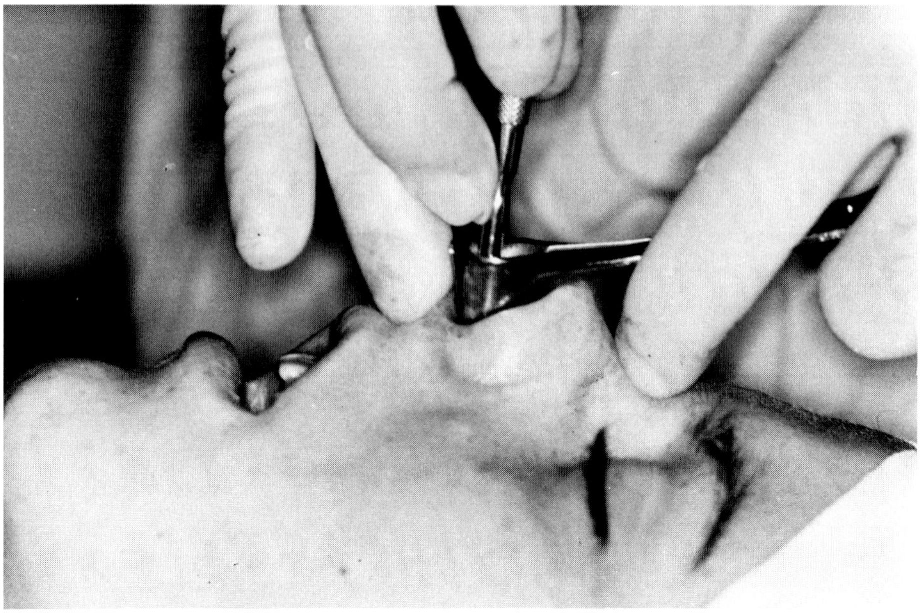

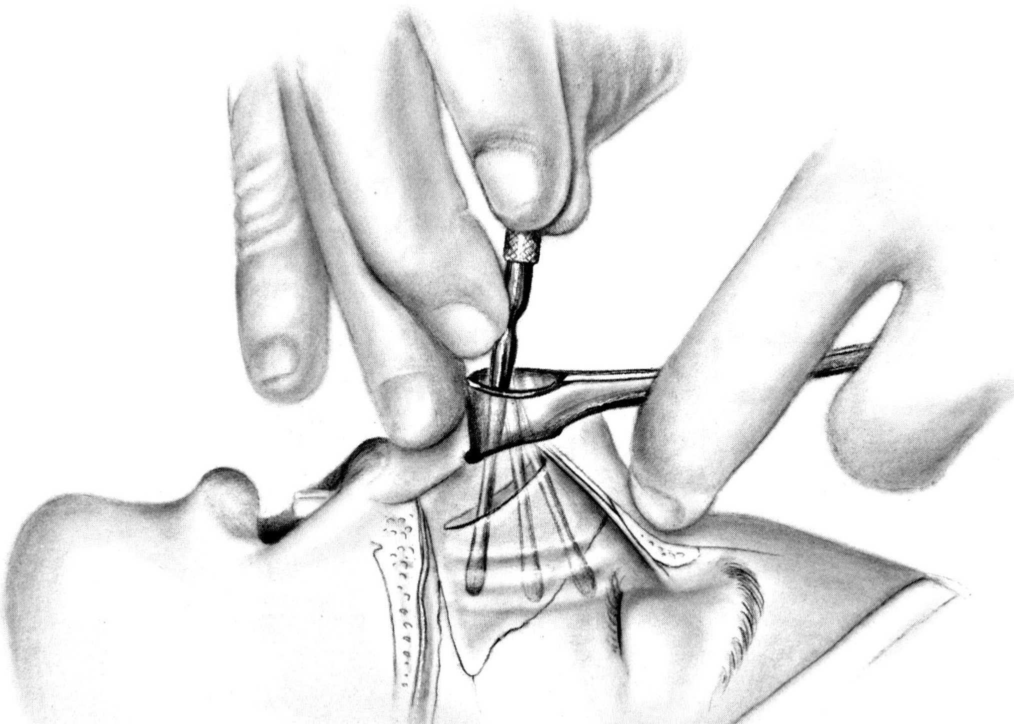

The entire mucoperichondrial flap is dissected away from the proposed site of resection.

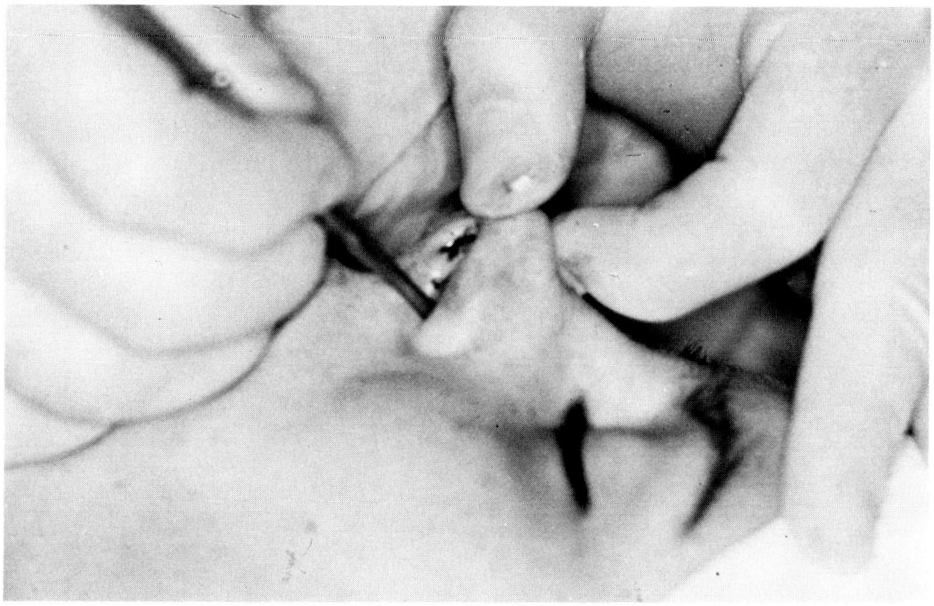

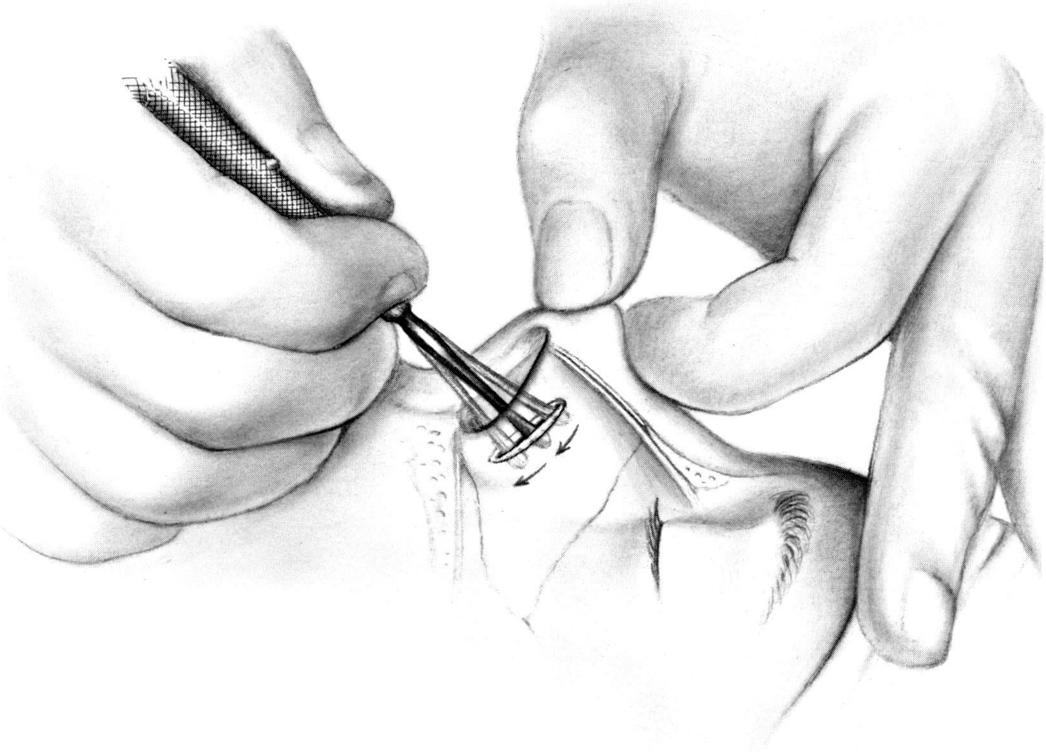

After dissection of one side of the mucoperichondrium, the sharp end of the Freer elevator is used to transect the septal cartilage at the site of the original mucosal incision. The sharp end provides enough cutting ability to transect the cartilage but is not so sharp that it will inadvertently go through the mucosa on the other side. Elevation of the perichondrium on the second side using the blunt end of the elevator covers the same area of dissection as the first side.

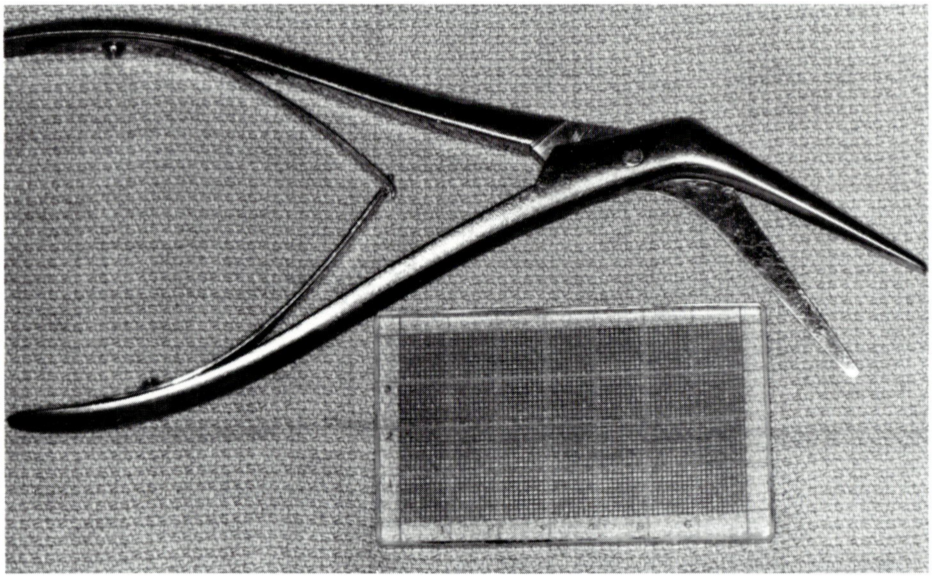

The key to this technique is the use of the Jackson turbinate scissors (nasal bone scissors). This instrument, originally designed for turbinate resection, has such a powerful mechanical advantage at its cutting edge that it is difficult to know when conchal bone is being cut. For this reason, the use of the instrument for turbinate resection was abandoned. However, the Jackson is excellent for harvesting septal material because it cuts through the osteochondral junction, thereby providing a long quadrangle of usable, intact cartilage and bone. The use of the Jackson turbinate scissors for septoplasty was introduced to me by Dr. Ira Tresley.

The placement of the jaws of the instrument so that both are inside the mucoperichondrial flaps is critical and can be tricky. As a jaw is being set on one side, the other has a tendency to slip out of the pocket. One must make certain that the instrument is inside both pockets before making the initial cut. Once the instrument is inside the pockets, the jaws are placed over the proposed site of resection parallel to the dorsum. The cutting edge must be at least 1.5 cm below the dorsal edge to preserve a substantial supporting strut. After the position of the instrument has been positively checked, the cut is made. A second cut is made approximately 1 cm inferior and parallel to the first cut.

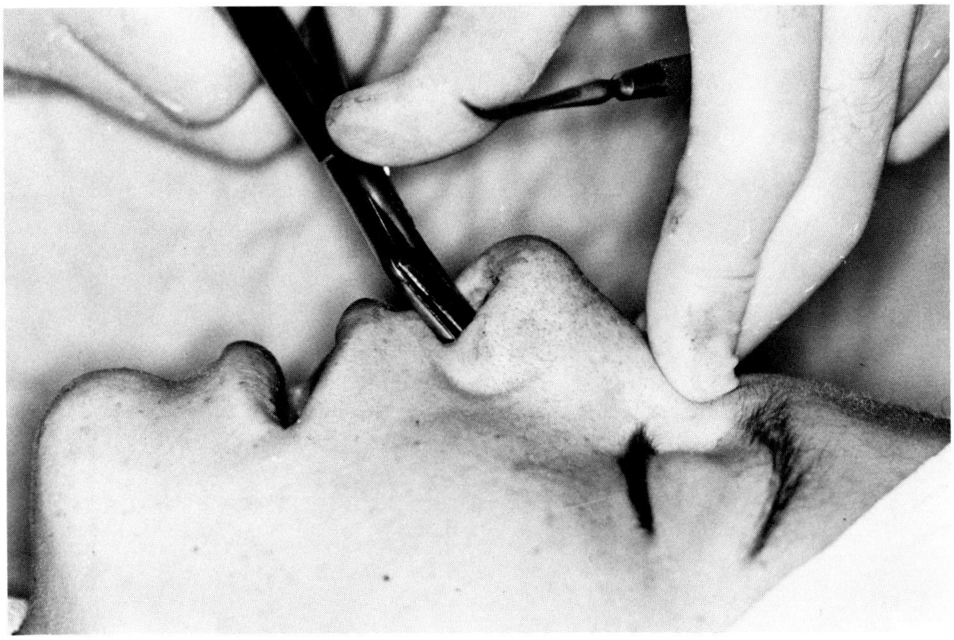

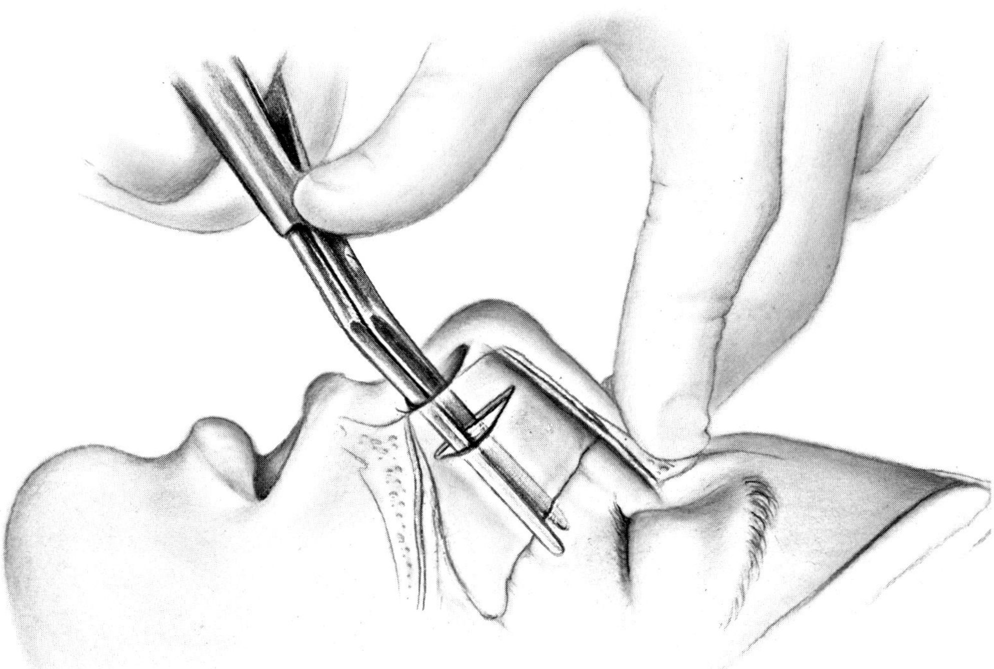

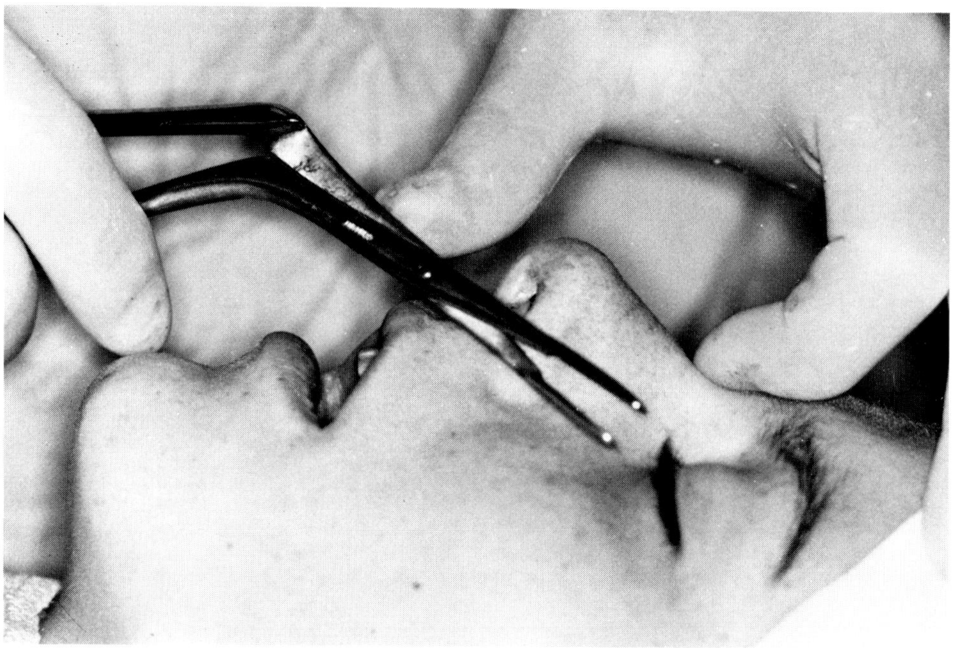

A pair of Killian septal forceps, with its long flat jaws, is ideal to extract the specimen intact.

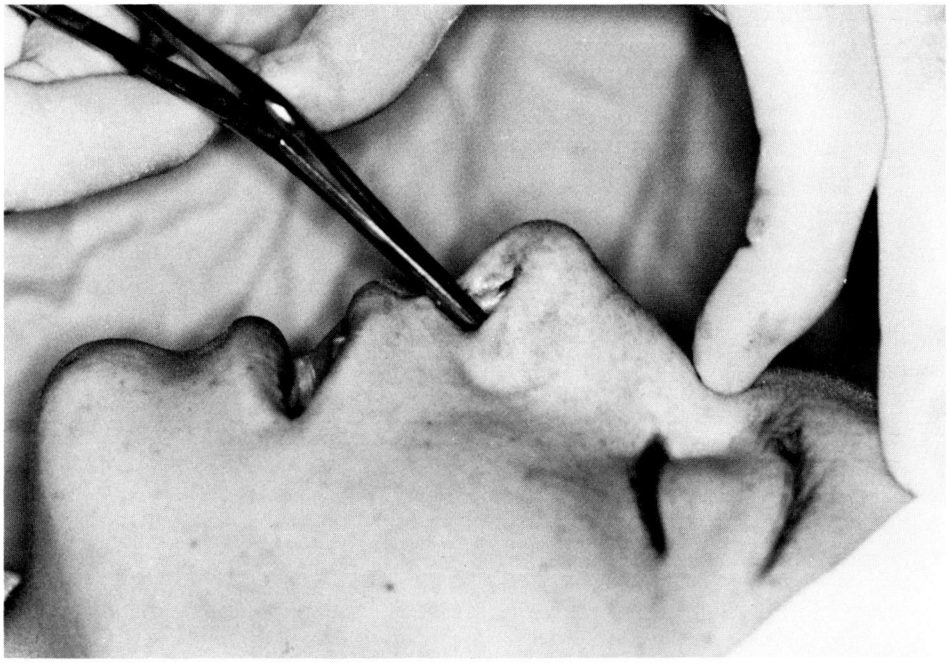

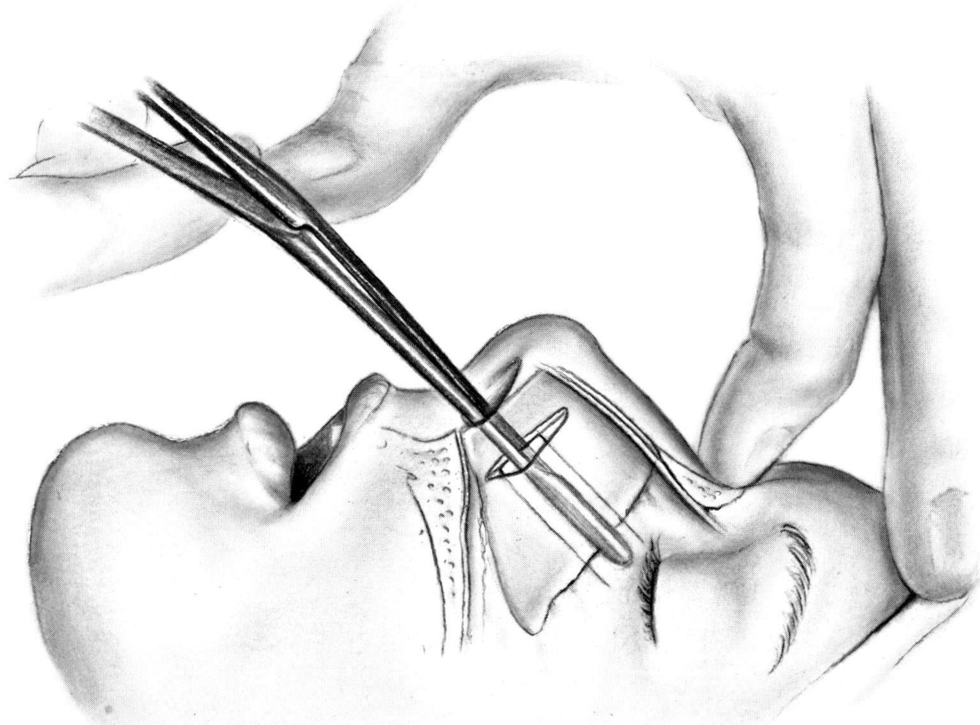

The septal forceps is placed deep within the pocket so that the jaws are well beyond the osteochondral junction. The perpendicular plate is then fractured using a slight twisting motion.

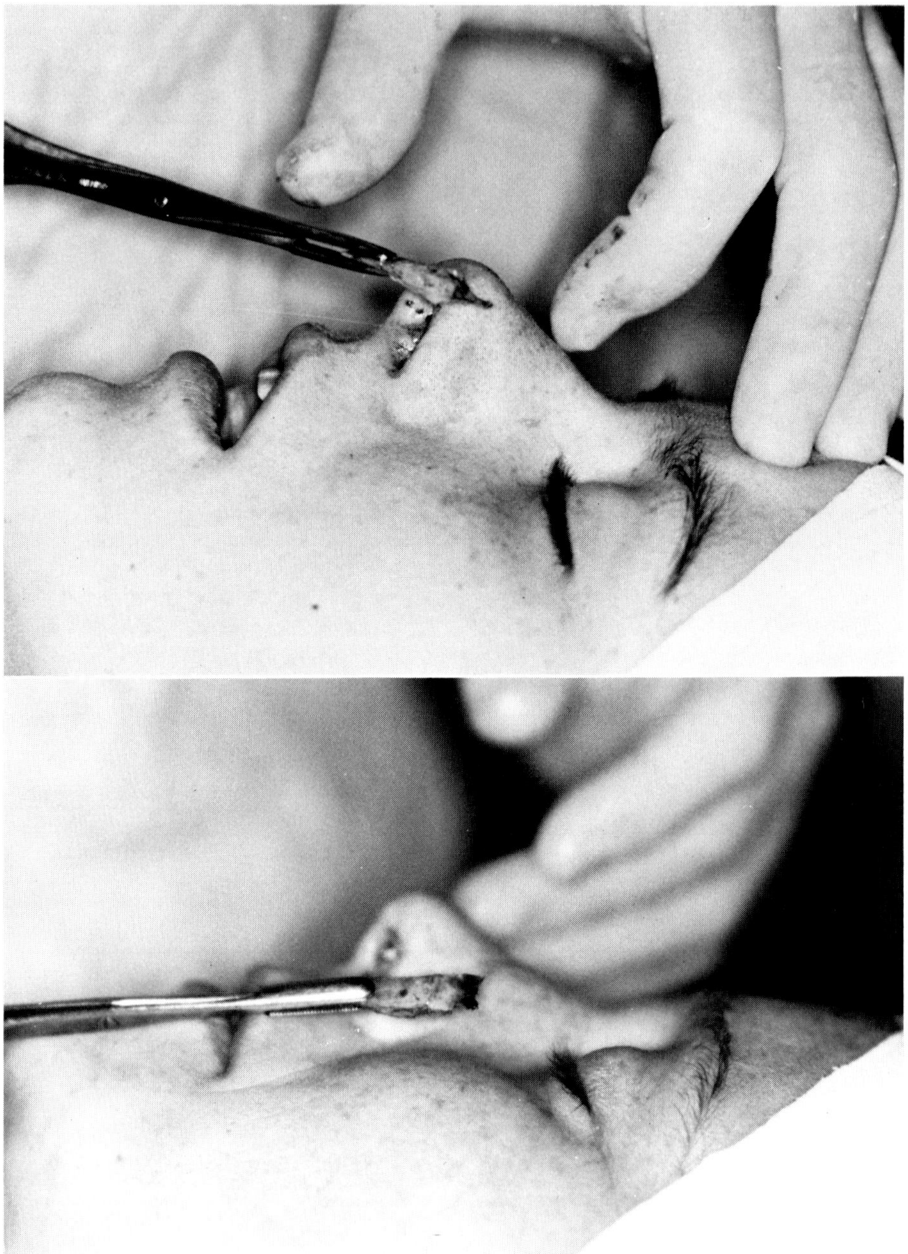

Following fracture of the ethmoid bone, the specimen is removed easily. This specimen shows the thinness of the perpendicular plate, which enables fracture by just a gentle twist.

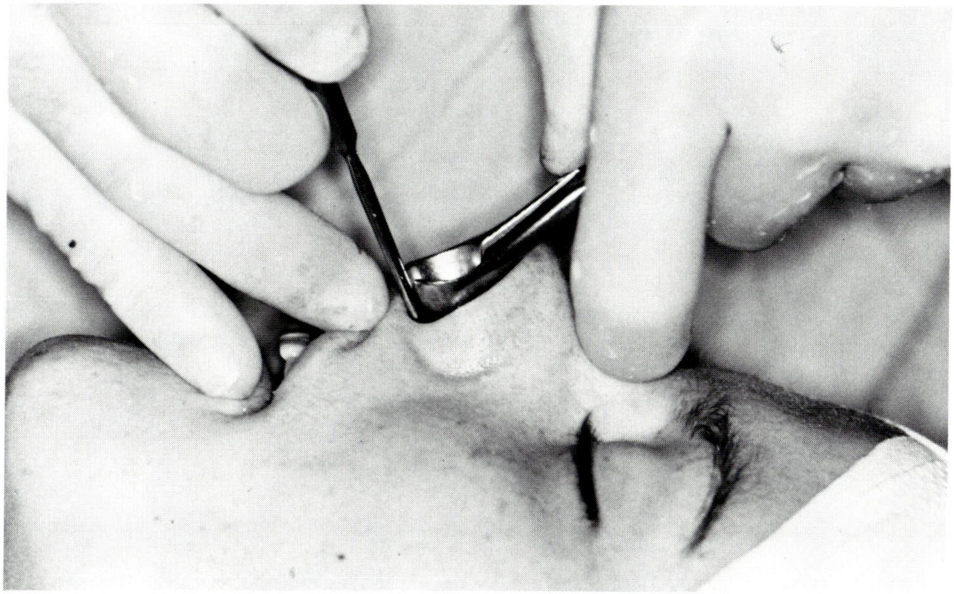

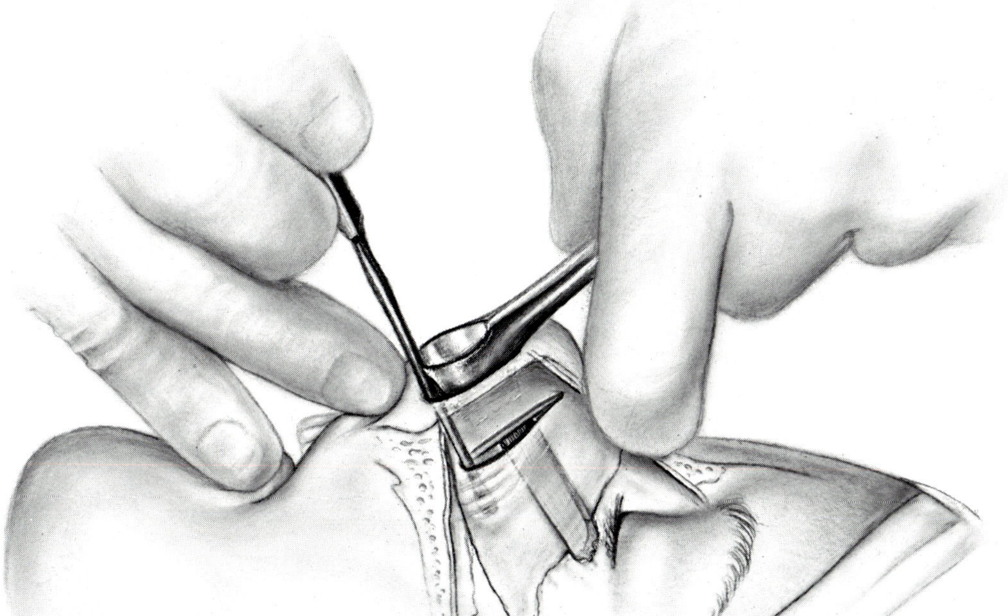

The resection of the central strip of cartilage provides access to the remaining septal skeleton. A Cottle perichondrial elevator is used for further dissection toward the vomerian groove. The sharp semicircular end of this elevator is excellent for dissecting tissues around septal irregularities or distortions of the vomer.

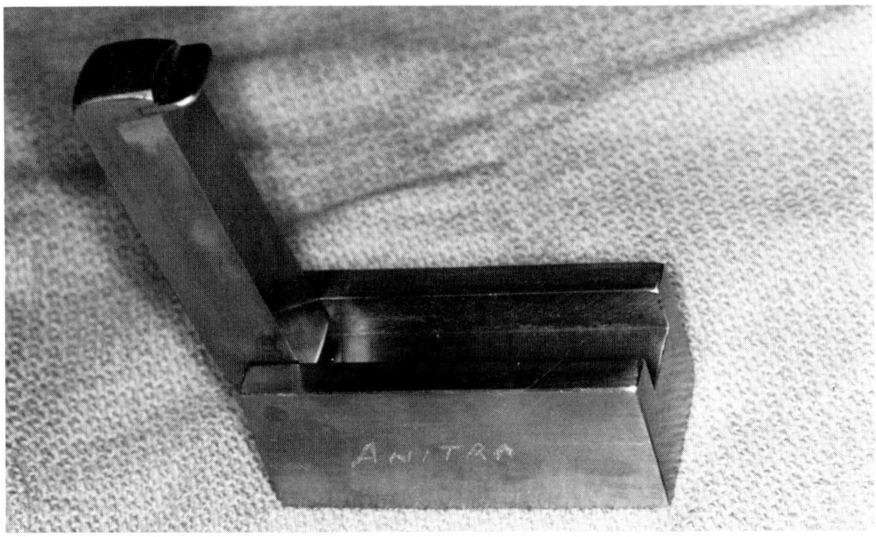

The Cottle cartilage crusher is useful for crushing cartilage or bone for grafting or reimplantation into the septal pocket.

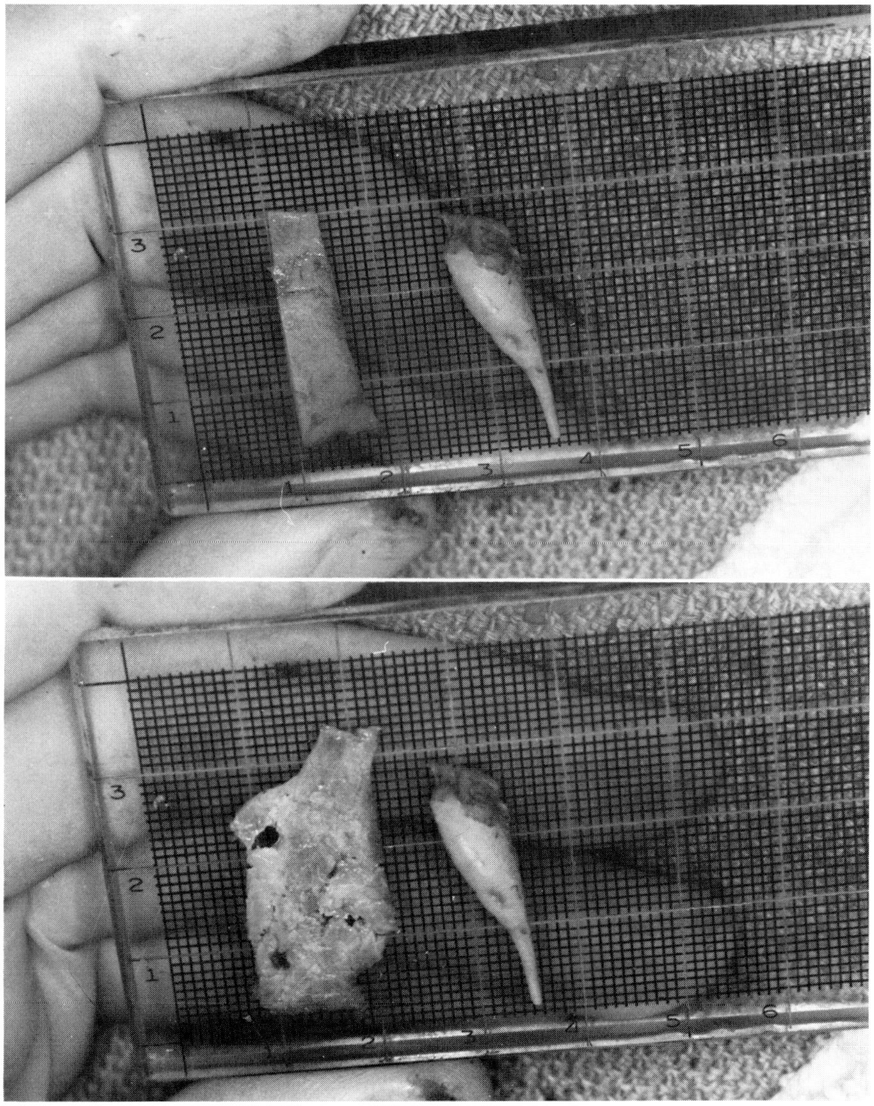

Cartilage specimen (on left side of grid) shown before and after it was crushed.

The procedure is completed by interrupted mattress sutures of 4-0 plain catgut to fix the mucosal flaps together and close the incision.

When the septum is repaired deep in the nasal recess, it is easy to place the needle through the mucosa, but it is not easy to retrieve it unless an instrument such as a bayonet forceps is used. The bayonet forceps allows the needle to turn as it is being retrieved so that it will not catch on the turbinate or other intranasal tissues.

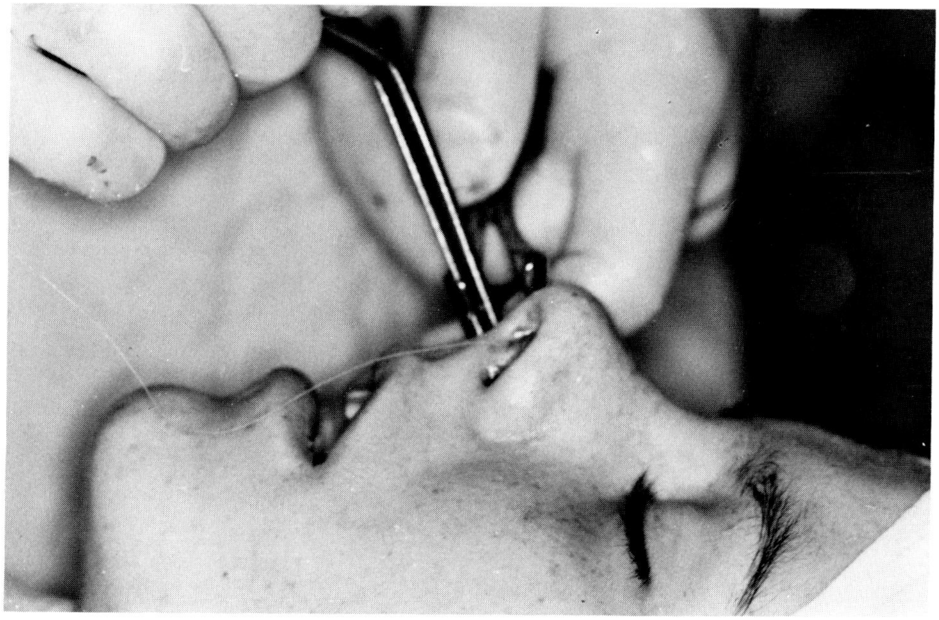

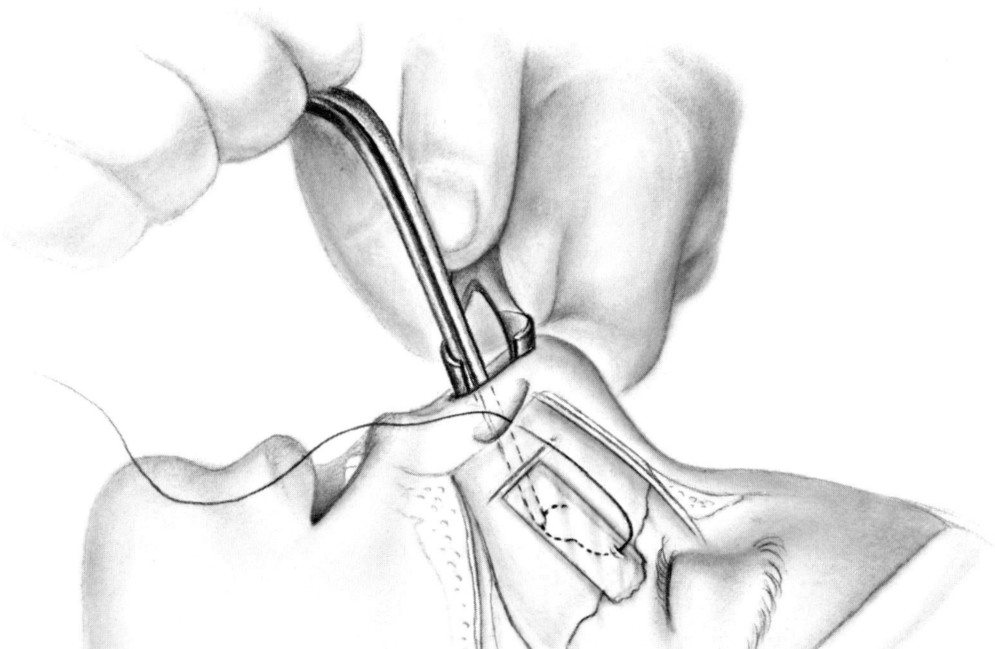

Septal cartilage banking

The idea of banking residual pieces of cartilage using the patient as the host bank was introduced to me in 1972 by Dr. Richard Webster. Since then I have moved his suggested site from the scalp to the more accessible postauricular sulcus. The banked cartilage has proved to be an invaluable and readily available source of graft material. The technique is rapid and simple.

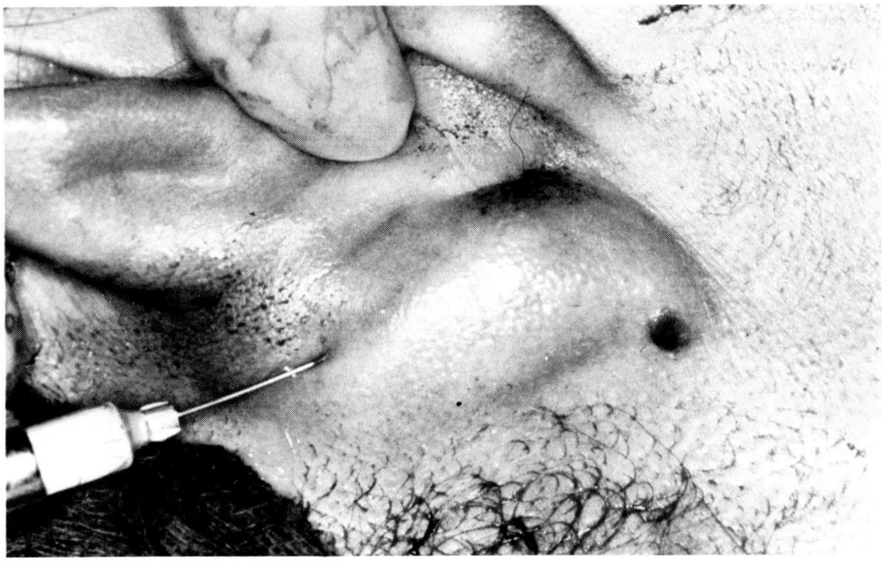

Following surgical preparation, 1% Xylocaine is used to raise a wheal in the postauricular sulcus.

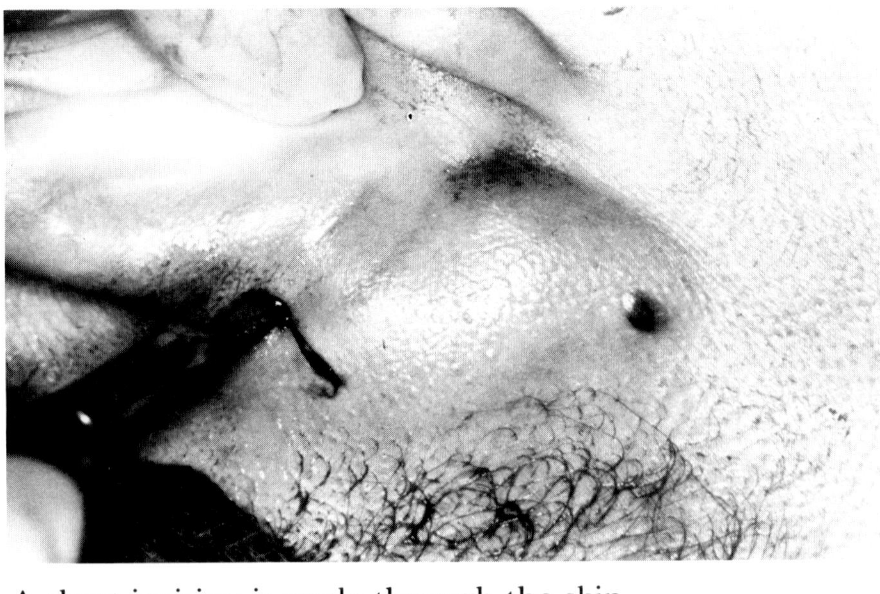

A short incision is made through the skin.

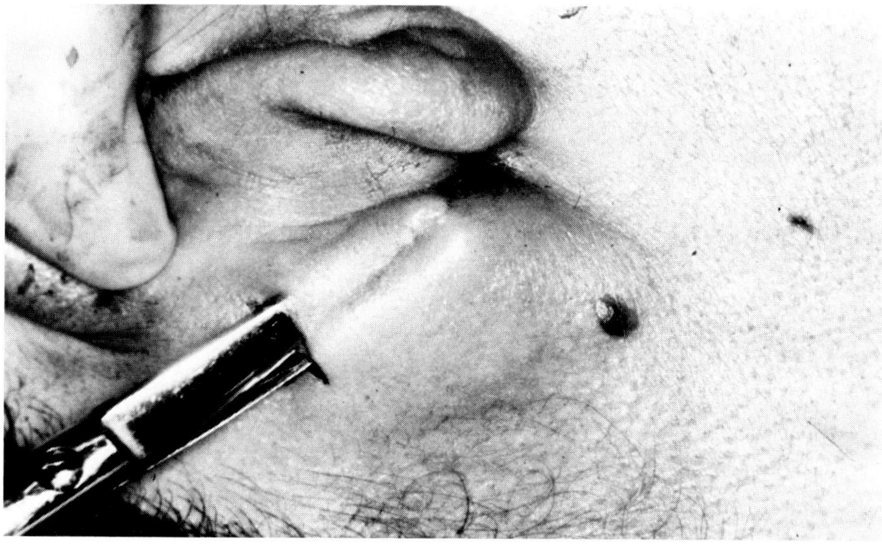

Then a subdermal pocket is dissected using a pair of Joseph scissors.

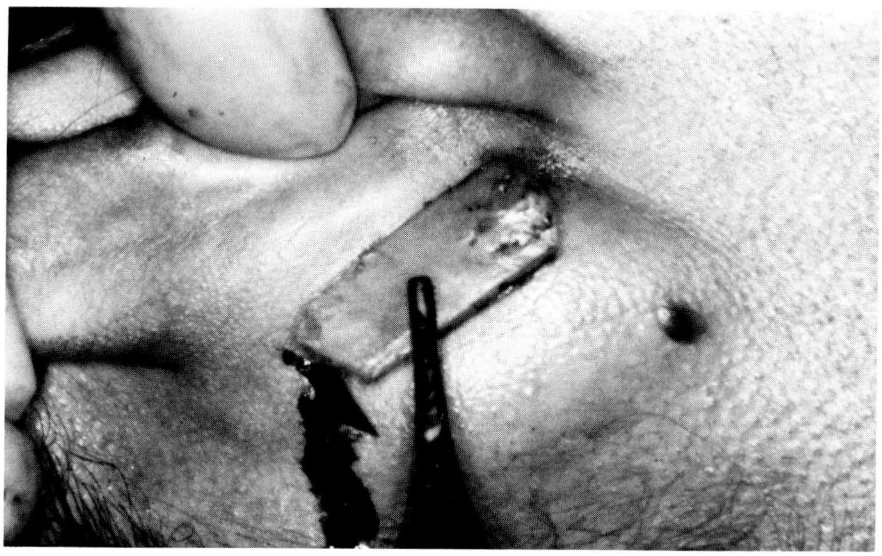

The pocket is made large enough to accept the specimen comfortably.

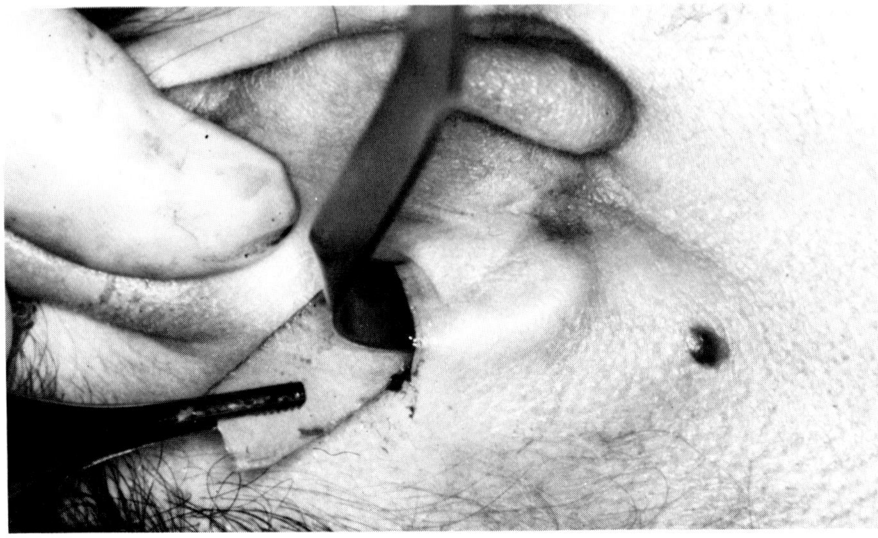

With the help of a Joseph retractor, the graft is slipped into the pocket.

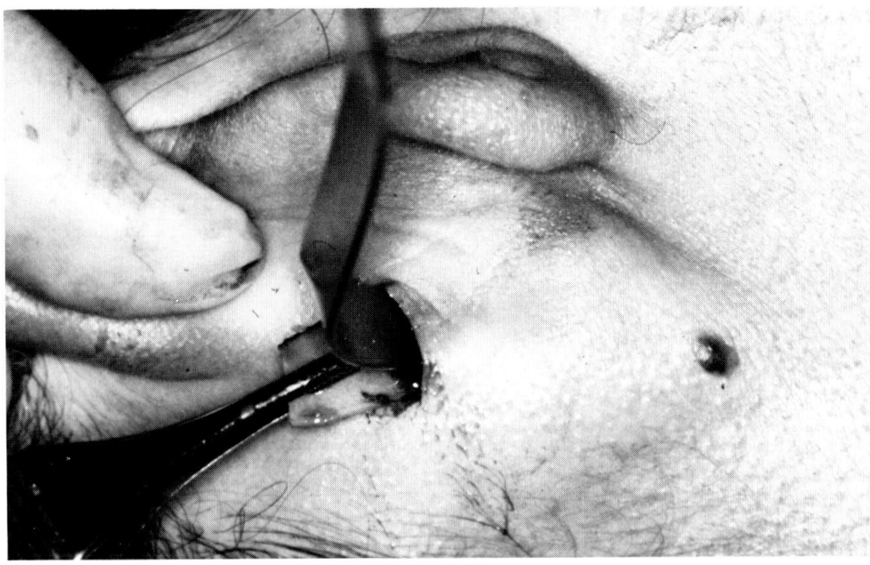

It should enter without tension on the tissues.

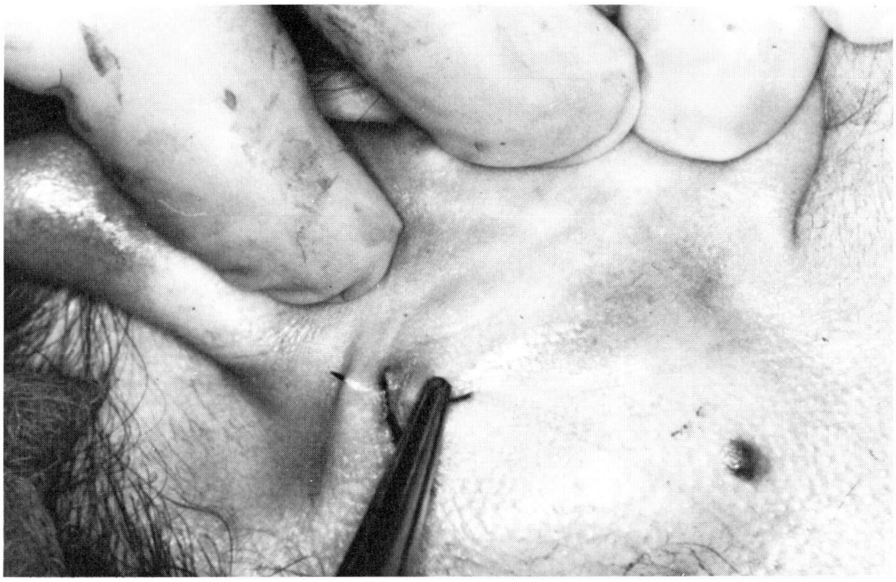

The wound is closed with interrupted sutures.

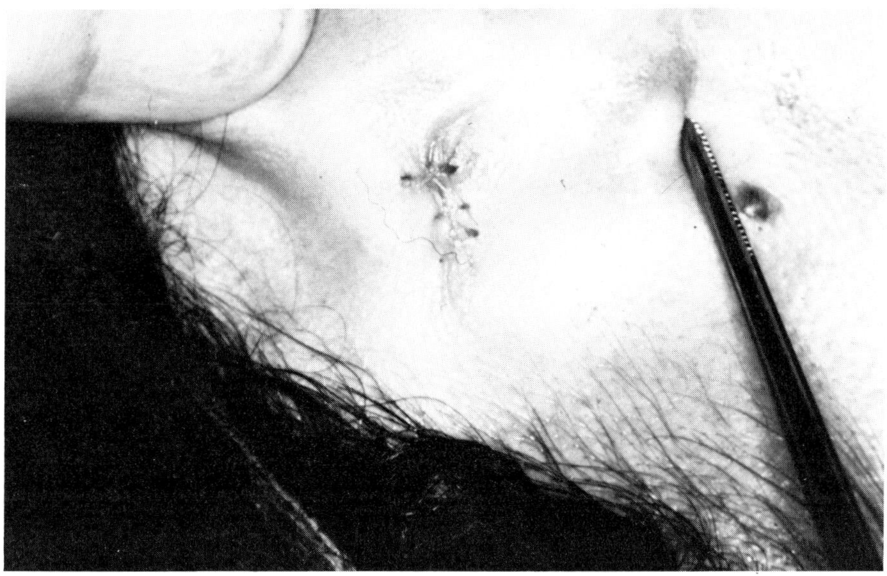

The graft is barely visible under the postauricular skin, but its edges can be palpated.

TURBINATE SURGERY

The treatment of airway obstruction due to turbinate hypertrophy can be undertaken safely and effectively at the time of rhinoplasty. Since the patient is already surgically prepared for nasoplasty, the surgeon has an excellent opportunity to correct the obstruction without an additional procedure for the patient.

In my experience, the best *long-term* treatment is partial resection of the offending turbinate. Inasmuch as crushing of the turbinate, steroid injections, and topical agents have proved to be ineffective over the long term, I now think they are not worthwhile procedures.

The following technique for partial resection of the turbinate is simple and effective. Although the incidence of postoperative bleeding is slightly higher than with rhinoplasty alone, it can be controlled by careful packing. The benefit to the patient is well worth this minimal risk.

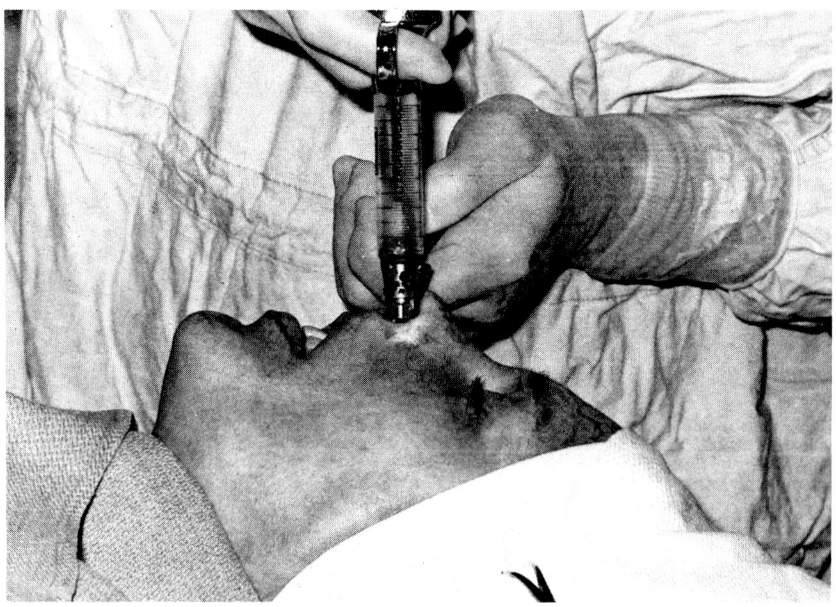

Surgical procedure

After cocaine-impregnated packs are removed, a 22-gauge 3½-inch spinal needle is inserted into the inferior margin of the inferior turbinate and then passed posteriorly.

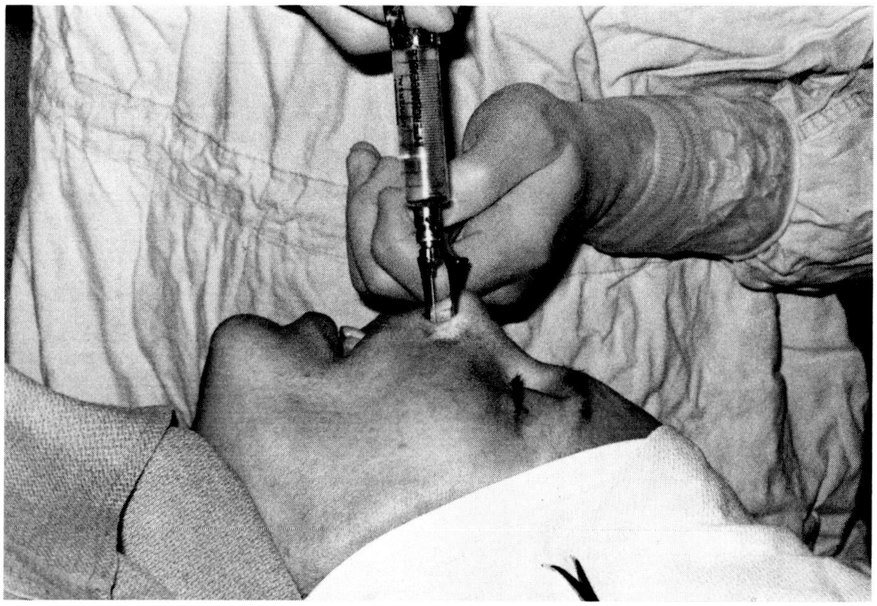

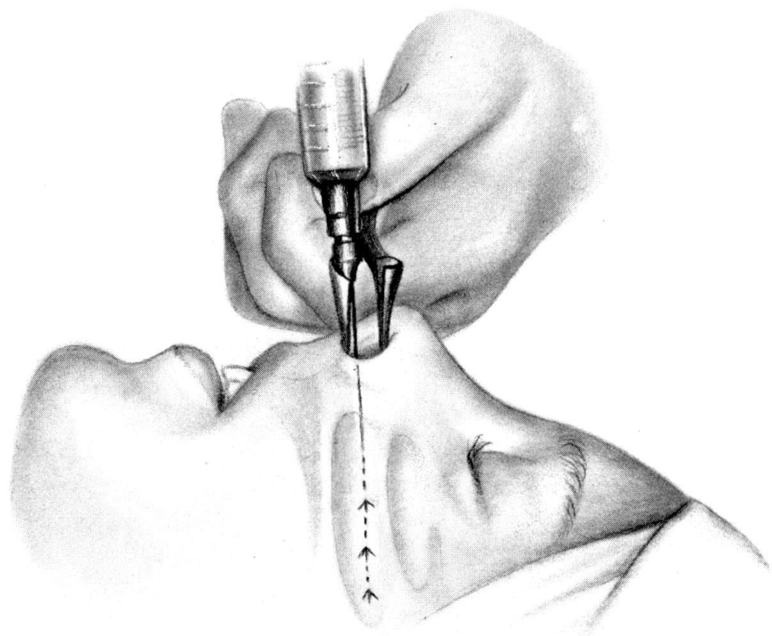

The needle is withdrawn slowly while a small amount of 1% Xylocaine with 1:100,000 epinephrine is injected.

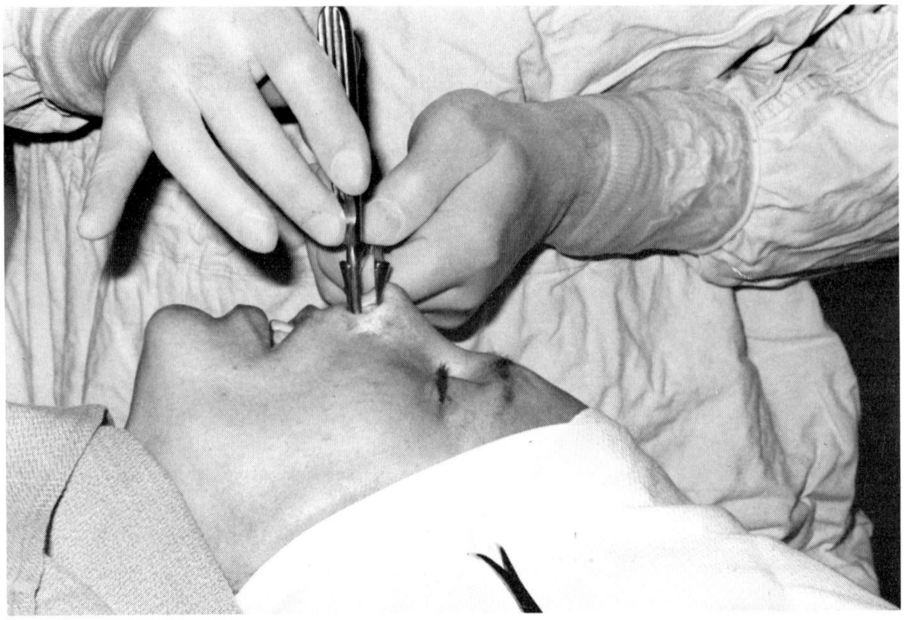

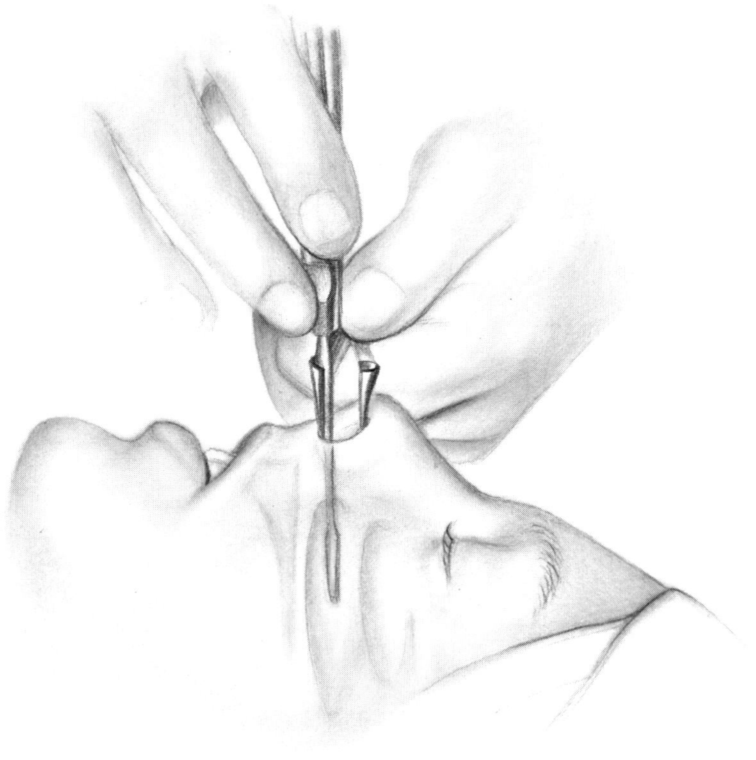

When the turbinate is impacted against the lateral nasal wall, a Joseph periosteal elevator is used to mobilize the turbinate. The tip of the elevator is placed at the lateral midpoint of the turbinate. The concha is fractured medially by slowly moving the handle of the instrument laterally. Only slight resistance is felt as the fragile conchal bone is fractured. Once the turbinate is moved away from the lateral nasal wall, the inferior part is in good position for resection.

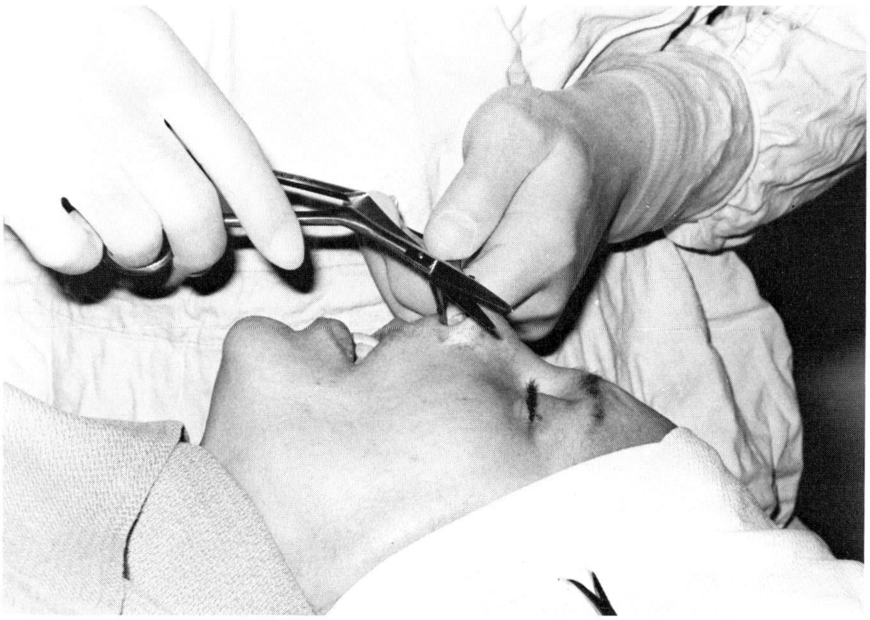

The Knight septal scissors is well suited for turbinate resection because it is long and heavy enough to cut through the turbinate and yet fine enough to enable the surgeon to recognize whether concha is being cut.

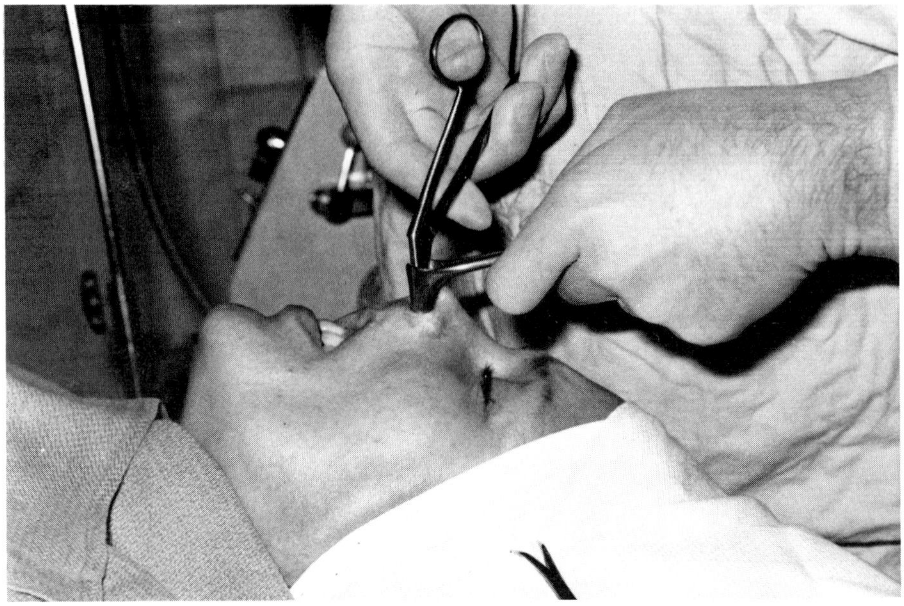

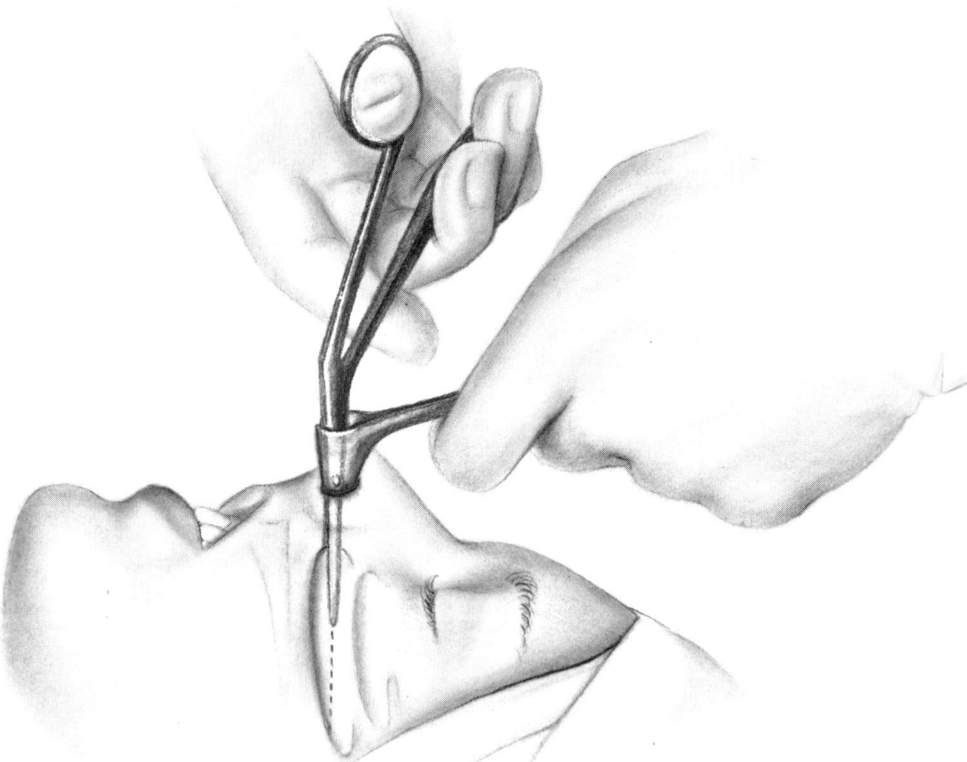

The surgeon can obtain the best view from the head of the operating table. Once the turbinate is in sight, the scissors is placed parallel to the plane of the turbinate.

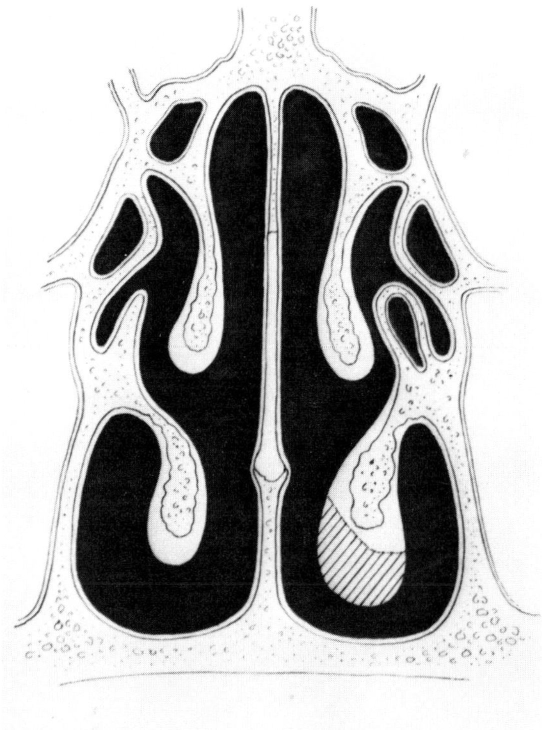

This schematic cross section shows the usual area of turbinate resection.

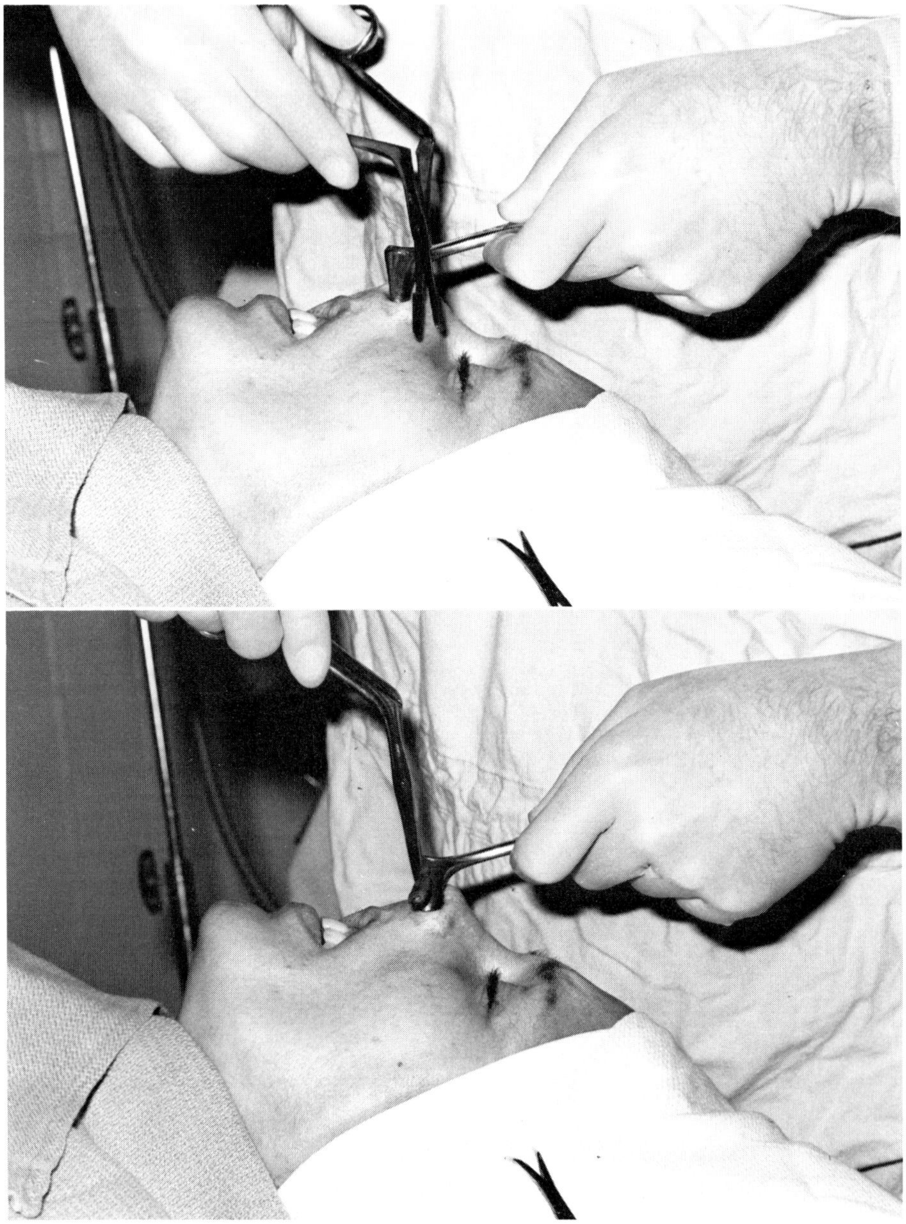

A pair of Killian septal forceps is used to retrieve the resected portion.

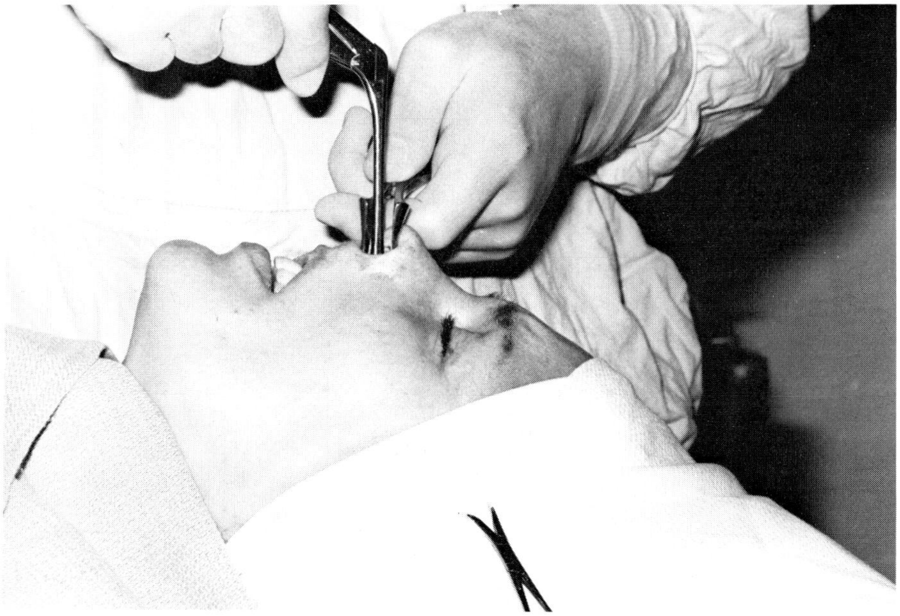

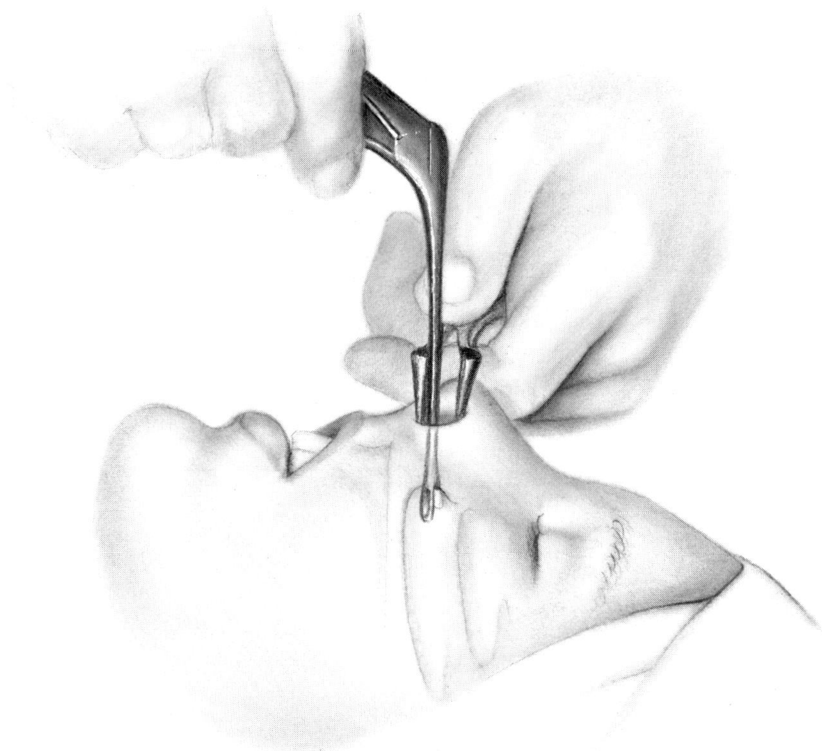

The leading edge or anterior part of the inferior turbinate is frequently the only obstructing portion. Segmental resection of the turbinate can be precisely controlled with a Gruenwald nasal forceps.

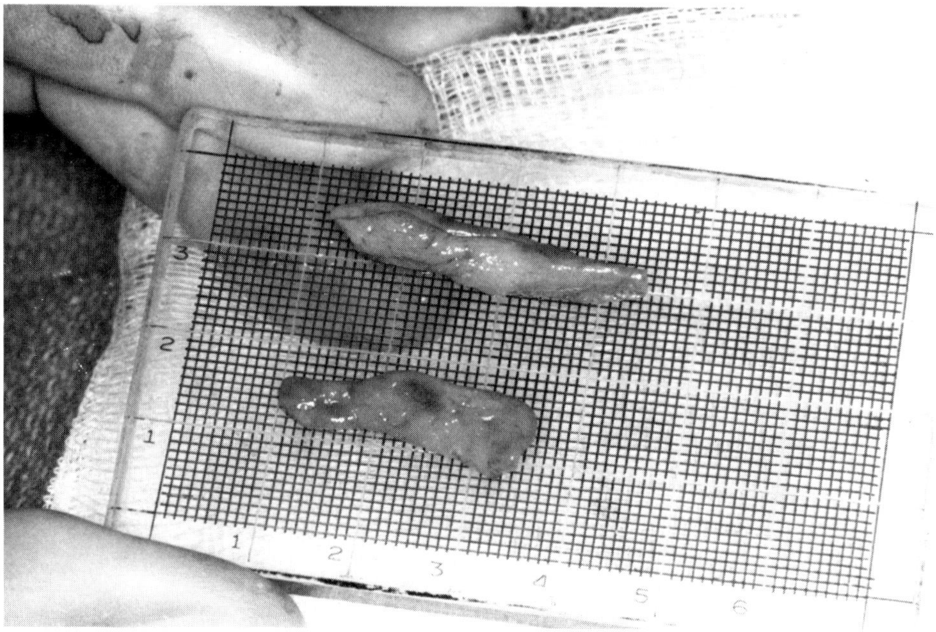

Typical specimens of the inferior segments of two hypertrophied inferior turbinates are shown on a cm/mm grid.

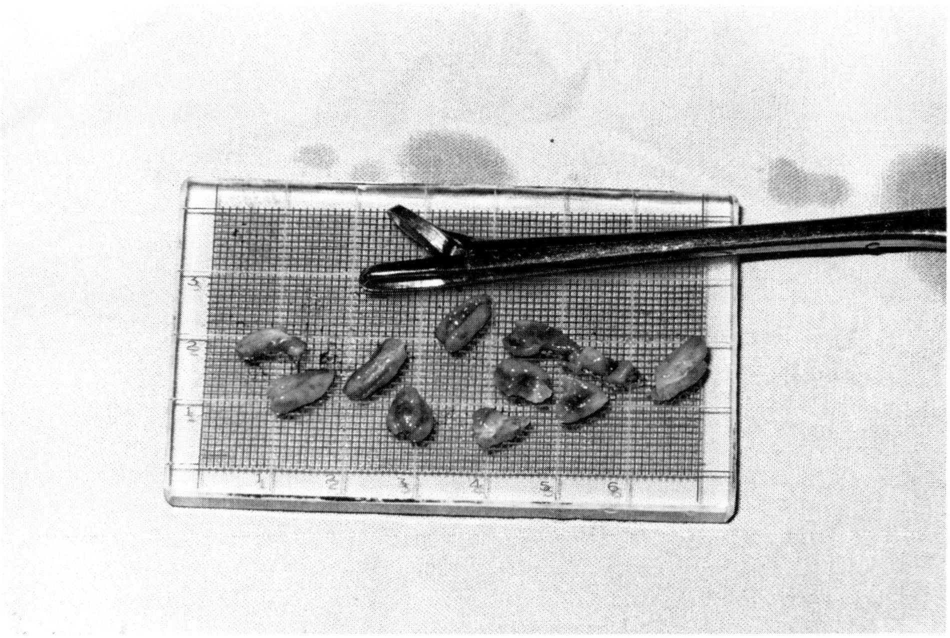

The cm/mm grid contains anterior segments of hypertrophied turbinates and a pair of Gruenwald nasal forceps.

Bleeding from the turbinate is usually venous. However, if there is arterial bleeding, it can be controlled by cautery using insulated forceps.

Following the procedure, Adaptic gauze covered with Bacitracin ointment is placed along the nasal floor, and successive packs of Adaptic gauze are layered over it. Overstuffing the nose is unnecessary and uncomfortable. The packs are left in place from 4 to 7 days. At 4 days the packs are checked. If they are mucus saturated, the top packs are removed very carefully. If there is adherence or slight bleeding the patient is asked to return in 3 days. At the end of a week, packs usually slide out without bleeding.

MAXILLARY AUGMENTATION

The general use of alloplastic materials in nasal surgery should be discouraged. However, the excellent long-term results of maxillary augmentation using alloplastics justify their use for this specific purpose. Although various types of Silastic can be used, my favorite material for maxillary augmentation is Supramid Extra Mesh because it is easy to insert and does not have firm edges that can be palpated under the skin. The primary disadvantage of the mesh is that it is difficult to remove.

Supramid Extra Mesh can be layered, folded, spindled, or rolled, depending on the required form and amount of augmentation. For augmentation of the entire anterior maxillary curve, a roll of mesh is placed just below the nasal spine in a horizontal plane, extending laterally past the alar-facial grooves. When just those areas under the alar-facial grooves require augmentation, a folded pad of mesh is placed under each alar lobule.

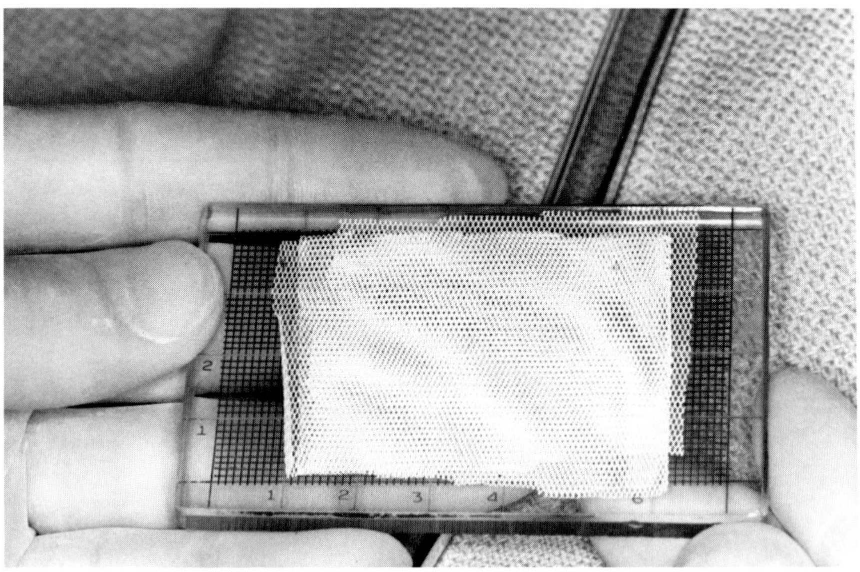

Preparation of a rolled implant

The mesh is measured depending on the amount of augmentation desired.

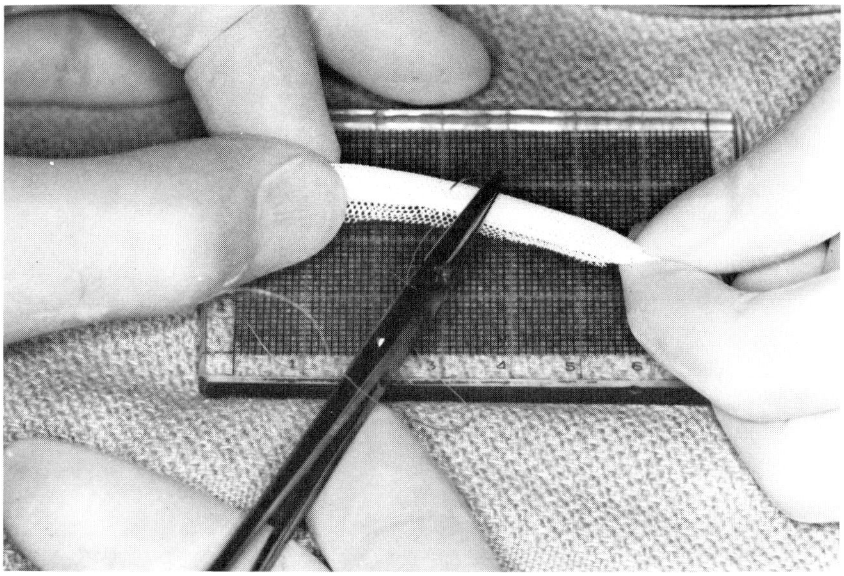

It is rolled as tightly as possible. As an assistant holds the ends, a 5-0 plain catgut suture is placed in the center.

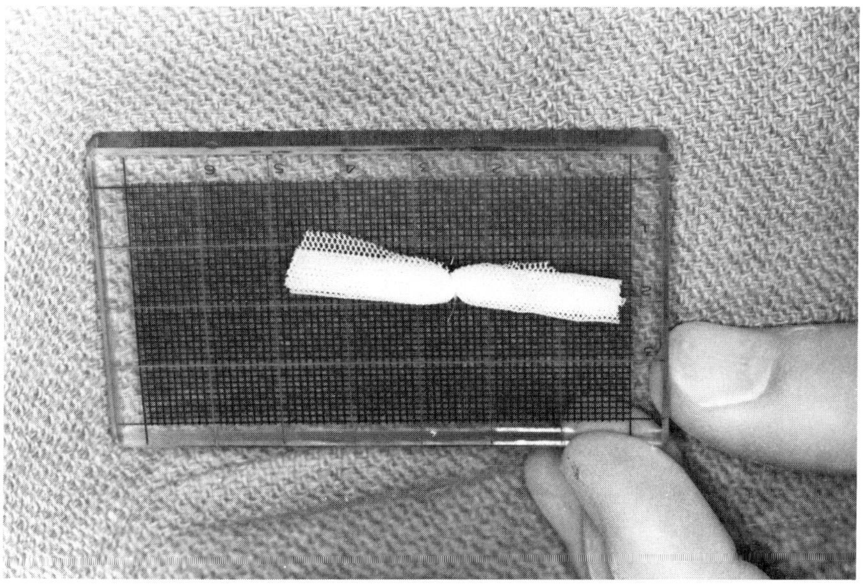

The ends are trimmed, and the implant is ready for insertion.

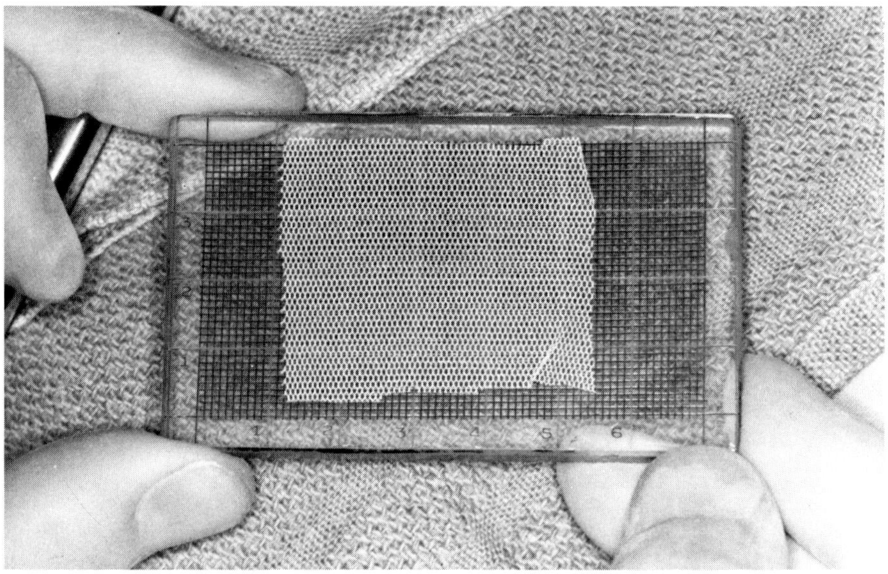

Preparation of lateral pads

The mesh pads are made the same size by measuring both at the beginning of the procedure.

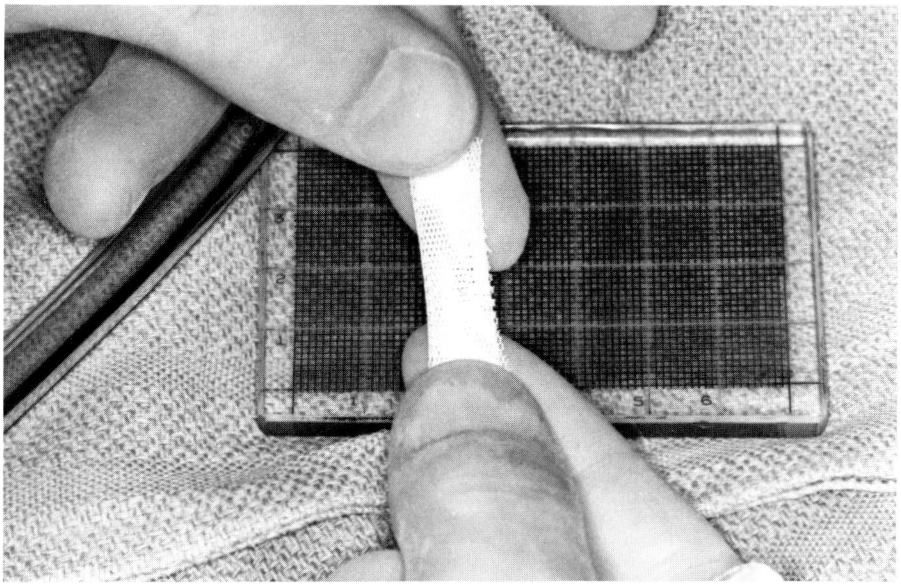

The mesh is folded, rendering a 7- to 8-mm wide strip of mesh.

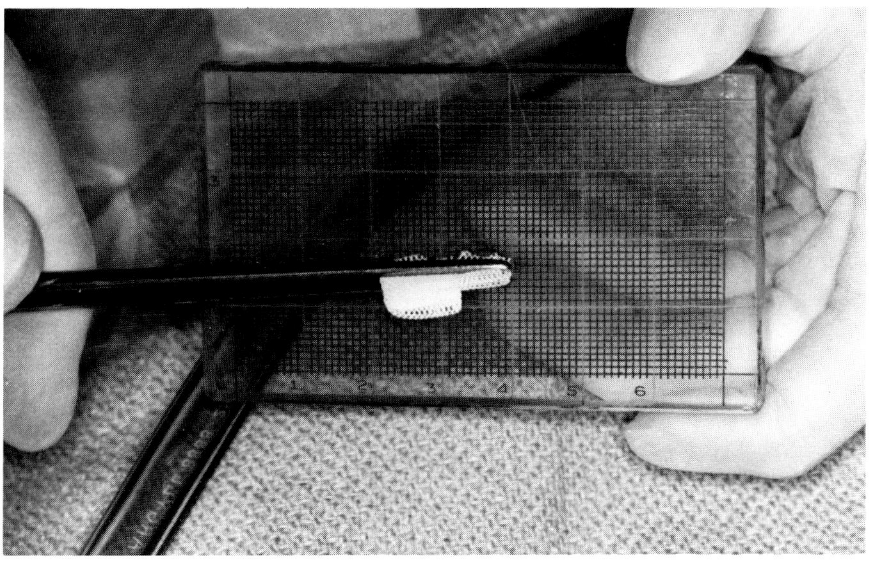

This strip is then folded to make a tapered implant so that the widest part can be placed just under the alar-facial groove.

Surgical procedure

Maxillary augmentation should precede intranasal surgery. The mesh is saturated with lincomycin hydrochloride (Lincocin) before its insertion.

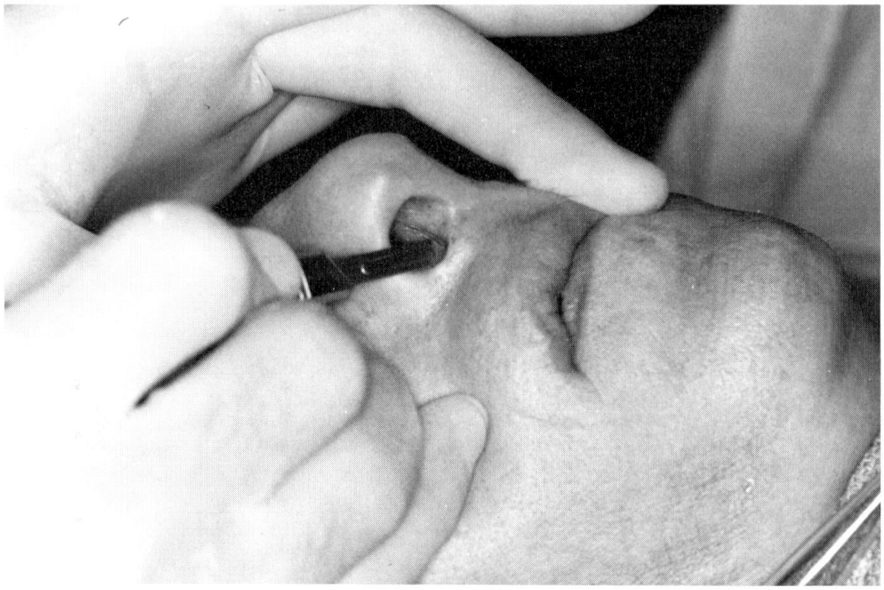

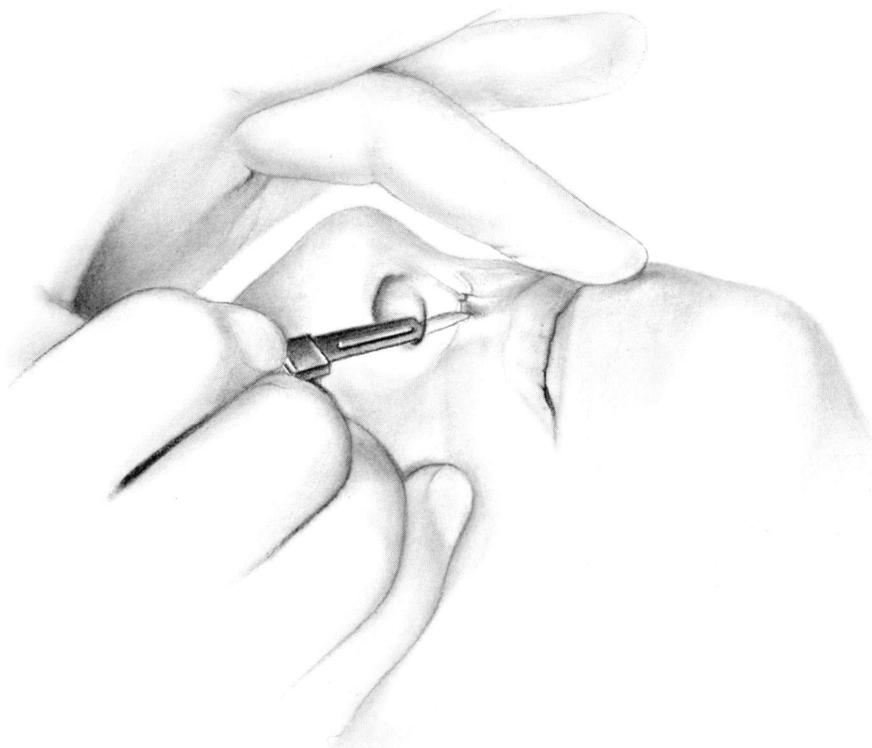

A stab incision is made in the vestibule, extending to the maxilla, just inferior to the nasal spine.

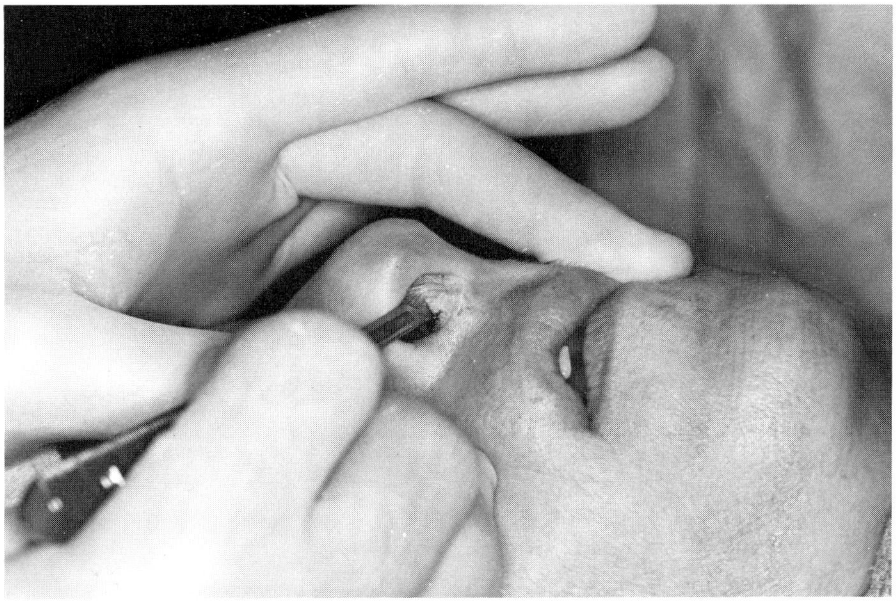

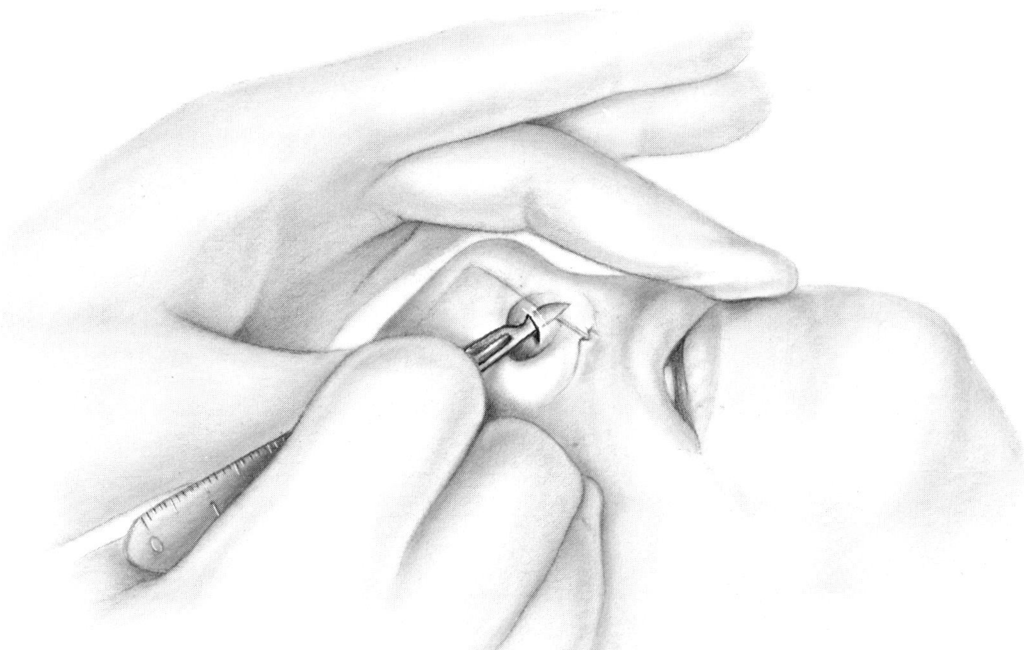

The incision is continued anteriorly along the caudal border of the septum.

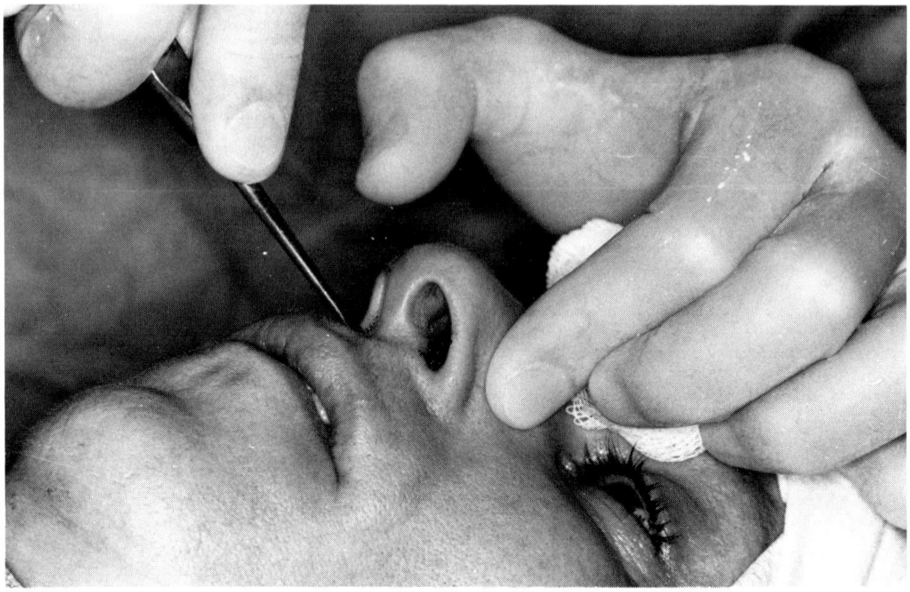

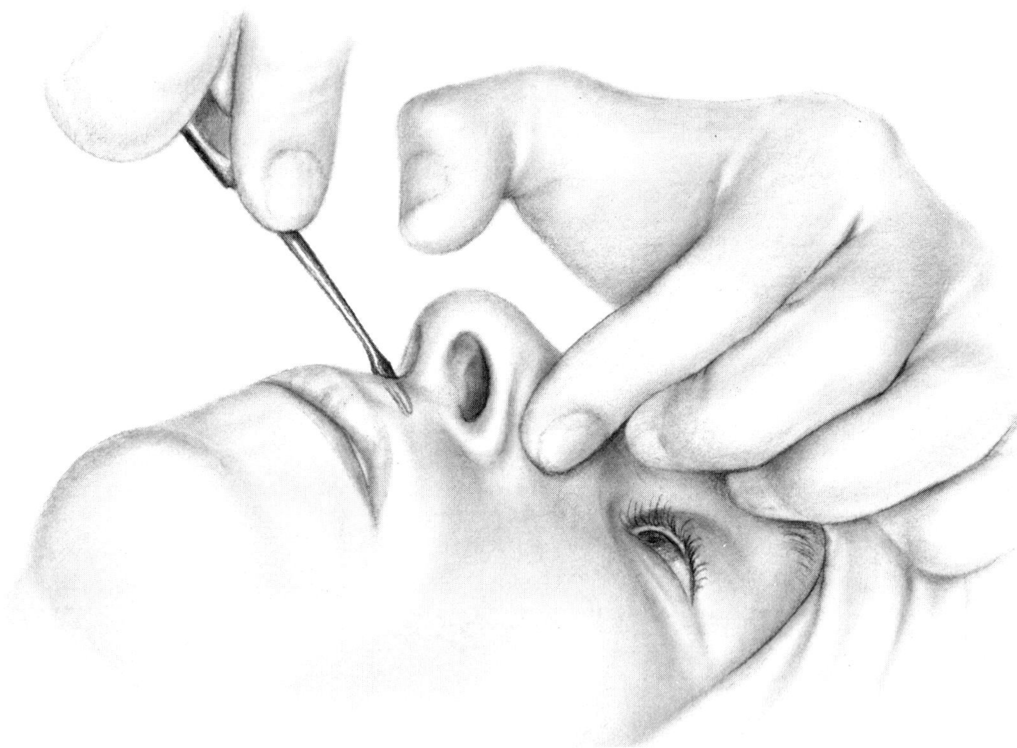

A Joseph periosteal elevator is placed firmly on the maxilla, and the tissues are dissected from the maxilla beginning at the spine and going laterally past the alar-facial groove. This is done on both sides.

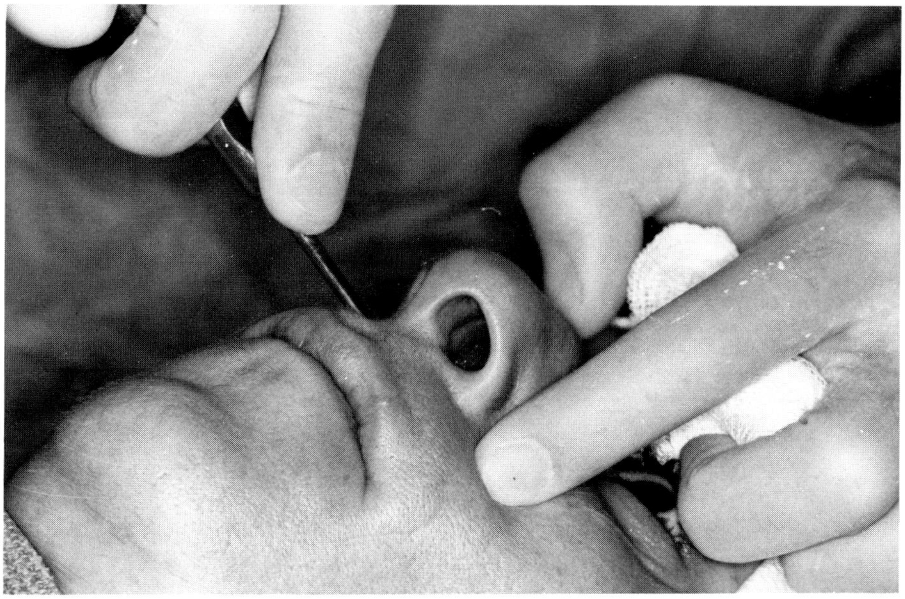

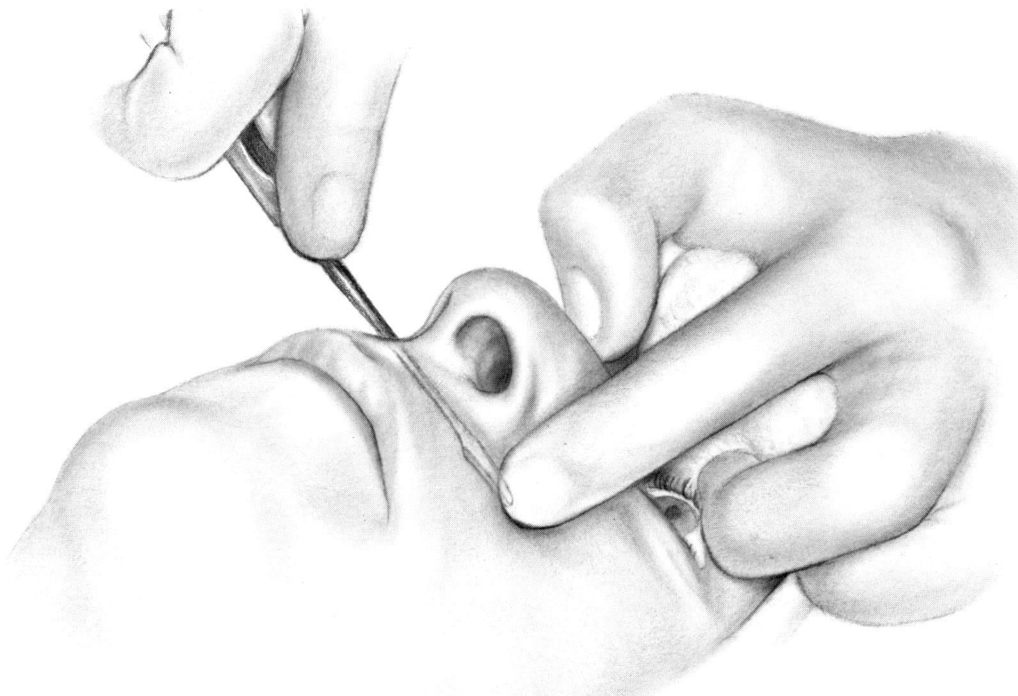

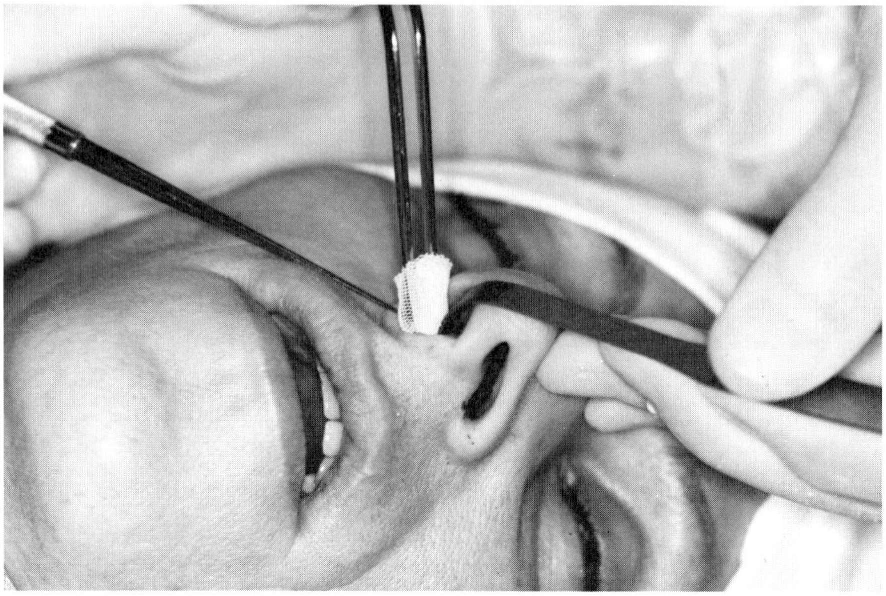

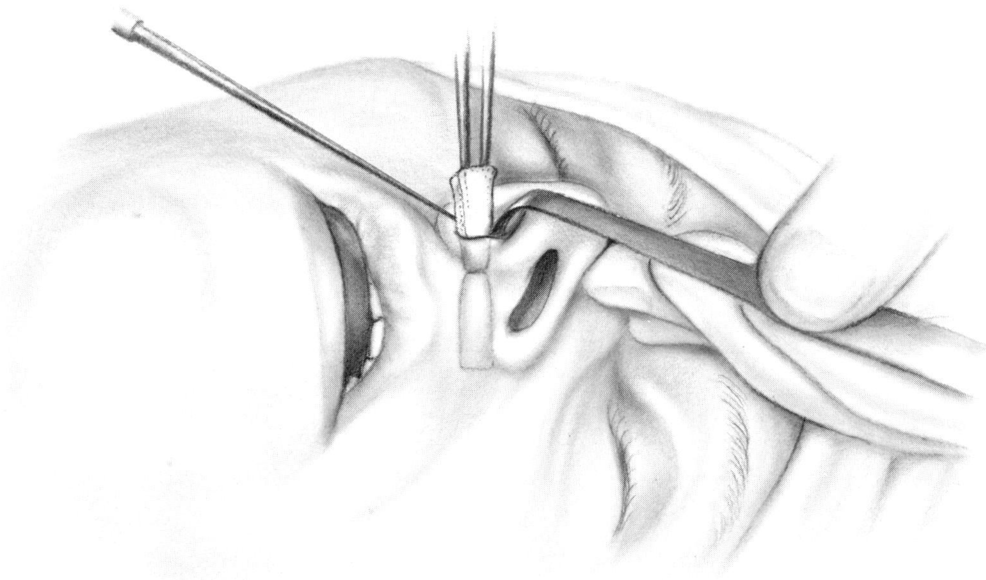

As an assistant retracts the nasal sill inferiorly, a Joseph retractor is placed in the wound, and the mesh is inserted into the pocket.

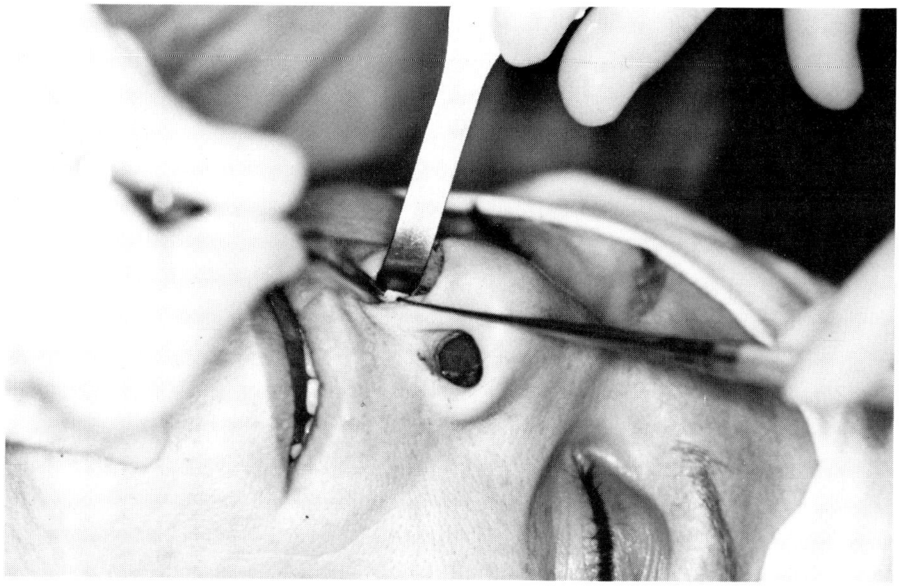

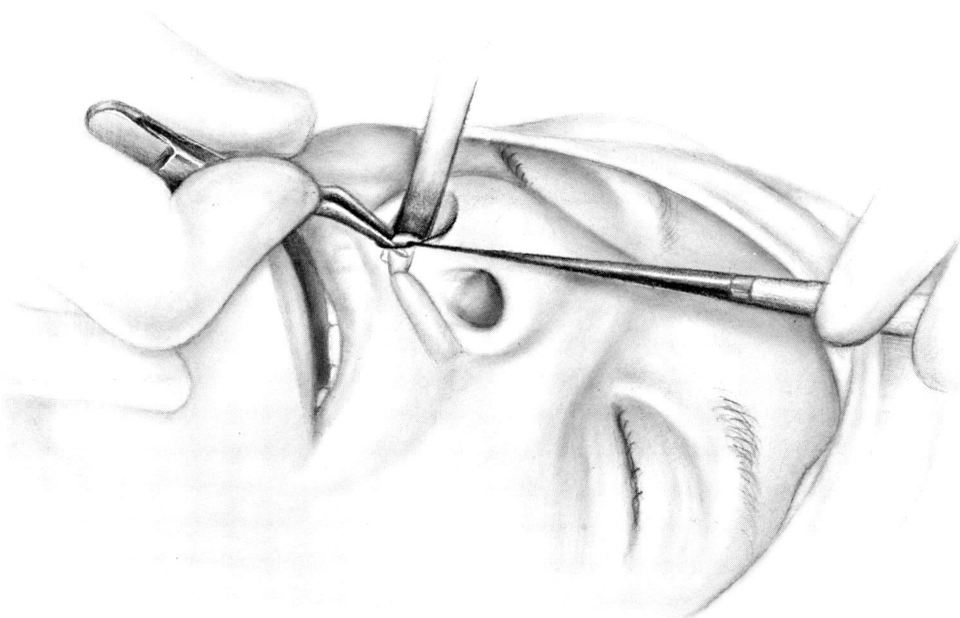

The opposite end of the implant is grasped with the bayonet forceps and placed in the opposite pocket. The center of the implant can be identified by the midline suture. Following insertion, the wound is immediately closed with a deep 4-0 plain catgut suture, retaining ample tissue cover. Wound closure is completed with interrupted 5-0 plain catgut sutures.

Case examples

This patient had a slightly retrusive maxilla, which gave her lip a posterior inclination. Postoperatively, following maxillary augmentation with bilateral Supramid mesh pads, the lip has been moved anteriorly. She has also had a primary "finesse" rhinoplasty with alar wedge resections.

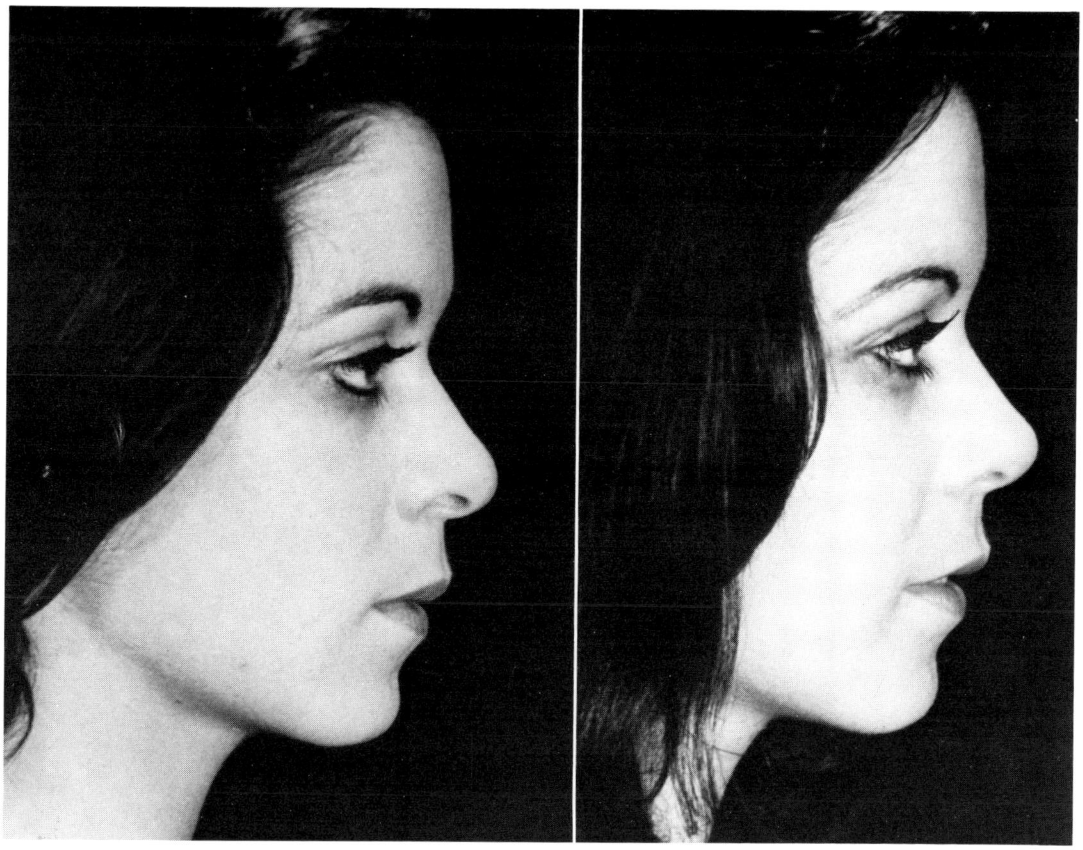

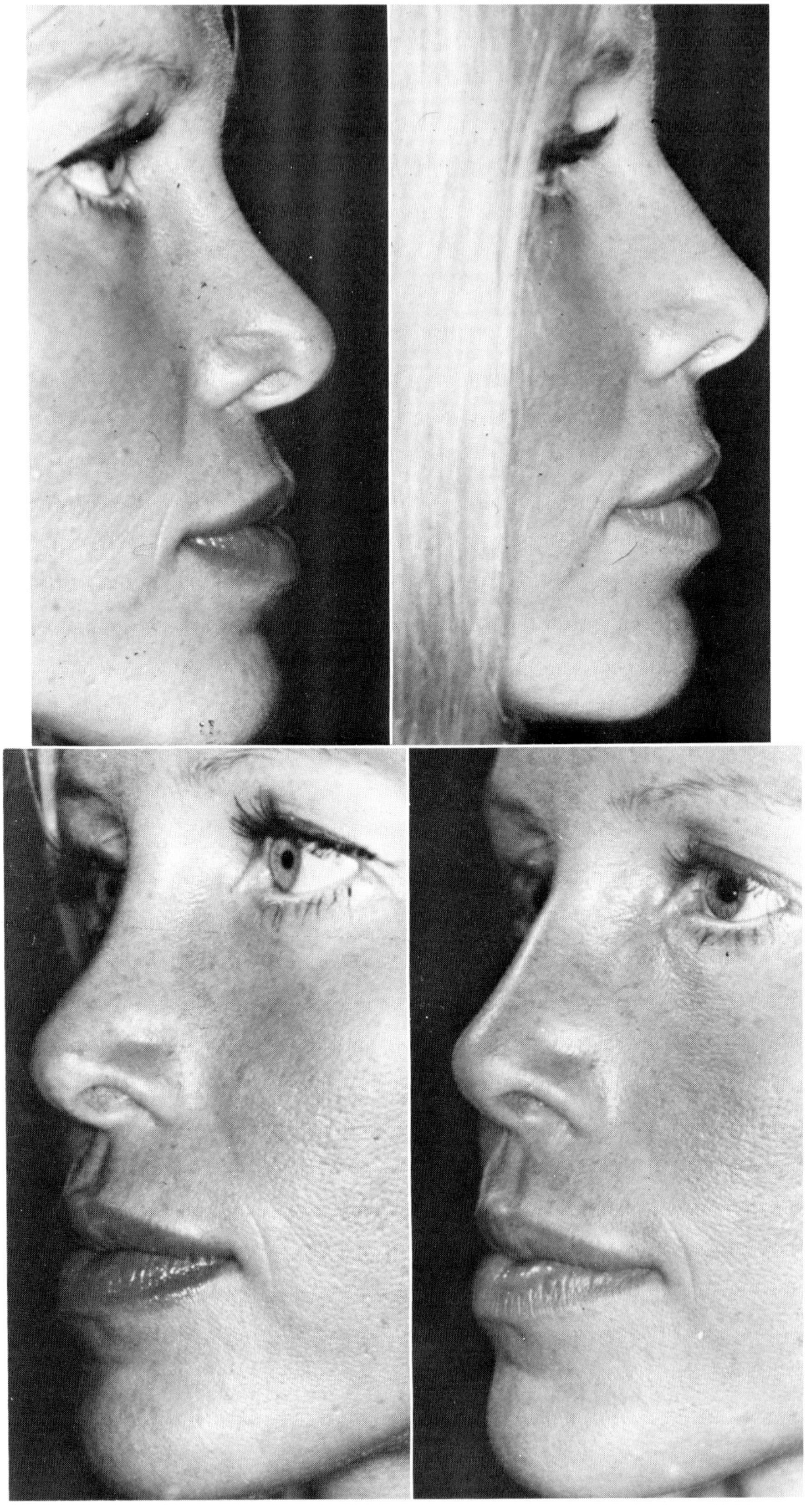

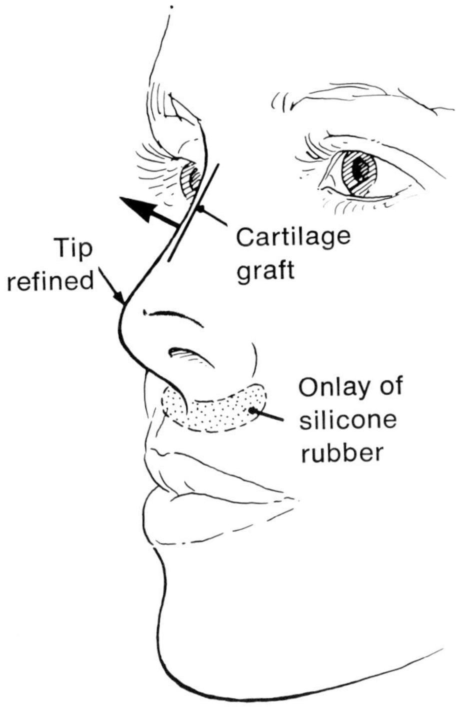

This patient's unsatisfactory primary rhinoplasty was accentuated by retrusion of her maxilla. Secondary correction consisted of a dorsal graft of septal cartilage, tip refinement, and maxillary augmentation using a carved piece of Silastic rubber.

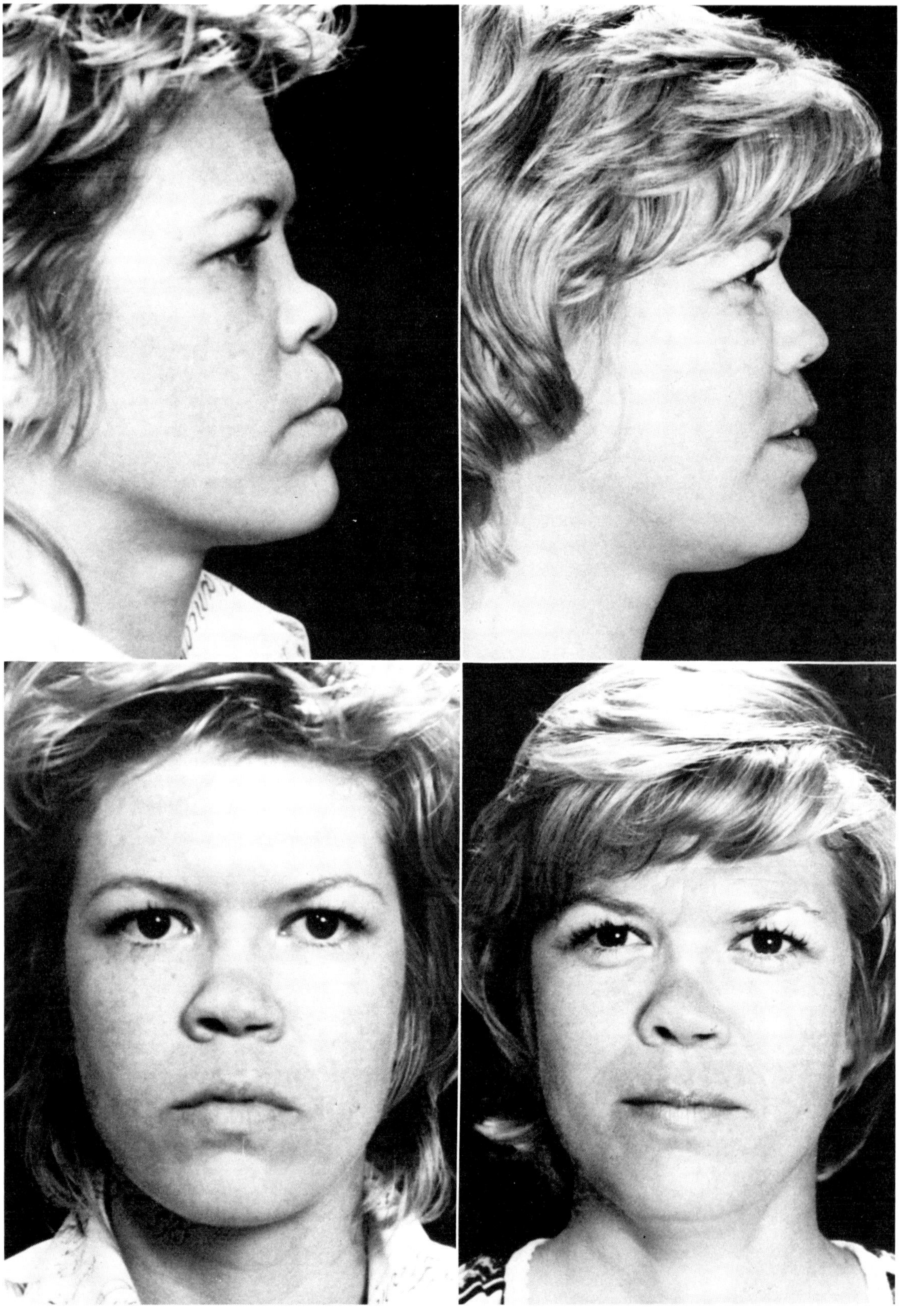

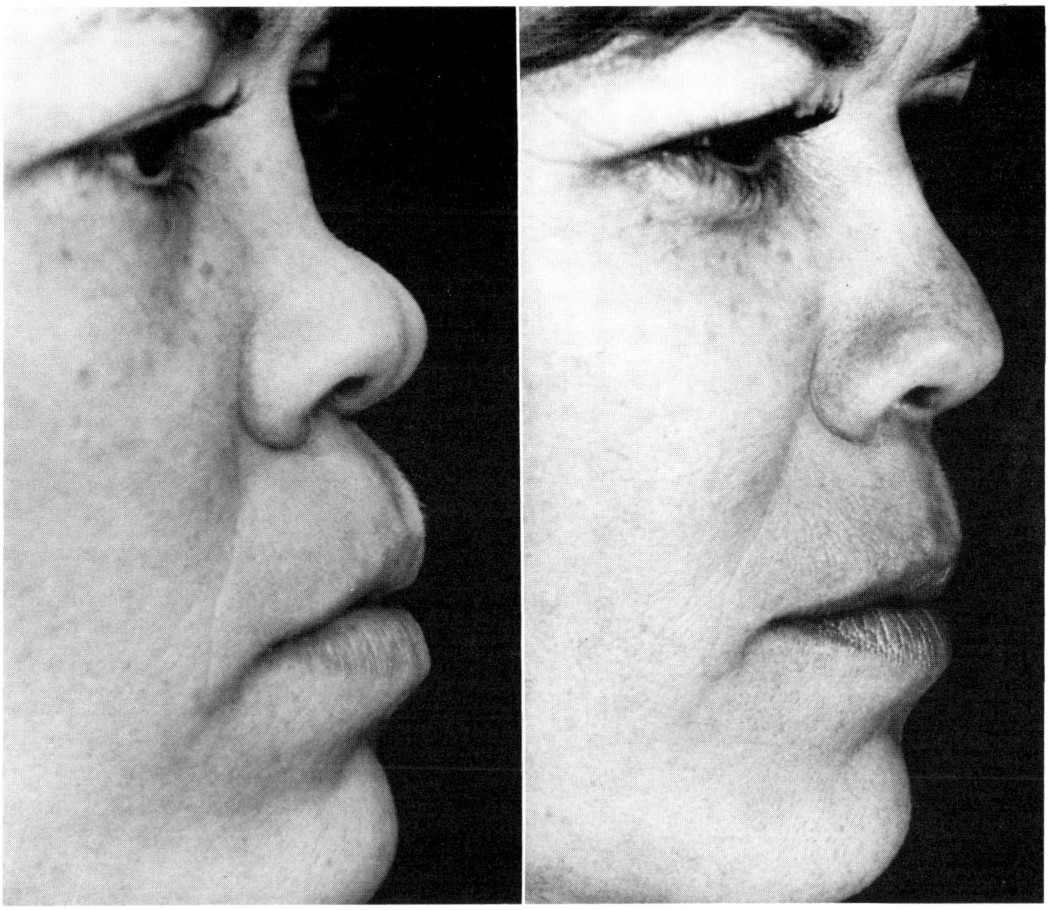

Under the condition of normal occlusion, congenital or post-traumatic midface retrusions can often be successfully corrected by augmentive techniques. This patient is shown preoperatively and 4 years following maxillary augmentation with a roll of Supramid Extra Mesh (6 mm in diameter). Primary rhinoplasty was also done.

ALAR RESECTION

As with rhinoplasty in general, the key to alar resection is individualization. Because of the various basal configurations, a simple wedge resection cannot be sufficient for every case. The purpose of alar resection also varies with each case. It may be to narrow the nostril, to reduce a large alar lobule, or to thin a heavy alar rim. Whatever the purpose, it should be well conceived because irreversible deformity can result.

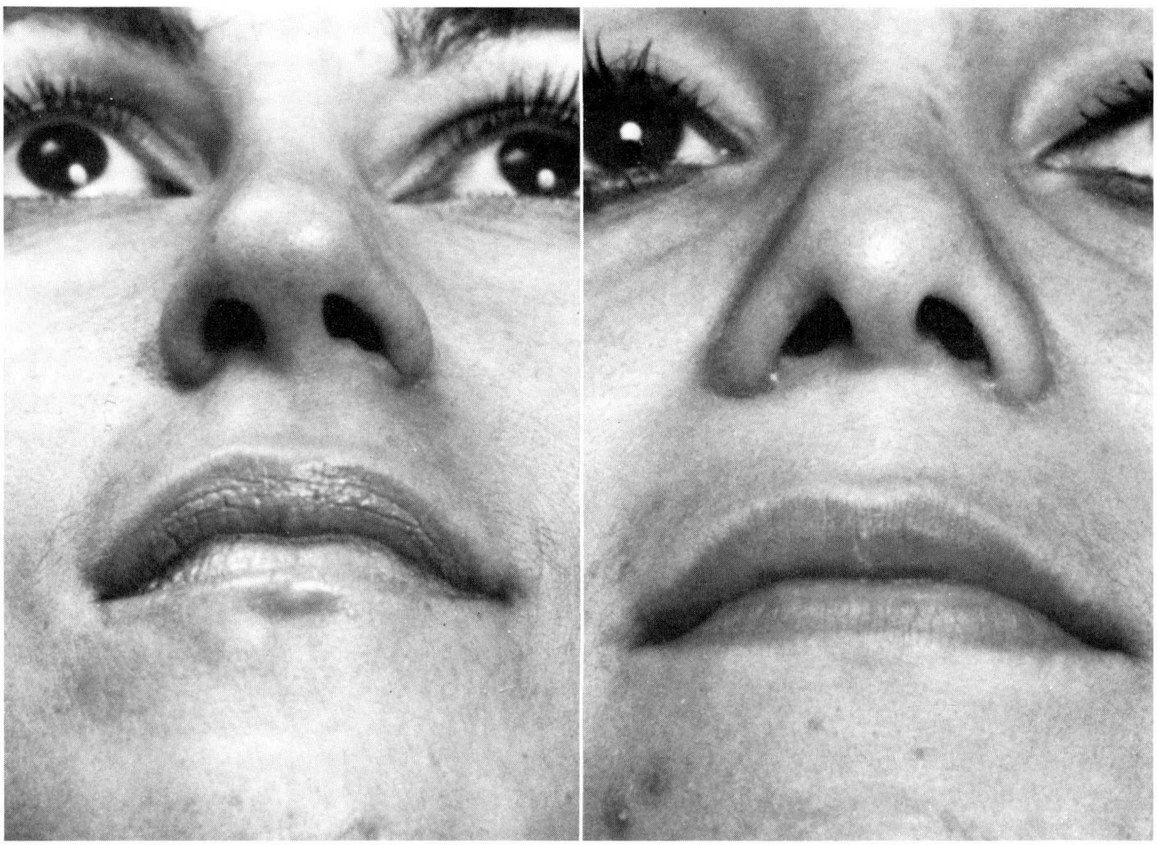

Common evidence of alar resection is a notch at the area of incision in the base of the nostril, as seen in these patients. The nasal base appears unnatural because the smooth contour of the nasal sill has been interrupted. This telltale notching has been virtually eliminated by a technique that preserves a small triangular flap that includes some of the medial nasal sill. This technique is discussed first because it is used in all resections involving vestibular skin.

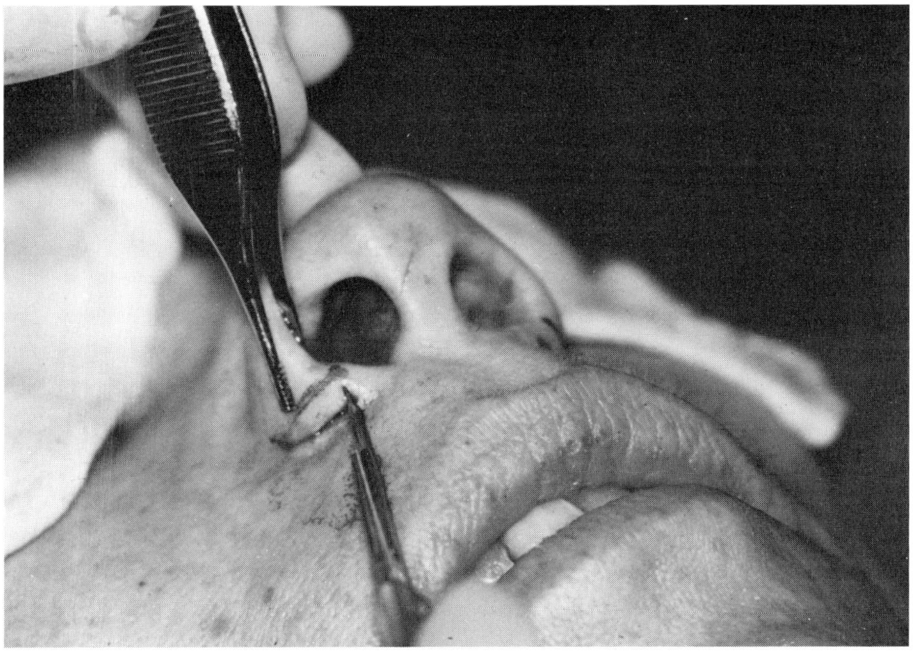

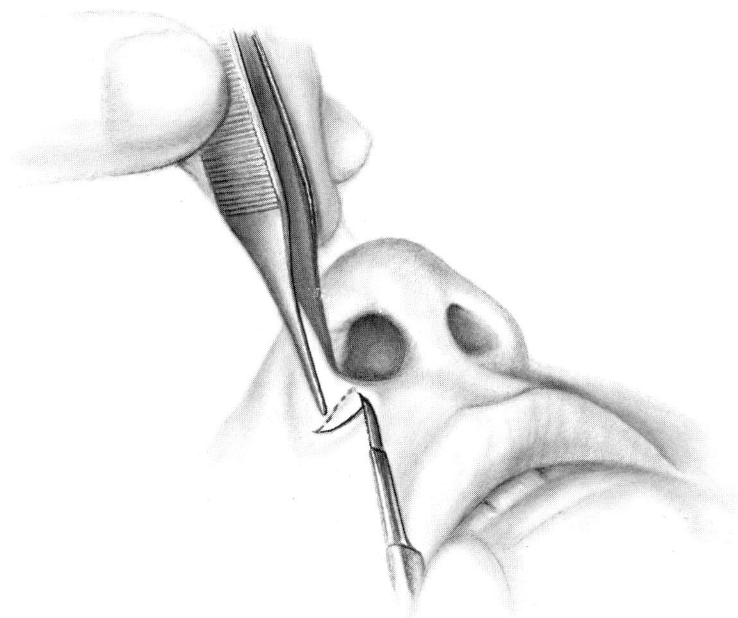

Surgical procedure

After the planned excision has been marked, an incision is made with a No. 11 blade, extending medially along the alar base and stopping short of the last 2 to 3 mm.

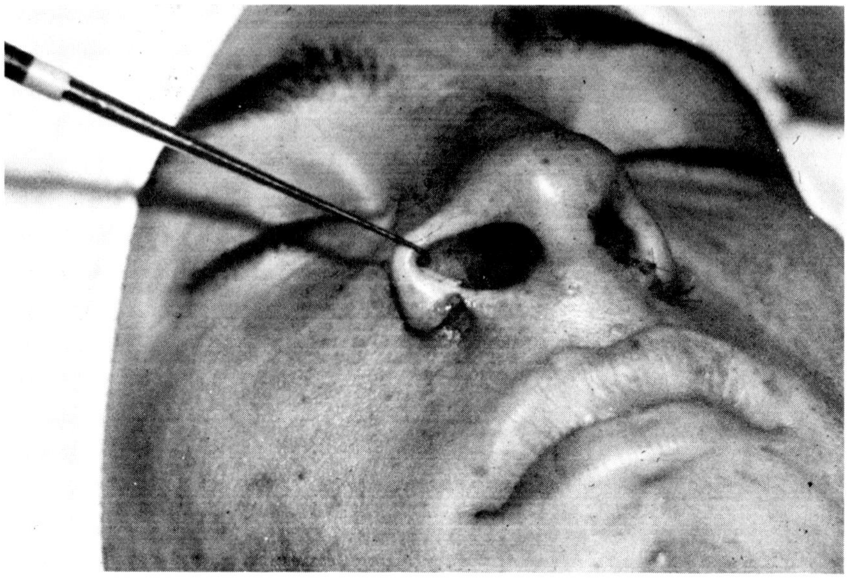

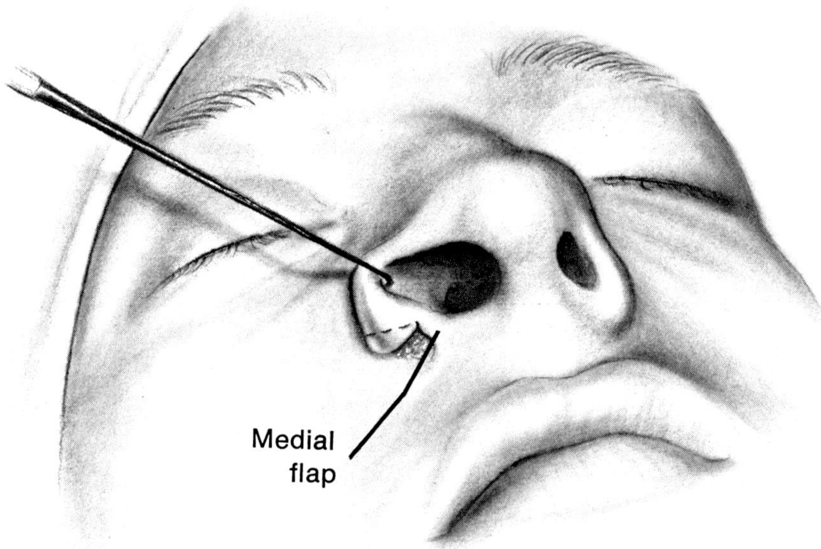

At this point a back cut that preserves a small triangular flap (which I shall refer to as the medial flap) is made. Except for a small segment of the nasal sill, the inferior cut has been made. The nostril is being pulled laterally to demonstrate the medial flap.

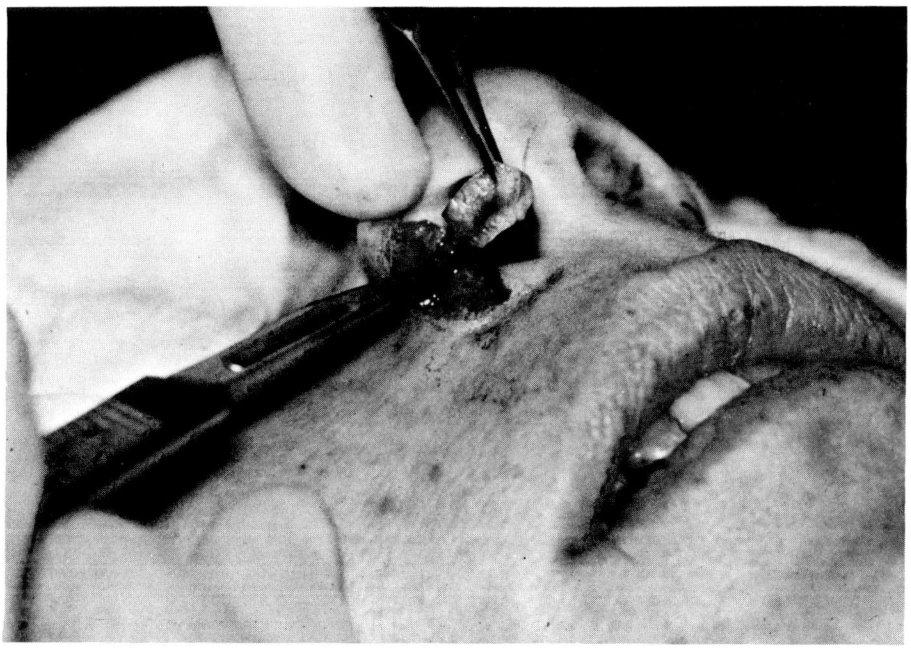

The superior cut is made, excising the wedge of tissue. The retained medial flap can be seen.

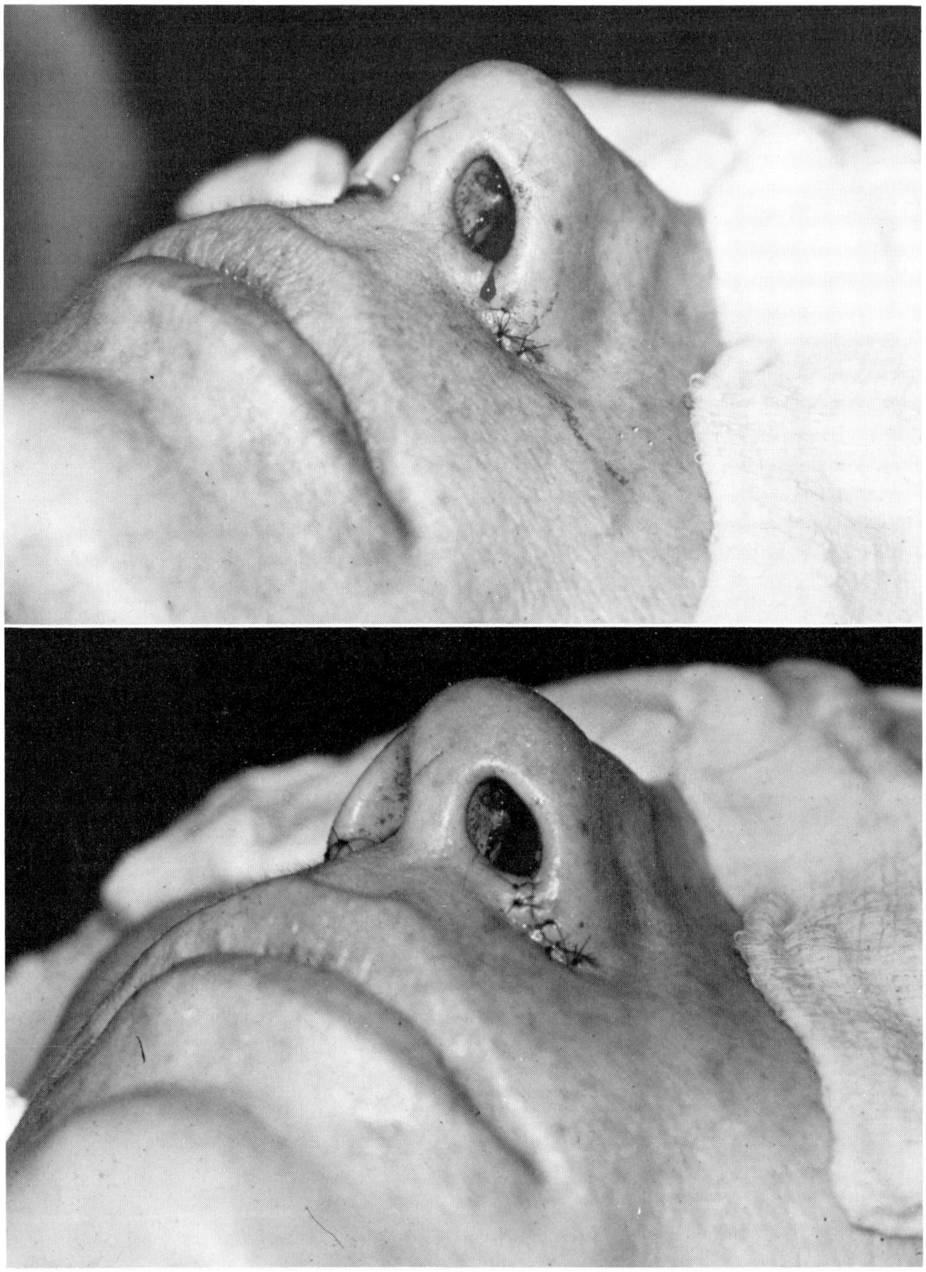

This patient's nasal sill has a natural continuity because of preservation of the medial flap. The flap is shown before and after suture placement.

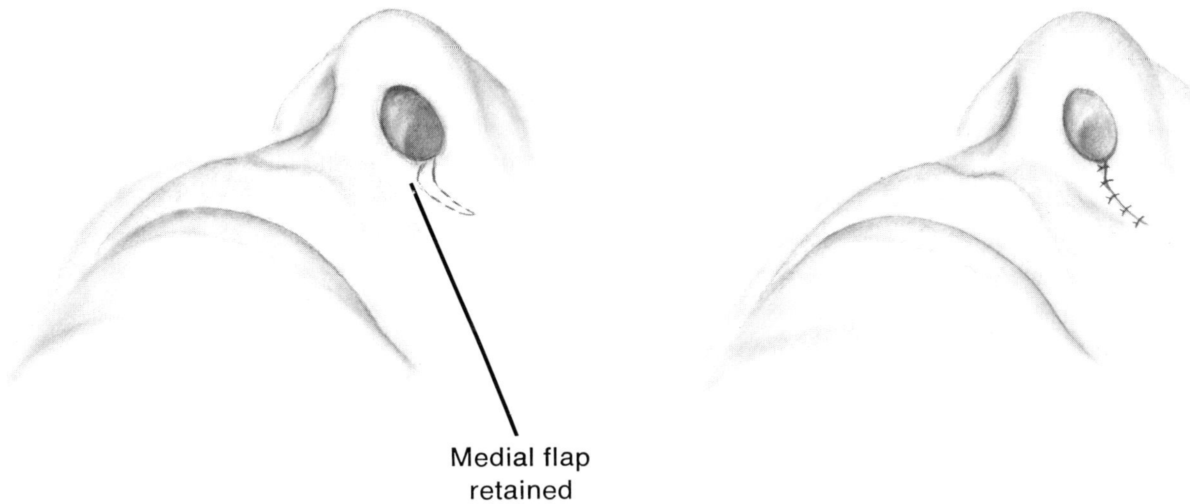

The use of a medial flap produces a natural-appearing nasal sill in all cases where vestibular skin is resected.

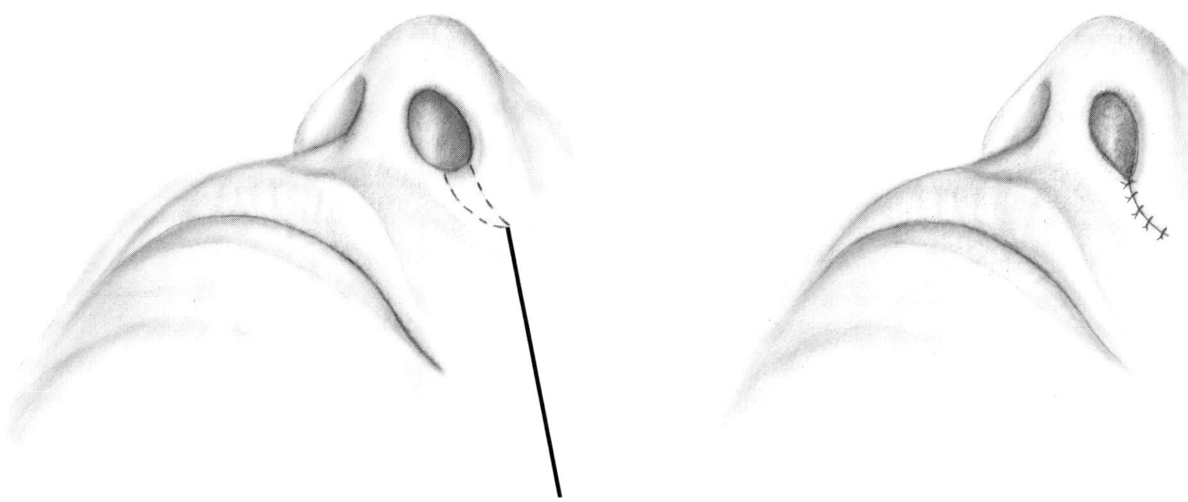

In comparison, if the tissues are resected, there is an unnatural, surgical notching of the nasal sill.

Types of alar bases

In planning alar wedge resections, the surgeon must consider the modification of two surfaces: vestibular and cutaneous. The width of tissue resected on the vestibular side changes the perimeter of the nostril, whereas the width of tissue resected on the cutaneous side modifies the contour of the alar lobule.

It is helpful to classify the three general types of alar bases to understand the importance of the two-surface concept in alar resection.

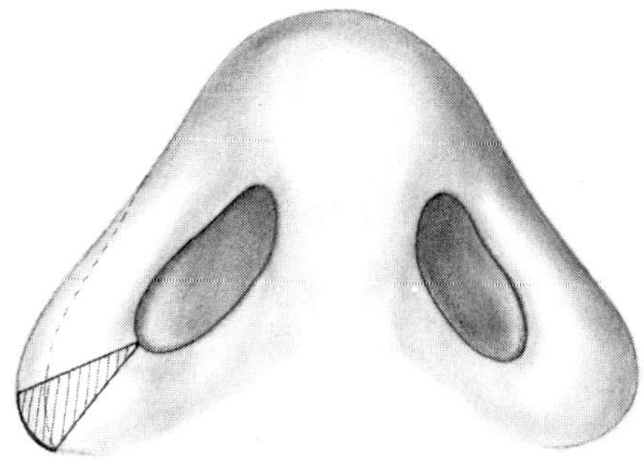

Category I patients have appropriately sized nostrils but excessive alar lobules. Only the lobules should be reduced without excising the vestibular skin.

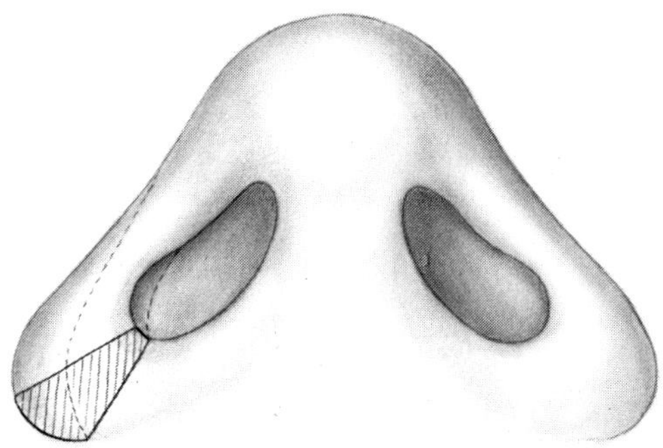

Category II patients have large nostrils that are less excessive than the alar lobules. Correction of these involves a greater resection of lobular skin than vestibular skin.

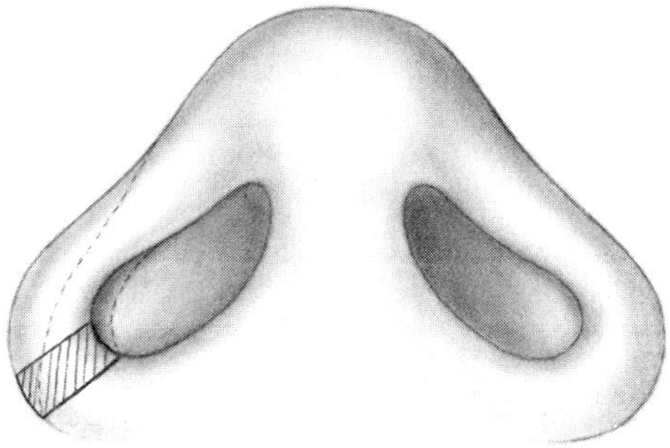

Category III patients have nostrils and alar lobules that are equally redundant. Reduction is achieved by equal resection of lobular and vestibular skin.

CASE REPORT 1: CATEGORY I

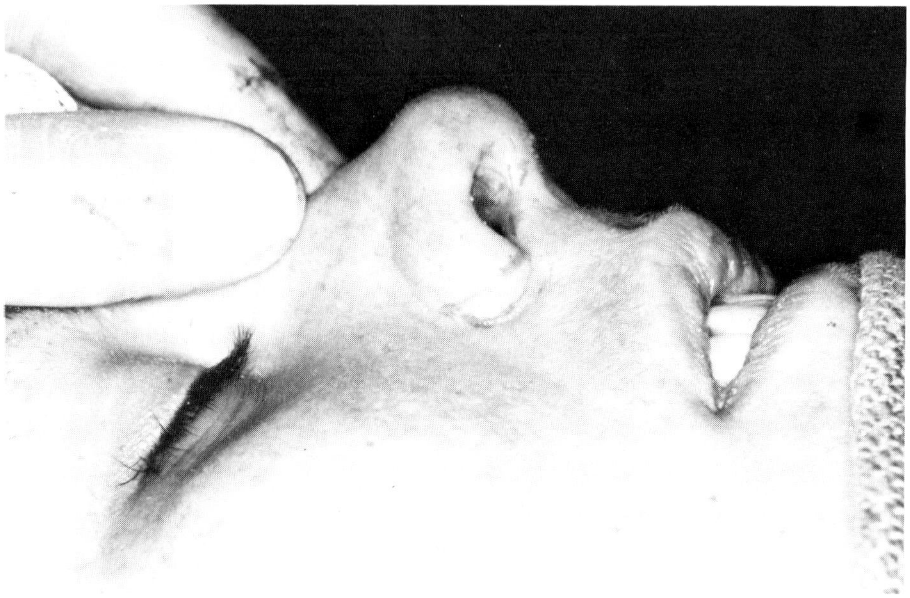

This patient has oversized alar lobules that tend to arch downward because of their breadth, placing the insertion of the lobule below the insertion of the columella. The nasal sill is sharply delineated from the insertion of the alae. Because the nostril size is good, the surgical plan is to reduce the lobule without incising the vestibular skin.

The skin is marked as shown, with the inferior incision just above the alar-facial groove.

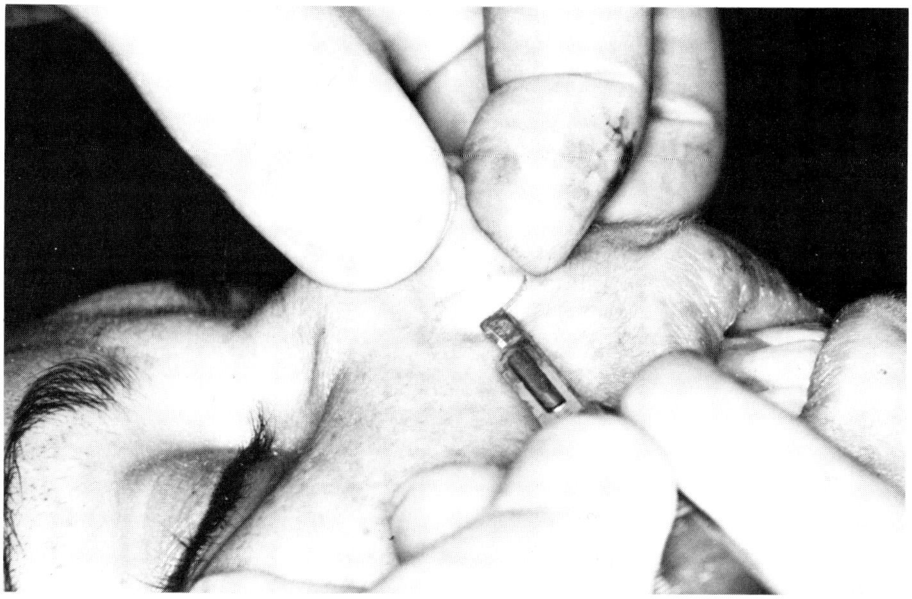

The incision is made using a No. 15 blade, beveling the cut so that the deepest edge will be just to the vestibular skin.

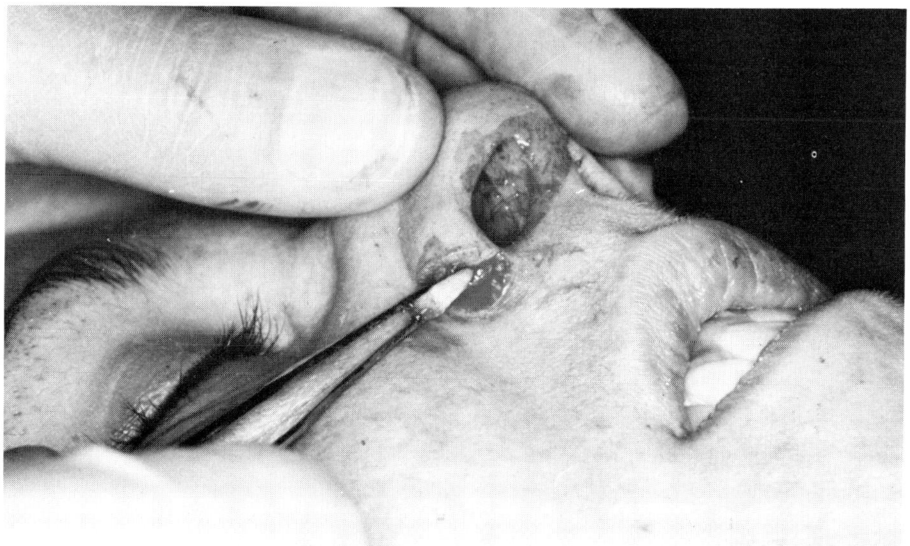

The wedge, measuring approximately 3 mm on the cutaneous side, is removed. The vestibular skin is intact.

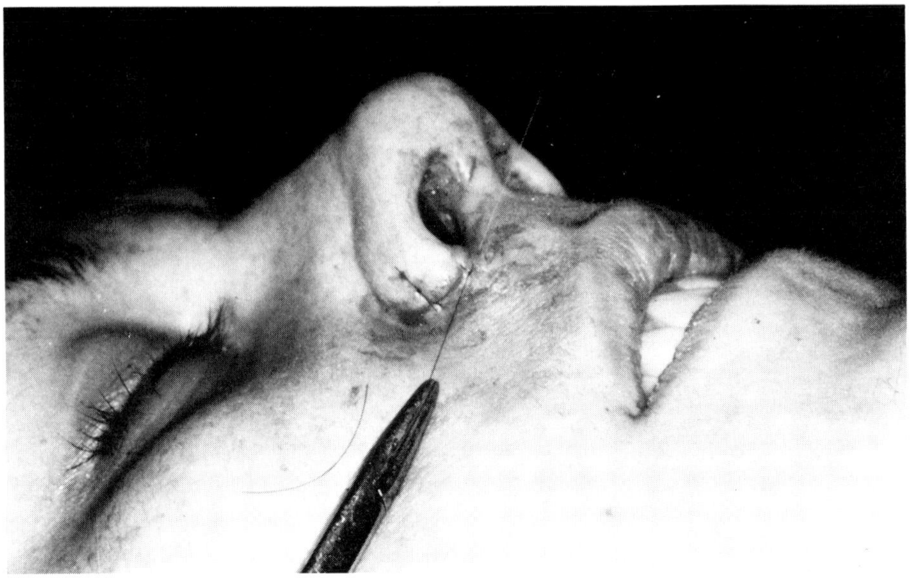

The skin is closed with interrupted 6-0 nylon sutures.

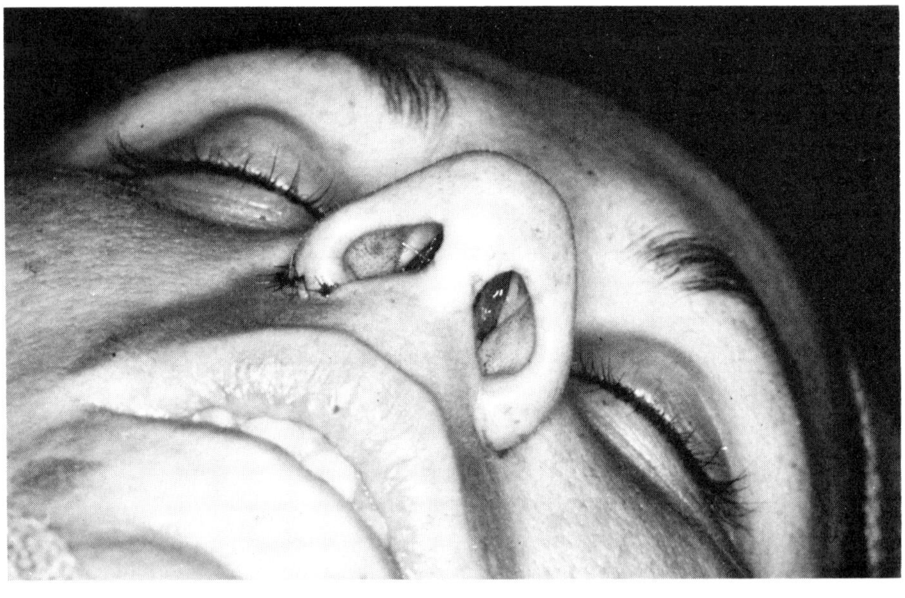

The minimal resection has re-formed the base without jeopardizing the symmetry of the nasal sills.

CASE REPORT 2: CATEGORY II

Most patients requiring reduction of the nasal base also require some reduction in the size of the nostril.

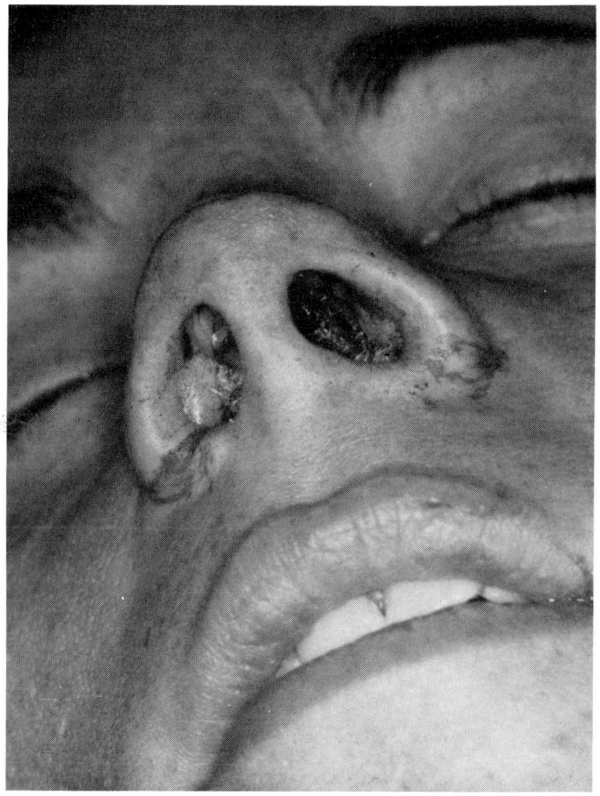

This patient's nostrils are slightly flaring; the moderately large alar lobules are rotated laterally. To rotate the lobule medially, more lobular skin than vestibular skin must be resected.

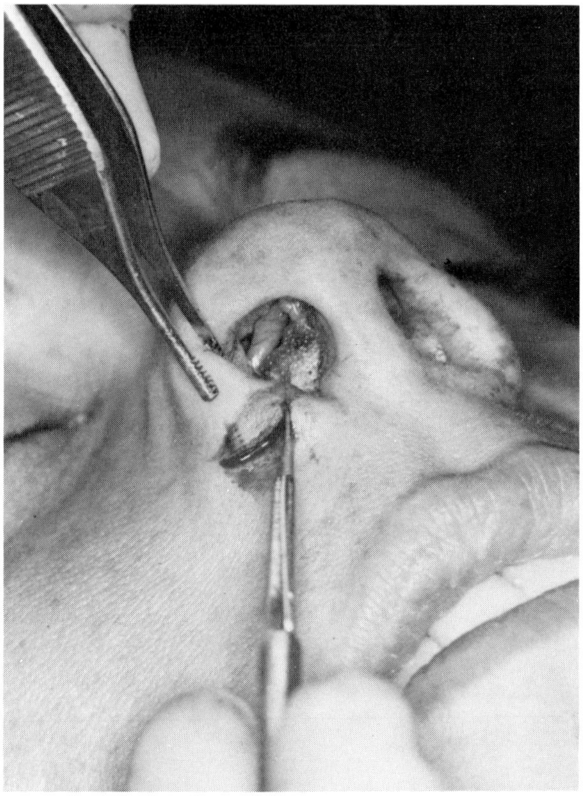

The initial cut begins just above the alar-facial groove. The medial flap can be seen. Note the angle of the No. 11 blade, which ensures resection of less vestibular than lobular skin.

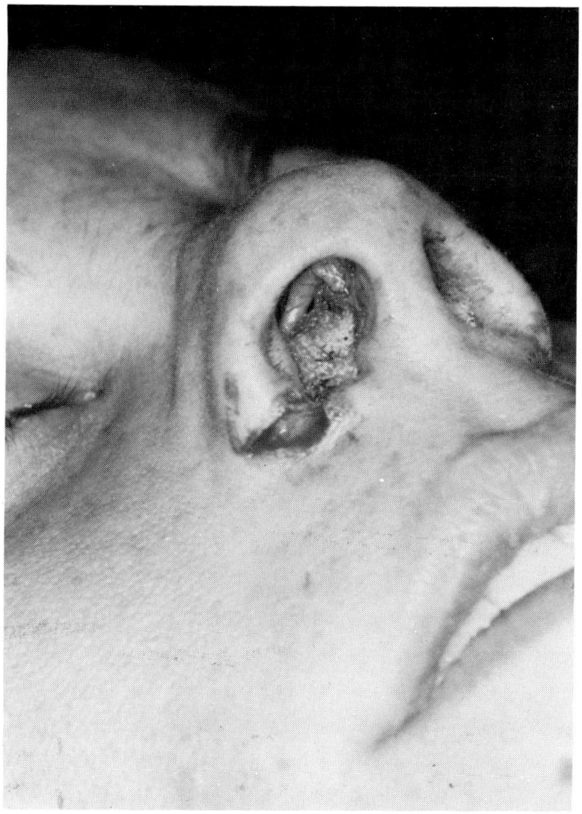

Following resection of the tissues, the vestibular defect measures approximately 3 mm at its widest, whereas the lobular defect measures approximately 7 mm.

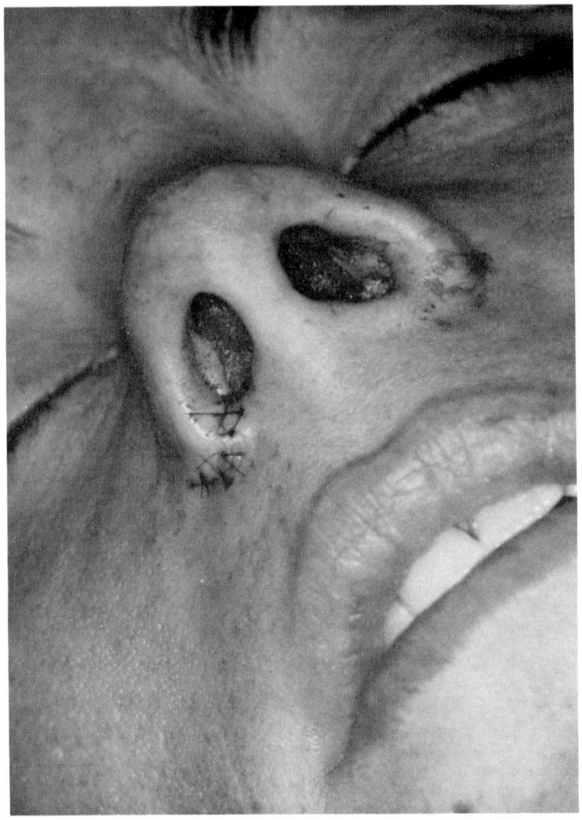

The desired effect of medially rotating the alar lobule and modifying the size and position of the nostril has been accomplished while maintaining natural continuity of the nasal sill.

CASE REPORT 3: CATEGORY III

In category III, the least common of the three, the curvature of the nostril and the contour of the alar lobule are parallel.

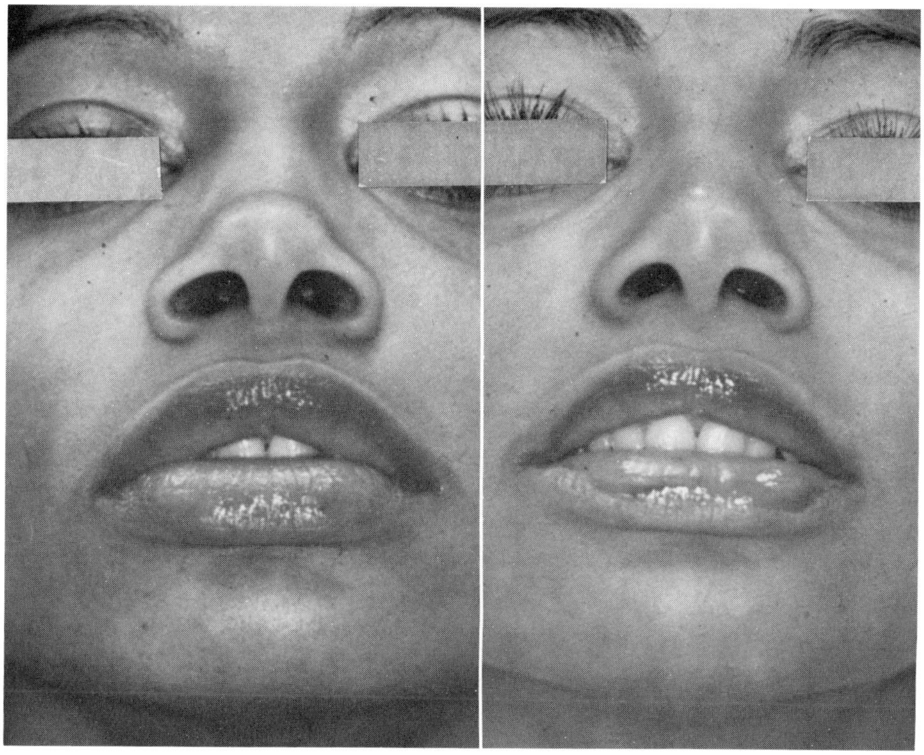

This patient illustrates exceptionally thin alar lobules. The nostril curves around and enters the nasal sill without the usual lobular thickening. Such patients present special problems because the latitude for error is small. The surgeon must resect tissues with special conservatism. Postoperatively, the continuity of the nasal sill on basal view is good, although there is a slight notch on the patient's left nostril at the point of resection. The medial flaps are preserved.

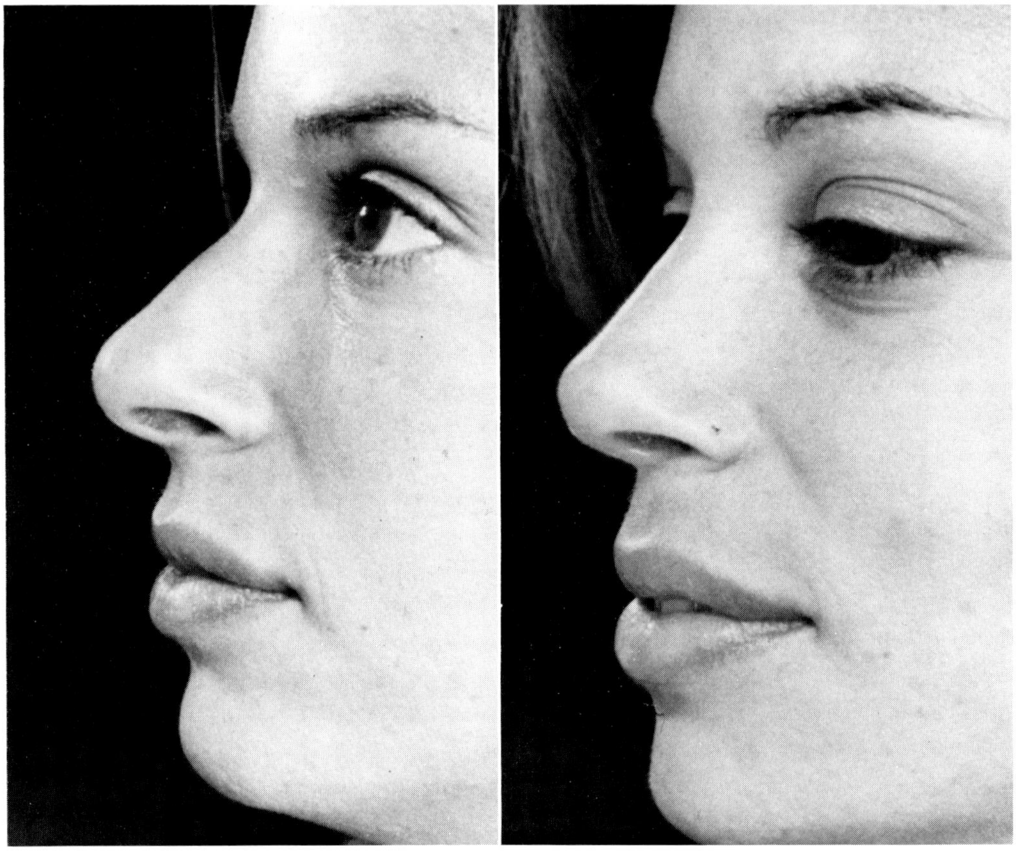

Effect of alar resection on nostril length

The proportion of the length of the nostril to the tip lobule is a concept that is discussed in Chapter 2. This patient's nostrils are too long for the tip lobule. Postoperatively, the nostril-tip proportion has been improved by the resection of 1.5 mm of vestibular skin and 2 mm of lobular skin. She is a category II patient.

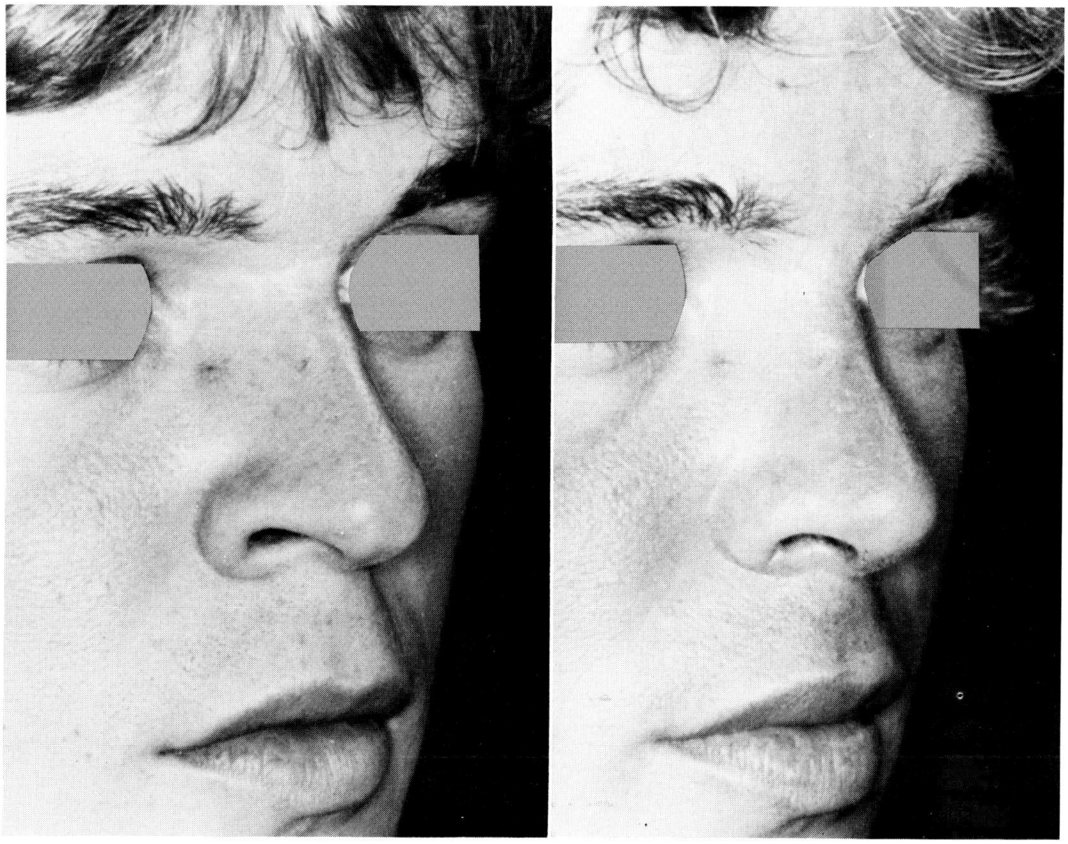

Nostrils that arch up and insert below the columella give the definite impression of a snarl. This unpleasant aspect of this patient's nasal base was corrected by effectively decreasing the length of the nostril. Nostril shortening was accomplished by resection of 2 mm of the vestibule and 3 mm of the lobule.

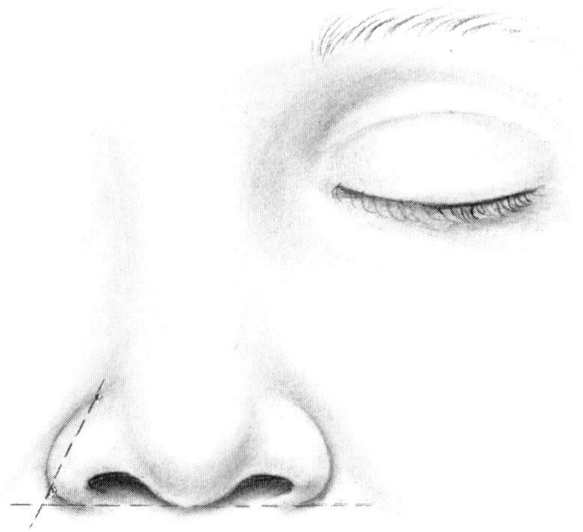

Plane of the alar lobule

An important consideration in planning alar resection is the position of the vertical plane of the alar lobule relative to the horizontal plane of the nasal base. Ideally the lobular plane should not be perpendicular to the basal plane but should slightly diverge laterally. Extreme lateral divergence is evident in flaring nostrils that need to be moved medially.

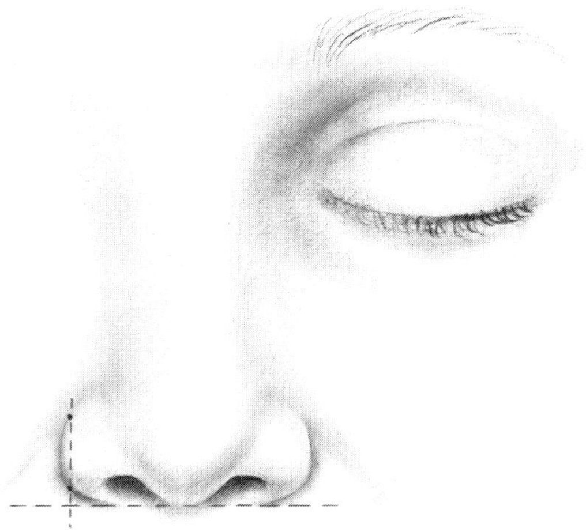

If the alar plane is perpendicular to the basal plane, alar resection should not be done.

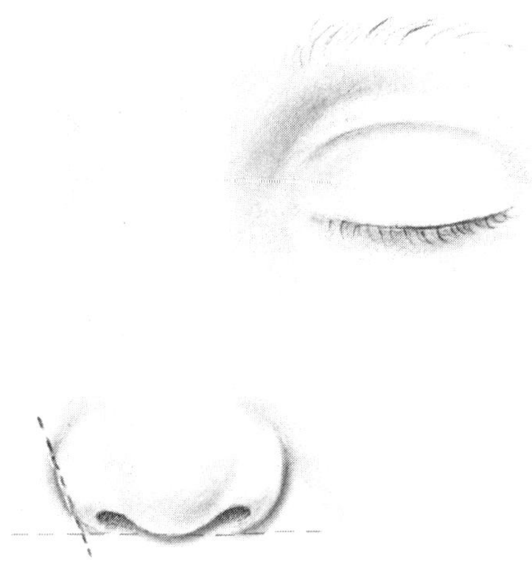

Wedge resections would cause a disproportionately narrow nasal base, resulting in a bowling pin appearance.

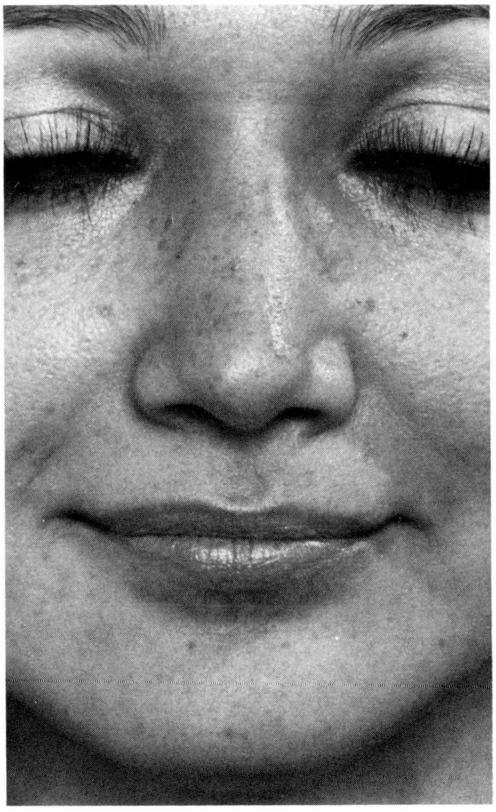

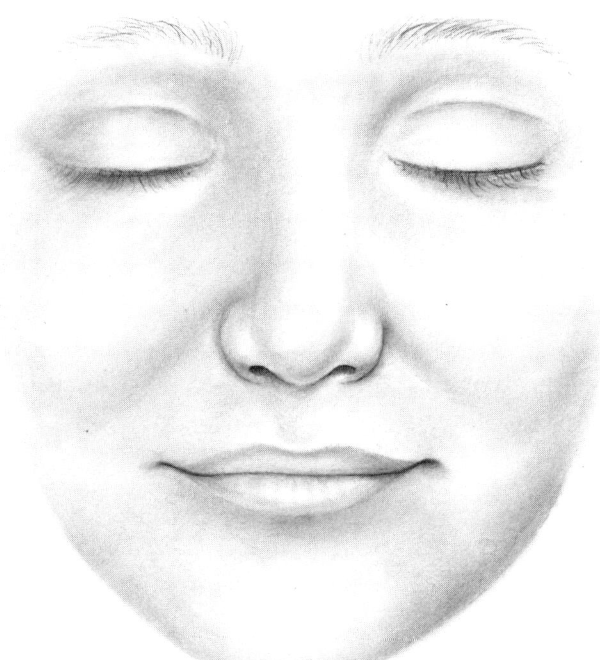

The nasal base that appears broad may have alar and basal planes that are perpendicular.

Though it may appear that alar resections would be beneficial, they probably would not. The drawing illustrates the likely aesthetic result if alar resections were done.

TIP GRAFT

Projection of the nasal tip past the dorsal line is one of the most common and difficult struggles in rhinoplasty. In primary rhinoplasty when the tissues are inadequate in substance or quantity, or in secondary rhinoplasty where supportive tissues are partially or wholly absent, augmenting or replacing the underlying structure of the tip becomes necessary. Without doing so, the aesthetic potential of many noses cannot be realized.

The use of an autogenous graft to the nasal tip has proved to be an effective and permanent means of achieving tip projection. Such grafts have been used and reported by surgeons for over 75 years. However, I do not think any graft previously reported has the efficacy of design and placement of the graft to be described.

An optimum result using a tip graft is contingent on the following:

1. *Mobility.* In animation, the nasal tip is brought toward the face by the action of the zygomatic muscles. This natural movement of the tip toward the maxilla should be preserved. A good tip graft must be free floating, with no dependence for support on the maxilla, thus eliminating a tent pole effect.

2. *Prime quality.* The graft material must be fairly rigid while allowing shaping with a scalpel or a bone-biting rongeur. It should not cause tissue reaction, absorb, or change shape after insertion. It must be suitable for areas with little tissue cover.

3. *Contouring potential.* A tip graft must achieve the desired end result of tip contour and projection without disturbing the delicate natural relationships of the nasal tip. The desirable angulation at the columellar-lobular junction must be preserved.

The material best suited to meet these criteria is septal cartilage. Although tip grafts of septal cartilage are not always successful, they are frequently the only hope for an otherwise unacceptable aesthetic result.

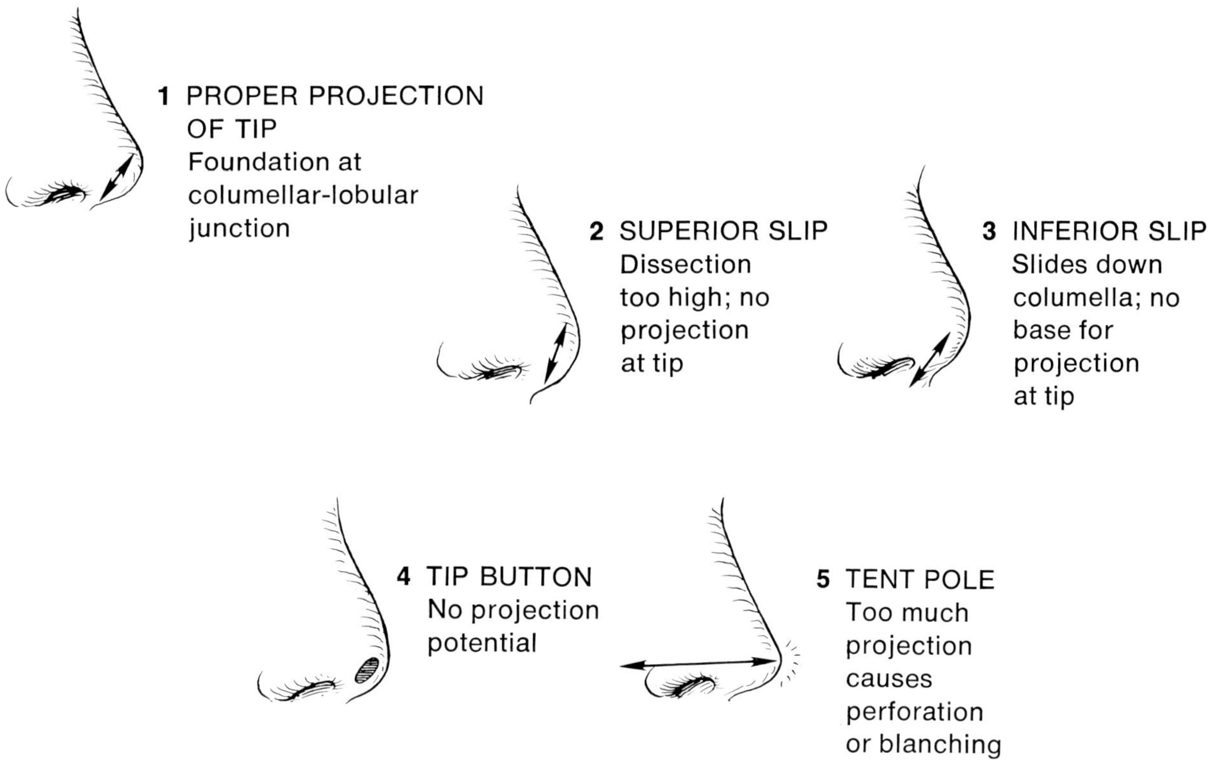

Tip graft placement

Note the various possibilities of tip graft replacement.

1. A properly designed graft should be placed high on the columella or at the columellar-lobular junction with a slight (35-degree) cephalic tilt. This potition places the internal points of stress at the tip and the columellar-lobular junction.
2. No projection results if the graft is allowed to slide too far superiorly. There is a tendency toward superior slippage if the lower lateral cartilages have been dissected free.
3. Unless the graft is based on the columellar-lobular junction, it tends to slide inferiorly, thus losing its footing.
4. The tip button has been advocated to fill out the tip contour and is an effective graft for that purpose. However, it does not have any projection potential.
5. Finally, a long strut in the columella obliterates the desirable break at the columellar-lobular junction. If it is long enough to be effective, it usually causes blanching. Moreover, if good judgment is not exercised with regard to length, the strut can perforate the skin of the nasal tip.

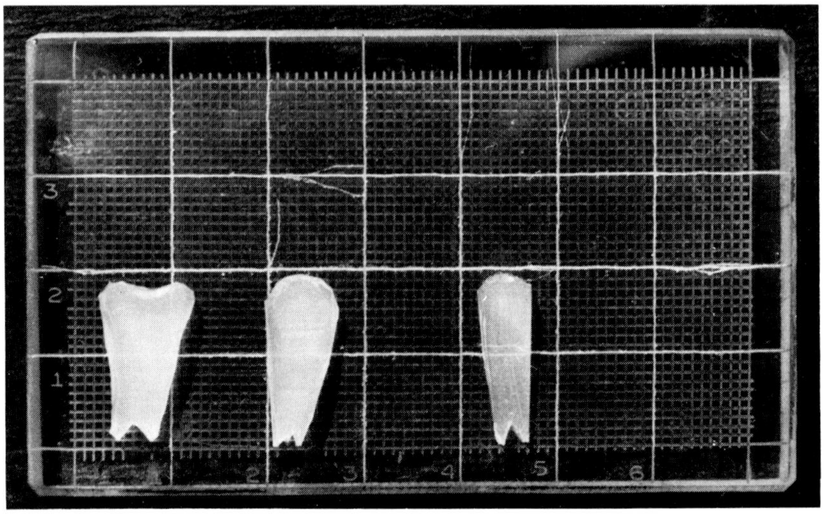

Tip graft design

The design of the tip graft as originally conceived had a broad, undulant superior surface to re-create the domes of the lateral crura. This graft design served well in noses with supple tissues but did poorly in tips scarred by multiple procedures. In these cases, improved results have been obtained by narrowing the superior end of the graft to decrease the mechanical advantage of that part over the base. With a narrow graft, there is less chance for the graft to be forced inferiorly. However, a narrow graft produces a single pointed tip, which, though undesirable, must sometimes be a compromise in order to attain tip projection.

These models demonstrate the most frequently used designs for tip grafts.

Tip graft problems

The following may be tip graft problems:

1. Malposition of the graft, with resultant asymmetry
2. Blanching of the tip, caused by a narrow graft or very thin tissues
3. Overprojection, resulting in an artificial appearance
4. Vascular compromise leading to tissue necrosis, caused by an oversized graft
5. Late disappearance of the graft, caused by slippage or partial absorption

The incidence of these complications varies with the experience of the surgeon and the condition of the tissues. However, the only complication resulting in permanent deformity is the perforation of tissues. With all other complications the result is reversible, since the tip graft simply can be modified or removed.

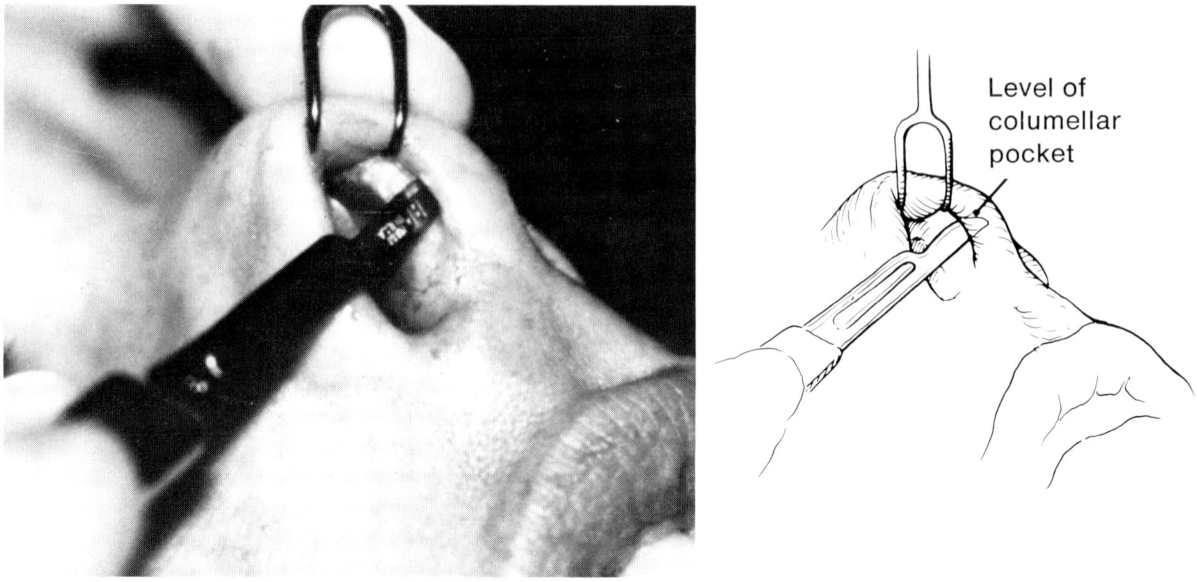

Surgical procedure

After the preliminary version of the graft has been rendered, an incision is made lateral to the columella—*never in the midline*. The incision begins no lower than the columellar-lobular junction and continues along the caudal border of the medial crus of the lower lateral cartilage.

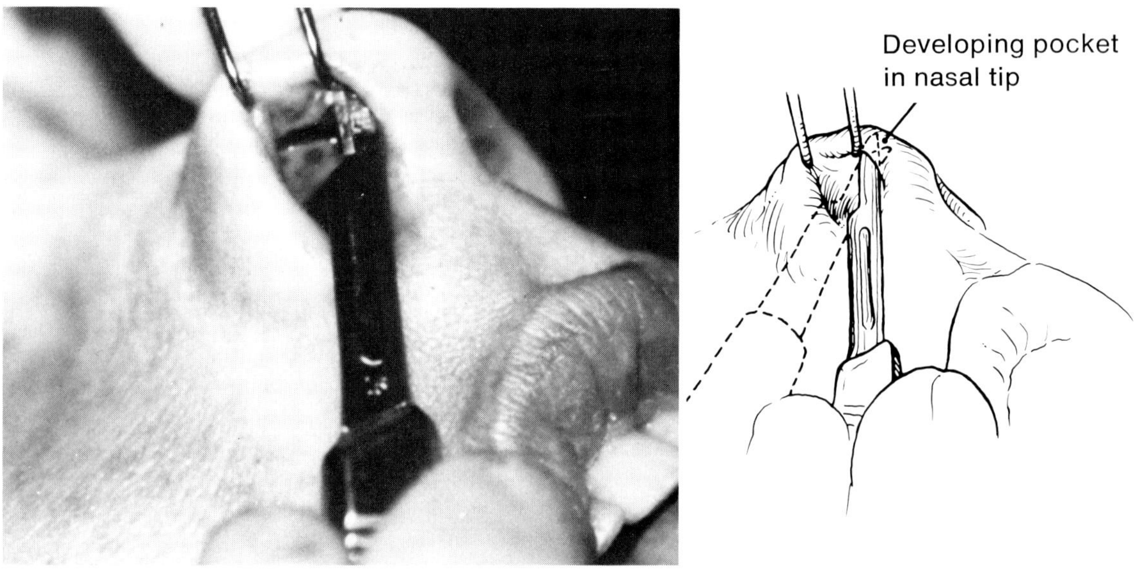

The incision is swept superiorly, anterior to the cartilage into the lobule. It is then swept laterally, staying close to the caudal reflection of the lower lateral cartilage. The pocket in the lobule is made with a scalpel or a Joseph scissors.

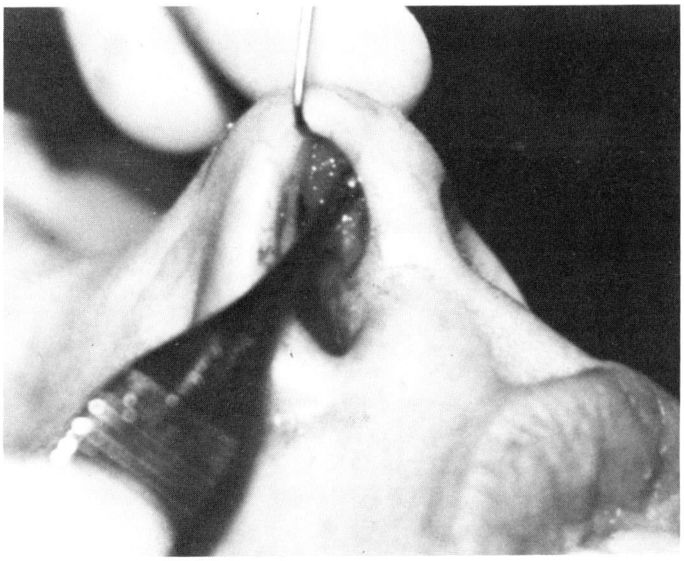

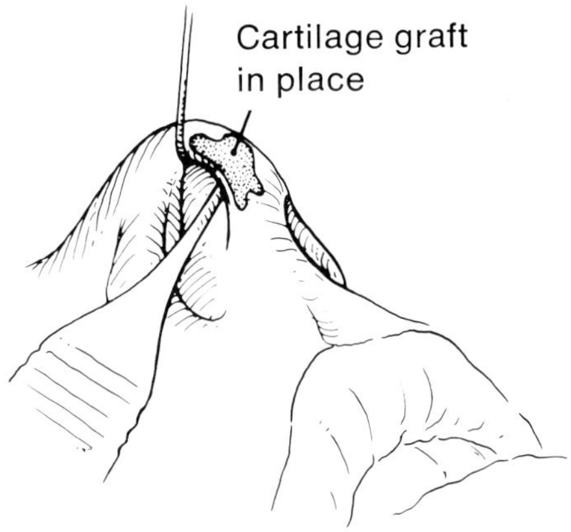

The graft is carefully placed in the pocket. If difficulty is encountered in placing the graft, the wound is opened laterally—never inferiorly—so that the foundation for the graft is not disturbed. Following insertion of the superior end of the graft, a judgment is made concerning the length. Obviously, it is wise to err on the long side. After the correct length has been determined, the inferior end of the graft is notched and then seated into the columella with the help of a single hook. The wound is closed with interrupted 5-0 plain catgut sutures. The position is secured by placing a tape dressing over the dorsum and tip as is done following the usual rhinoplasty. The dressing is left in place for 1 week.

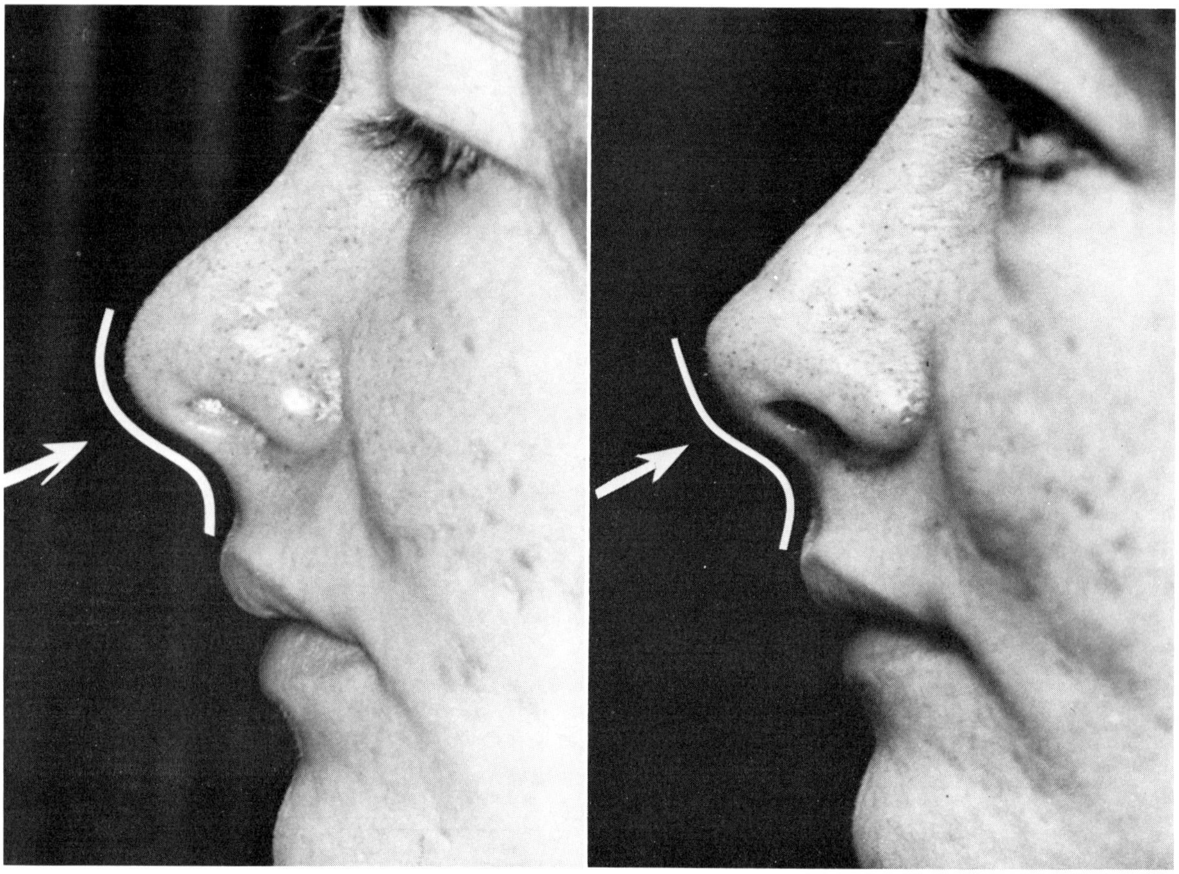

Correct placement of a tip graft provides the illusion of lengthening by providing an endpoint to the dorsal profile. It also provides the break at the columellar-lobular junction. Note the effect of lengthening and the effect on the columellar-lobular angle. This patient also had dorsal augmentation.

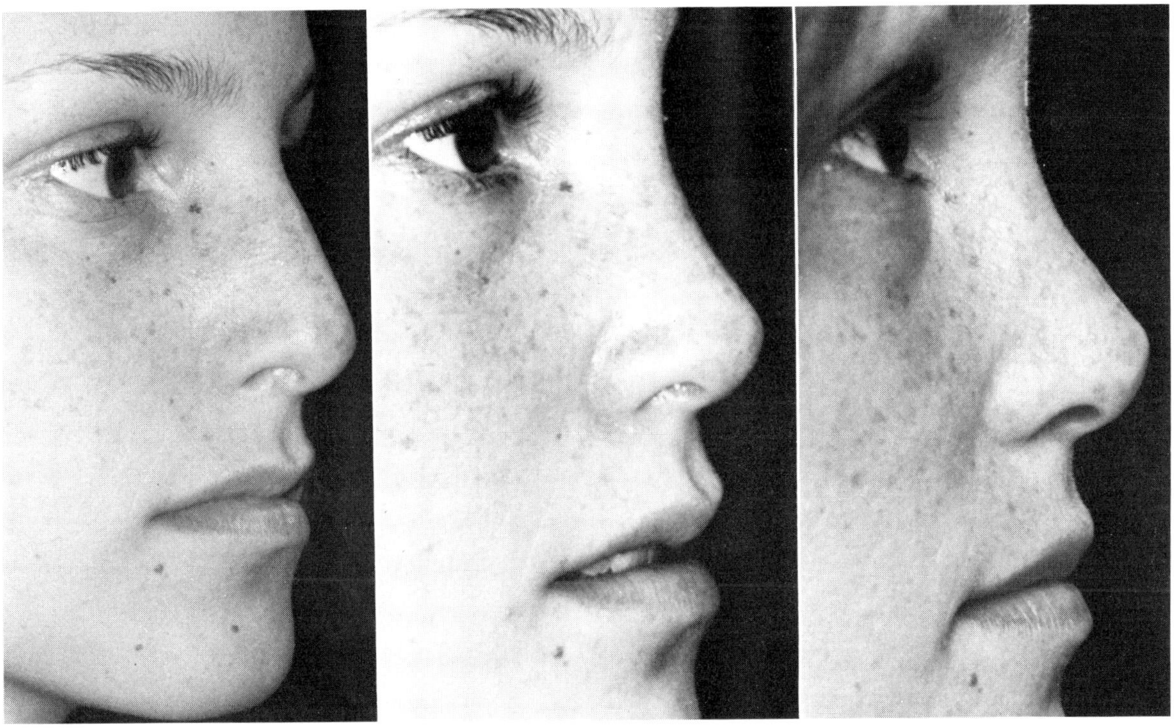

These are comparative photographs of a patient before surgery and then 1 year and 4 years after tip graft placement. Virtually no change has occurred in the projection of the tip 4 years after surgery.

EAR CARTILAGE GRAFTS

The cartilage from the concha of the ear is a high-quality autogenous reconstructive tissue that is available in substantial amounts. It is an excellent material for nasal reconstruction not only when septal cartilage is lacking, but when a smooth, convex surface is required. For example, the convex surface of the concha re-creates an excellent dorsal contour without irregularities. Other uses for conchal cartilage include tip grafts and vestibular atresias.

The total resection of the concha through an anterior approach leaves minimal deformity and is simpler than the posterior approach. The following technique was introduced to me by Dr. Burt Brent.

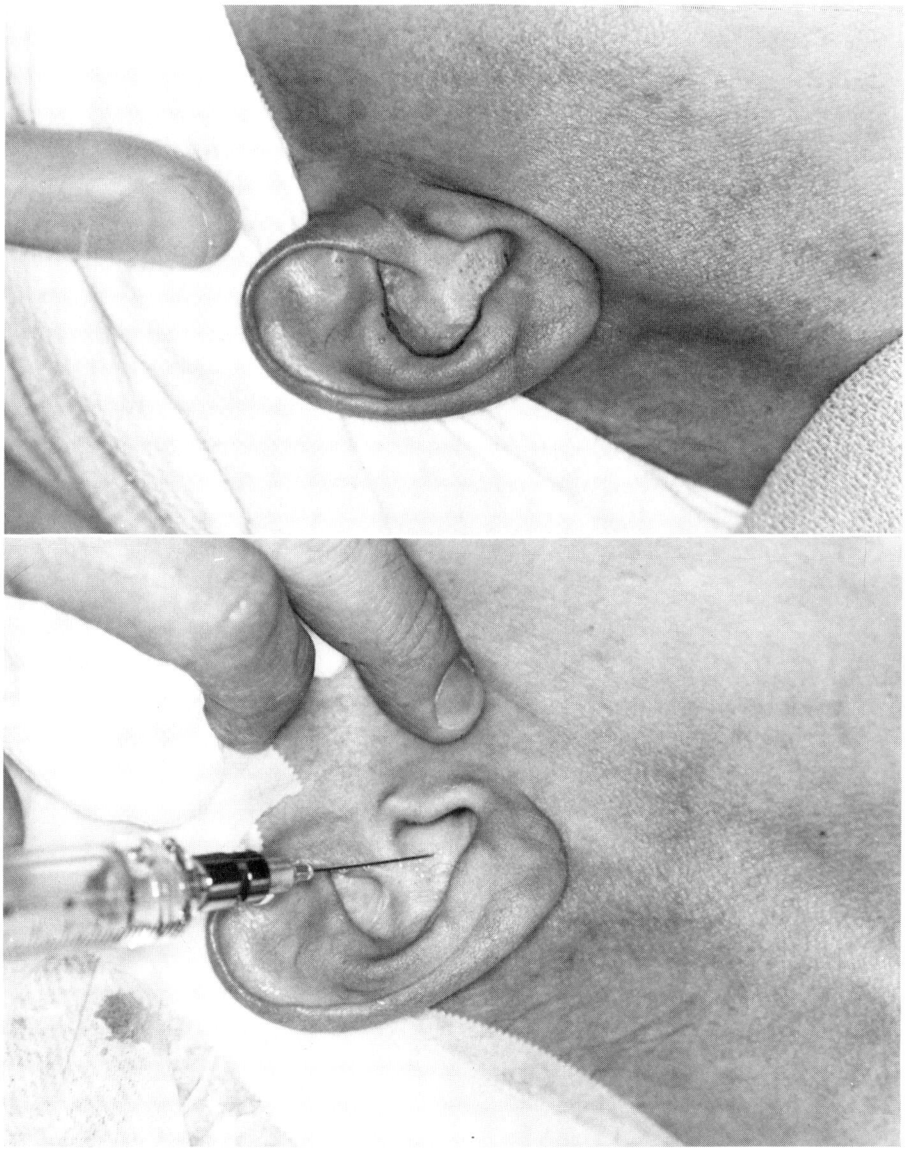

Surgical technique

Following the usual preoperative preparation, the line of incision is marked, extending from the farthest point of the inferior crus, around the antihelical curve, and ending just below the external auditory canal. The skin and perichondrium are then infiltrated with 1% Xylocaine with 1:100,000 epinephrine, elevating the perichondrium anteriorly. The cartilage is pierced to enable posterior infiltration.

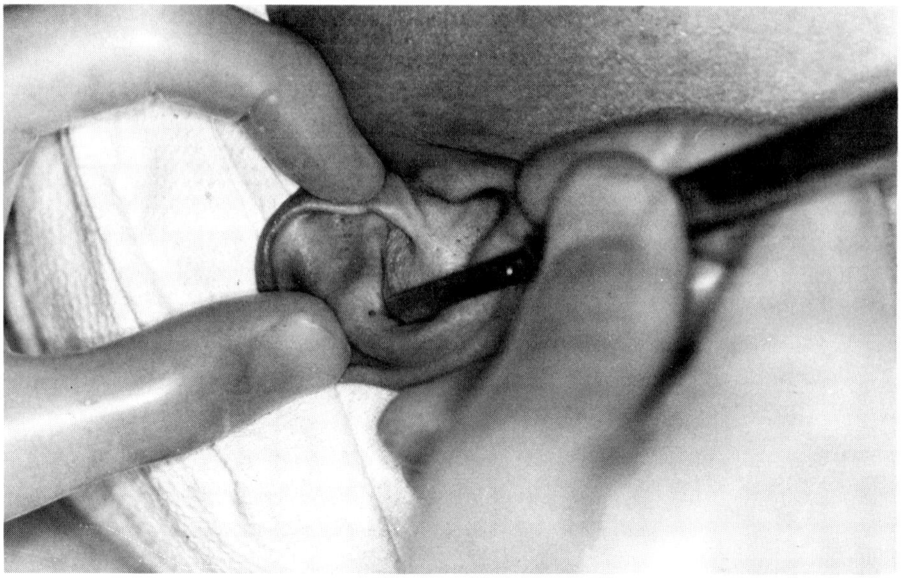

A No. 15 blade is used to incise along the area marked, with the incision going into but not through the conchal cartilage. Incising into the cartilage facilitates dissection of the perichondrium from the anterior surface.

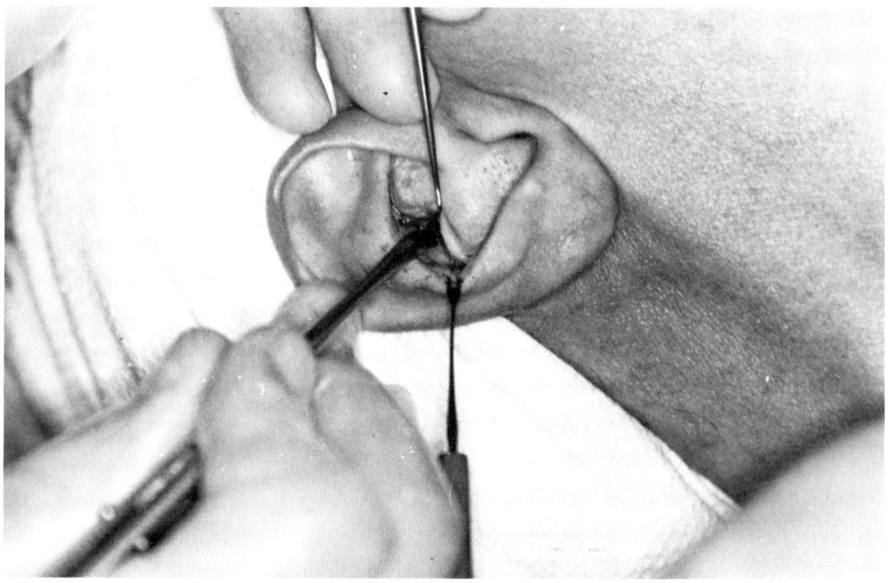

The anterior flap is retracted with a hook while the ear is stabilized with a small double hook. A Freer elevator is used to dissect into the subperichondrial plane.

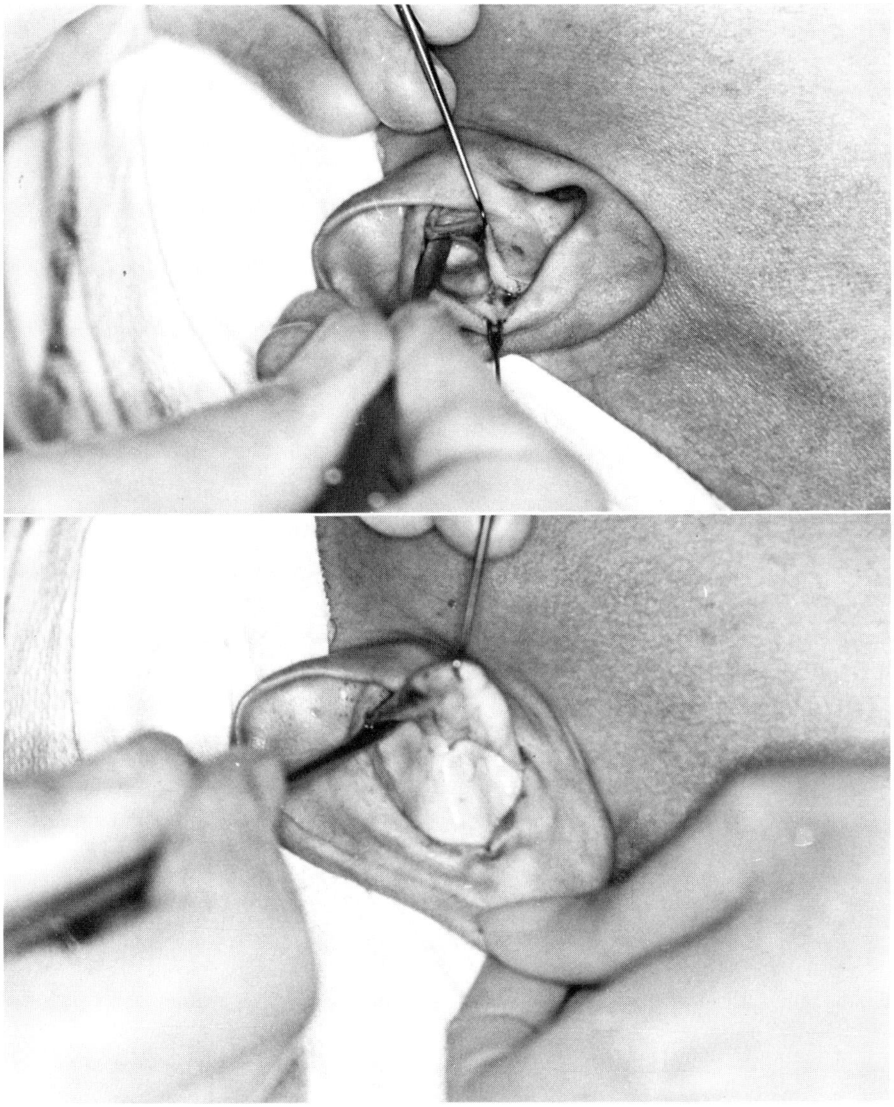

The dissection is continued with the blunt end of the Freer elevator. Care is taken not to fracture or tear the conchal cartilage during the course of dissection. The dermal perichondrial flap is retracted while the dissection is completed.

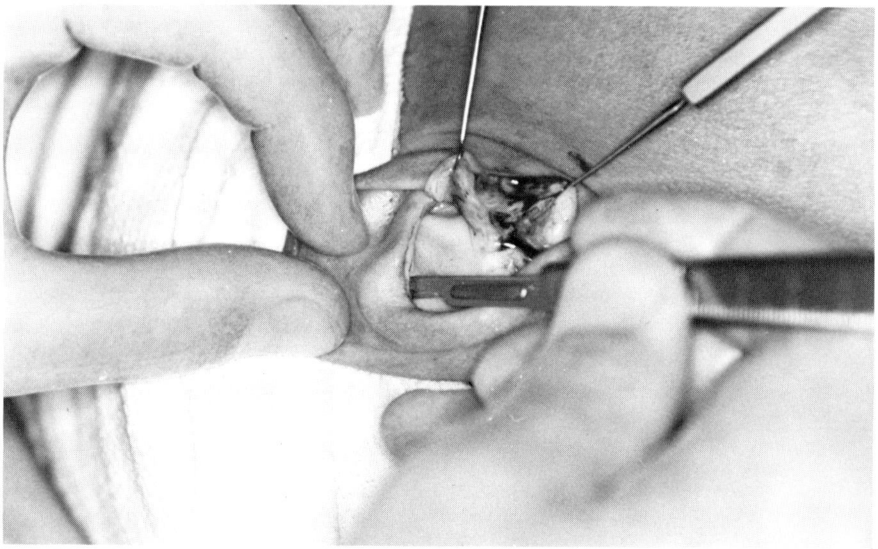

The cartilage is incised along the entire perimeter of the wound, extending through the perichondrium. The perichondrium ensures the survival of the free-cartilage graft, but it also provides needed substance for the remaining concha. Because of the benefit to both donor and recipient sites, the anterior perichondrial layer is preserved for the donor site, and the posterior layer is resected with the graft.

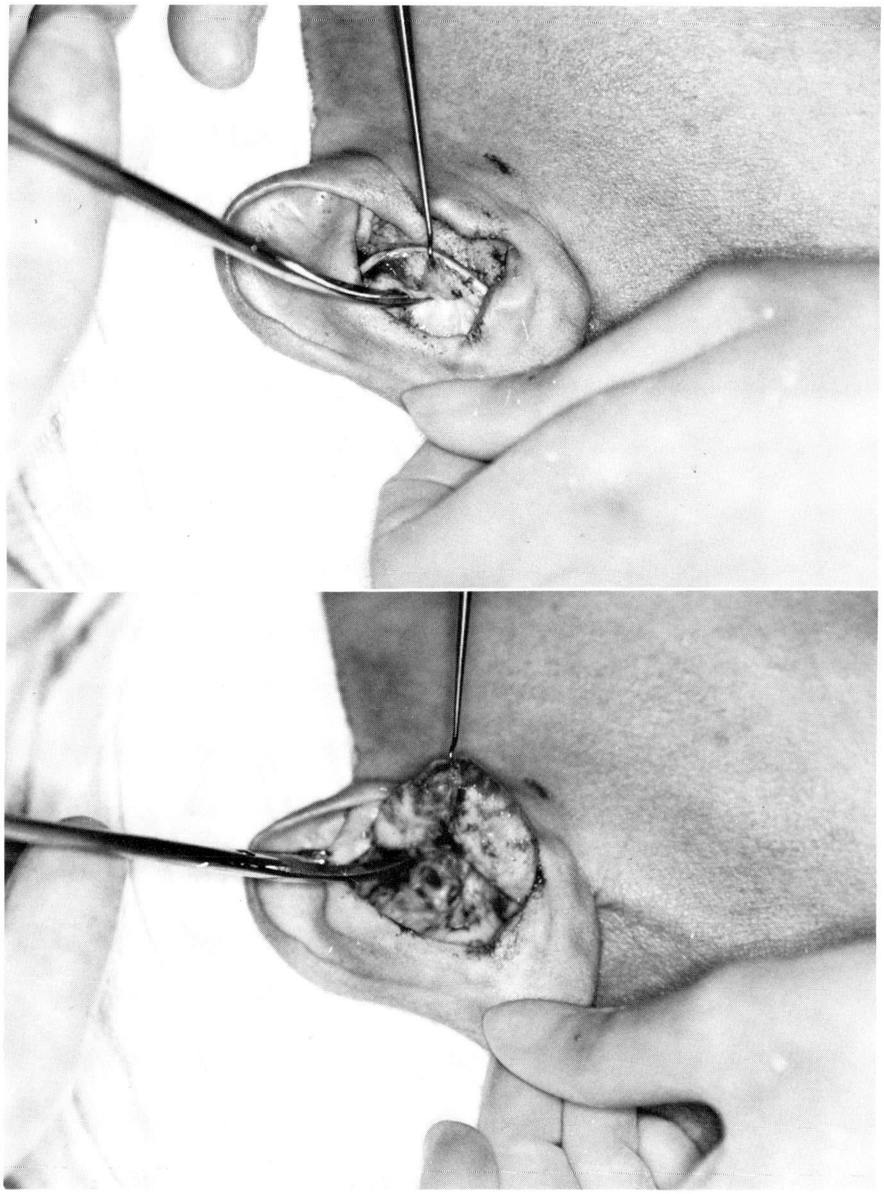

A single hook is used to gently retract the cartilage forward while a curved Joseph scissors dissects along a subperichondrial plane to free the entire conchal cartilage.

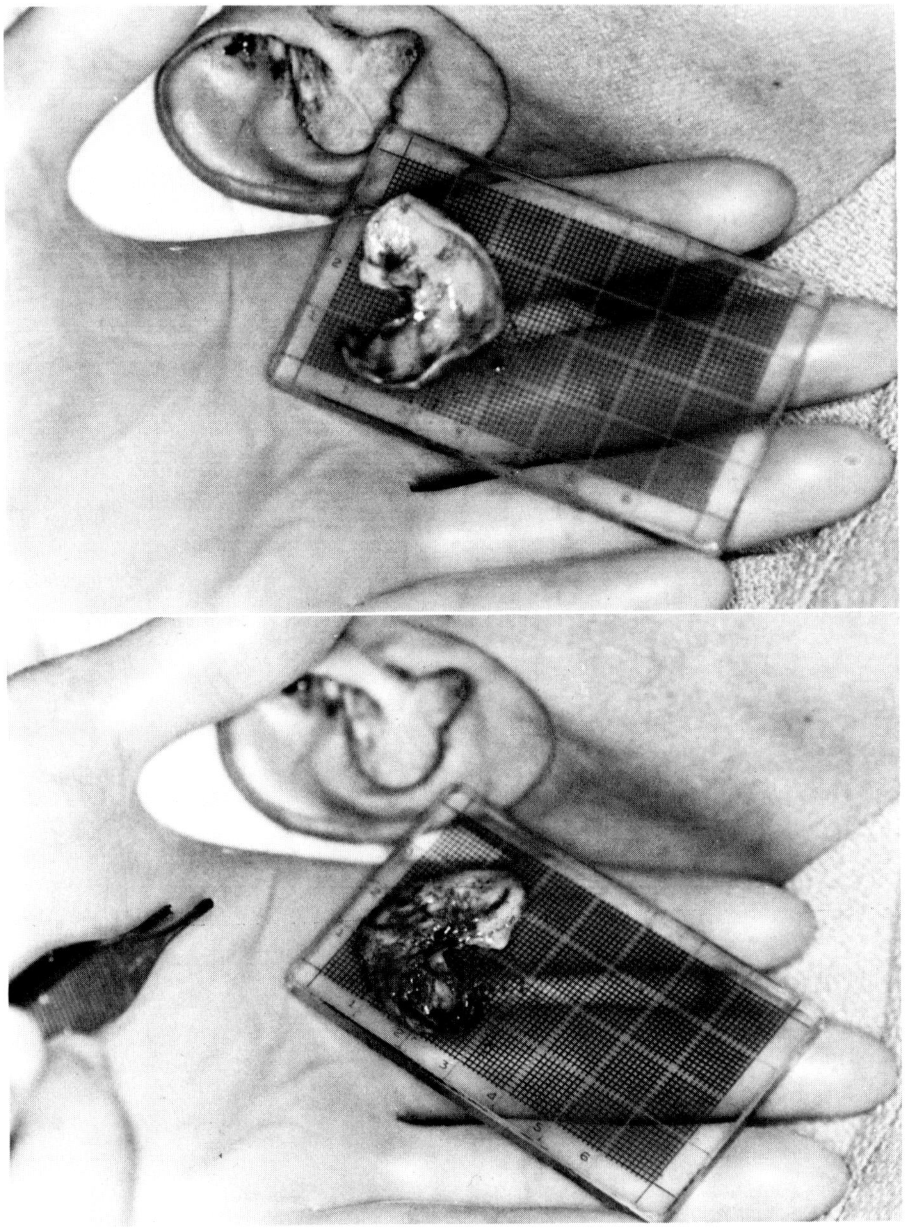

The specimen is placed on a cm/mm grid with the anterior surface void of perichondrium and the posterior surface with perichondrium attached.

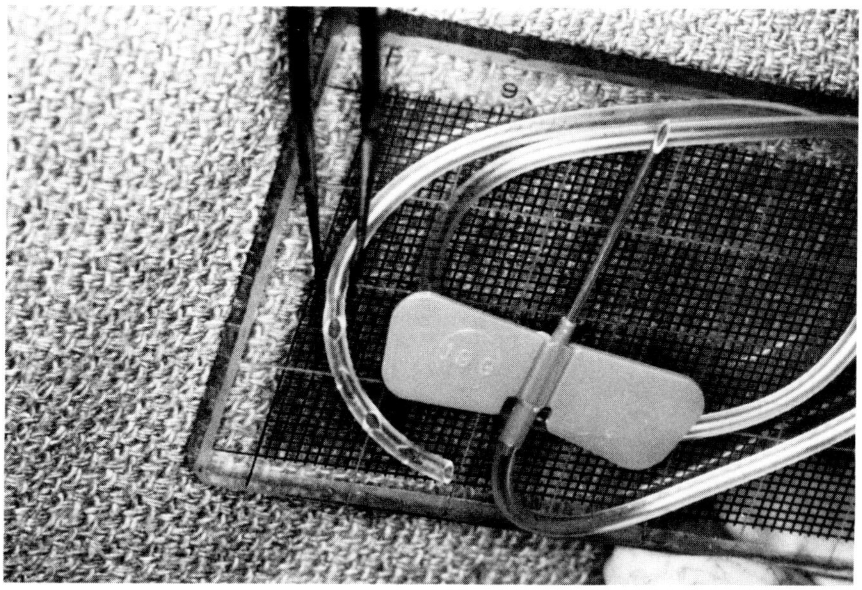

A 19-gauge butterfly infusion set is prepared by cutting off the connector and notching three or four holes along the distal 2.5 cm.

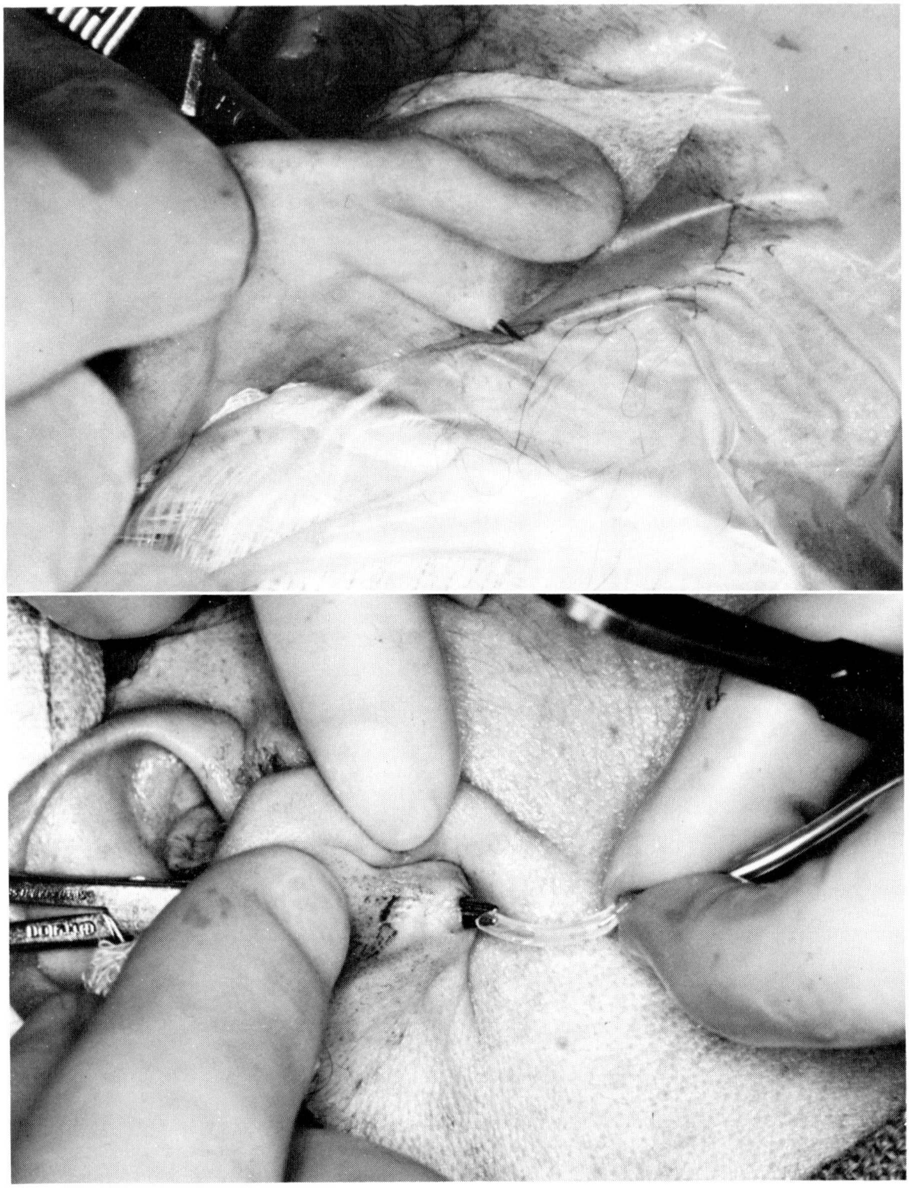

A small hole is placed through the inferior pole of the concha, and the prepared distal end of the tubing is drawn through the wound.

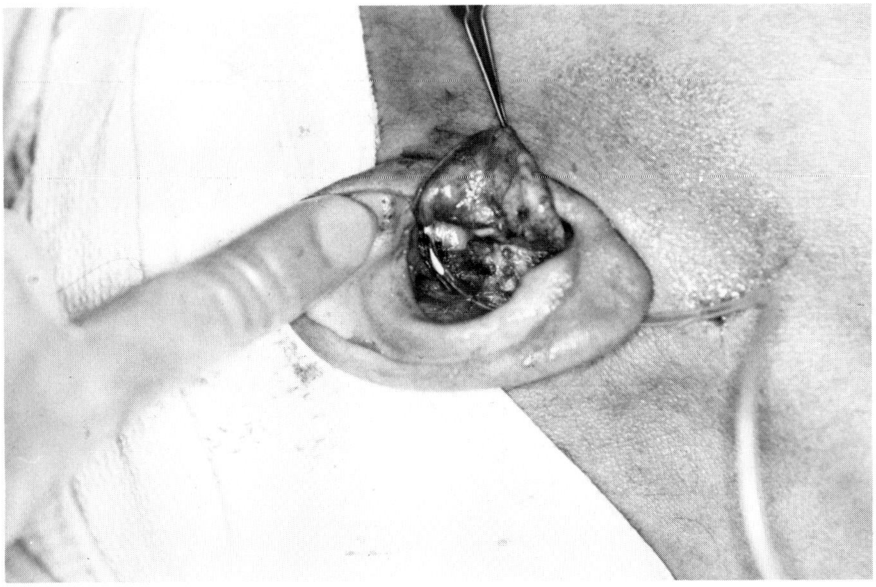

The end of the tubing is fixed to the floor of the concha by a single 7-0 chronic suture. The tubing is secured externally by fixation sutures of 5-0 plain catgut.

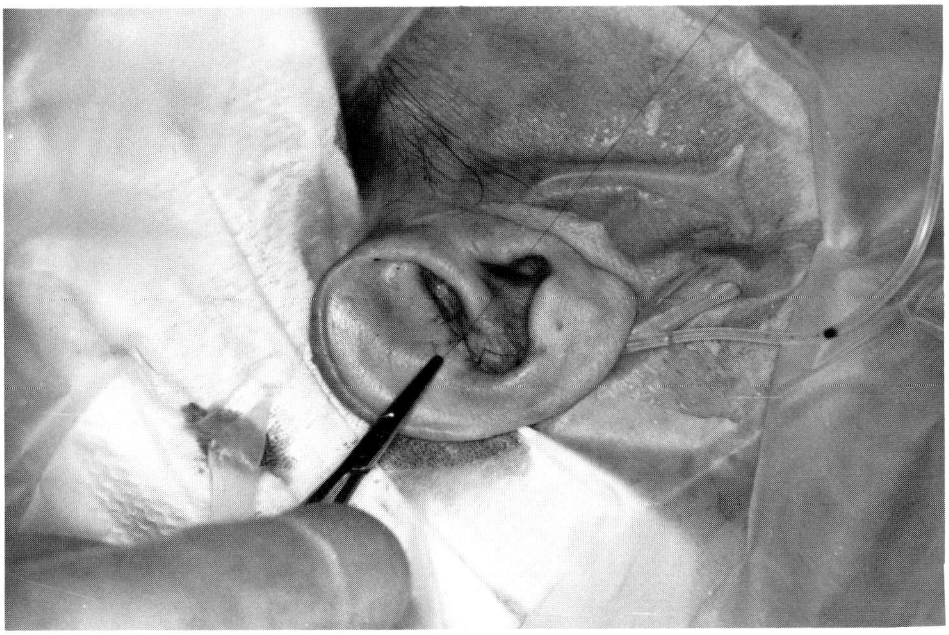

The wound is closed with a running lock suture of 7-0 chromic catgut.

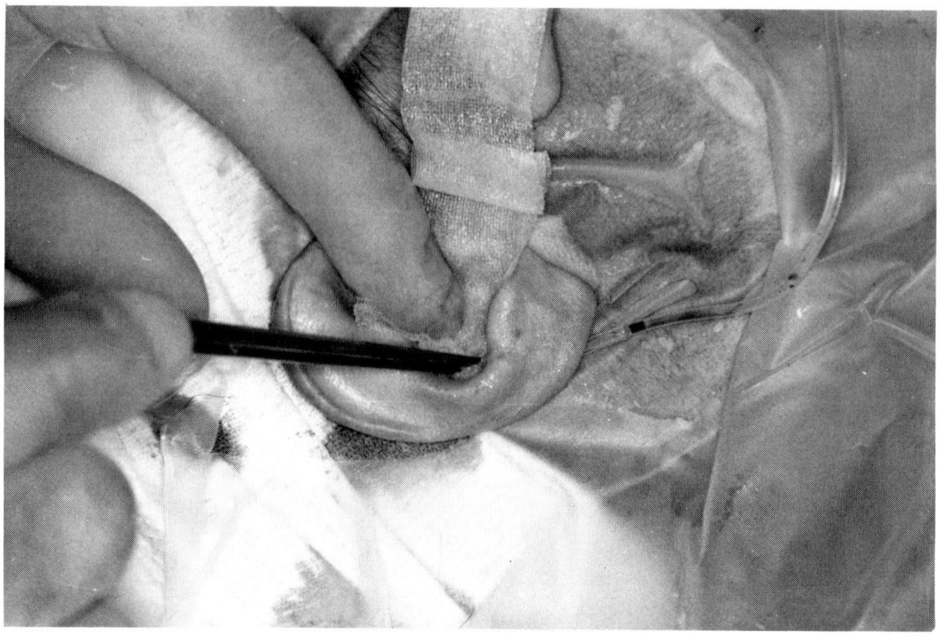

Vaseline gauze is gently packed into the concha.

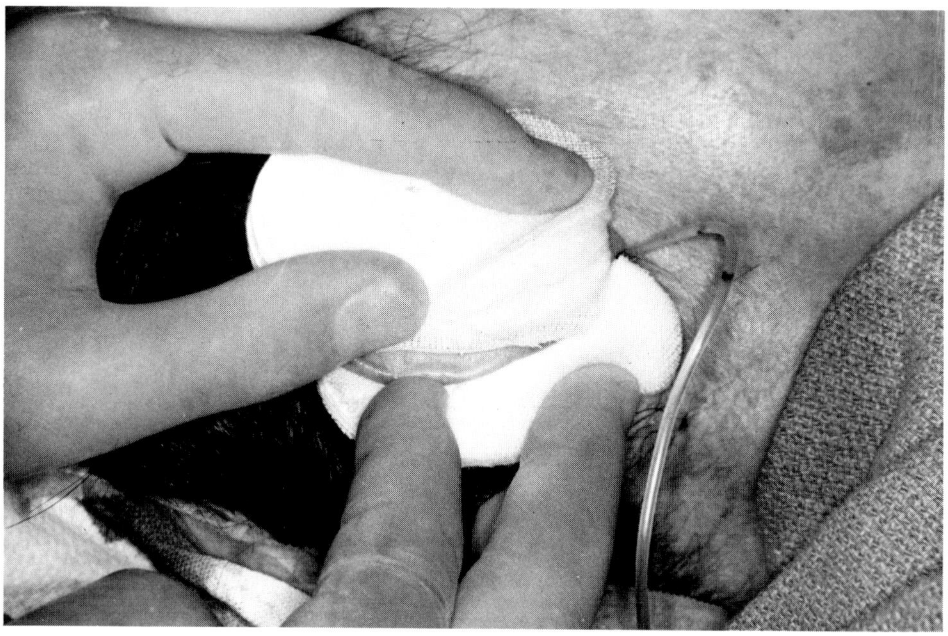

The ear is covered with an eye pad, and another is placed behind the ear.

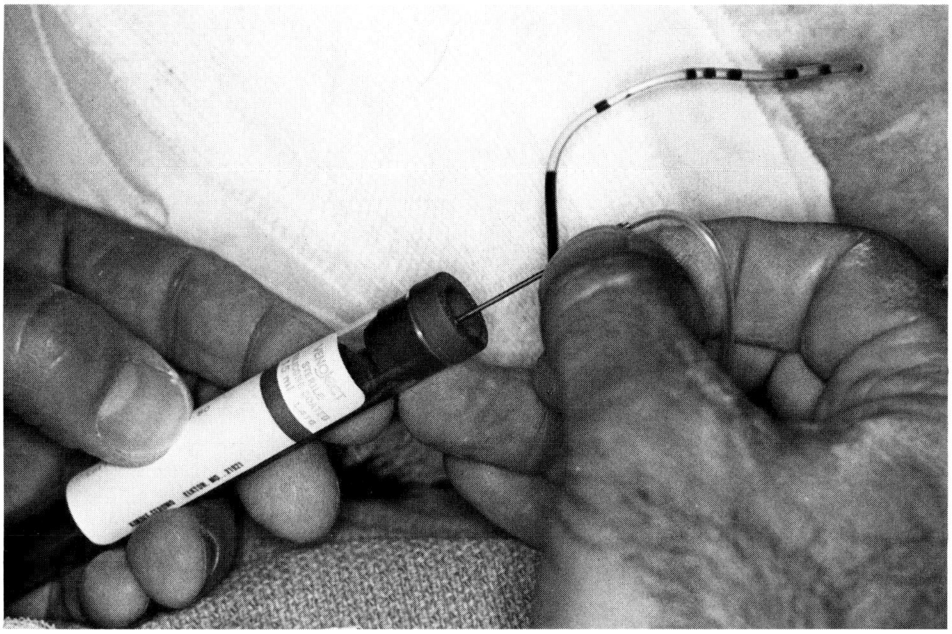

The butterfly needle is inserted into a blood collection vacuum tube.

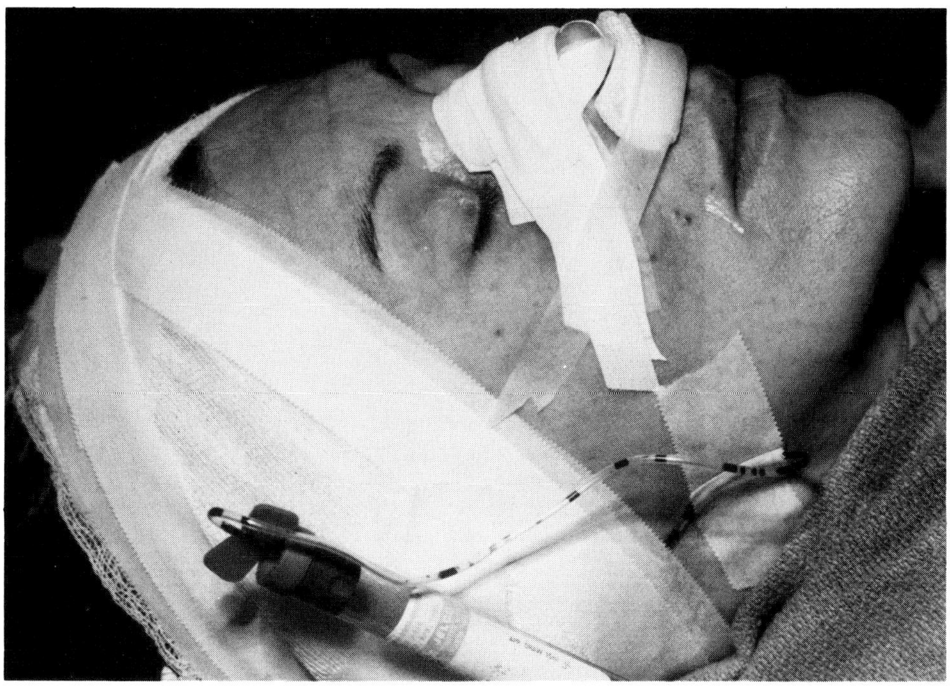

A circumferential Kling dressing completes the procedure.

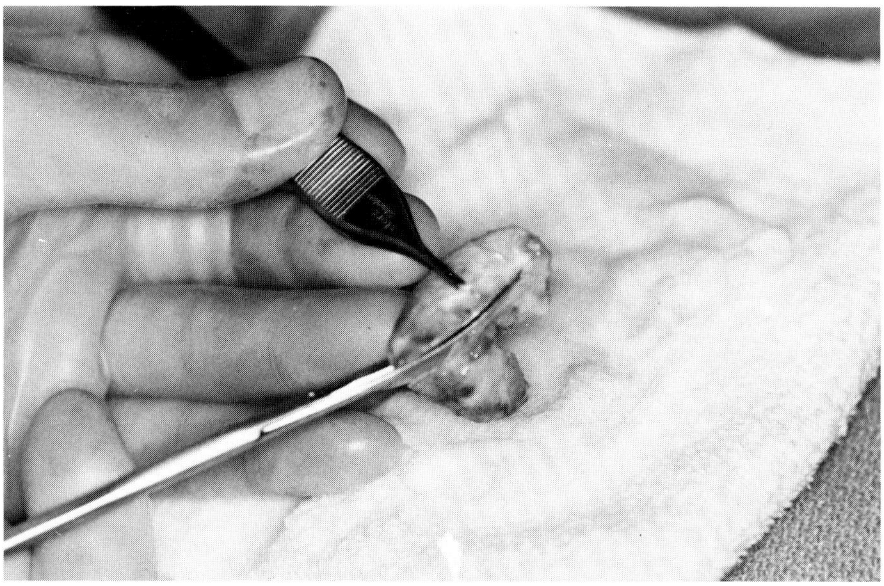

Conchal cartilage for dorsal grafts

The natural curve of the conchal cartilage makes a superb dorsal graft. The planning of the initial cut is crucial if the maximum length is to be obtained.

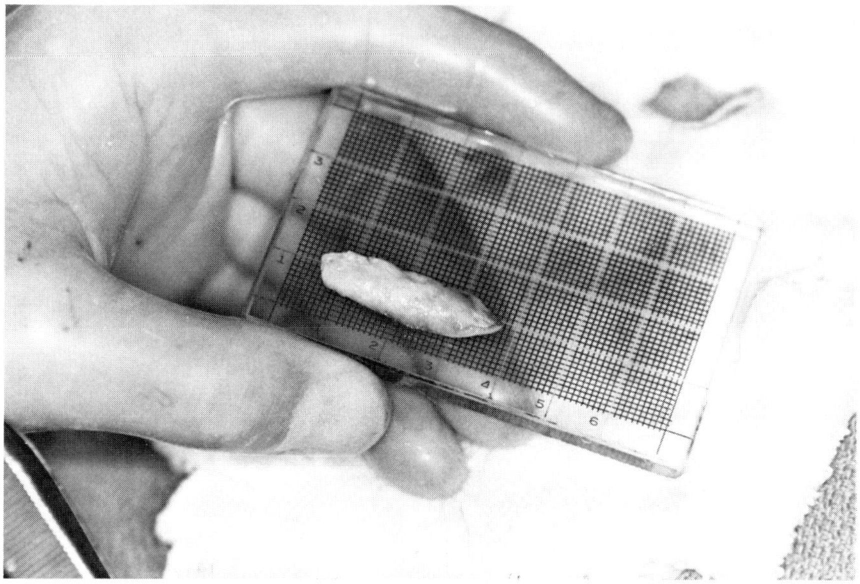

The prepared dorsal graft illustrates the excellent dorsal reproduction.

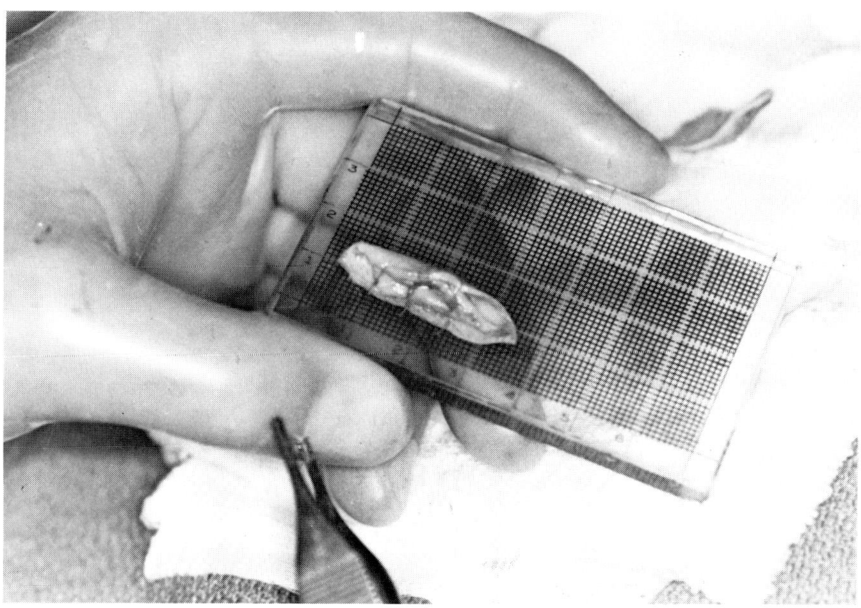

The graft is filled with residual pieces of cartilage and fixed by three 5-0 Dexon sutures.

CASE EXAMPLES

A dorsal graft from resected conchal cartilage was used in the nasal reconstruction of the patient below who had undergone five prior surgeries. In addition to the obvious disfigurement, there was total ablation of all usable cartilage and bone from the septum (see pp. 495-511).

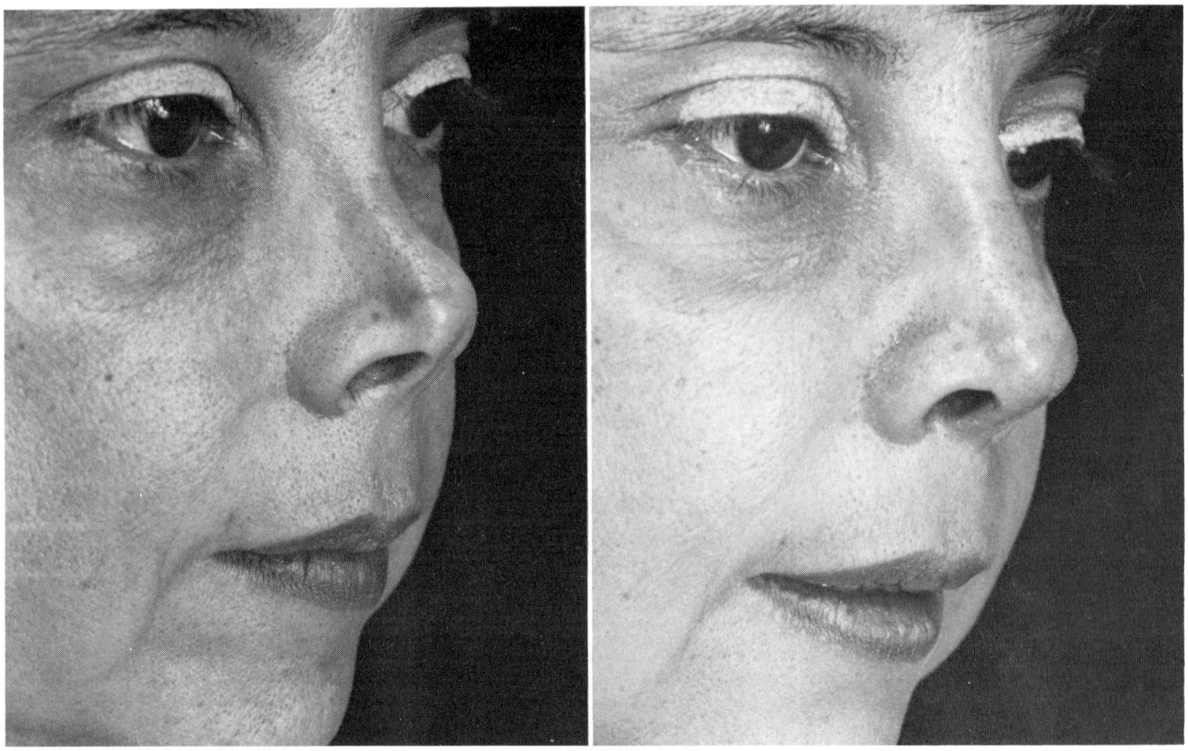

The patient on p. 253 blamed her long-standing psychiatric history on a loss of ethnicity subsequent to a primary rhinoplasty. Therefore, it was her adamant desire that her nose be restored. The patient specifically requested the return of her preoperative dorsal irregularity. With this in mind, conchal cartilage from the ear was selected as a dorsal graft because the natural curve of the cartilage so closely duplicates the normal fullness at the caudal end of the bony vault. Intentionally, the conchal cartilage graft was made slightly full in the middle third to re-create the preoperative contour.

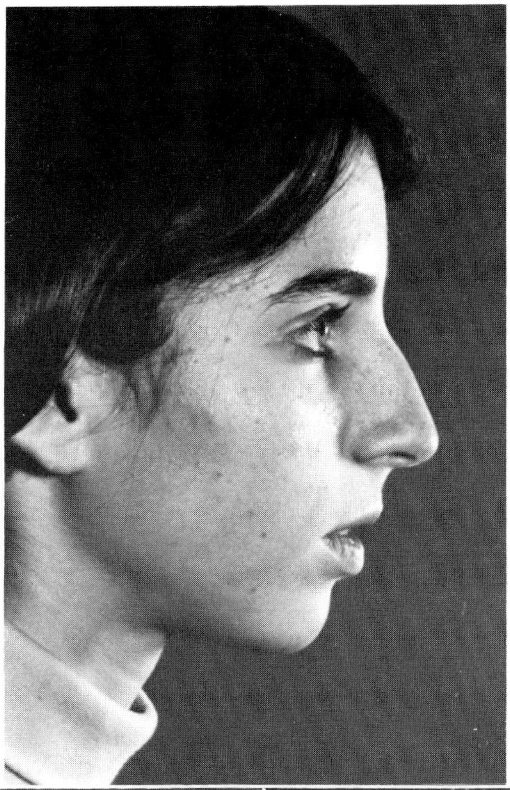

Preoperative view of patient

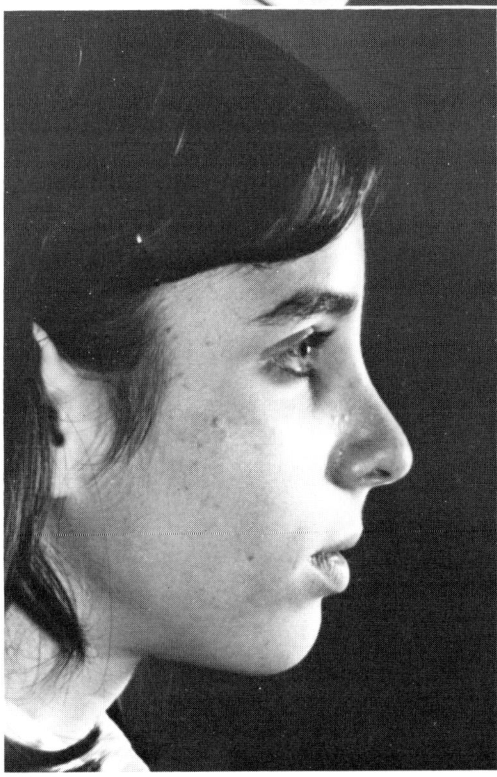

Postoperative result following primary rhinoplasty

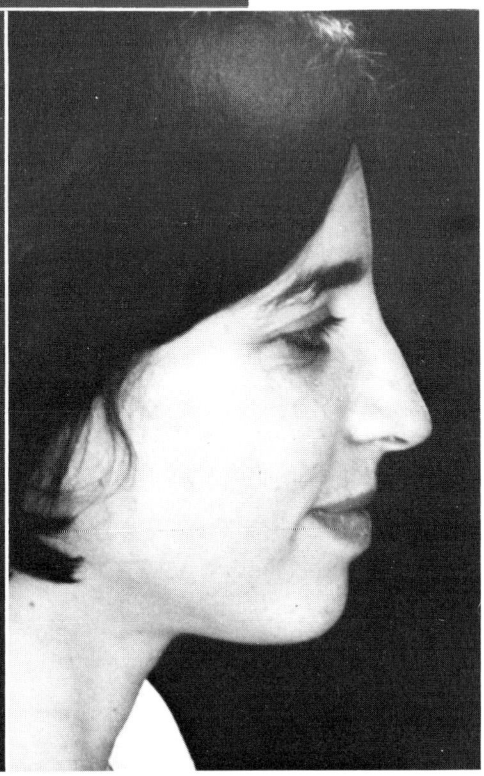

Secondary rhinoplasty result, an approximation of the primary nose

Conchal cartilage for tip grafts

Excellent material for tip grafts can be obtained from the inferior pole of the concha (cavum conchae) where the cartilage is thick and relatively flat.

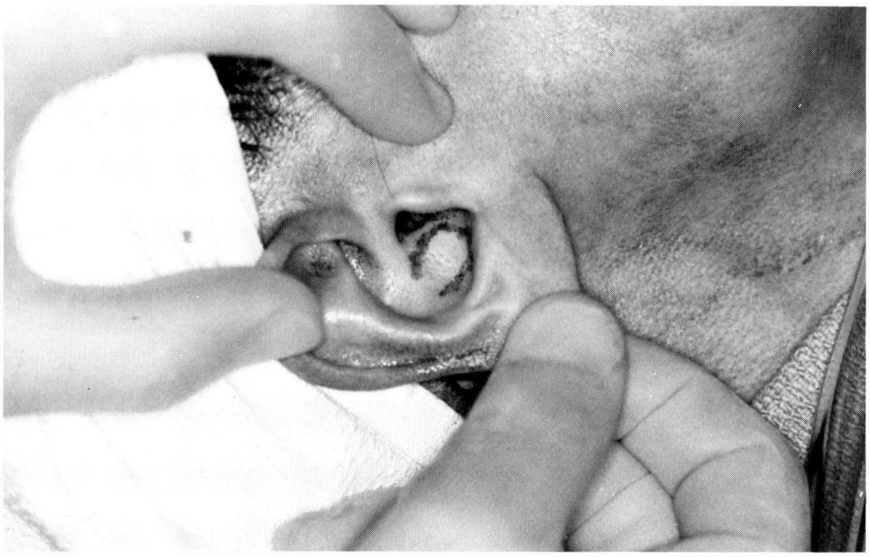

SURGICAL PROCEDURE

Following the usual preparation, the area of the graft is marked with gentian violet. The tissues over the area of dissection are infiltrated with 1% Xylocaine with 1 : 100,000 epinephrine. The cartilage is pierced with the needle, and the anesthetic is injected into the posterior surface.

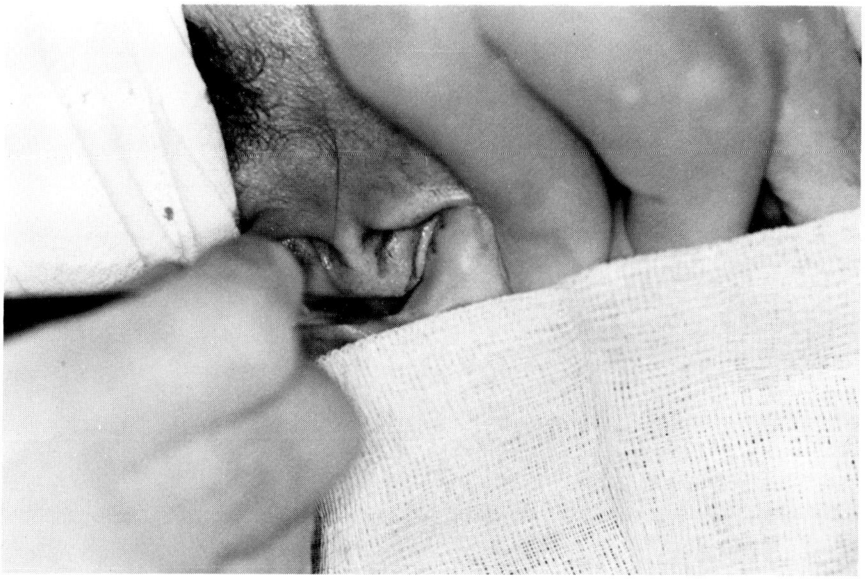

A crescent-shaped incision long enough to give access to the cartilage is made just below the antitragal protruberance.

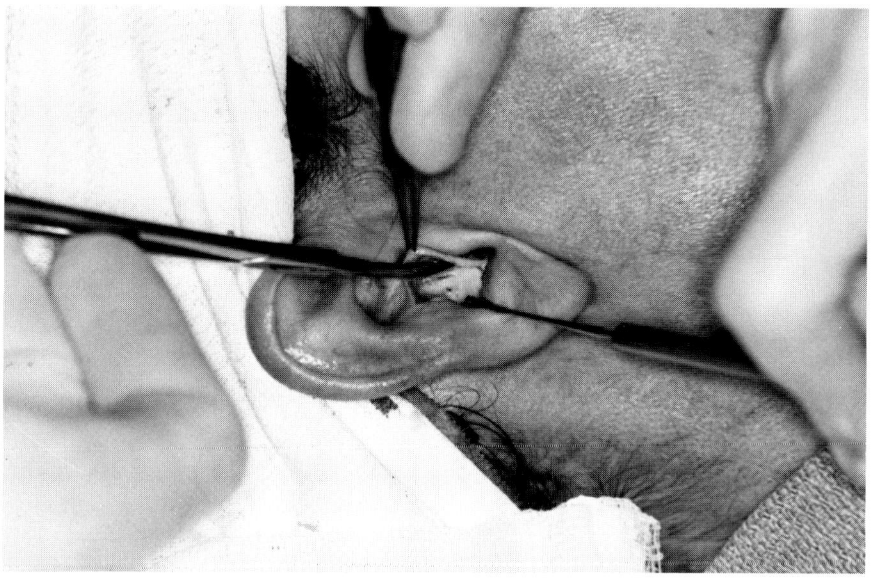

The anterior skin with perichondrium is dissected away from the cartilage.

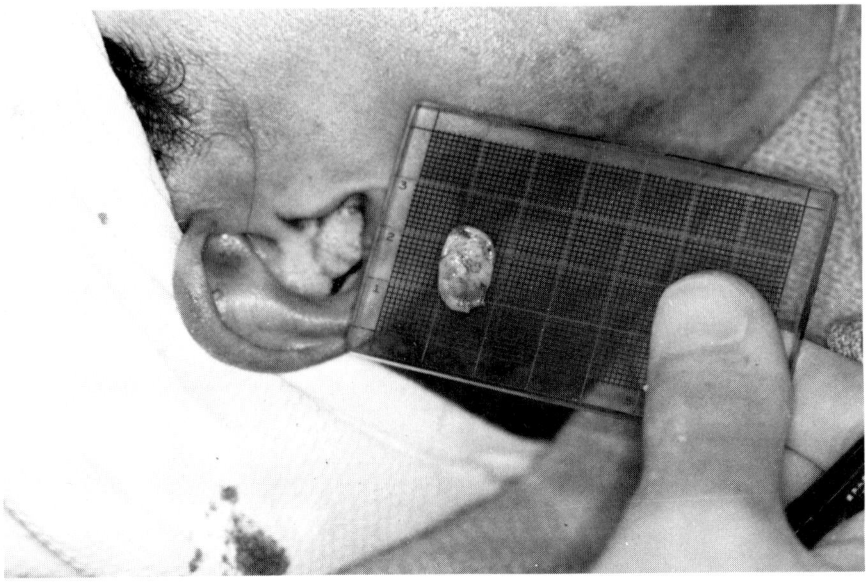

The cartilage is dissected out. The graft is shown following resection. It measures 10 × 16 mm and is over 1 mm thick. The posterior surface of the graft has perichondrium attached.

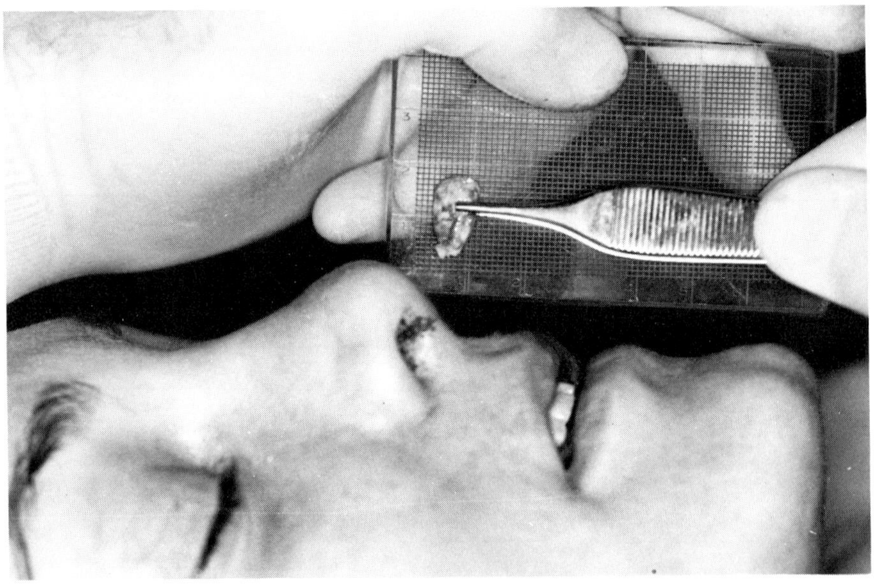

The graft is now ready for insertion.

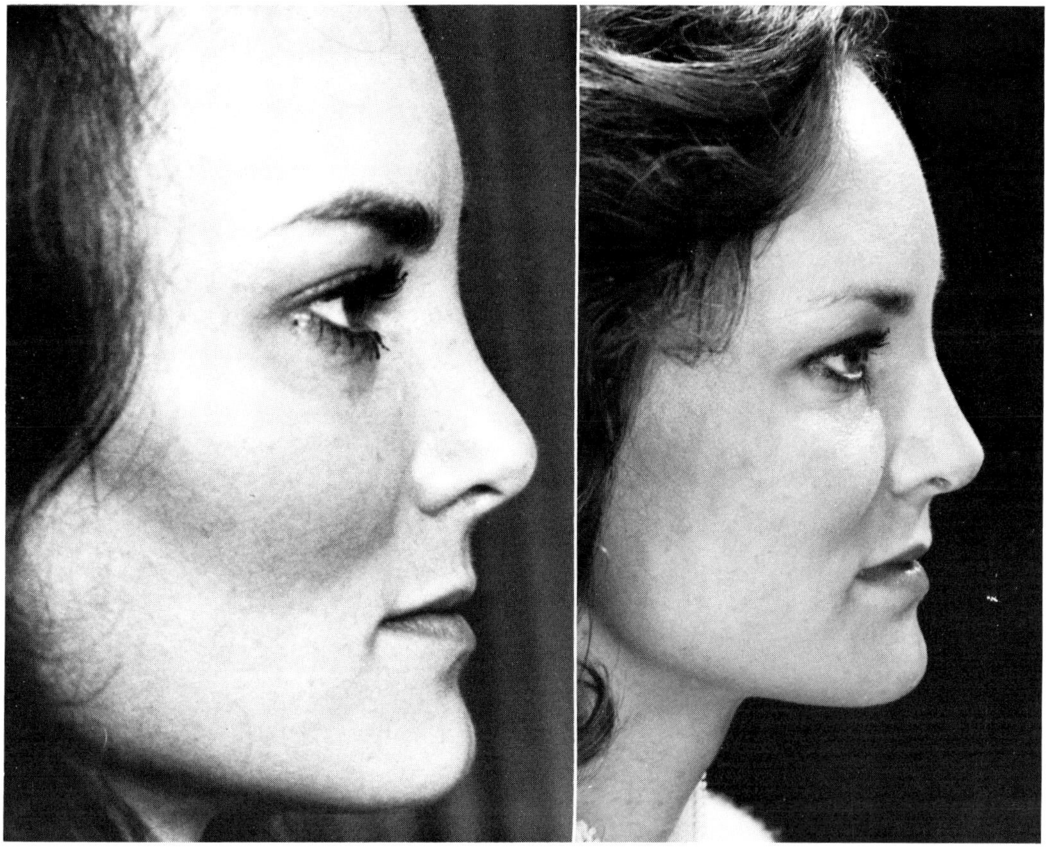

CASE EXAMPLE

This patient received a conchal cartilage graft to the nasal tip. She also had dorsal augmentation with remnants of septal cartilage.

Conchal cartilage for vestibular atresias

The correction of vestibular atresias is a notoriously frustrating problem because the forces of constriction are unrelenting. Full-thickness grafts contract unless the patient religiously and painstakingly wears an obturator for a protracted period of time. Even then, success is questionable. In general, local flaps provide good results for minor atresias (grades I and II), depending on the location of the atresia. However, for severe atresias the use of a composite graft from the anterior surface of the ear is a feasible and effective means of correction.

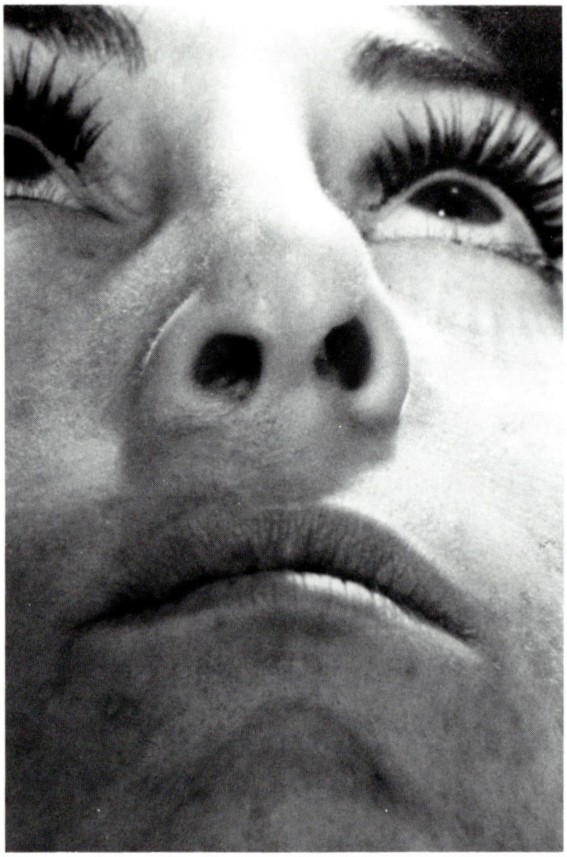

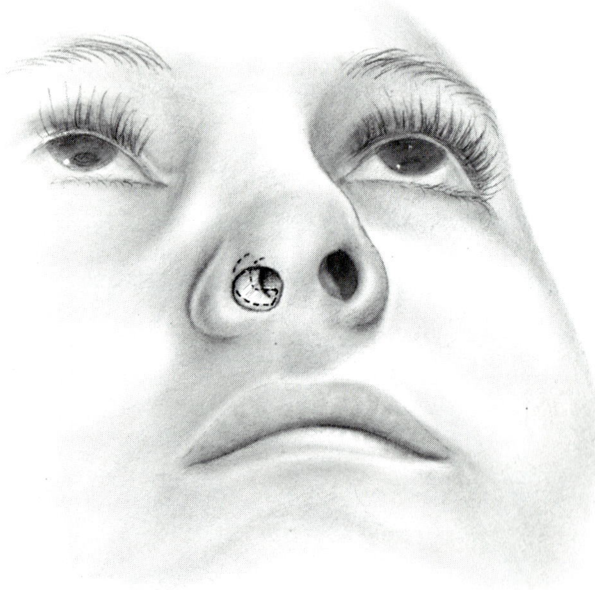

CASE REPORT

This patient has a cleft lip nasal deformity with a grade III vestibular atresia on her right. There had been one unsuccessful attempt to correct the atresia.

Parallel cuts were made bordering the synechial web, extending from the floor of the nose to the apex of the vestibule. These two cuts were joined at the distal end of the flap by an incision made on the nasal floor.

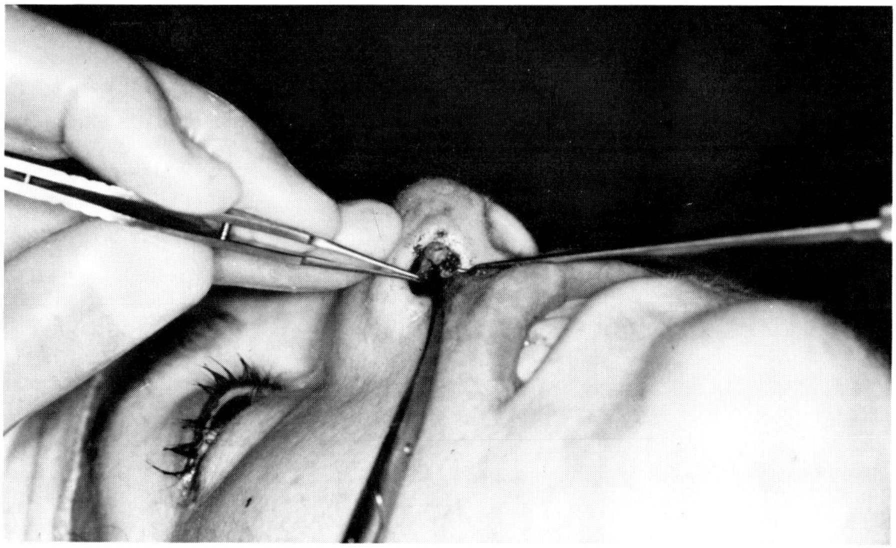

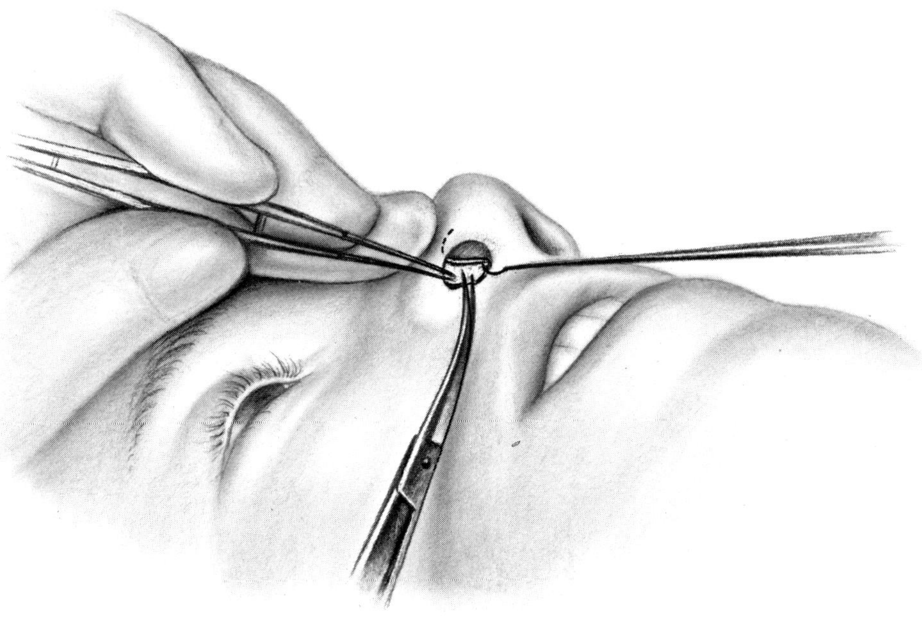

The flap was gently retracted with a single hook, and the thick scar tissues were dissected from the undersurface of the flap. The wide dissection and elevation of the flap left a large defect in the nasal wall and vestibular floor.

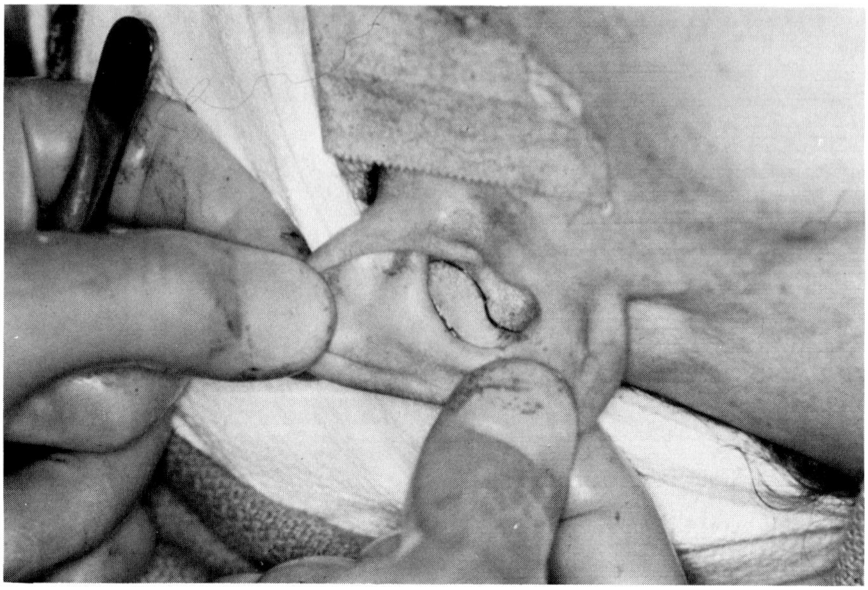

The graft size was estimated slightly larger than the defect.

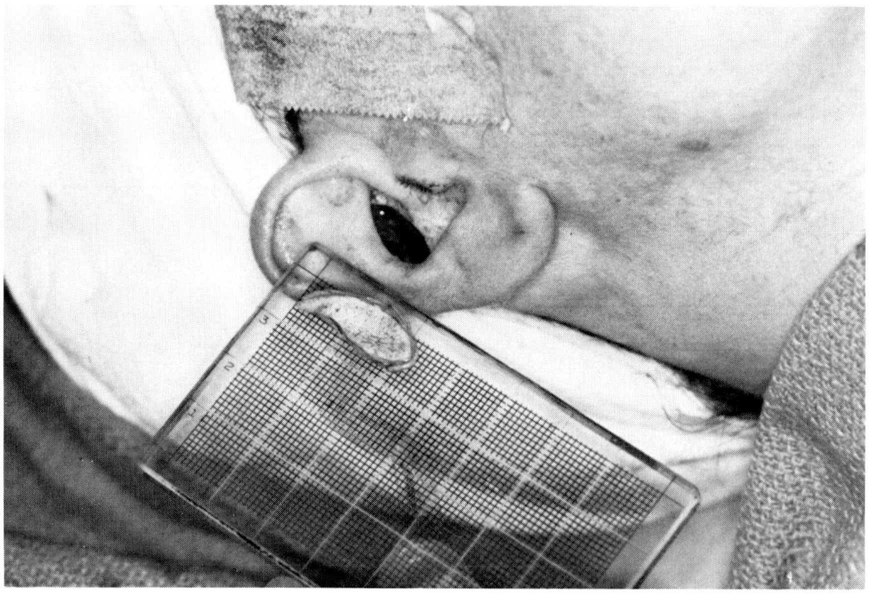

The specimen was resected with the perichondrium attached to the posterior surface.

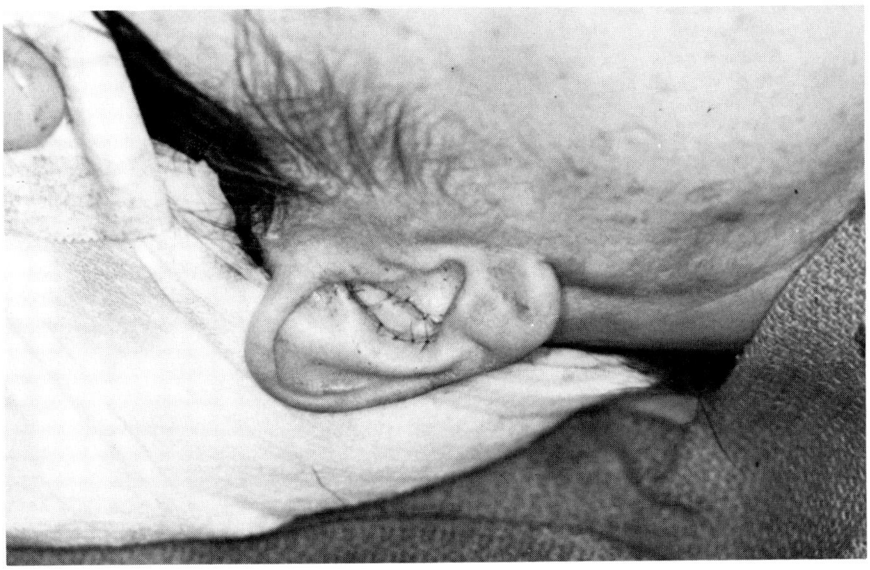

The defect in the ear was repaired with a full-thickness postauricular graft.

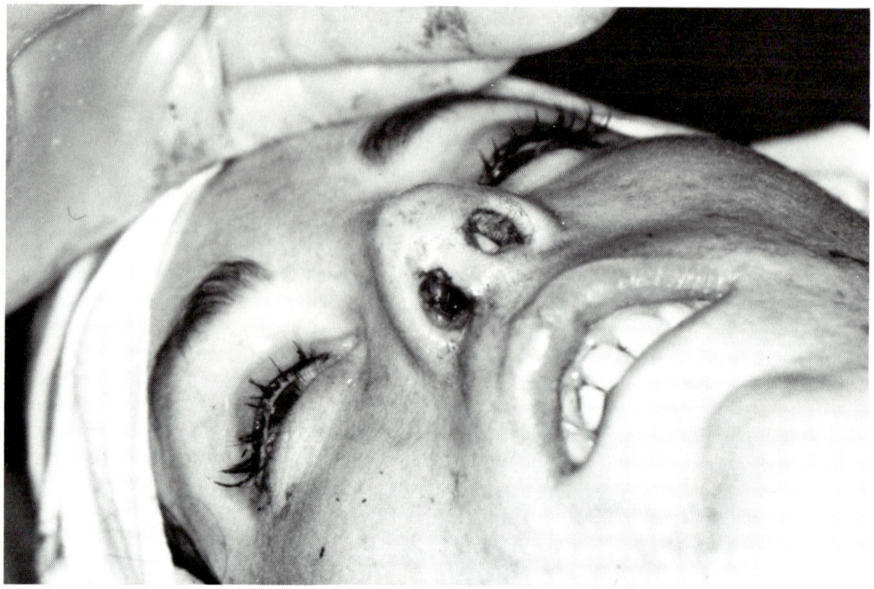

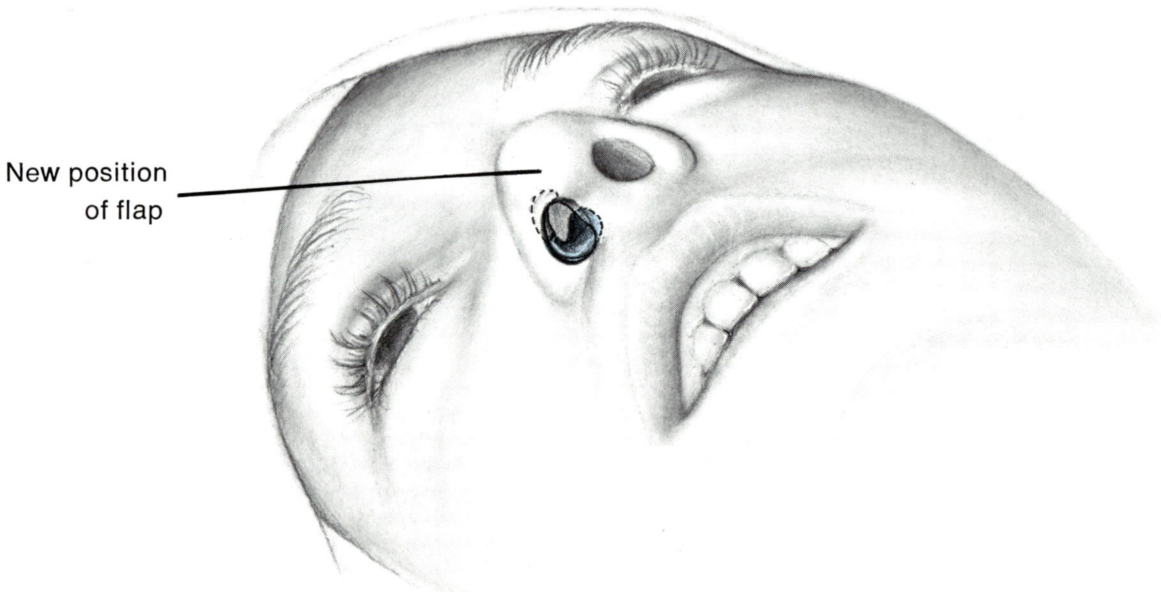

The large end of the graft was placed along the floor of the nose, and the narrow end was extended up the lateral nasal wall. The graft was meticulously sutured with 7-0 chromic catgut. Adaptic gauze was used to pack the nose before the usual nasal splint and dressing were applied.

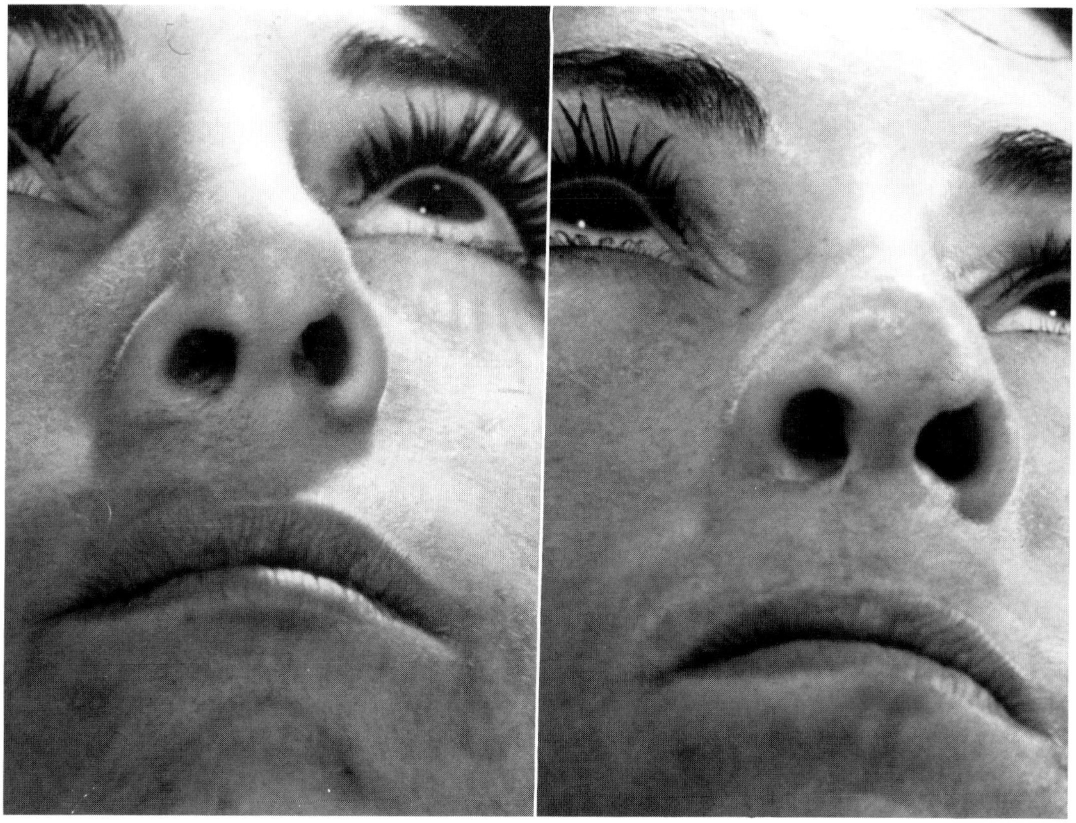

Postoperatively, there is a significant increase in the nasal airway. The floor of the right nostril has been elevated by grafts of bone and cartilage over the maxilla. A secondary rhinoplasty with a tip graft was also done.

Correction of alar rim

In this patient notching of the right ala was corrected by an elliptical composite graft from the anterior surface of the ear. The graft, which measured 12 mm long and 3 mm wide (maximum), was placed into an opening made 4 mm above the nostril and parallel to it. The graft was well secured with interrupted 7-0 chromic catgut sutures. The defect in the donor ear was covered with a full-thickness postauricular graft.

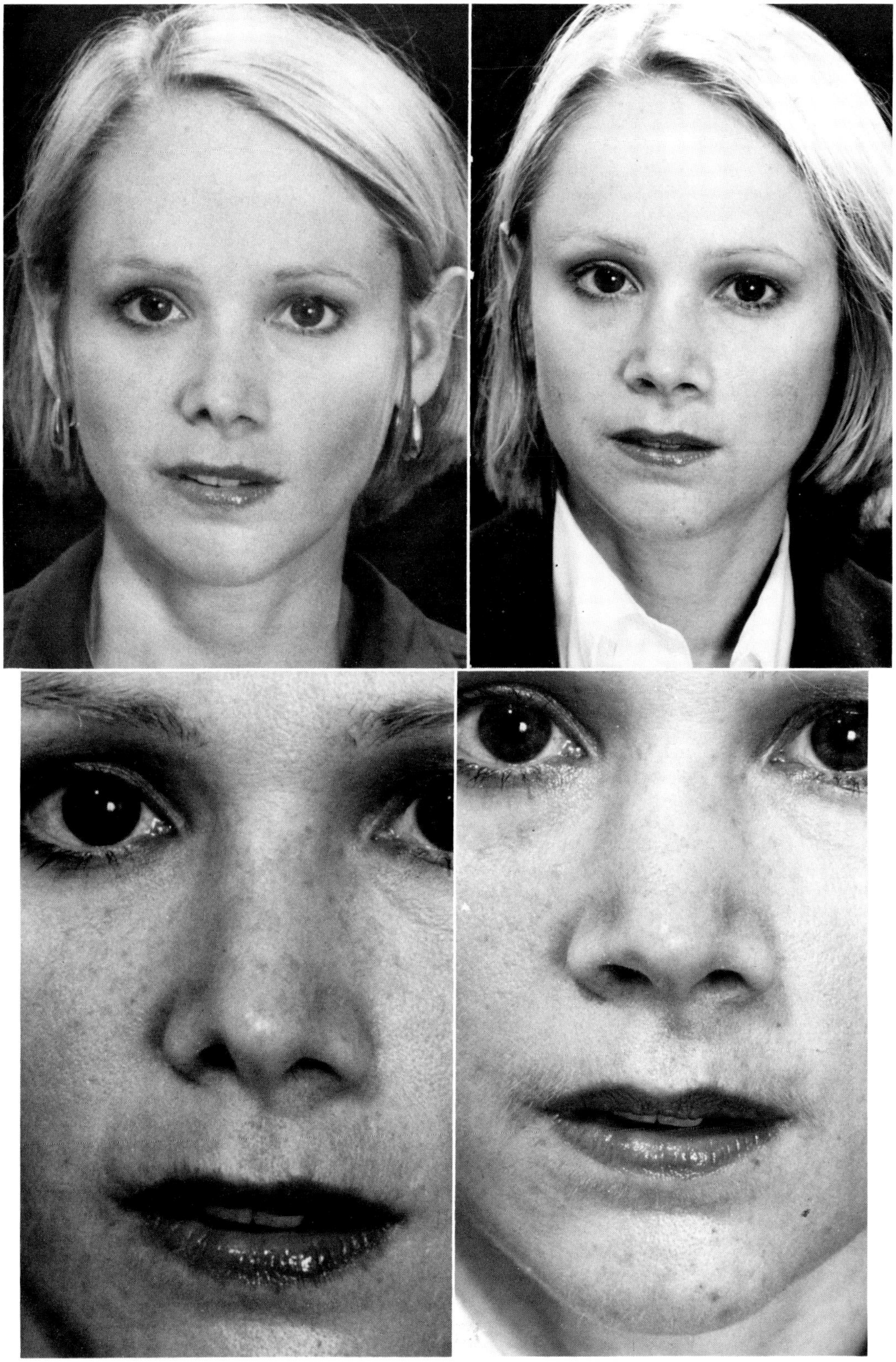

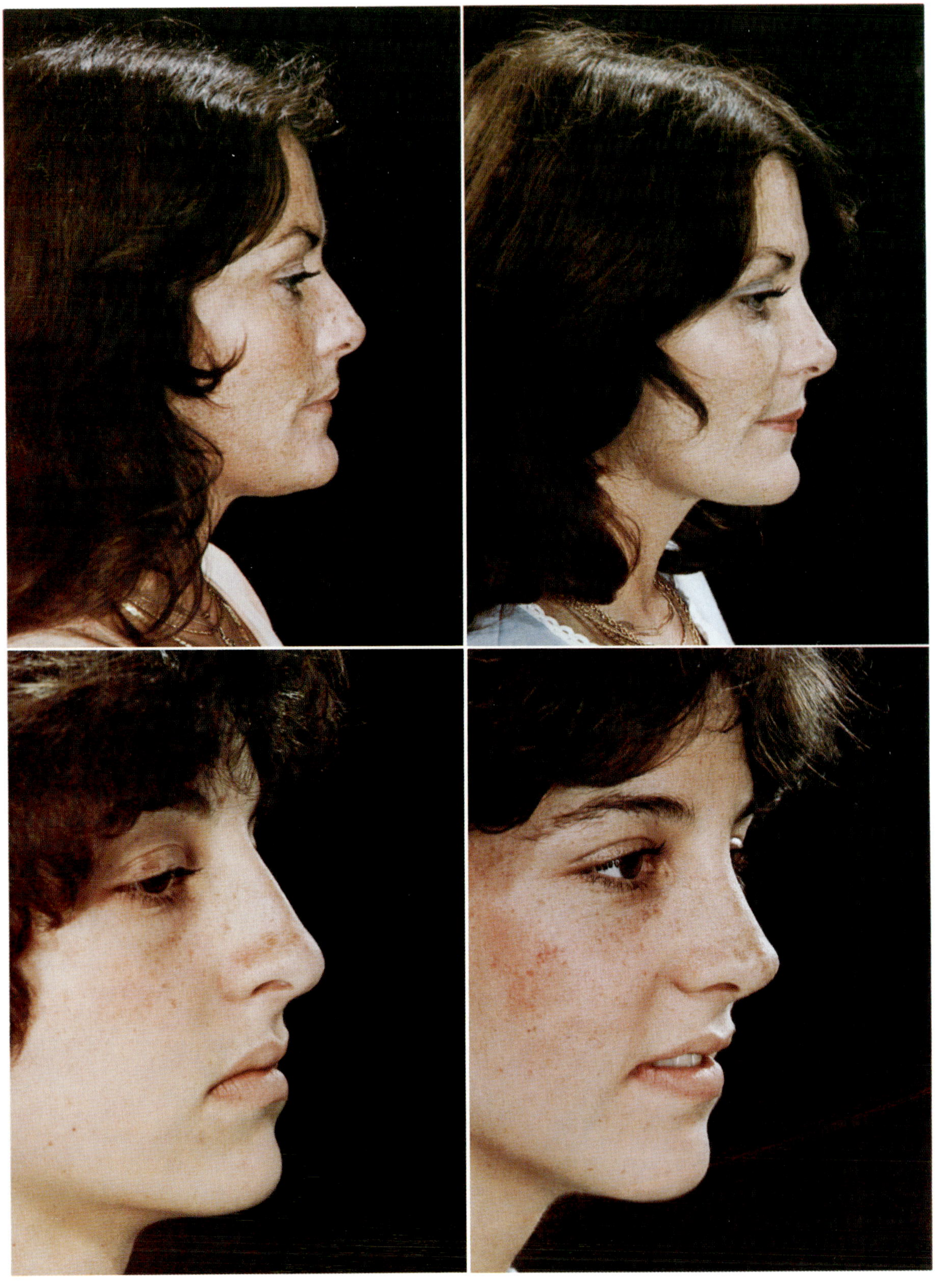

CHAPTER 5

Finesse in rhinoplasty

Case reports

1: Preservation of frontal contour
2: Preservation of lateral contour
3: Overall refinement
4: Conservation of the stately nose
5: Limited rhinoplasty—the basal complex

Rhinoplasty was originally designed for those patients whose nasal configuration fell outside their cultural standard of beauty. Surgery usually involved the nose with the gargantuan hump with a low-hanging tip and a patient who would state, "I don't care what you do; anything would be better than this."

With the growing publicity of rhinoplasty and the desire for physical perfection, patients now consult plastic surgeons regarding noses that are aesthetically acceptable—at times, nearly ideal. These patients embody a new sophistication and discernment in their expectations, which require results that are remarkably subtle and artistic. These patients have little to gain and potentially much to lose.

The finesse, or minor correction, is a relatively new concept. In 1904 Nalaton and Orbredonne published a textbook, *La Rhinoplastie,* in which they stated: "The surgeon cannot pretend to correct a slight malformation. If a nose be slightly deviated or humped, or show a slight saddle deformity, these are unfortunate defects, but we do not believe that the correction of such defects can be achieved by surgery."

In today's aesthetic surgical practice, the plastic surgeon cannot refuse the challenge of the minor distortion, even though its correction is often most difficult and the outcome often imperceptible.

Minor distortion does not necessarily mean minor rhinoplasty. A subtle change may require modification of all nasal parts, if only to a slight degree. Thus, the difficulty in the finesse is in judging what to modify, and the danger is in judging how much.

CASE REPORT 1: PRESERVATION OF FRONTAL CONTOUR

A strong, but attractive nose is sometimes not acceptable to the patient. This patient wanted a general reduction of the nasal contour but repeatedly stressed that she wanted "the same look." The finesse required a general but slight reduction of all nasal parts to effect an inconspicuous change.

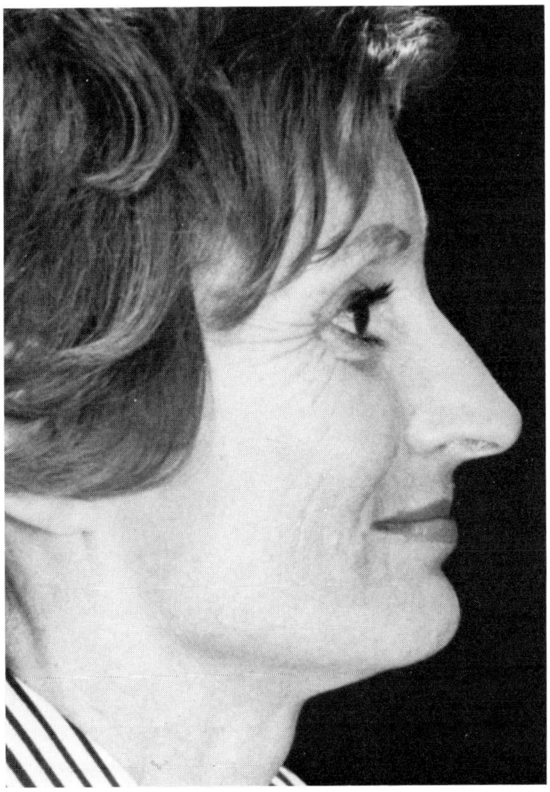

The dorsum is slightly high, but the radix and supratip areas are in fairly good relationship to the strong and projecting tip. The bony pyramid is excellent, the skin cover is fine and soft, and the tip cartilages are of excellent character. The columella is slightly low, and the subnasion is full.

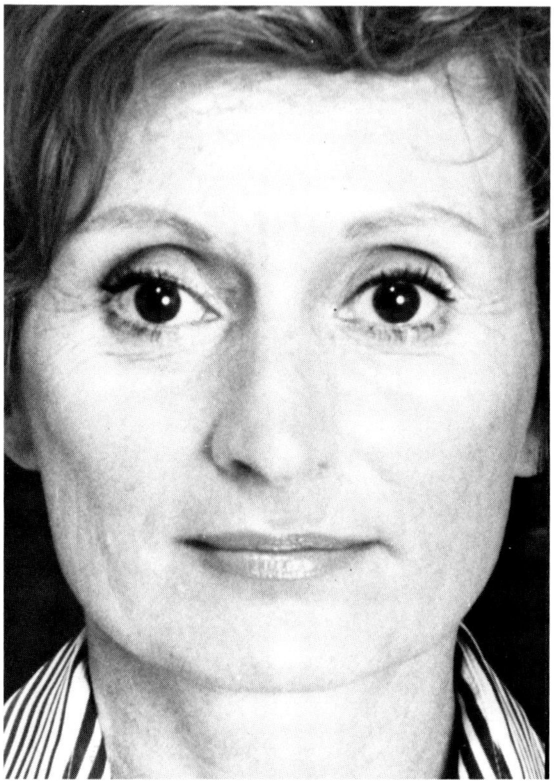

The patient was especially pleased with her appearance on front view and emphatically requested that no changes be made on that view. On palpation the nasal pyramid was found to be of normal length and in excellent relation with the other nasal parts. She was advised that there would be a slight increase in the show of her nostrils, which would occur with the necessary shortening of her nose. The difference in the right and left nostrils was pointed out, and she was told that this would remain unchanged.

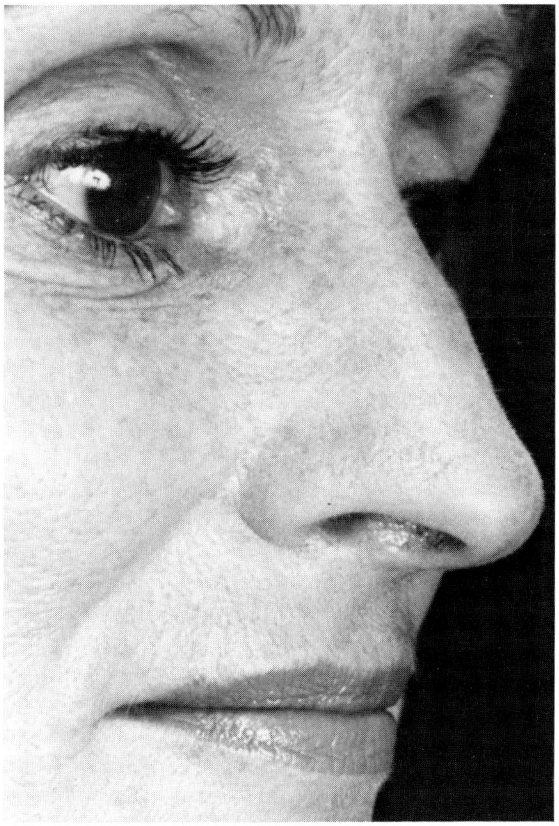

The right and left oblique views are symmetrical. In the right oblique view, there is minimal caudal projection of the bony pyramid. The upper cartilaginous vault is well structured, with good continuity to the bony vault. The lateral projection of the lower lateral cartilages is excellent, as is the general tip configuration. The nostrils are thin and long—*a warning of possible notching or collapse in the event that too much lateral crura or mucosal lining is resected.*

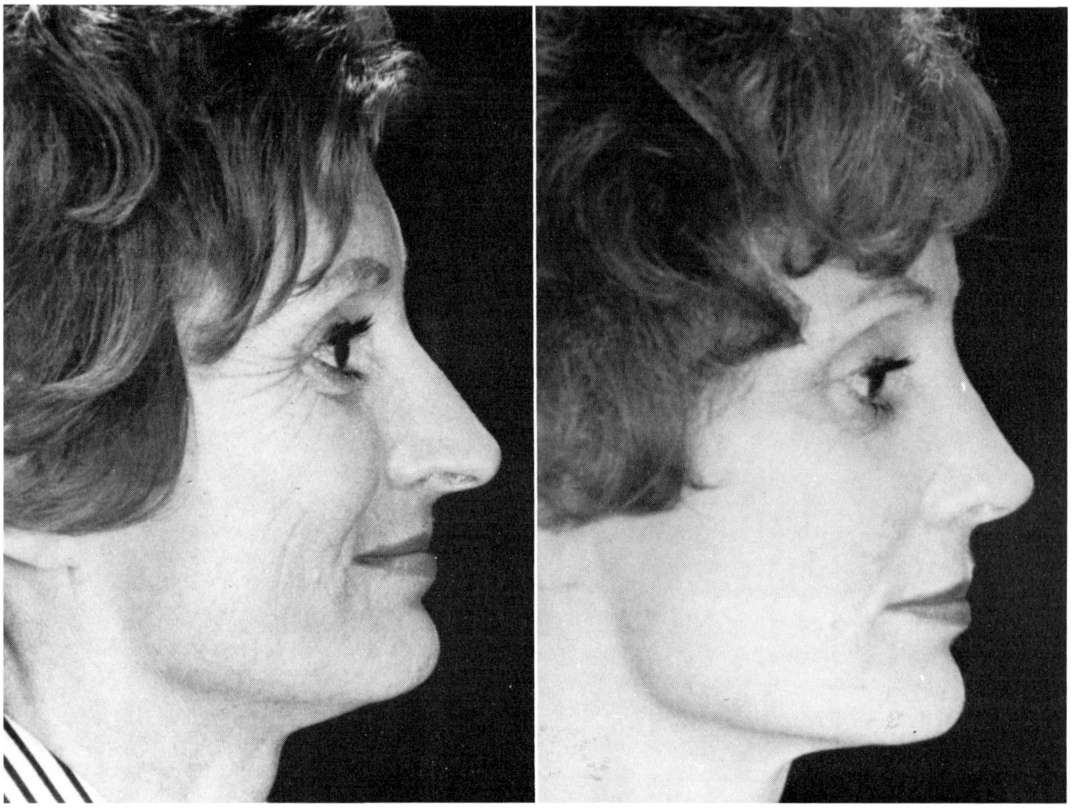

Postoperatively, the visual change was minimal even though all nasal parts were modified. The nose was shortened by a 2-mm resection of the caudal septum. The nasal spine was conservatively reduced, which provided slightly more lip length to balance out the still strong nasal profile.

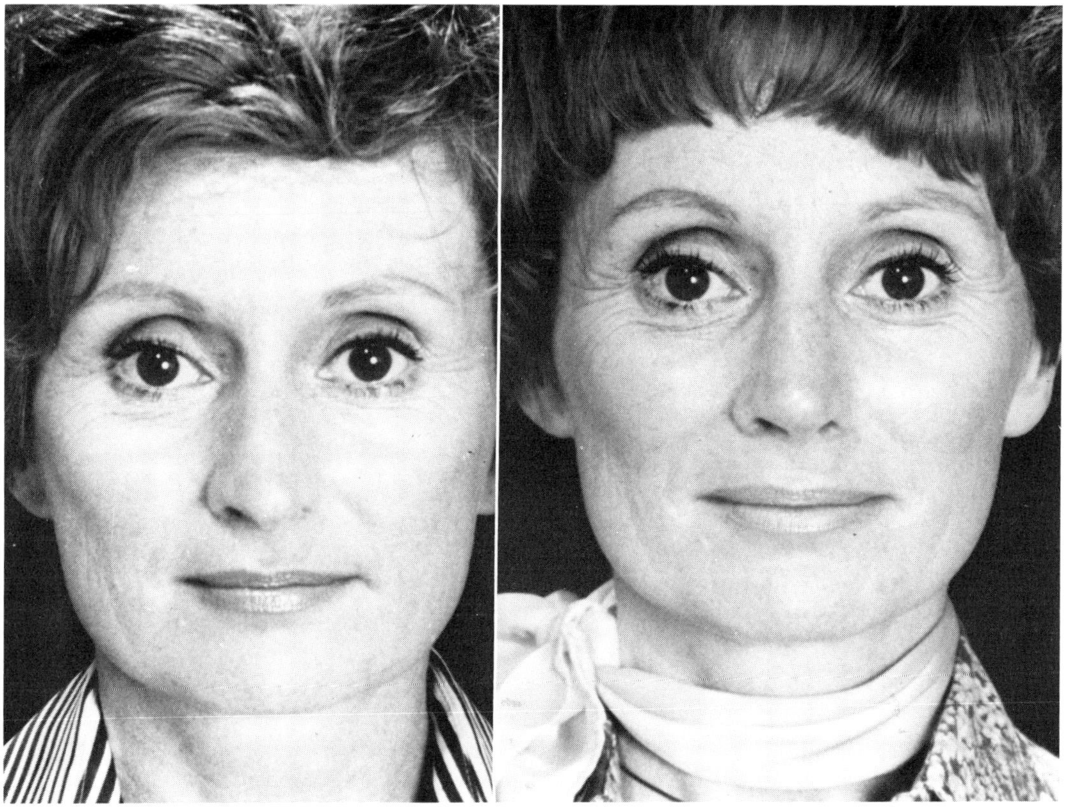

On front view, the preoperative character of the nose has been preserved in spite of shortening, reduction of tip projection, and narrowing. The visibility of the nostrils caused by the shortening has made the preexisting difference in their contour more apparent.

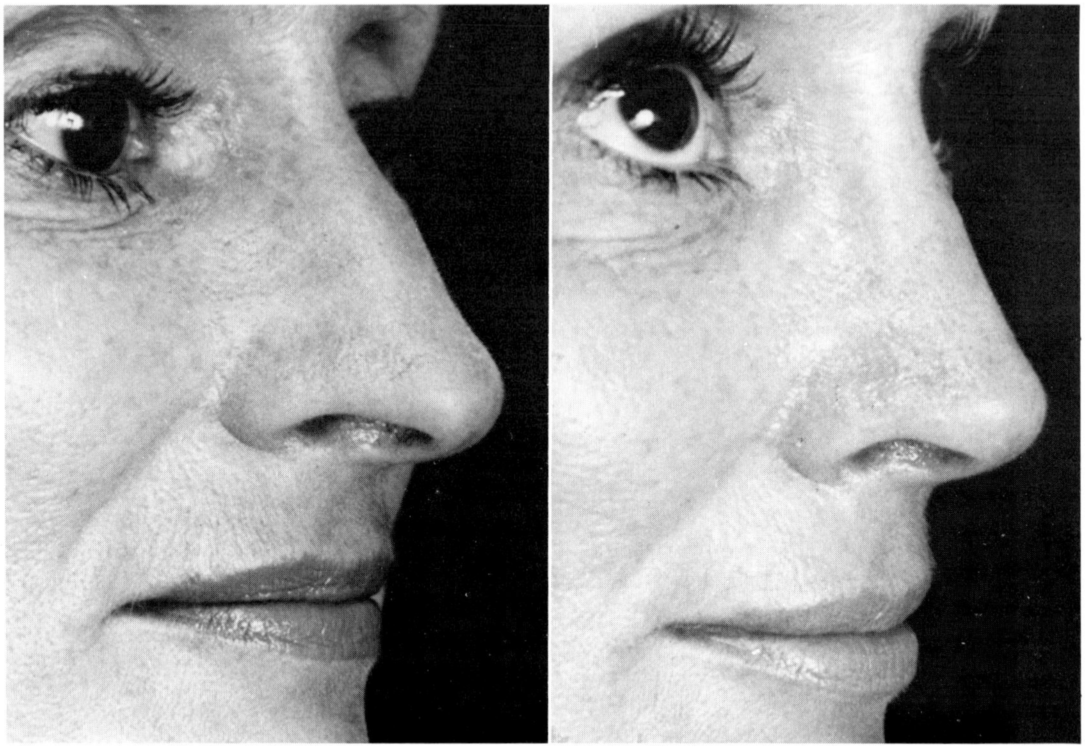

On right oblique view, there is some evidence of narrowing, which is seen as a concavity along the malar groove. A slight lateral displacement of tissues remains at the caudal edge of the bony vault. The relationship of the supratip area to the tip has been maintained, as well as the preoperative definition of the tip.

Summary of surgical procedure

1. Limited skeletonization over the bony vault, wide skeletonization over the upper cartilaginous vault
2. Transfixion incision to the nasal spine
3. Conservative resection of the nasal spine
4. Minimal reduction of the bony dorsum with Foman rasp
5. Reduction of the height of the roof of the upper cartilaginous vault, leaving the mucosa intact
6. Delivery of the lower lateral cartilages through rim incisions
7. Cephalic trim of the lateral crura (leaving a 5-mm width of cartilage) and resection of 2 mm from the dome areas
8. Lateral osteotomies only, with repositioning of the nasal bones
9. Two-mm trim of the caudal septum, including the mucosa
10. Submucous resection of the caudal ends of the upper lateral cartilages, no mucosal resection

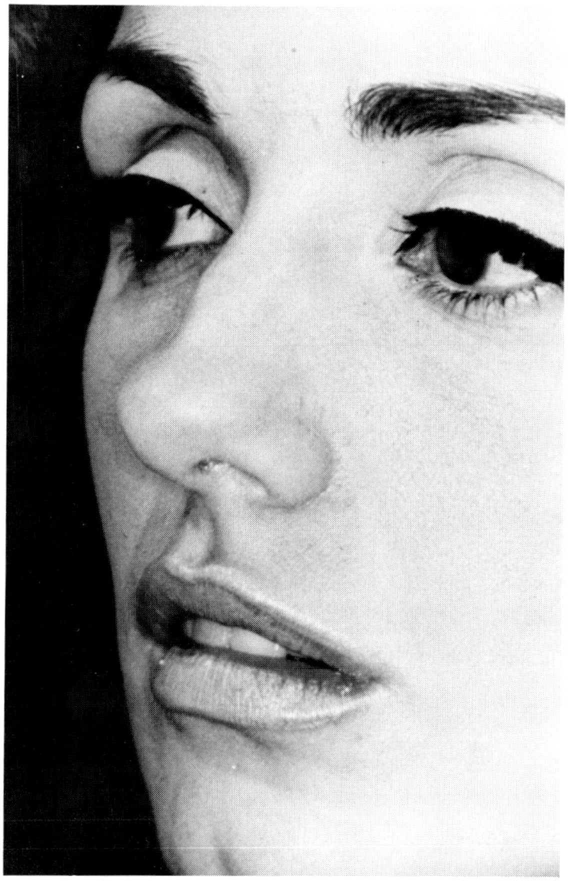

CASE REPORT 2: PRESERVATION OF LATERAL CONTOUR

Although this patient was happy with her nose in most areas, she felt that on oblique view it looked like a "boxer's nose." The right and left oblique views are symmetrical. On left oblique view, the severe irregularity of the nasal line is manifest. The lateral projection of the caudal end of the bony vault is exaggerated by a poorly supported upper cartilaginous vault and a hypertrophied lower lateral cartilage.

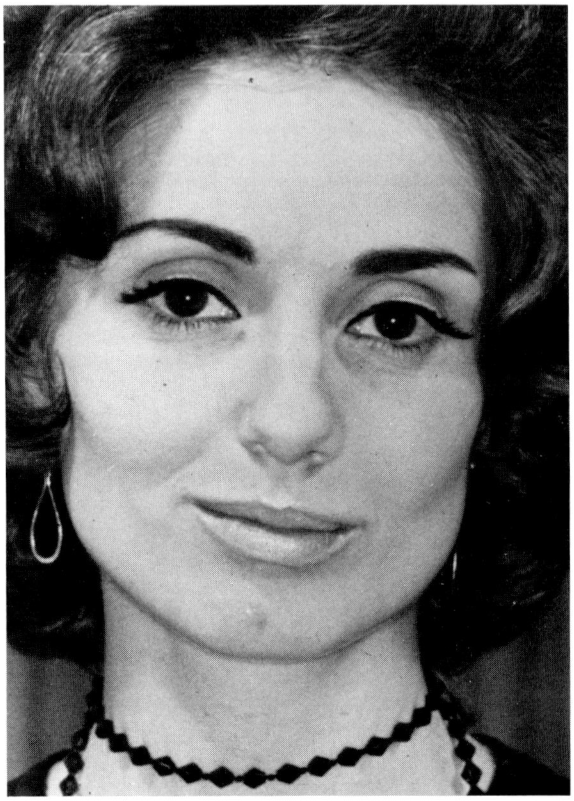

On front view, the irregularity of the nasal contour is evident but is not as distracting as it is on oblique view. The hypertrophied lower lateral cartilages have a slight cephalic malposition, which gives the tip a round, or ball-like, appearance and simultaneously gives the illusion of shortness to the nose because of the break in the flow of lines from radix to tip.

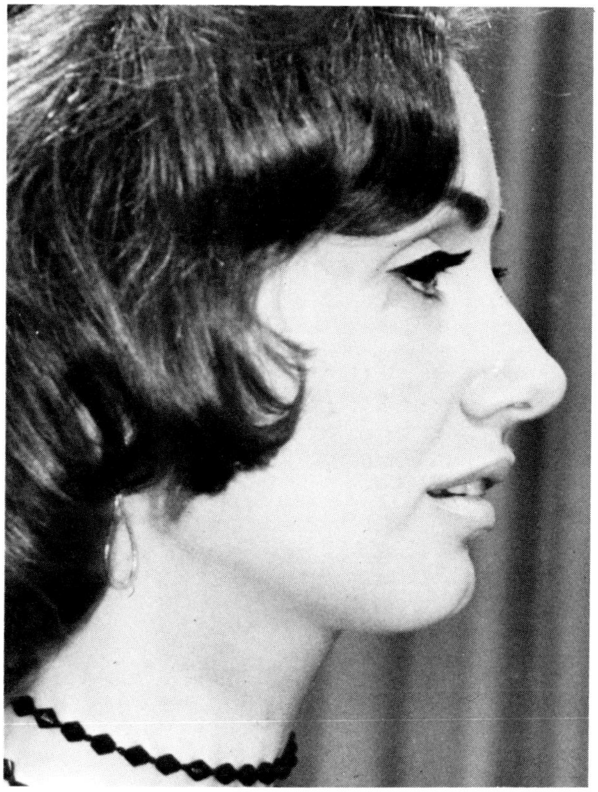

On lateral view, the nasal silhouette is excellent. The tip is slightly overprojecting. The upper lip is short, which exaggerates the appearance of nasal prominence. With a profile as good as this, the margin for error is dangerously small.

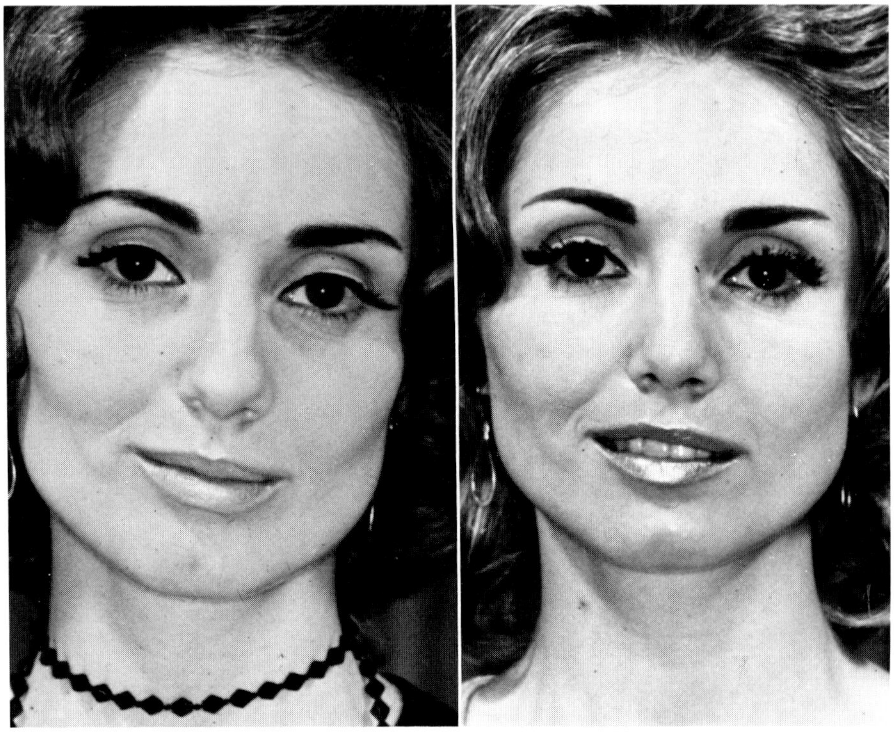

Postoperatively, there is virtually no change in the width of the nasal pyramid at the radix and only slight narrowing caudally. The relationship of the width of the bony pyramid to the base of the nose is correct. Further narrowing could cause a disproportionate narrowness of the upper vault.

The irregular line from the radix to the nasal tip has been improved. The grooves just above the alar lobules (slight malposition of the lower lateral cartilages) are diminished following reduction of the cartilage mass by cephalic trim. The nostrils are more evident postoperatively because the nose was shortened.

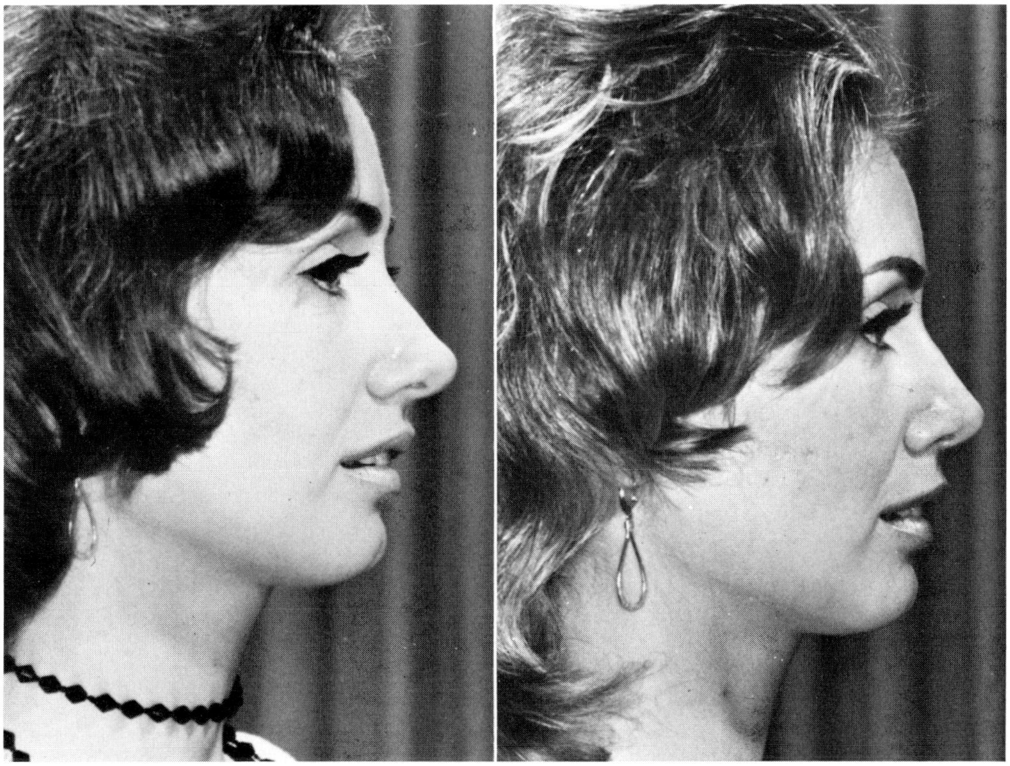

On lateral view, the change in the nasal aspects is negligible. The dorsal line was not altered, and yet the nasofacial angle appears to have been reduced. This illusion of change is a result of a reduction of the tip mass, slight resection of the nasal spine, and minimal trim of the caudal septum and mucosa.

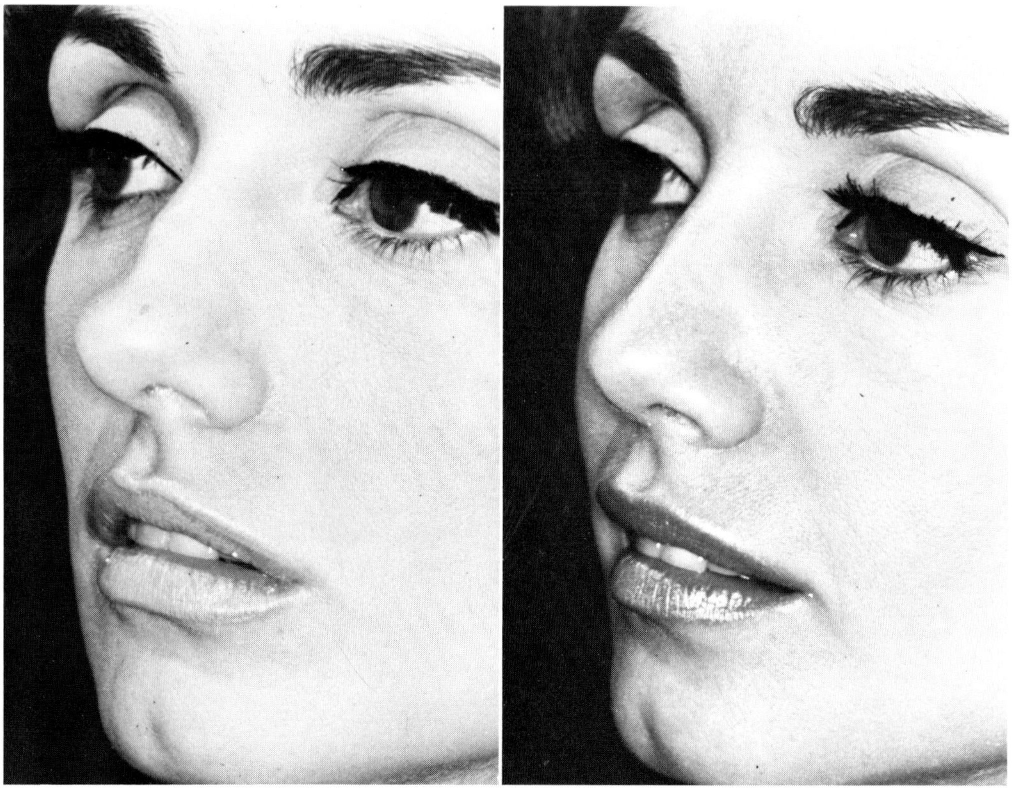

Improvement of the oblique view involved only tissues lateral to the dorsal line. Skeletonization over the bony vault extended just to the lateral projections of the caudal end of the bony pyramid, which then was reduced with a Foman rasp. Lateral osteotomies with cautious repositioning of the bony pyramid helped to reduce the lateral disparity between the upper cartilaginous vault and the bony vault. This irregularity was further improved by placement of grafts, using the cephalic parts of the alar cartilages, over the upper lateral cartilages.

Summary of surgical procedure

1. Minimal skeletonization over the bony vault, moderate skeletonization over the upper cartilaginous vault
2. Transfixion incision to the nasal spine
3. Conservative resection of the nasal spine
4. Trim of the membranous septum and caudal mucosa overlying the cartilage, but with no resection of the cartilage
5. Rasp of the bony vault for reduction of the lateral projections, but with no reduction in dorsal height
6. Lateral osteotomies to narrow the bony pyramid
7. Delivery of the lower lateral cartilages through rim incisions
8. Trim of the cephalic excess (leaving a 5-mm caudal segment) and resection of 1 mm of dome
9. Onlay of resected lower lateral cartilages over the depressed upper lateral cartilages, with the cut edges placed along the dorsum
10. Conservative submucous resection of the caudal edges of the upper lateral cartilages, with preservation of all mucosa

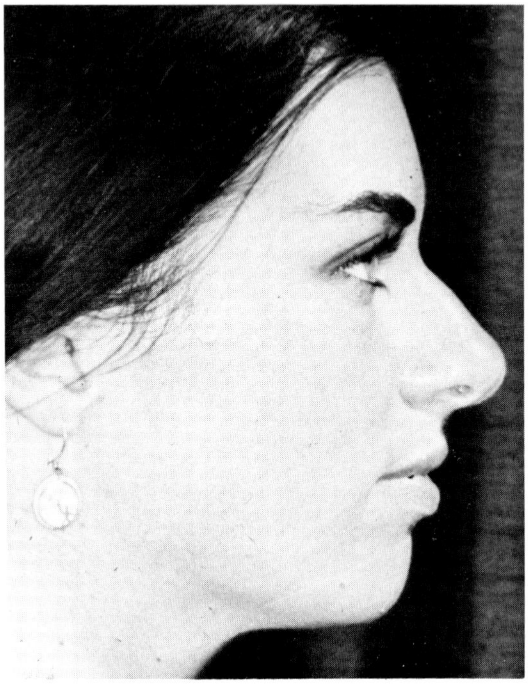

CASE REPORT 3: OVERALL REFINEMENT

The nasal facial relationships of this patient are favorable, and yet the nose gives an overriding impression of bulkiness and unrefinement. On lateral view, there is a very small dorsal hump. The dorsal line is interrupted by the emergence of the supratip area. The tip contour forms a semicircular outline from the supratip to the insertion of the columella. The lack of an end point at the tip contributes to the impression of bulkiness. The low columella and rounded tip give an inordinant prominence to the base of the nose. This prominence and slight dorsal hump produce an illusion of a downward tilt of the tip in spite of an open nasolabial angle.

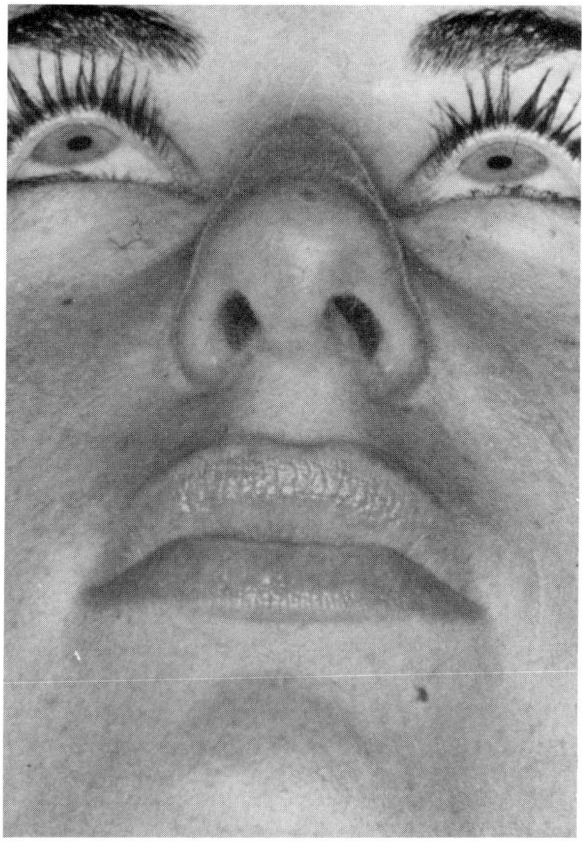

Instead of being triangular, the basal perimeter is almost square, and the nostrils are perpendicular to the plane of the lip.

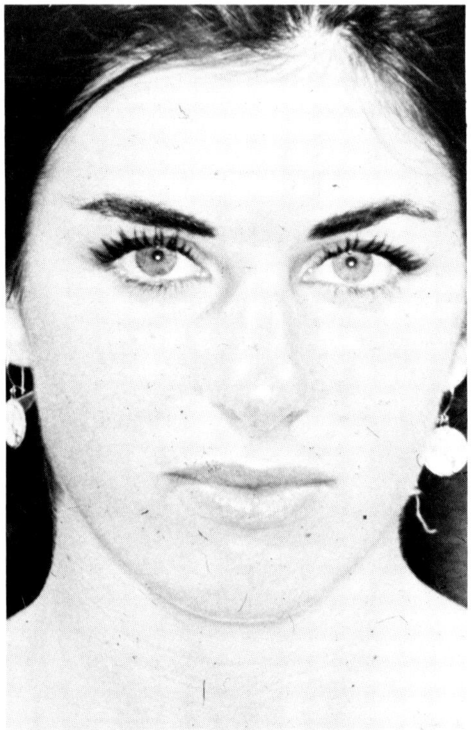

On front view, the nose appears too broad for the central third of the face. The nasal tip reflects a wide light reflex pattern. The low columella appears to shorten her lip. The bony pyramid is of good length; the upper cartilages are substantial and in good alignment with the bony vault, producing a smooth lateral line from root to base.

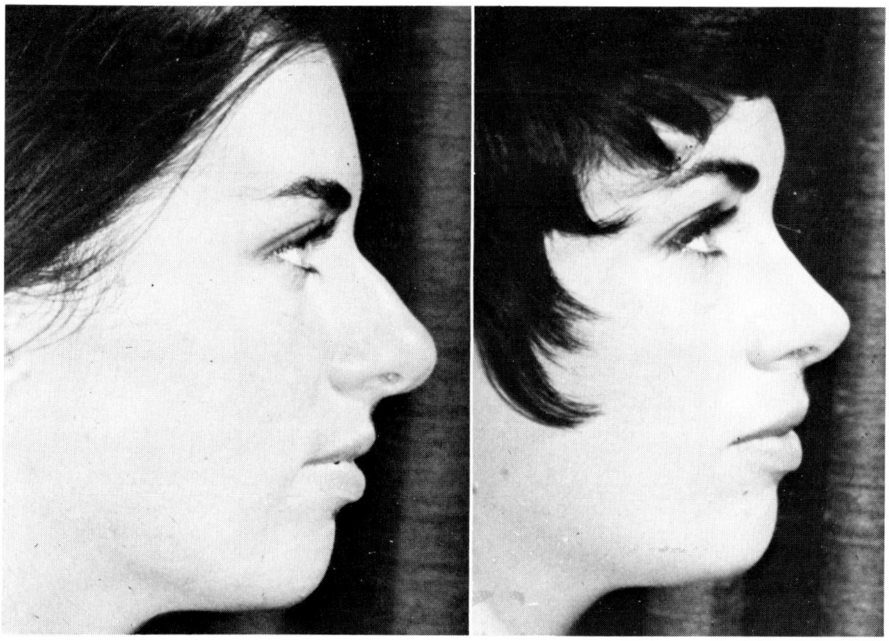

Minimal changes in all nasal parts have produced a considerable change in the nasal gestalt. Though the nose is actually shorter, it has the appearance of being longer because of the uninterrupted line from the root to the tip. This effect was obtained from the reduction of the dorsal hump and tip delineation. The deeper subnasion created by partial resection of the nasal spine has achieved a separation of the lip from the nose, placing the midface in better accord.

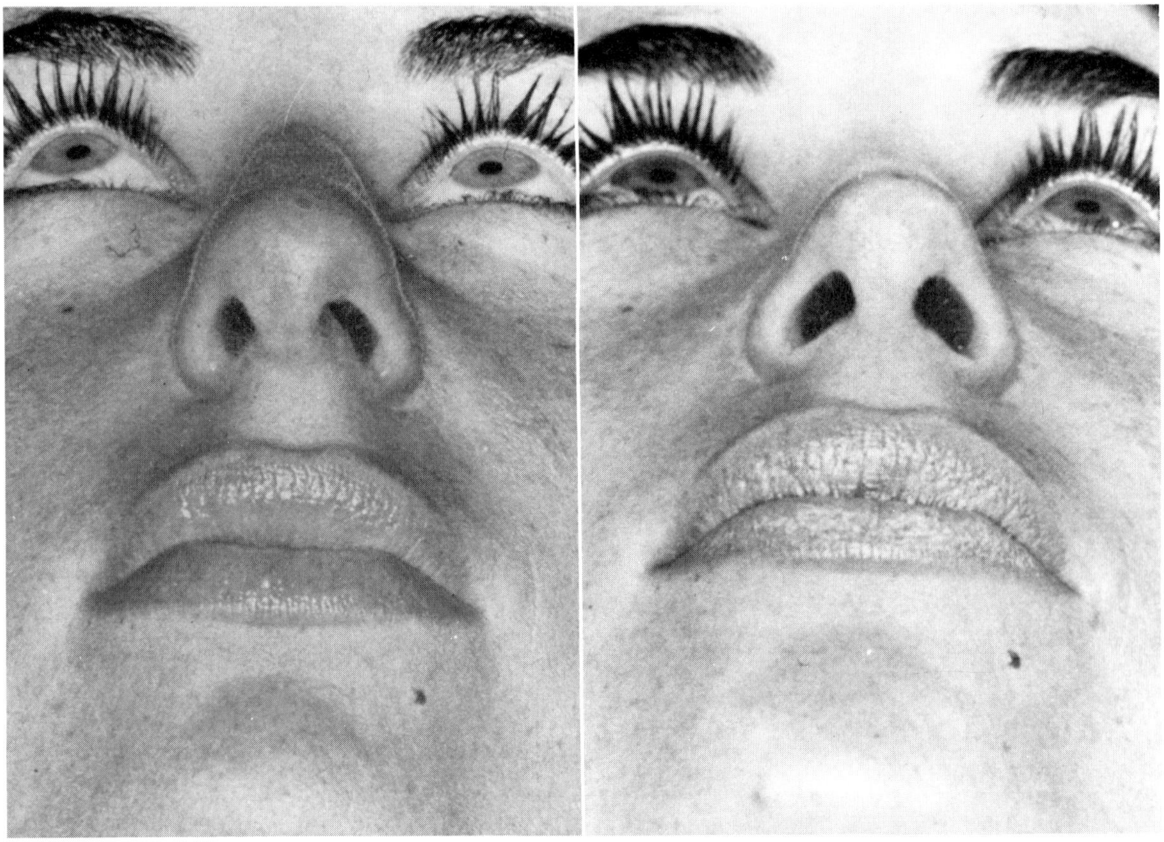

The square basal outline was converted to a softly triangular one, with the nares inclining toward the tip. The tip cartilages were delivered through rim incisions. Following a cephalic trim (leaving a 4-mm width of lateral crura), the dome areas were attenuated with interdigitating scoring incisions, which produced an increase in the height of the arch of the lower lateral cartilages.

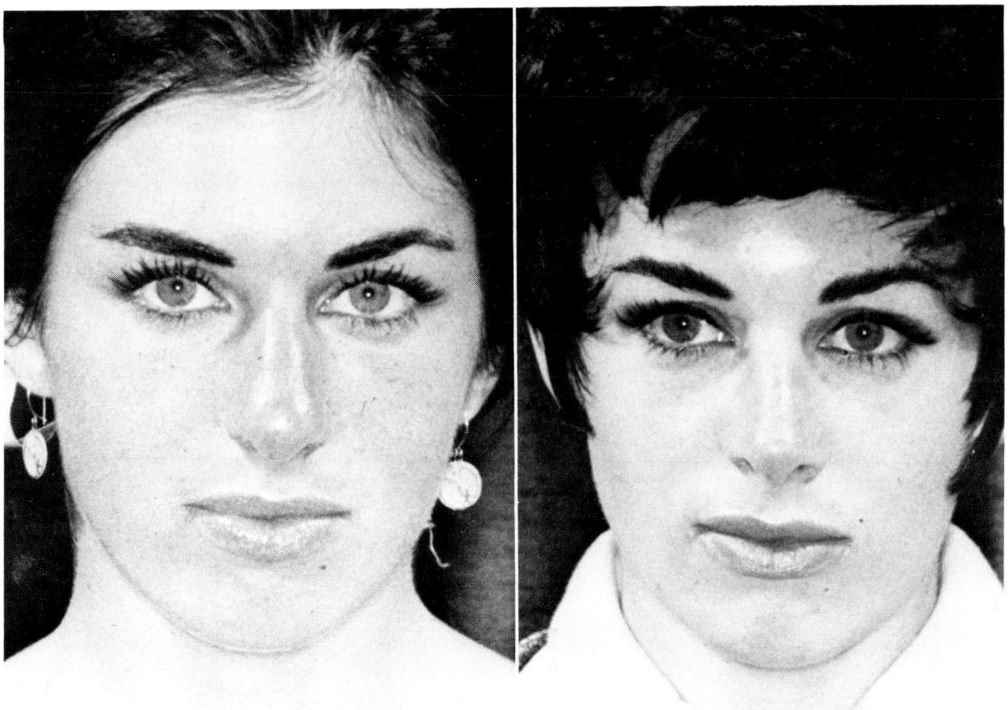

On front view, the prominence of the midface has been improved by the slight narrowing of the bony pyramid, adjustment of the inferior caudal septum, and tip refinement. The lateral nasal contour forms symmetrical lines from the superciliary ridges to the three-point reflex at the tip.

Summary of surgical procedure

1. Moderate skeletonization of cartilaginous and bony vaults through intercartilaginous incisions
2. Transfixion incision to nasal spine
3. Slight reduction of the nasal spine
4. Trim of the posterior two thirds of the caudal septum
5. Reduction of the bony hump with Foman rasp
6. Scalpel trim of the roof of the upper cartilaginous vault, mucosa still intact
7. Delivery of the tip cartilages through rim incisions
8. Trim of the cephalic edges (leaving a 4-mm width of lateral crura) and attenuation of the dome areas with interdigitating scoring cuts
9. Lateral osteotomies only, with repositioning of the bony pyramid
10. Submucous resection of the caudal ends of the upper lateral cartilages, no mucosal resection

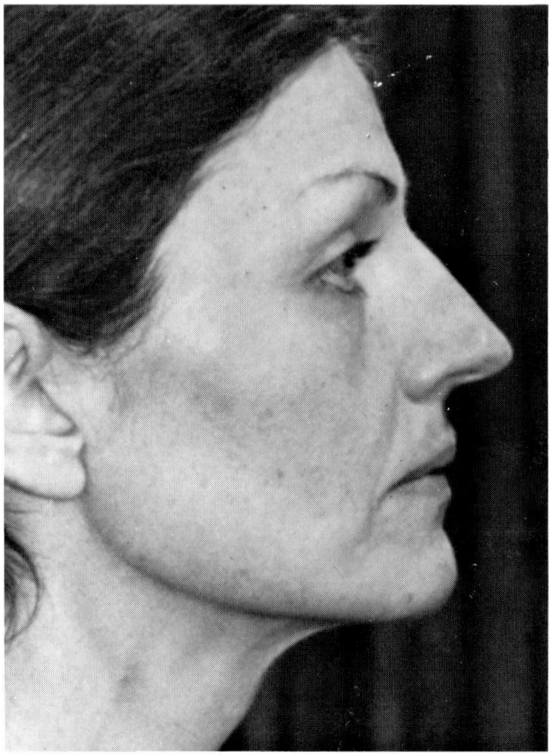

CASE REPORT 4: CONSERVATION OF THE STATELY NOSE

This patient, who is a 5-foot 11-inch professional model, wanted to maintain the look of stateliness that her large nose had provided during her professional life. She was concerned about the less attractive way her nose appeared in photographs over the past few years but was adamant that she did not want a small nose.

On lateral view a large and elegant nose is seen in harmony with the face. There is a slight dorsal hump. The tip is lower than the dorsum by 2 mm, which is enough to give the tip configuration a downward look in spite of the open nasolabial angle. The break at the columellar-lobular junction is imperceptible, which adds to the illusion of tip droop. The alae insert lower than the columella, which gives her face a look of displeasure.

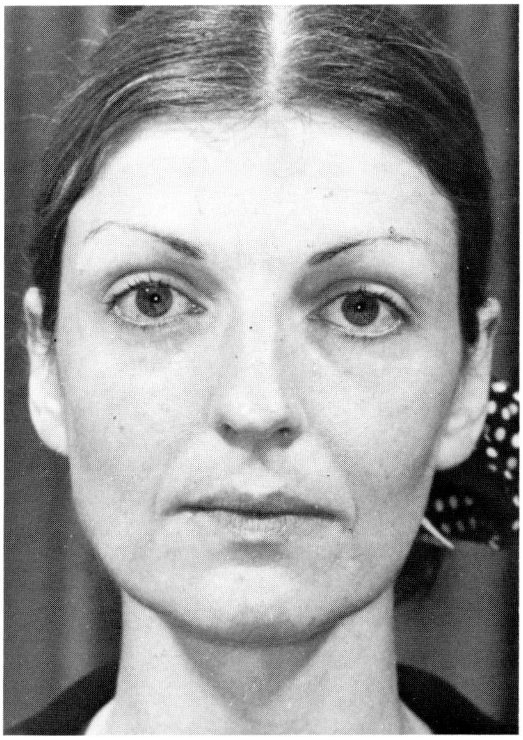

On front view, there is an unevenness to the lateral nasal lines that cannot be camouflaged with makeup. There has been a progressive flattening of the nasal tip over the past 10 years.

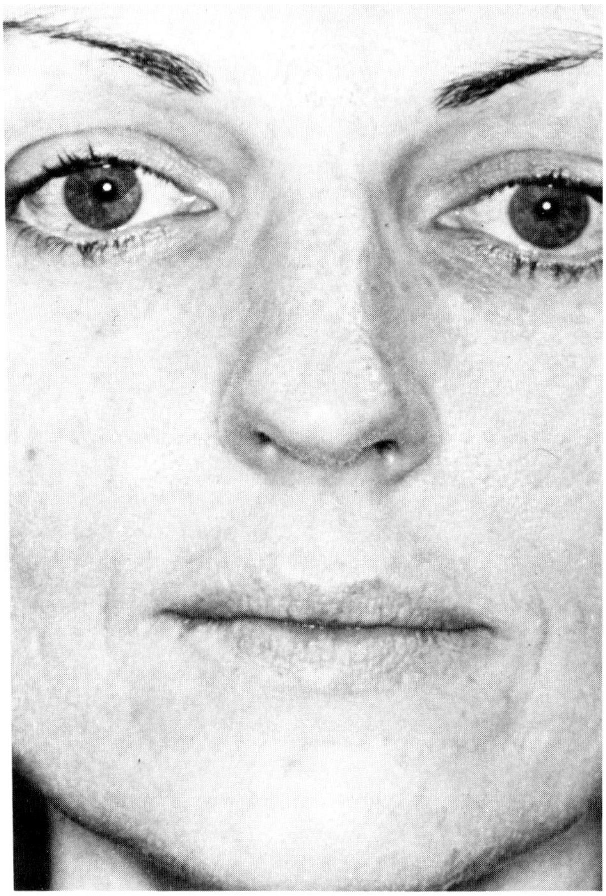

On close-up front view, the bony vault is slightly broad, flowing into a narrower upper cartilaginous vault and finally into a very broad and flattened tip complex. The nose appears shortened because the lateral dorsal line ends at the point of tip differentiation.

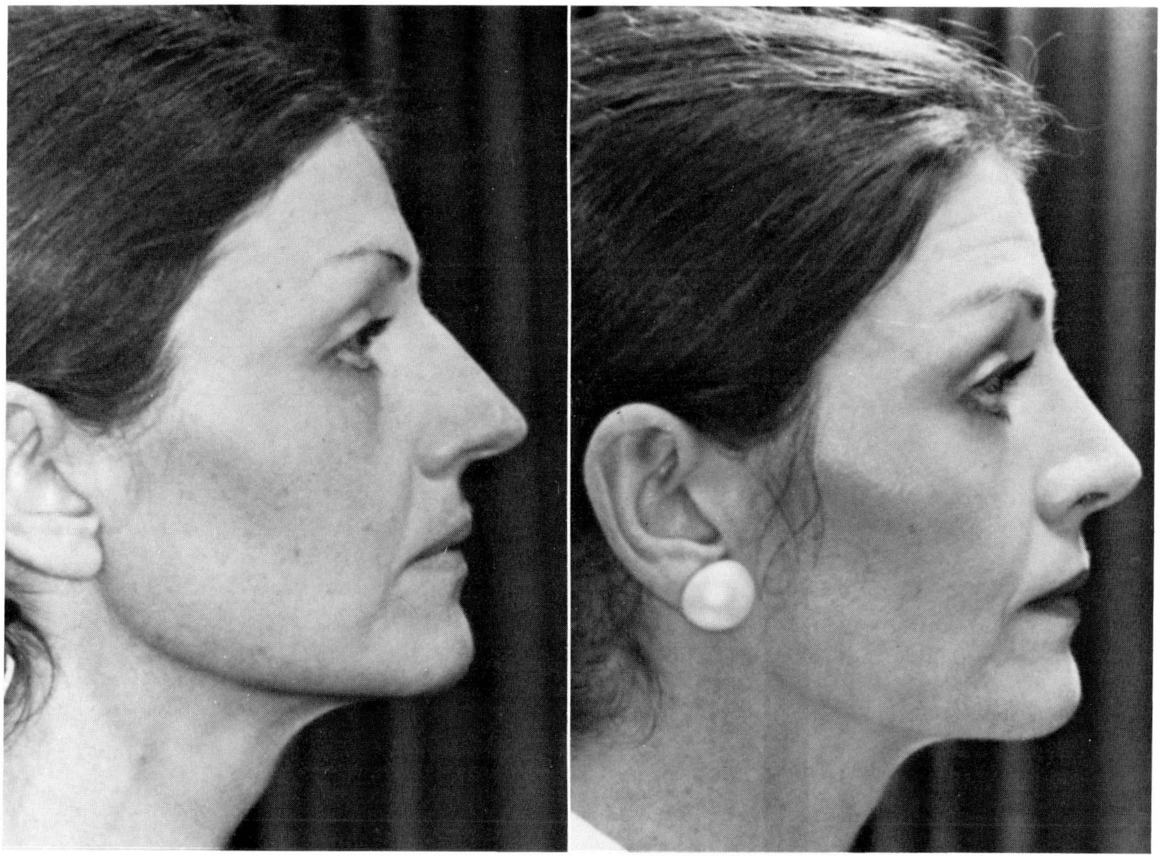

Although it was important that the nose not be shortened, it was necessary that the tip be rotated cephalad to achieve the prior, youthful position of the tip. Because of this, wide skeletonization over the upper cartilaginous vault was done, followed by limited skeletonization over the bony vault. The membranous septum was incised to the spine, with a resection of redundant mucosa over the caudal septum. No cartilage or spine was resected from the caudal edge.

A minimal reduction of the bony dorsum with a Foman rasp was followed by a careful manicure of the roof of the upper vault to match the level of the reduced bony vault.

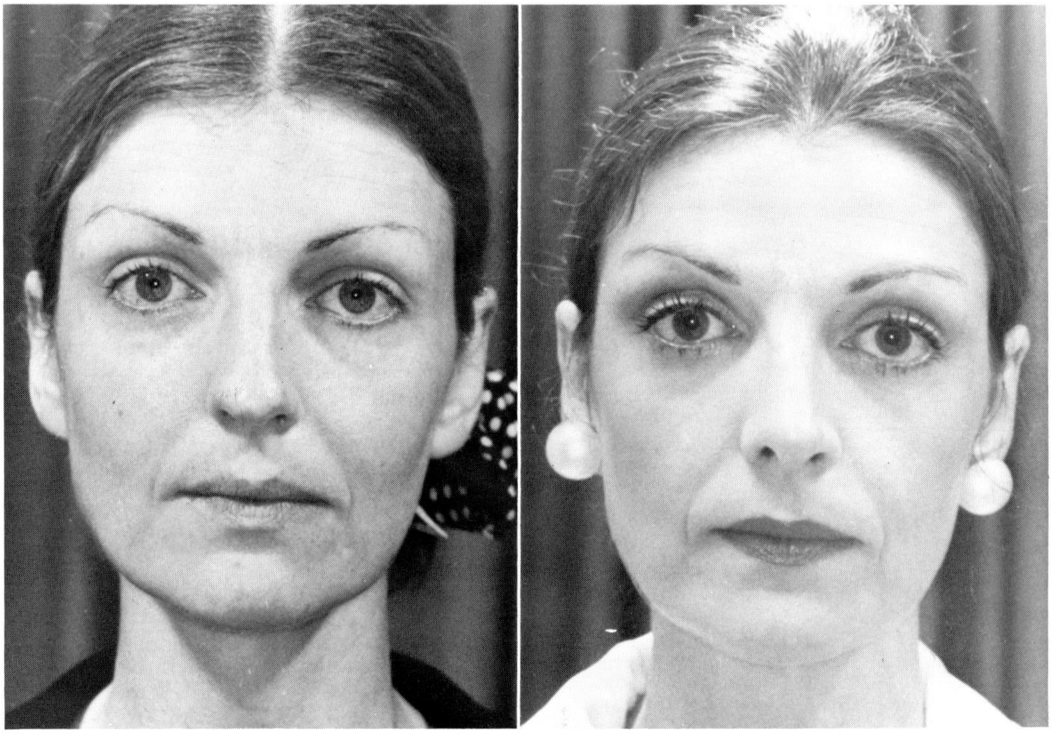

Following the rotation of the tip cephalad, the lower lateral cartilages were delivered through rim incisions. Because of the excessive arch of the tip cartilages, a 2-mm segment of cartilage was resected from the dome of each lower lateral cartilage, allowing the tip to narrow and converting the square basal perimeter to a more triangular one. The change in the architecture of the tip cartilages produced a longer-appearing nose even though it is actually shorter. This illusion is created by the uninterrupted line from the root to the end point at the tip.

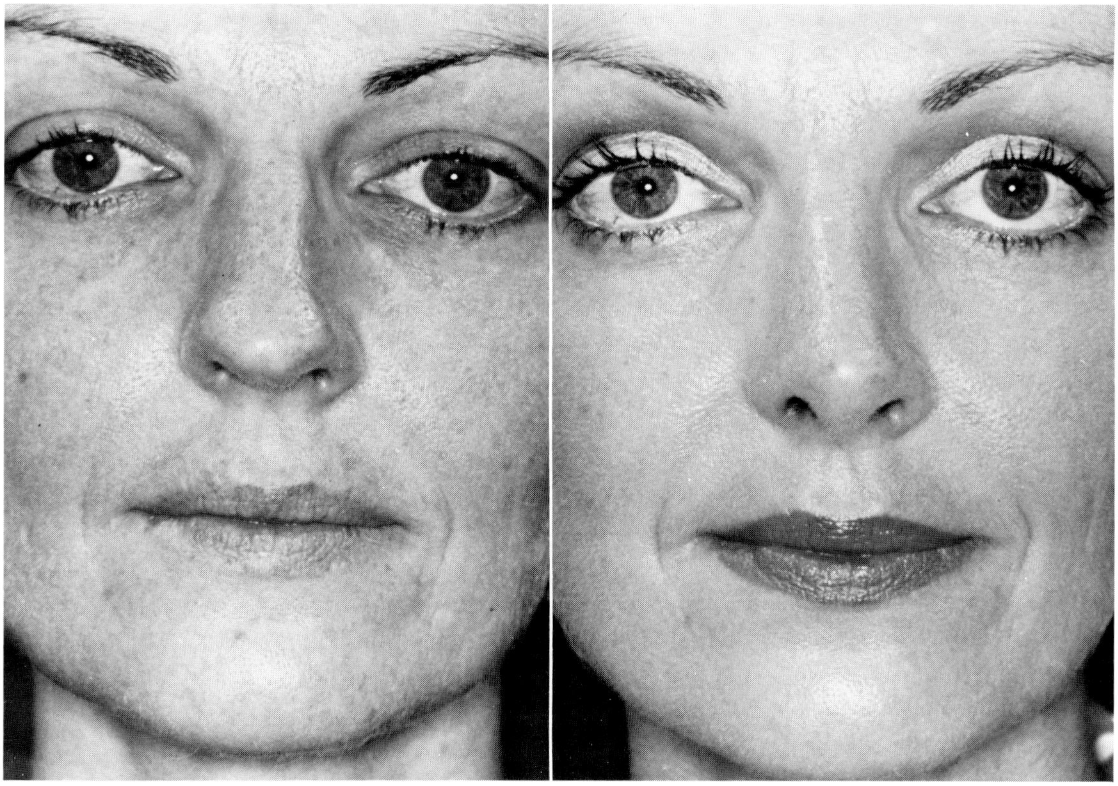

The highest point of the tip has been moved cephalad by upward rotation of the soft tissues and modification of the lower lateral cartilages. Lateral osteotomies with repositioning of the nasal bones have maintained the flow of the bony and upper cartilaginous vaults, resulting in smooth lateral nasal walls.

Summary of surgical procedure

1. Wide skeletonization of the middle vault through intercartilaginous incisions, limited skeletonization over the bony vault
2. Transfixion incision to the nasal spine
3. Resection of the redundant membranous septum without resection of the cartilage
4. Reduction of the bony hump with Foman rasp
5. Trim of the cartilaginous roof over the upper vault (mucosa still intact)
6. Delivery of the lower lateral cartilages through rim incisions
7. Cephalic excess trimmed from the tip cartilages, preserving 5 mm of lateral crura
8. Two mm of cartilage resected from the domes of both lower lateral cartilages
9. Lateral osteotomies only, with repositioning of the nasal pyramid

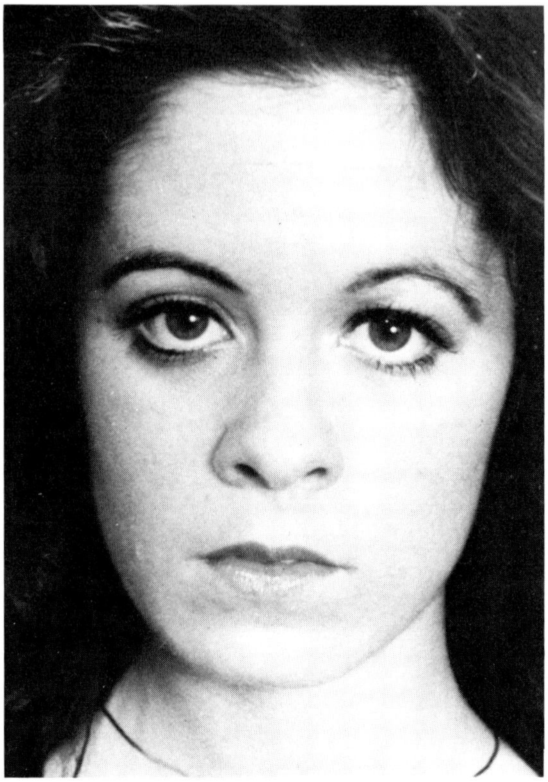

CASE REPORT 5: LIMITED RHINOPLASTY—THE BASAL COMPLEX

Both osteotomy and reduction of the dorsum may be unnecessary if good aesthetic relationships are present.

This patient illustrates a finesse that involves only the basal complex. On front view, the nasal pyramid is symmetrical. The bony vault is narrow for the comparatively broad tip, which is flattened and appears bulbous. The nostrils are visible and flaring. The lip is long.

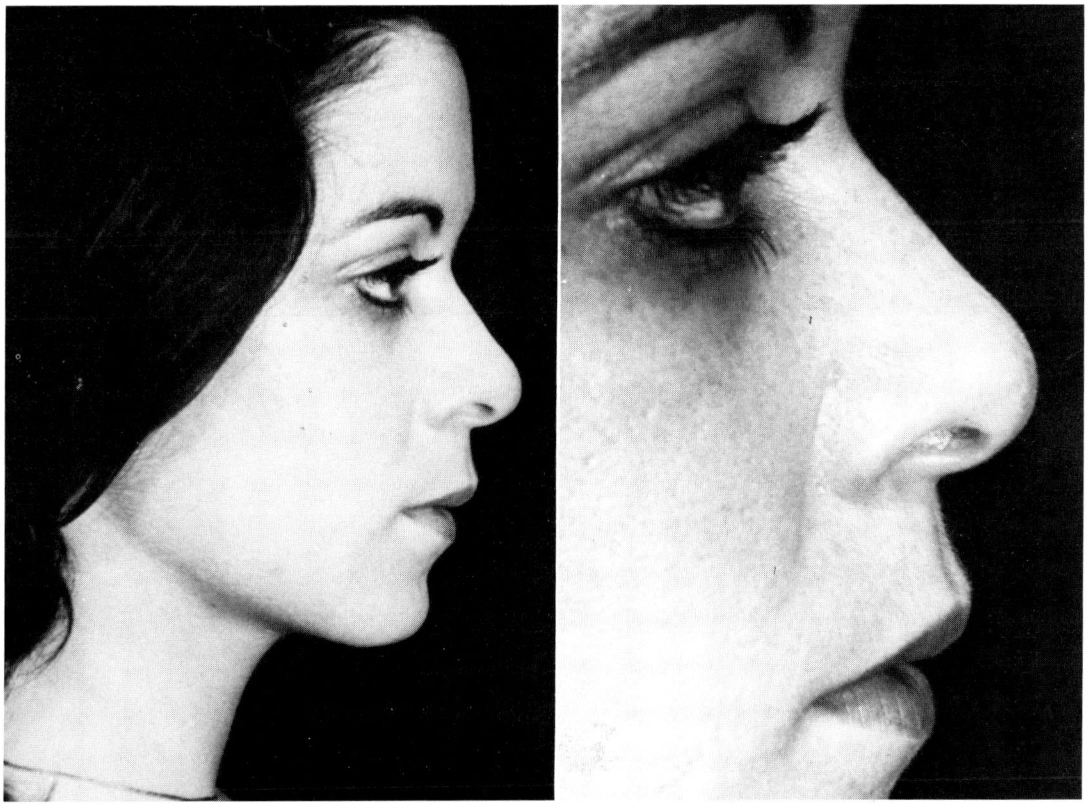

On lateral view, the dorsum is straight, ending in a poorly defined tip, which is, nevertheless, the highest projecting part. The columella is low in relation to the alar rim. The alar rim arches up and inserts below the insertion of the columella, producing an unpleasant expression. The nasolabial angle is open, but the subnasion is retrusive, the consequence of a small maxillary spine.

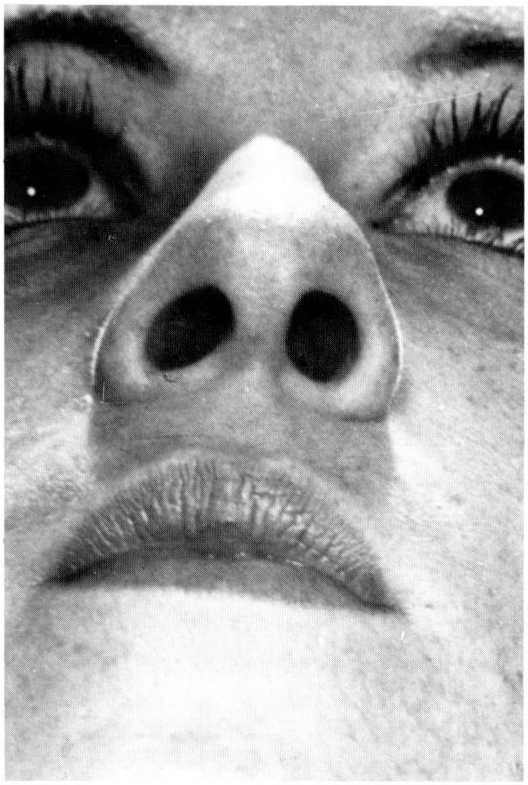

On basal view, the almost round nostrils, combined with the bulbous tip, produce a basal contour that is too broad and too flat.

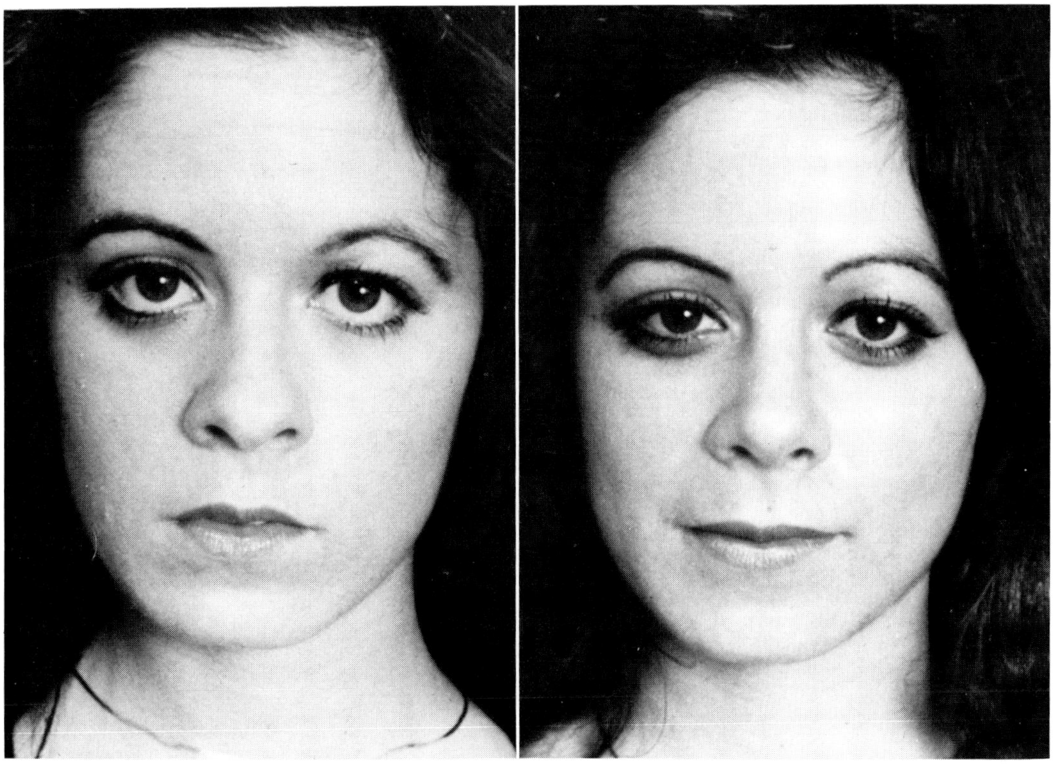

Following surgery, which involved only the lower third of the nose, all of the nasal parts have come into balance. The nose appears longer because of tip sculpturing, which included a cephalic trim (leaving a 5-mm wide lateral crus) and attenuation of the dome with scoring incisions. The base is narrower following alar wedge resection.

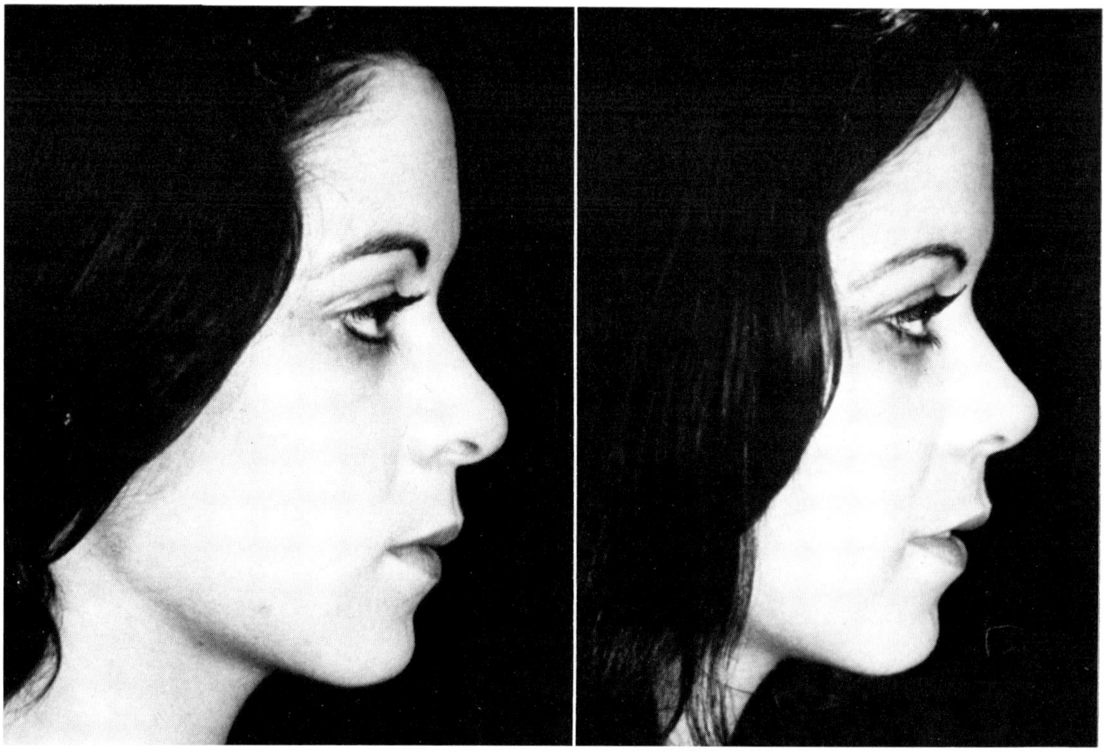

On lateral view, the dorsal line has been preserved. The tip is more projecting and less bulbous, which refines the appearance of the nose by the illusion of lengthening. The maxillary augmentation (4-mm wide roll of Supramid Extra Mesh 30 mm long) has softened the subnasion and eliminated the retrusion. The effect of maxillary augmentation on the nasolabial angle and the alar wedge resection have eliminated the unpleasant aspect of the nasal base. Transfixion of the membranous septum to the spine and generous skeletonization of the upper cartilaginous vault allowed rotation of the tip complex cephalad, which improved the relationship of the columella to the alae.

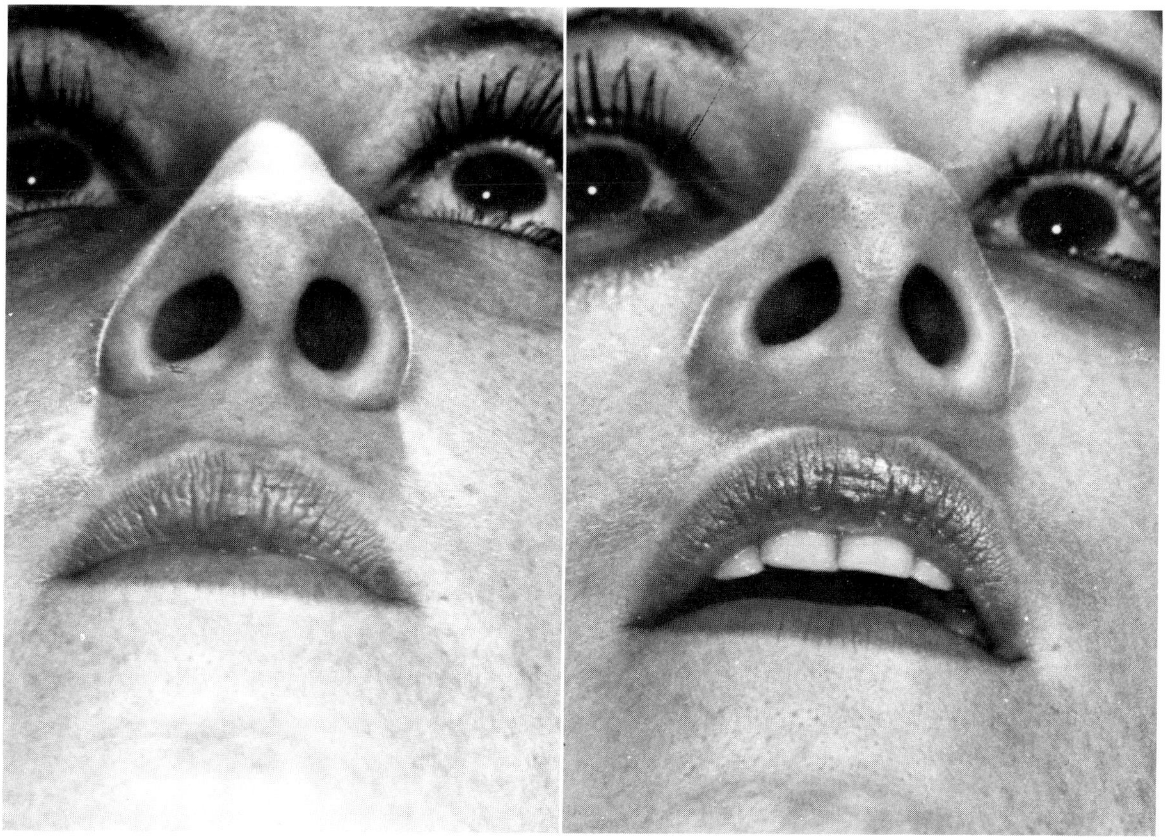

Alar wedge resection has changed the shape of the nostrils without producing notches in the nasal sill. This, in combination with tip refinement, results in a nasal base that is fine and natural.

Summary of surgical procedure

1. Skeletonization through bilateral intercartilaginous incisions, moderate skeletonization over the upper cartilaginous vault, and limited skeletonization over the bony vault
2. Transfixion incision to the nasal spine
3. Maxillary augmentation by the use of a tightly rolled Supramid implant measuring 4 mm in diameter and 30 mm long
4. Excision of a wedge of membranous septum from the caudal septum
5. The bony and upper cartilaginous vaults left intact
6. Delivery of the tip cartilages through rim incisions
7. Trim of the cephalic excess (leaving a 5-mm wide lateral crus) and attenuation of the dome area with interdigitating scoring incisions
8. Submucous trim of the caudal upper lateral cartilages, no mucosal resection
9. Bilateral alar wedge resection

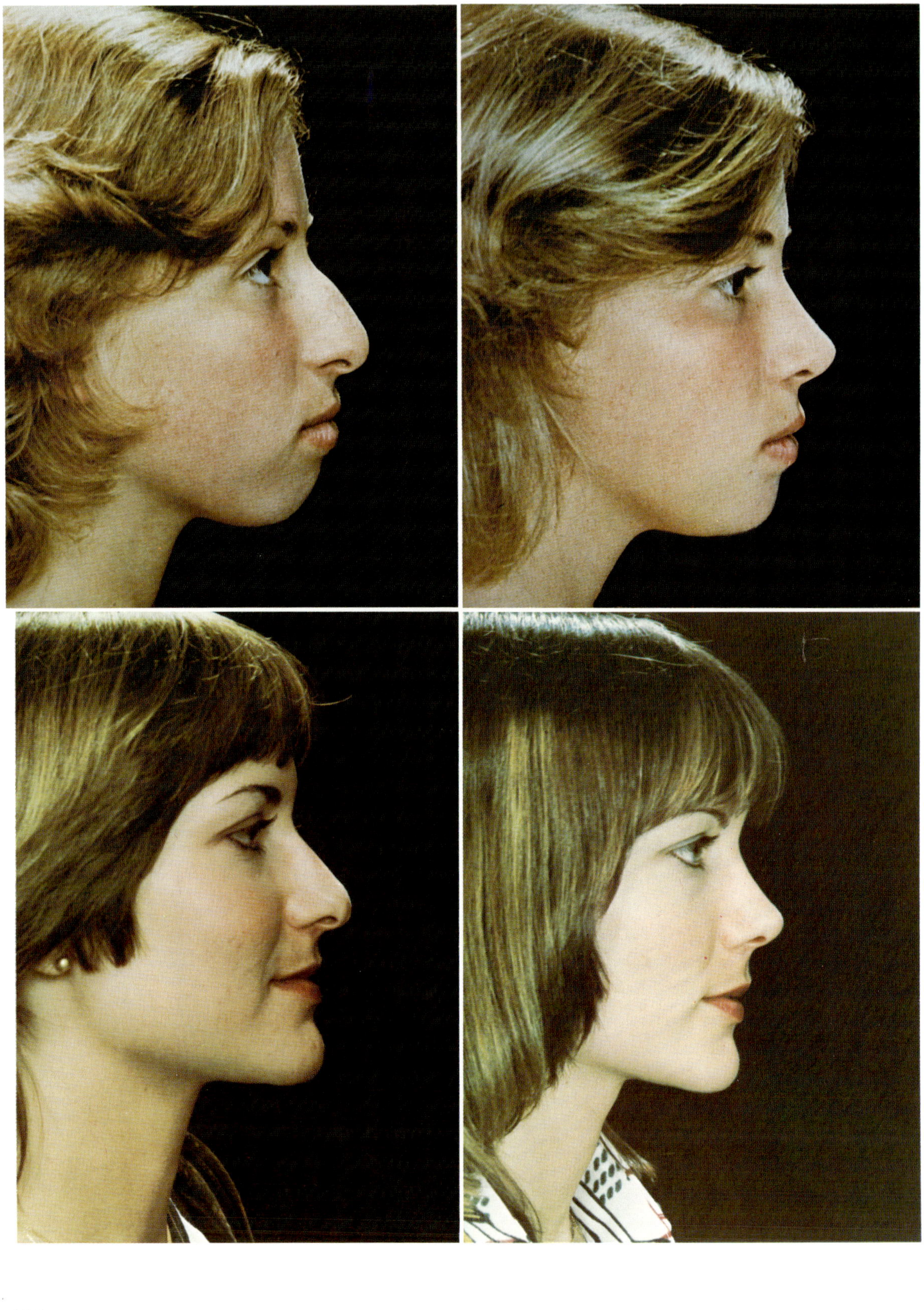

CHAPTER 6

Problem noses

Straight dorsum
Short nasal bones
Crooked nose
Tip with inadequate projection
Ultraprojecting tip
Malposition of the lower lateral cartilages

STRAIGHT DORSUM

The straight dorsum requires little or no reduction. Therefore, the margin for error, in judgment or technique, is negligible. The nose with a straight dorsum is a veritable pitfall because the danger of overresection frequently is unrecognized. Overreduction of the dorsum often sets up a progression of surgical errors as the surgeon reduces other nasal tissues in an attempt to bring the nose into proportion. The fact that a high percentage of secondary rhinoplasty patients' original noses were straight or nearly straight attests to the reality of this problem.

Technique is of particular importance in these cases because the surgeon who has not mastered a technique that will predictably lower the dorsal line just 1 or 2 mm will not be able to successfully treat the patient with a straight dorsum. Details of the surgical technique used in patients who are in this category are covered in Chapter 5.

The following illustrations demonstrate the need for recognition of the problem of the straight dorsum and the need for *minimal rhinoplasty* in these cases.

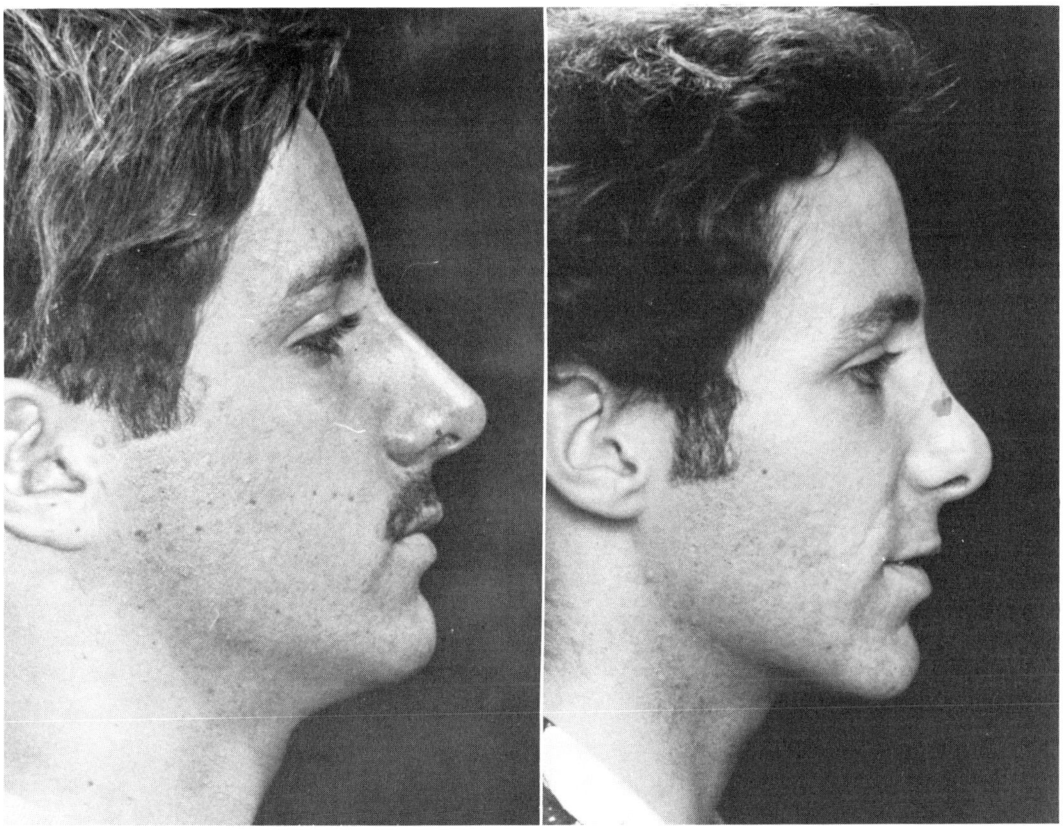

This patient was seen in consultation at age 17, at which time his request for rhinoplasty was declined. He returned 8 years later, 7 years following a primary rhinoplasty. He then requested that his nose be restored to its original configuration.

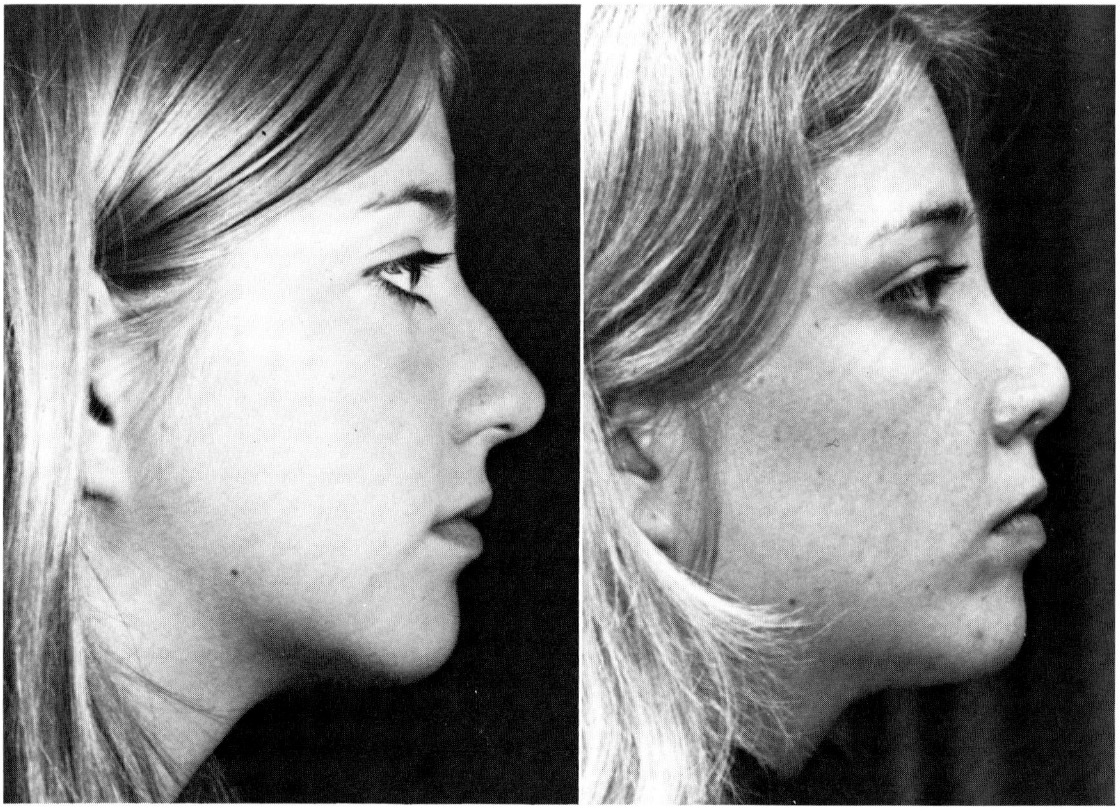

The nose with the small dorsal irregularity also falls into the category of the straight dorsum because the same danger exists. The nose requires *realignment,* not reduction. In this patient, over-reduction of the dorsum was followed by four subsequent surgeries for correction of the supratip fullness. The last "thinning" procedure resulted in vertical grooves along the nasal tip. The patient was told that she "formed scar tissue" and had "thick skin," which, sadly, became true after the repeated surgeries. The supratip fullness is not caused by scar tissue. It is caused by a loss of skeletal support.

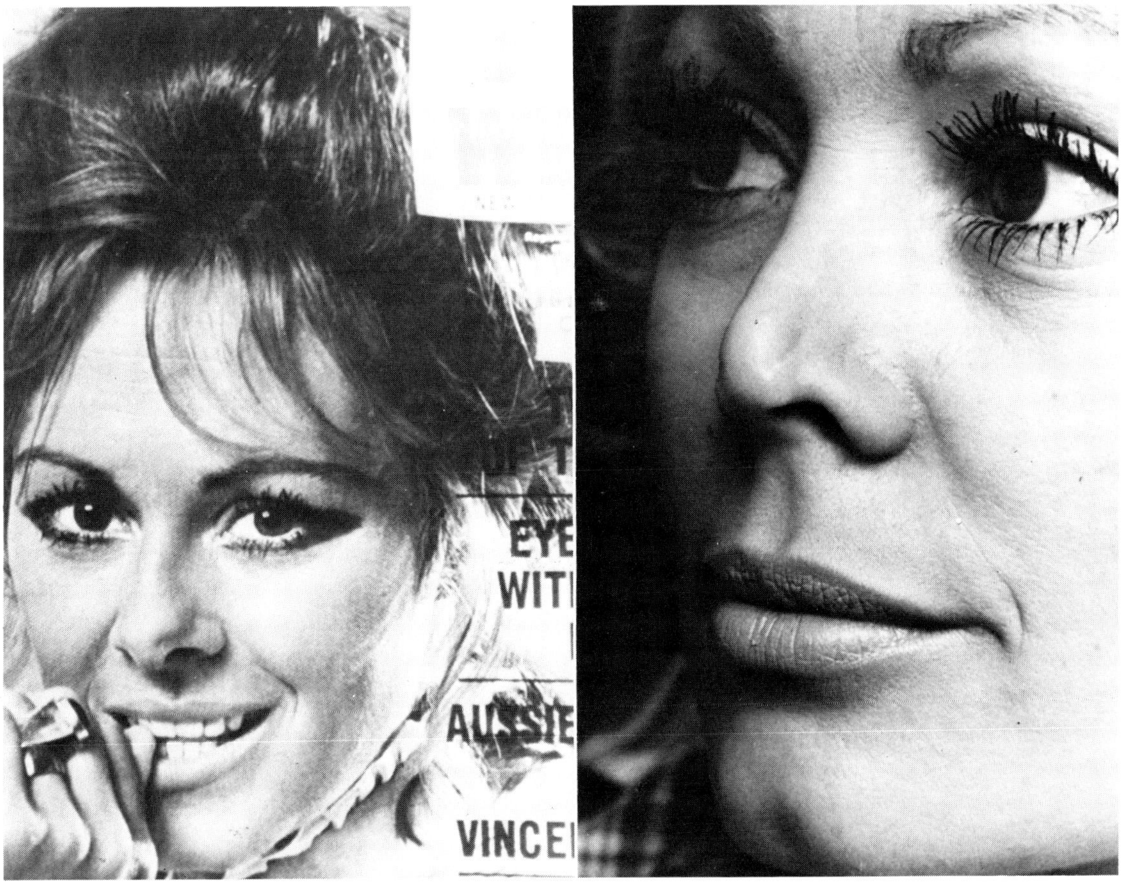

This professional singer was happy with her appearance, but she was told that her bulbous nasal tip was unattractive in photographs. She received a series of four rhinoplasties, which made her appearance progressively worse. This case demonstrates again that overreduction of the dorsum inevitably begins a series of surgical errors.

From what can be seen in the preoperative photograph, I think the original nose could have been corrected by limited skeletonization without transection of the membranous septum, a slight cephalic trim of the tip cartilages, and only a 1- to 2-mm reduction of the dorsum.

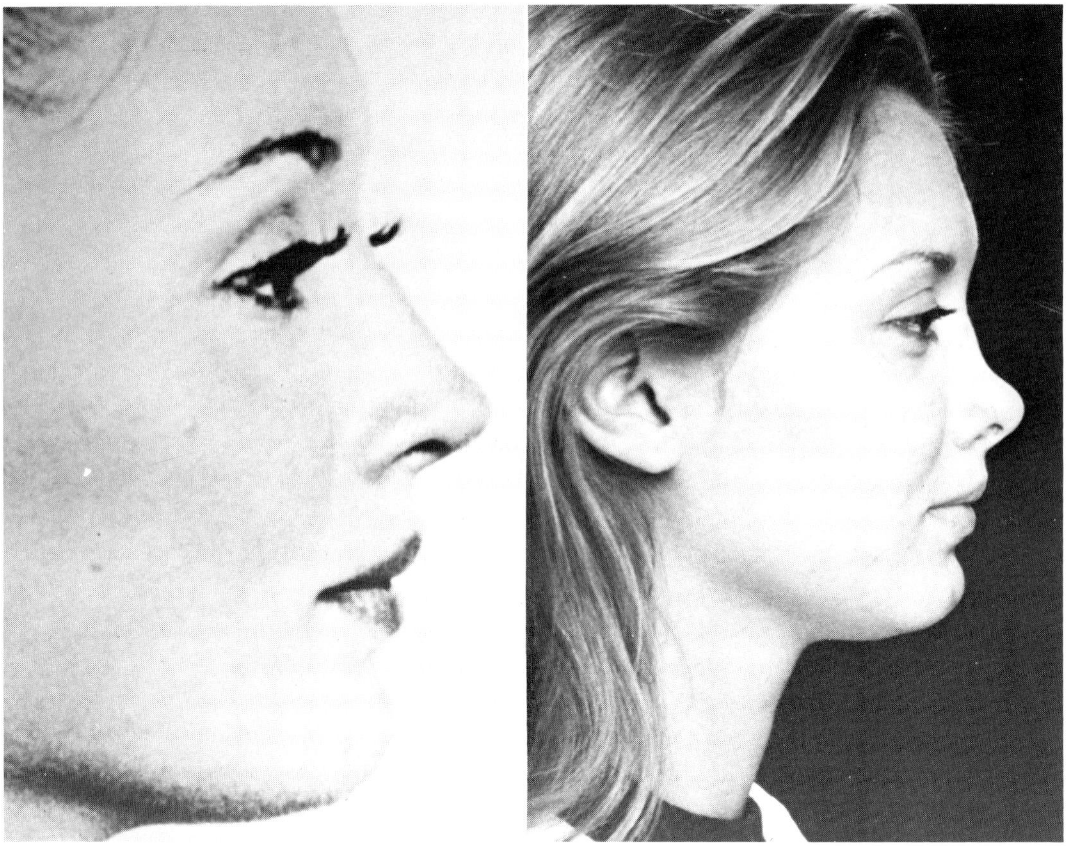

This model with an exceptionally good nose wanted only the small dorsal irregularity removed. Slight dorsal rasping with a Foman rasp would have been sufficient to remove the irregularity and preserve the elegant profile.

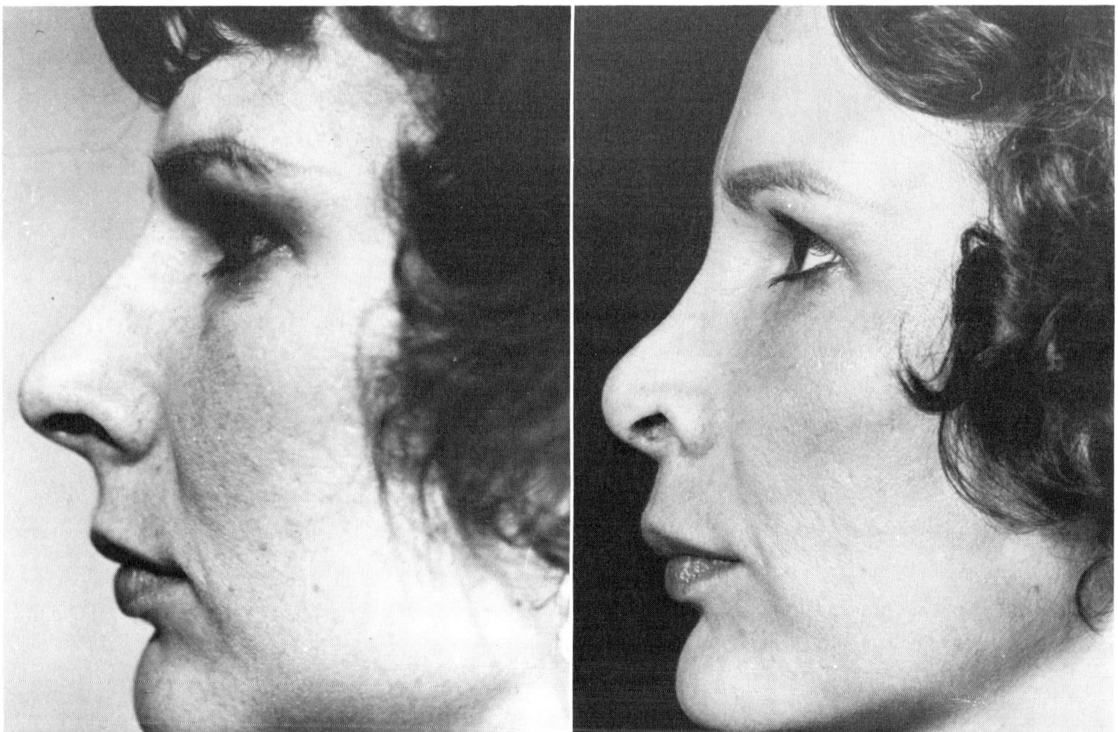

This patient, who had a straight dorsum, is discussed in Chapter 7.

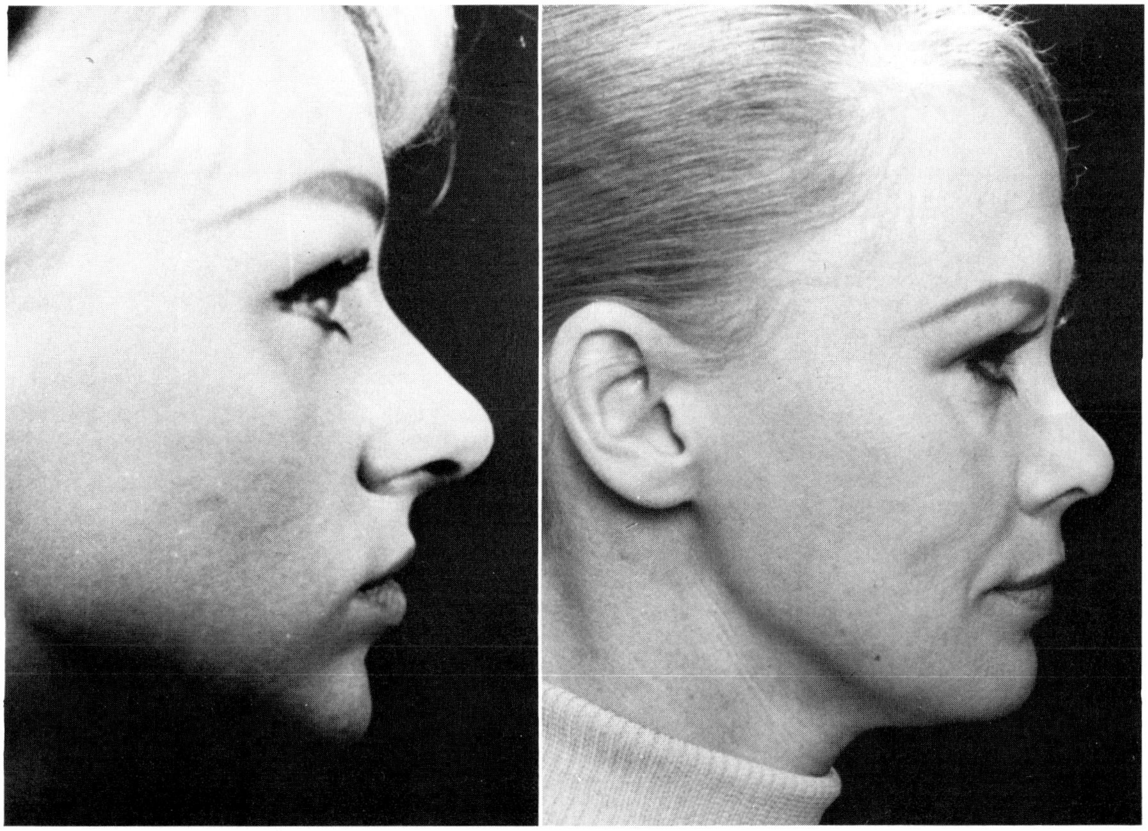

This patient had a straight dorsum, which was compounded by the additional problem of a short bony pyramid. She is discussed in detail in Chapter 7.

If the significance of the straight dorsum is recognized, the nose with a straight dorsum has exciting prospects. One of the most fascinating things about rhinoplasty is the dramatic change in the appearance of a nose that can occur with the very slightest alteration in its structure. This is usually apparent after conservative treatment of these patients.

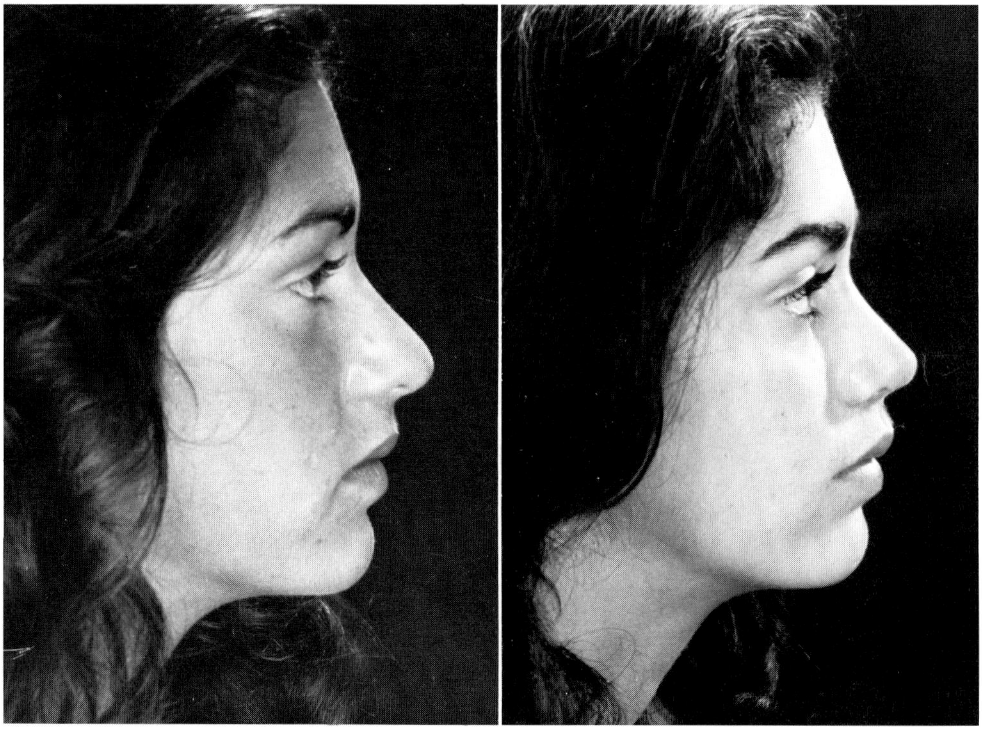

This patient was unhappy with the overall blunt appearance of her nose and with the downward inclination of the tip. The correction involved less than a 2-mm reduction of the dorsal height, modification of the lower lateral cartilages by cephalic trim, attenuation of the domes, and lateral osteotomies.

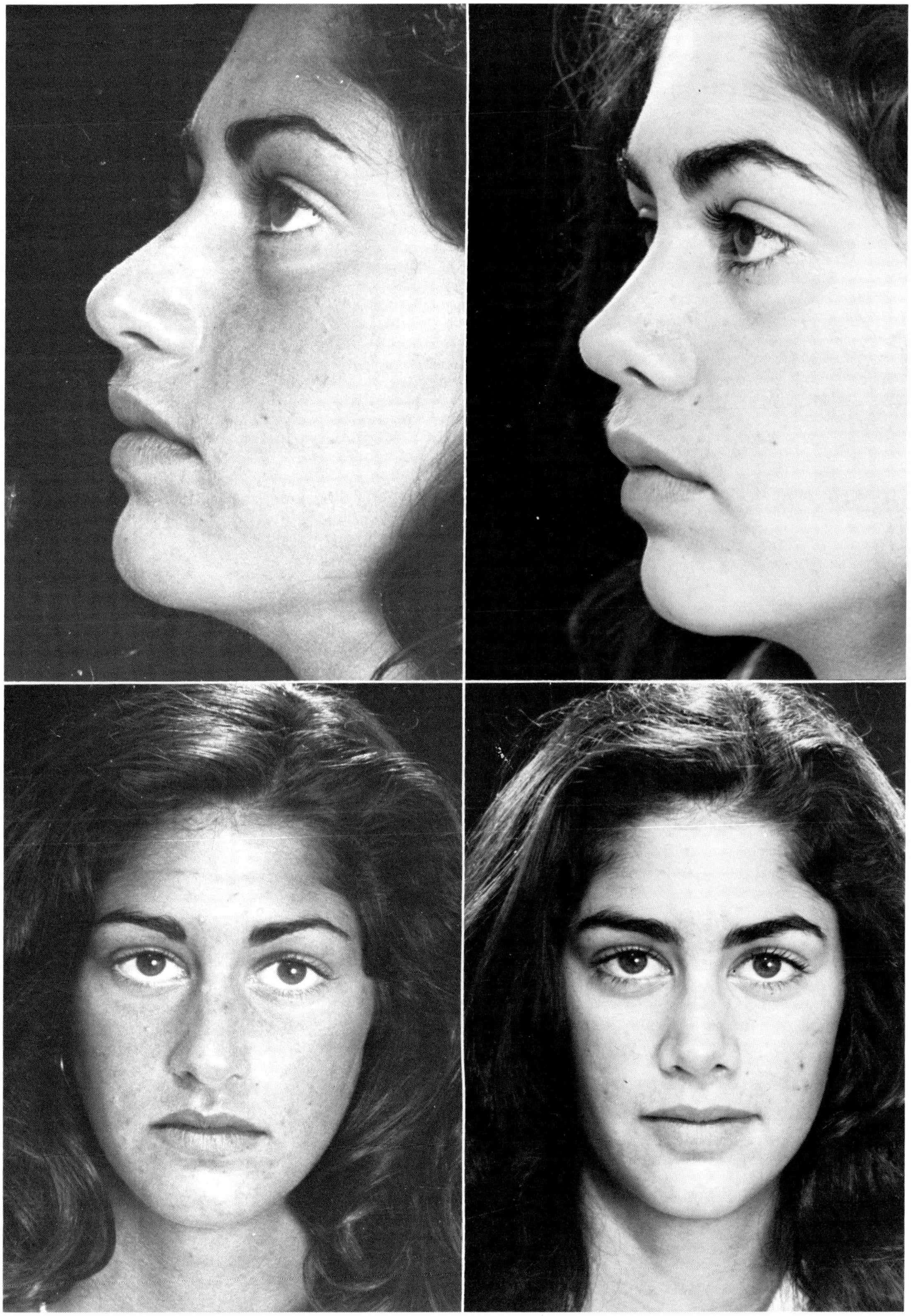

SHORT NASAL BONES

Anatomic variations in nasal bones are well known. Using his collection of skulls, Schaeffer demonstrated many osseous variations, ranging from elongated nasal bones that bound the lateral margins of the pyraform aperture to totally absent nasal bones that were replaced by the frontal processes of the maxilla. These are not merely anatomic curiosities. Structural differences in nasal bones can and do affect surgical outcomes, both aesthetically and functionally.

Nasal bones that are short have particular clinical importance in view of the major supportive function of the bony pyramid. When nasal bones are short, the support of the middle nasal vault is already precarious. If the bony dorsum is reduced and the nasal bones are fractured, as in routine rhinoplasty, it is likely that the lateral walls of the middle vault will collapse against the septum.

The normal bony pyramid extends approximately one-half the distance from the radix to the angle of the septum. The normal pyramid is of sufficient length to provide support to the upper lateral cartilages and to provide the necessary width to the middle third of the nose for a smooth pyramidal contour.

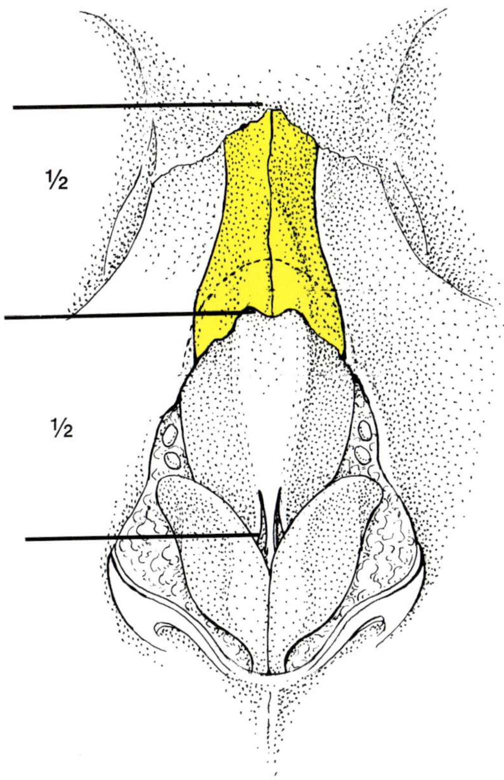
½
½

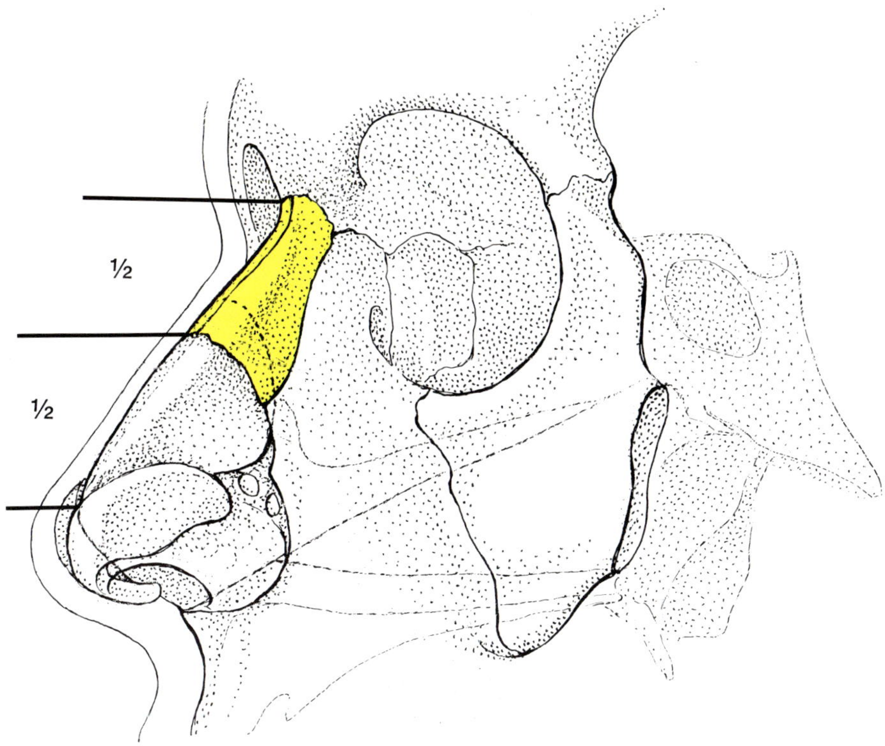
½
½

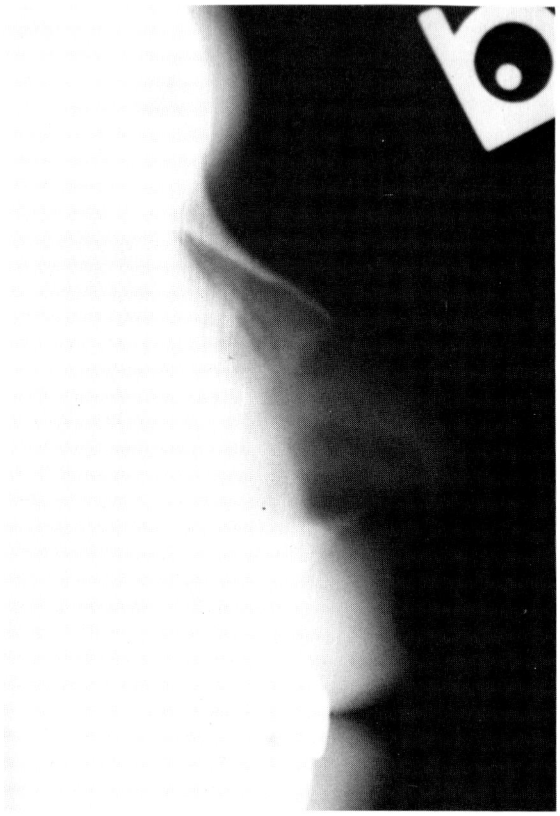

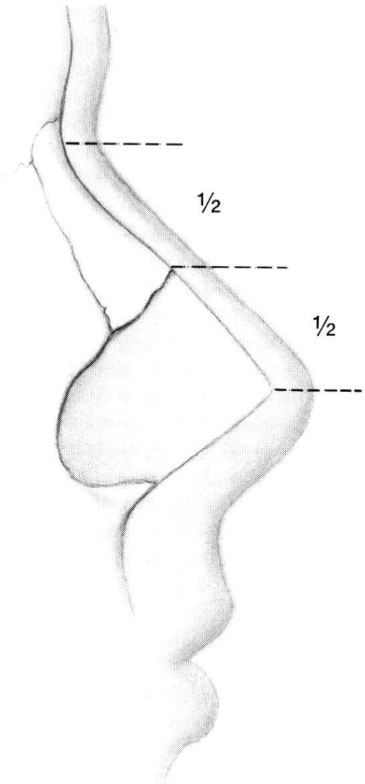

The x-ray film of a normal nasal bone illustrates the usual length in relation to the size of the nose. The reference points at the radix, the caudal end of the bony vault, and the angle of the septum are shown.

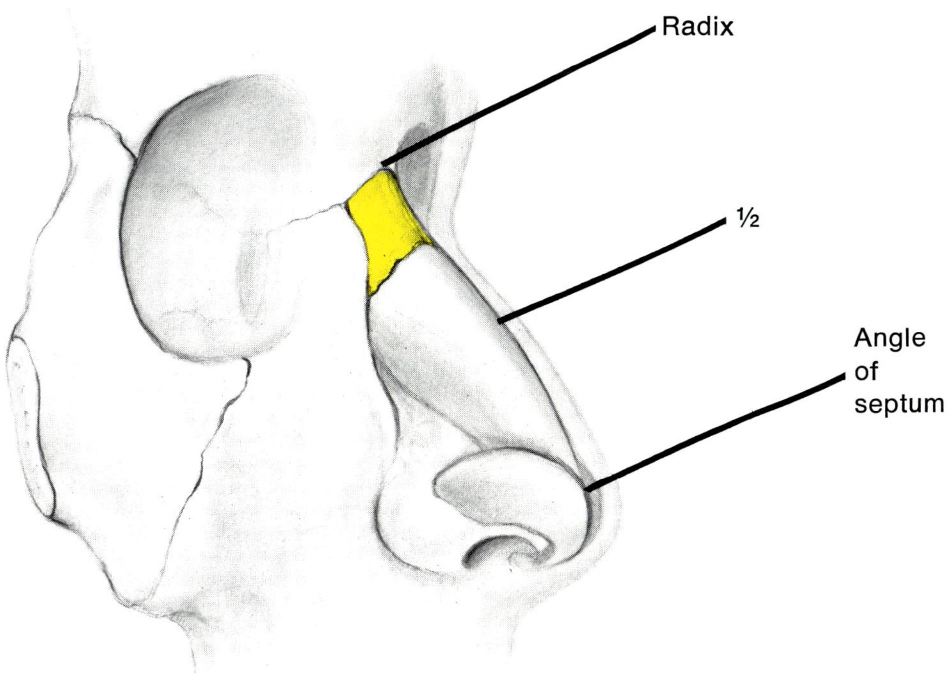

The short bony pyramid extends less than one-half the distance from the radix to the angle of the septum. Although the point at which short bones becomes clinically relevant varies, in general any bony pyramid spanning less than one fourth of the designated distance must receive special consideration.

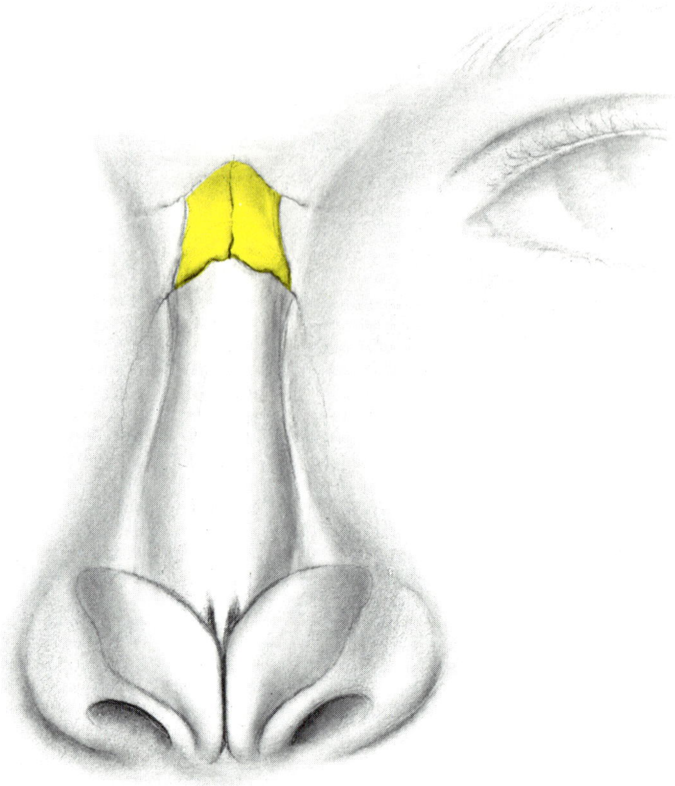

Because of inadequate bony framework, there are bilateral concavities in the frontal nasal contour preoperatively. This pair of concavities forewarns of short nasal bones.

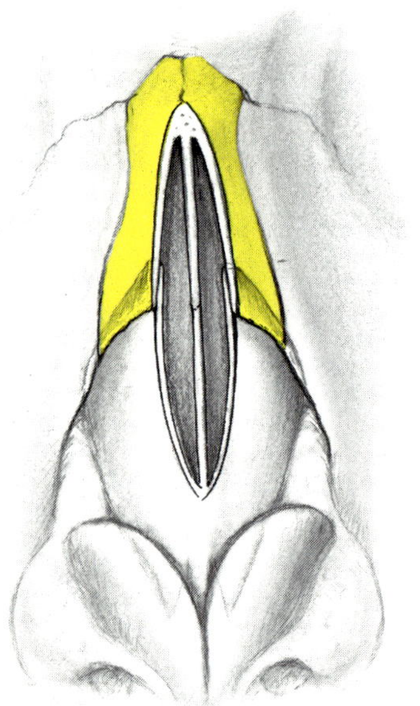

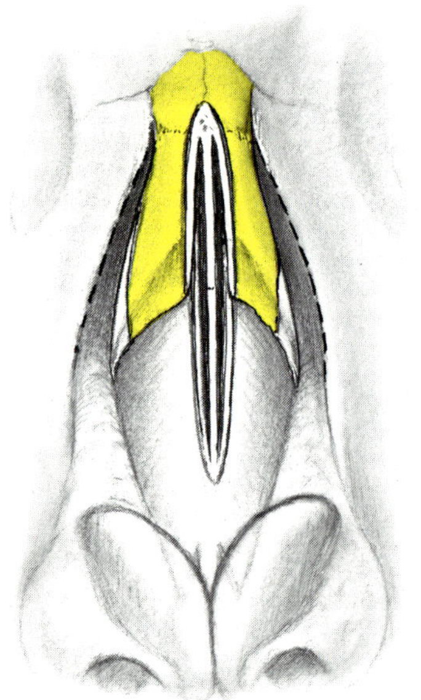

The nasal pyramid of normal length maintains support to the lateral nasal walls following resection of the roof and following lateral osteotomies.

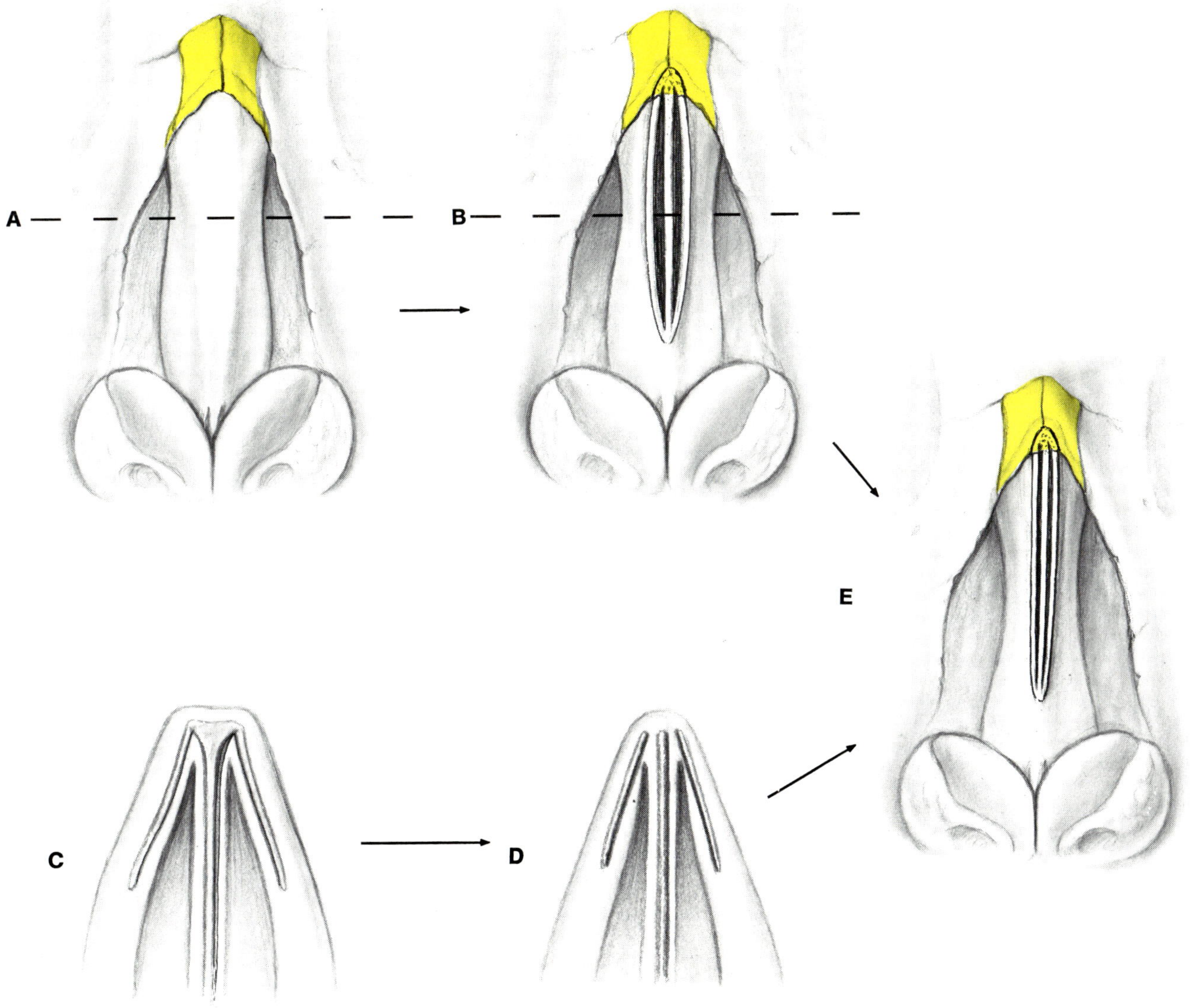

Section through **A** Section through **B**

In contrast to the significant bony hump present in many patients, the dorsal hump in patients with short nasal bones is almost entirely cartilaginous *(A)*. Resection of the roof during rhinoplasty *(B)* removes the principal lateral support of the upper lateral cartilages, that is, the top of the septal T *(C)*. This leaves only the remaining lateral attachments to the bony vault as total support and lateral distractors *(E)*. As a result, there may be an alarming narrowness to the middle third of the nose following dorsal reduction (*D* and *E*). In effect, the nose would be compromised aesthetically, but equally distressing is that the nose may be compromised functionally. Without the distraction and support of both the nasal bones and the anterior septal T, the upper lateral cartilages may act as a flutter valve, impeding nasal inspiration.

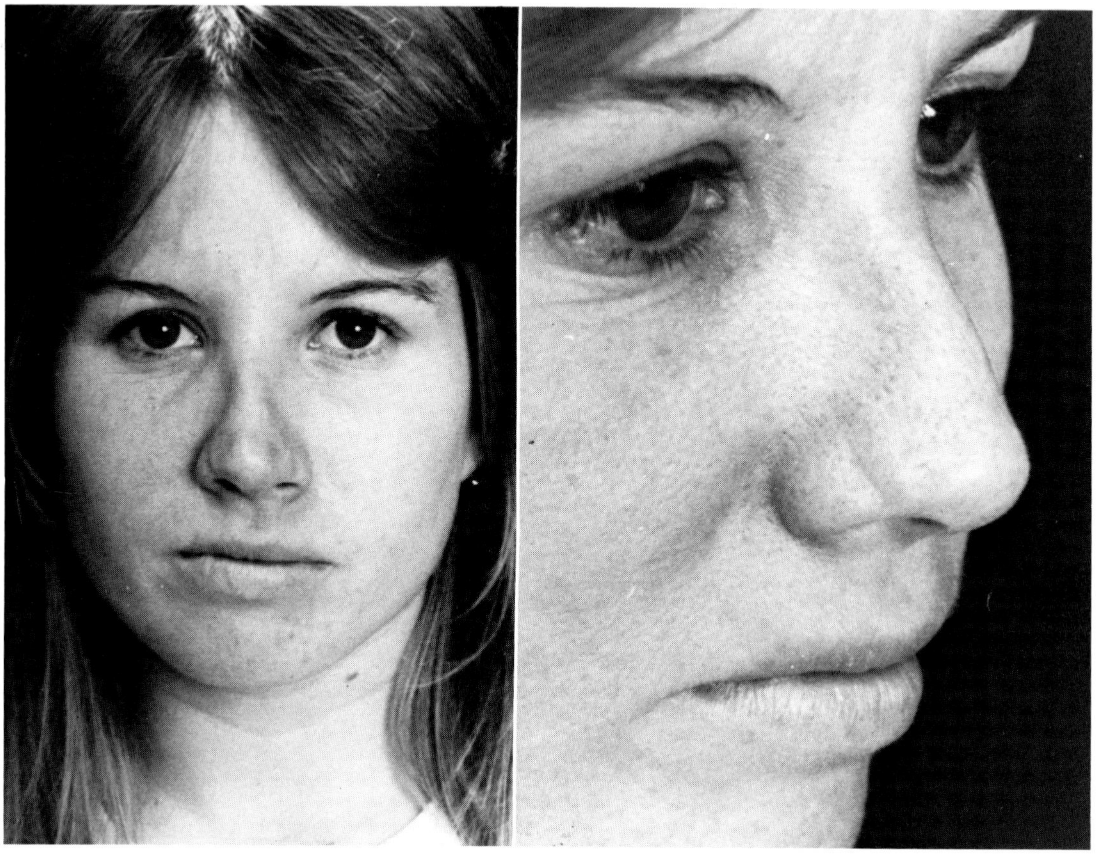

This patient with short nasal bones was seen following a conservative rhinoplasty. A small amount of hump was resected, and no fracture was performed. The central third of the nose is too narrow for both radix and base in spite of heavy tissues. On both views, the caudal edge of the bony pyramid is visible.

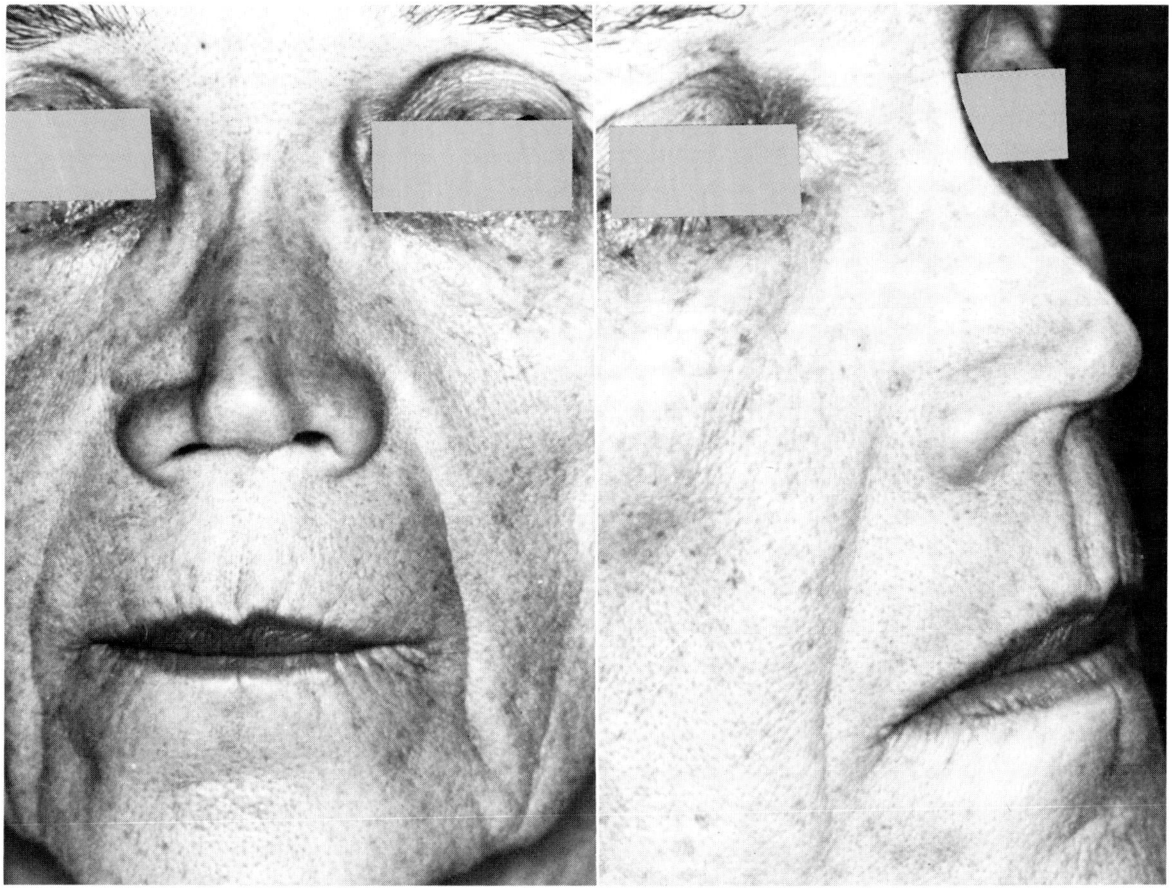

Thin tissues overlying a short bony pyramid may lead to a devastating result if the problem is not recognized. This patient had short nasal bones, extending approximately one-fourth the distance between the radix and the angle of the septum. During rhinoplasty, lateral and medial osteotomies were performed. Mobilization of the short nasal bones completely ablated the bony arch, leaving only the dorsal edge of the septum to provide support and contour to these very thin tissues.

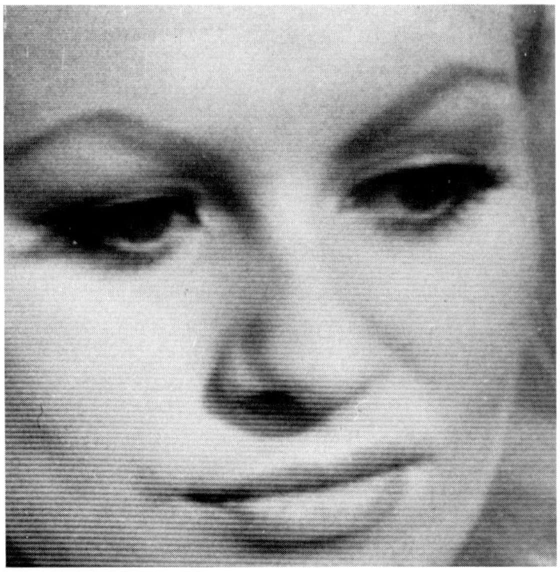

This patient's bony pyramid is best seen in a preoperative photograph of a television appearance. A cross light highlights the dorsal contour, effectively delineating the caudal border of the bony pyramid.

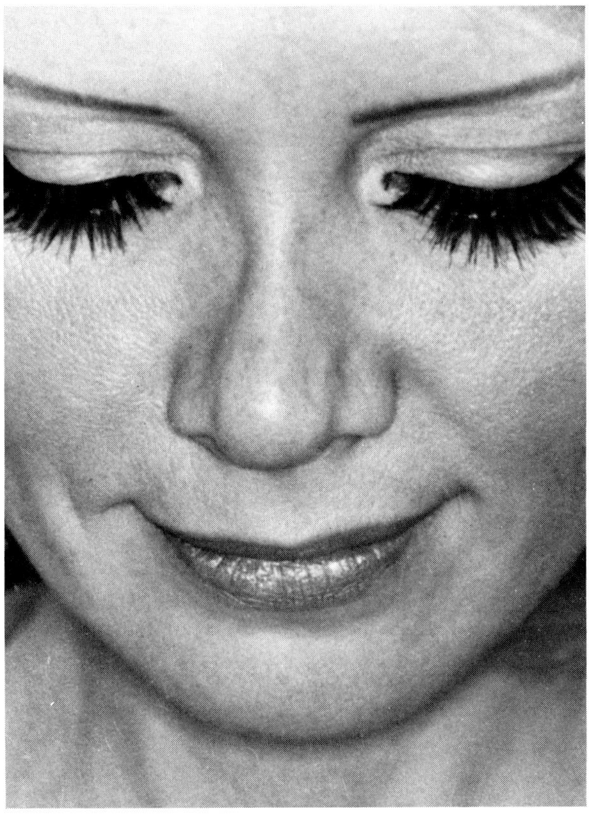

The patient is shown following two rhinoplasties.

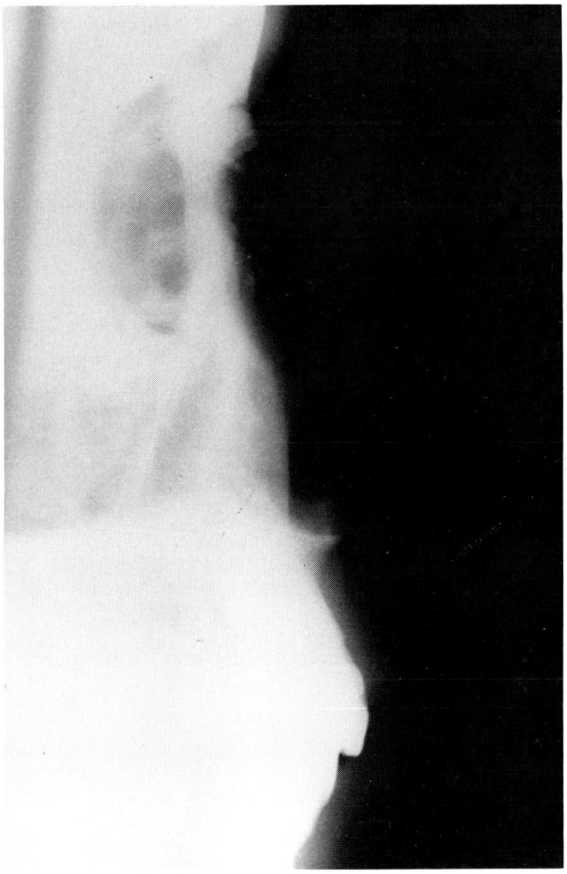

The x-ray film was taken before reconstruction and shows an extremely short bony pyramid. This patient is discussed in detail in Chapter 7.

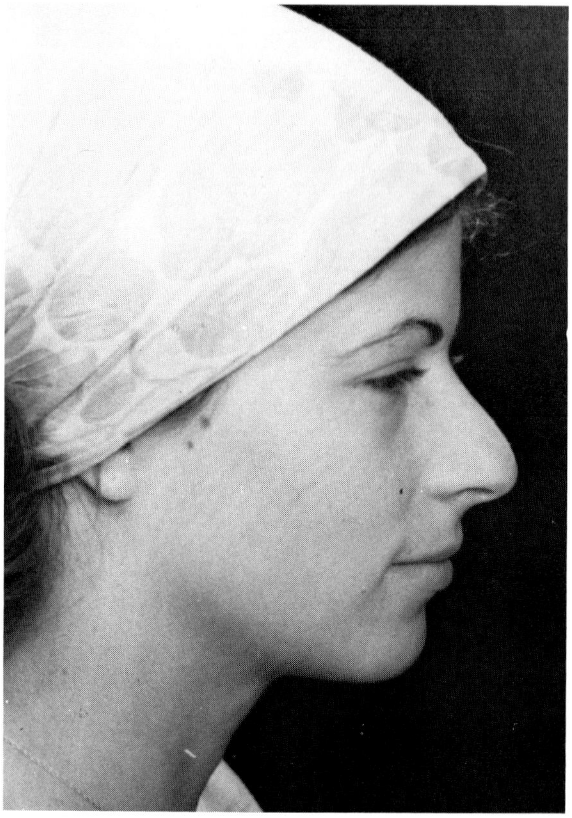

Case report 1: Reimplantation of resected dorsum

Patients with short nasal bones may have high dorsal profiles. There is little to warn of the impending problem on lateral view. Because of her high dorsum, this patient seems to be an ideal candidate for the standard Joseph rhinoplasty.

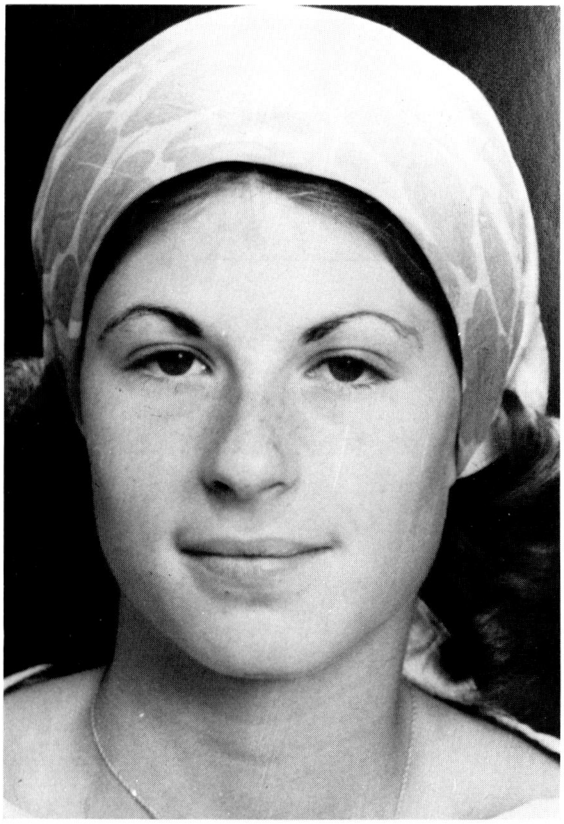

Characteristic of patients with short nasal bones is a narrow upper vault. This characteristic look should make the surgeon suspect a short bony pyramid.

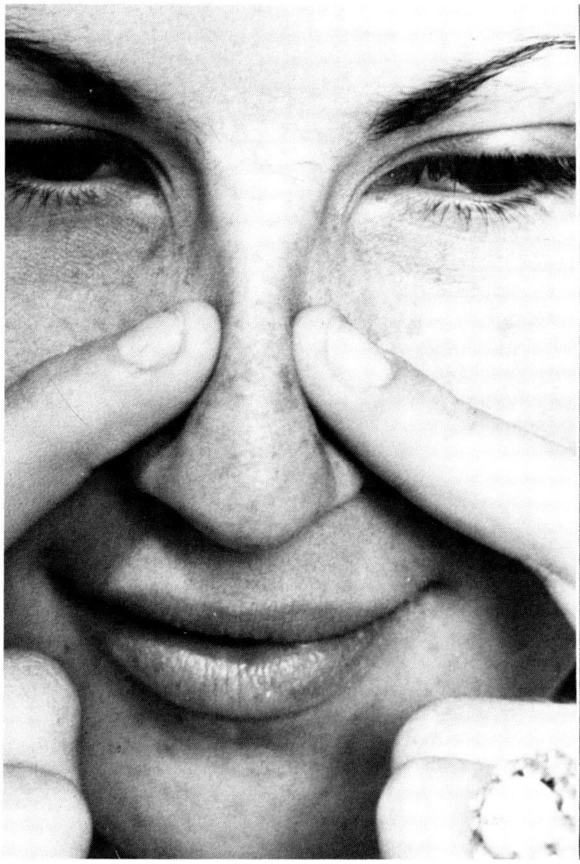

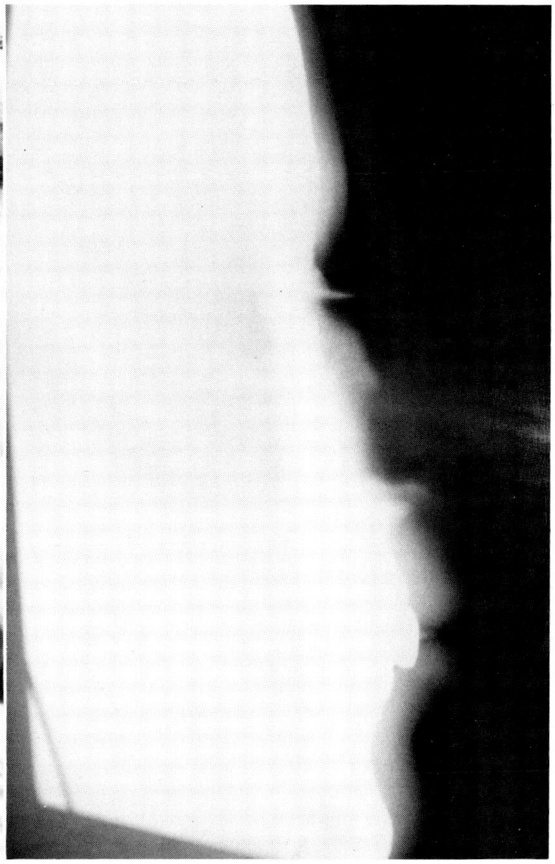

On palpation, the short bony pyramid is evident. The x-ray film confirms that the short nasal bones and the frontal process of the maxilla form the lateral border of the middle vault.

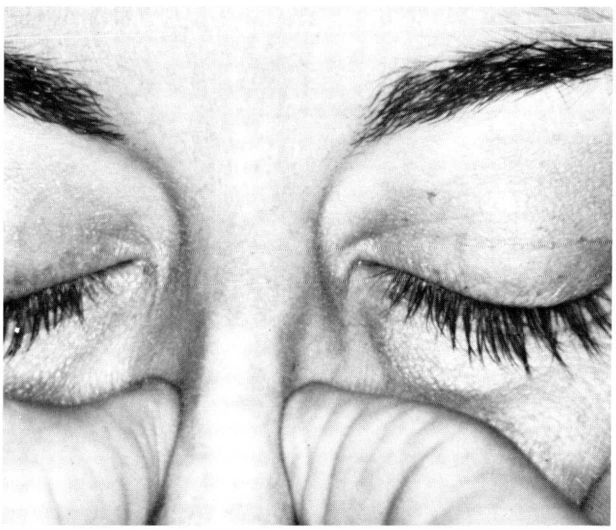

SURGICAL PROCEDURE

The nasal bones are palpated before surgery.

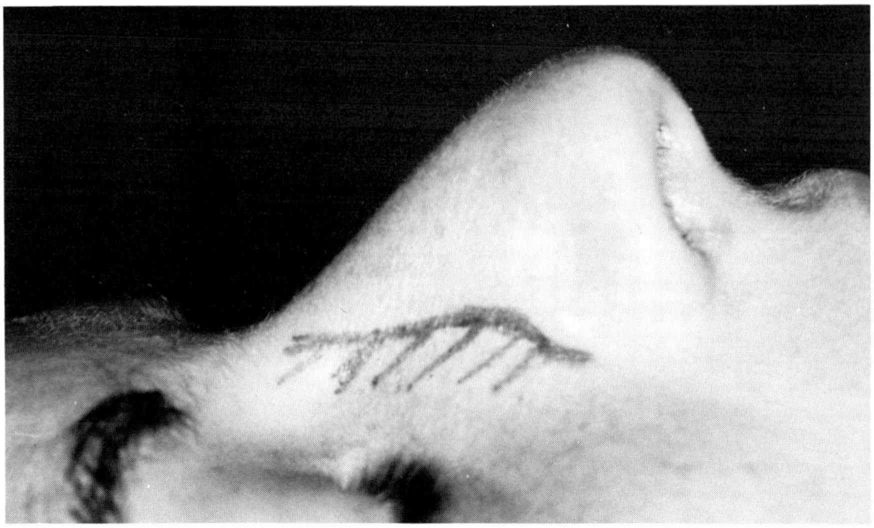

The contour of the frontal process of the maxilla as it extends to the nasal bones is marked.

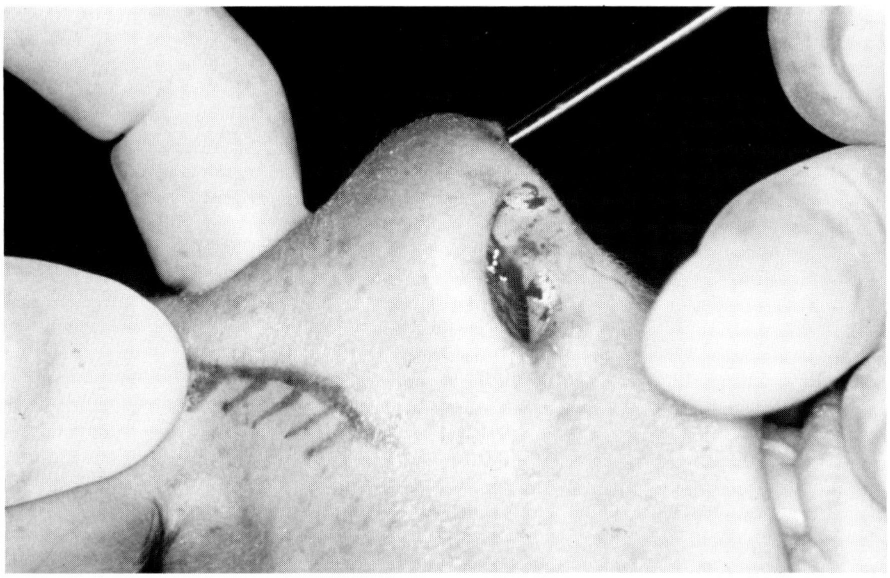

Skeletonization is limited over both the upper cartilaginous vault and the bony vault. A right-angle knife is used to skeletonize the dorsum to the angle of the septum.

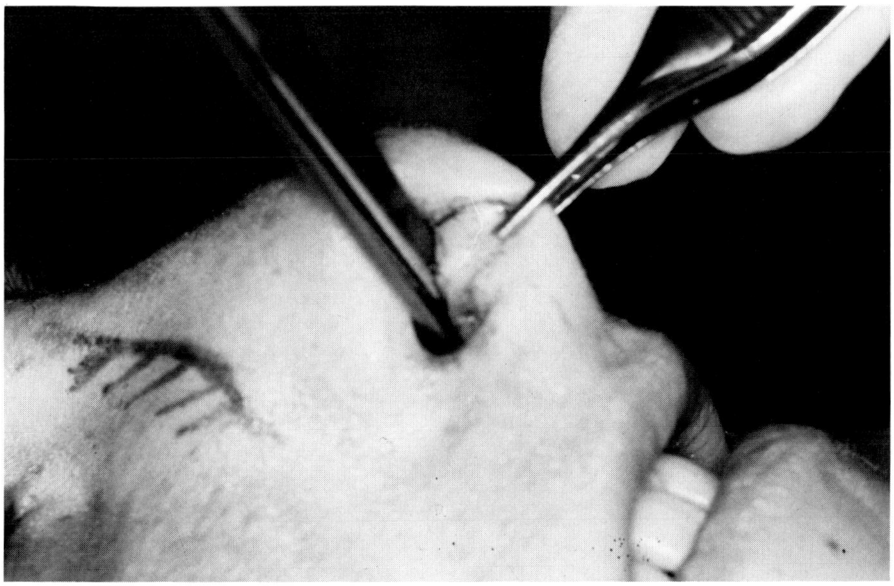

Transfixion of the membranous septum is done with a pair of Mayo scissors and extends to the nasal spine.

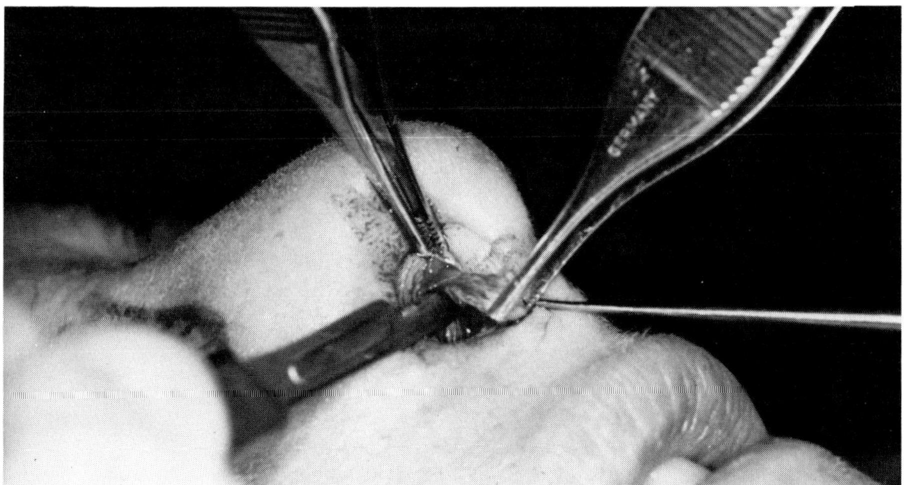

Following reduction of the nasal spine with a double-action bone rongeur, a triangular segment of caudal septum is resected. The widest segment of cartilage (base of triangle) is posterior, becoming narrower toward the angle of the septum.

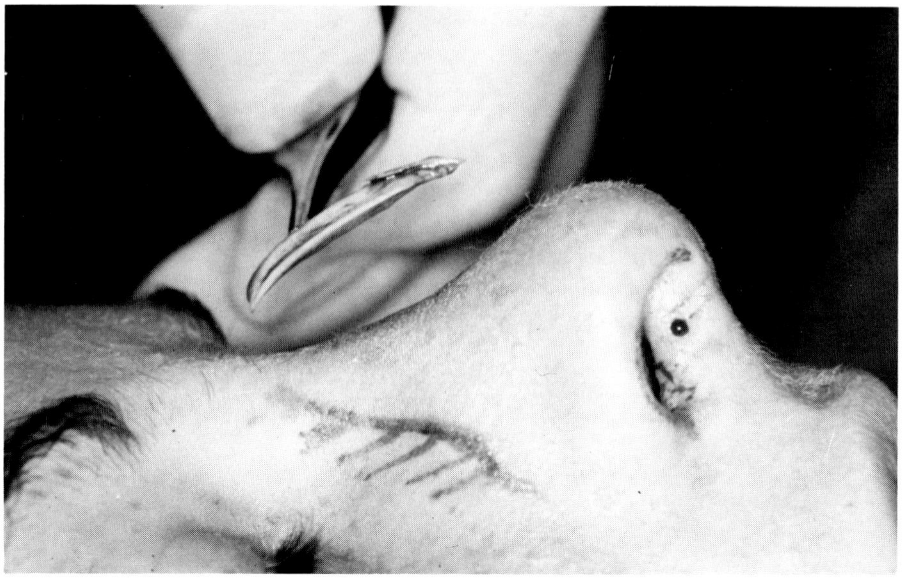

Because virtually all of the dorsum is cartilaginous, the entire dorsal segment is removed with a knife. Following resection, the position of the tip can be accurately assessed.

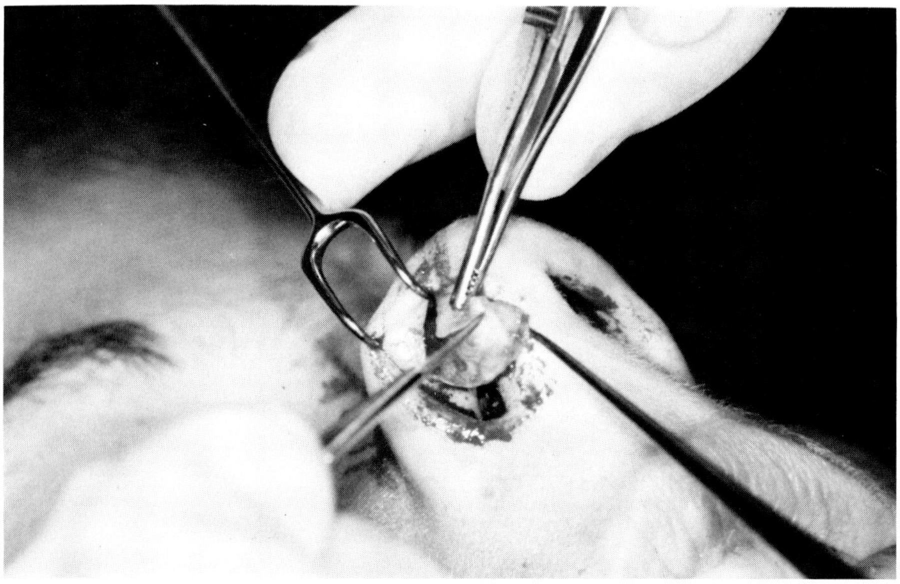

The lower lateral cartilage is delivered through a rim incision and the cephalic part trimmed. A substantial caudal part is preserved.

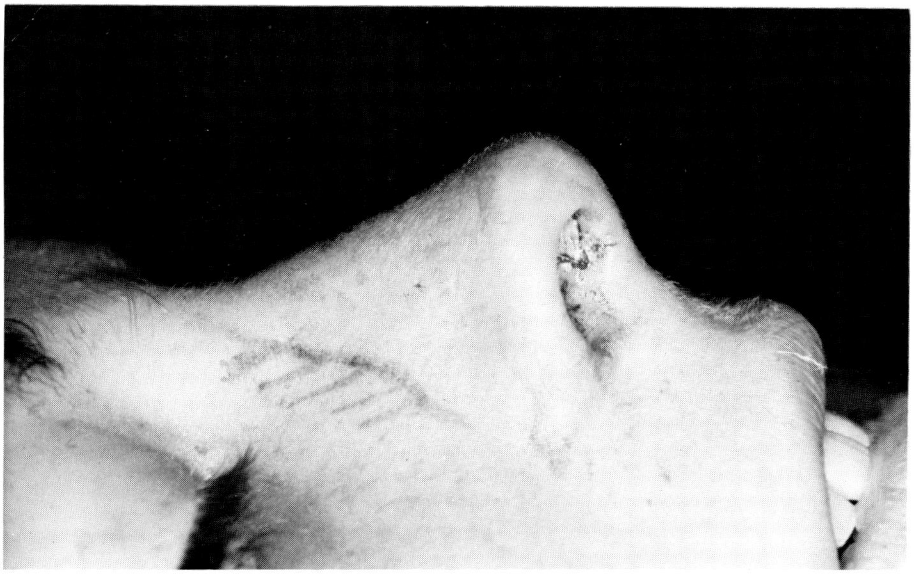

A dorsal graft using the resected dorsal cartilage (Skoog technique) re-creates a smooth dorsal contour. A dorsal graft is necessary to cover the open roof following dorsal resection and to provide support to the middle vault.

Summary of surgical procedure

1. Limited skeletonization
2. Transfixion to the nasal spine
3. Reduction of the nasal spine
4. Reduction of the caudal septum
5. Resection of the cartilaginous dorsum
6. Delivery of the lower lateral cartilages through rim incisions
7. Cephalic trim of the lateral crura without modification of the dome areas
8. Replacement of the trimmed dorsal cartilage as a free graft

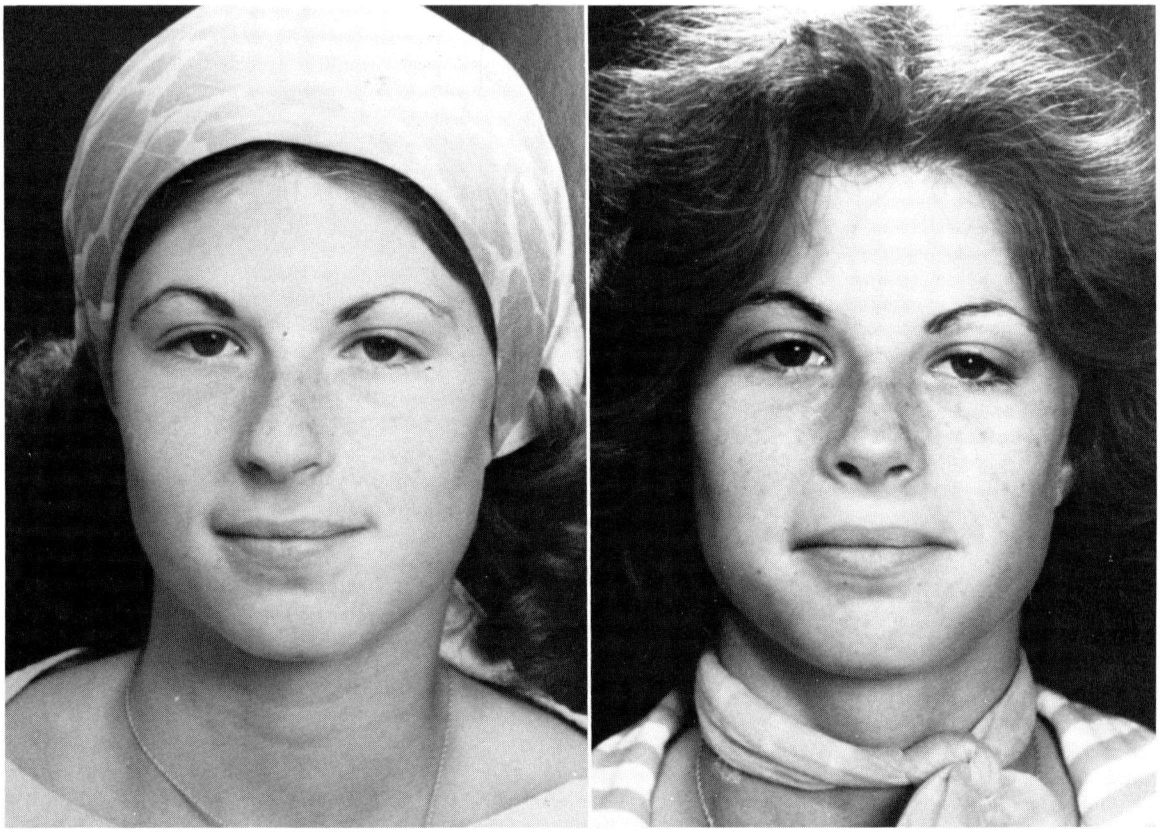

POSTOPERATIVE RESULTS

Postoperatively, the central third of her nose appears slightly broader because of the reduced height of the dorsum. The tip refinement is manifest by a light reflex that delineates the tip. If one closely examines the preoperative nose, it is easy to imagine the visual effect of excessive narrowing of the upper and middle vaults that would necessarily result from osteotomies.

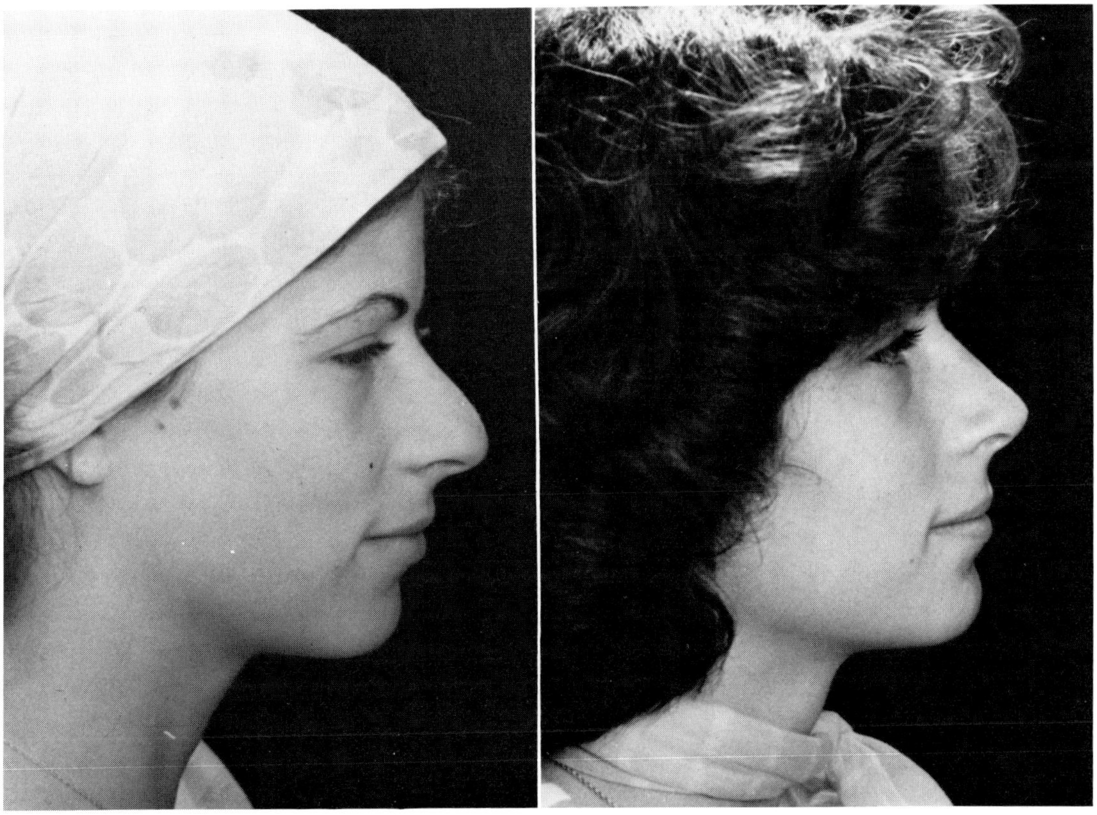

On lateral view, the dorsum is straight, and the tip is the highest point in the nasal profile. Resection of the spine and caudal septum has increased the length of her upper lip.

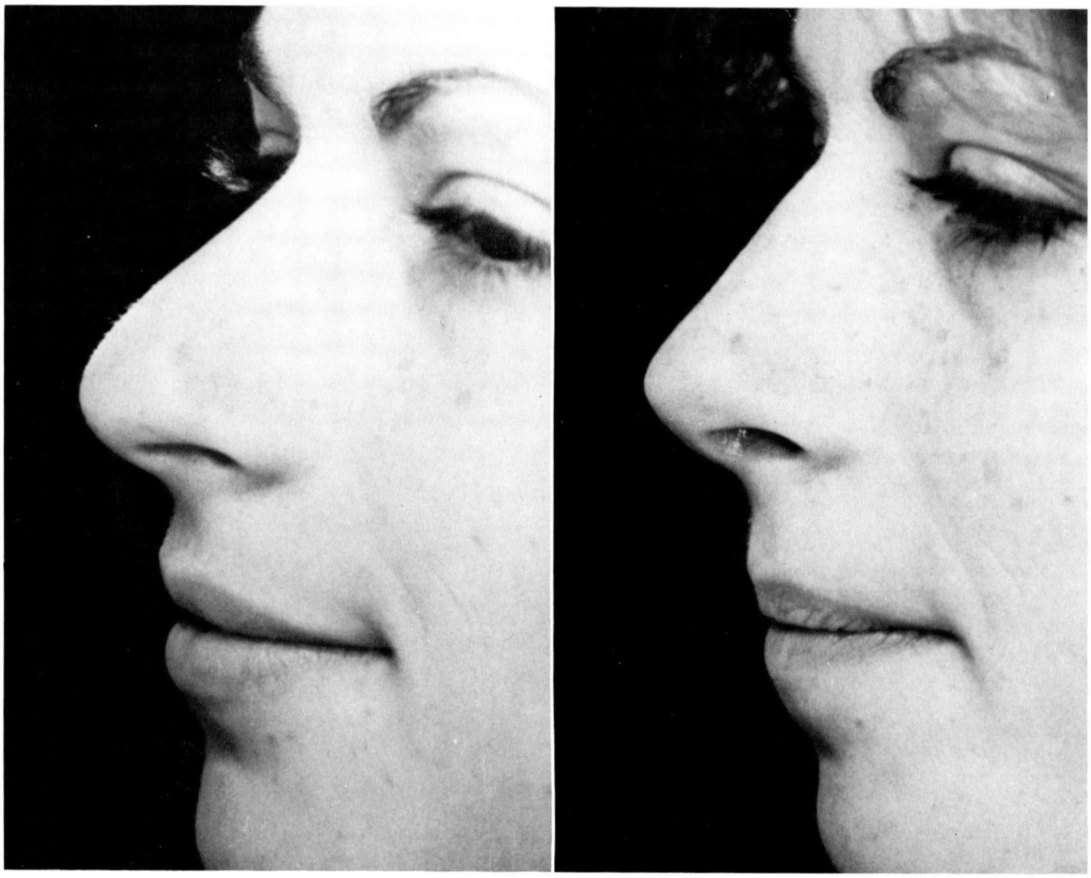

On left oblique view, the nose has a nonsurgical appearance and good definition of its parts. The projection of the graft near the radix provides a natural irregularity that is well accepted by this patient.

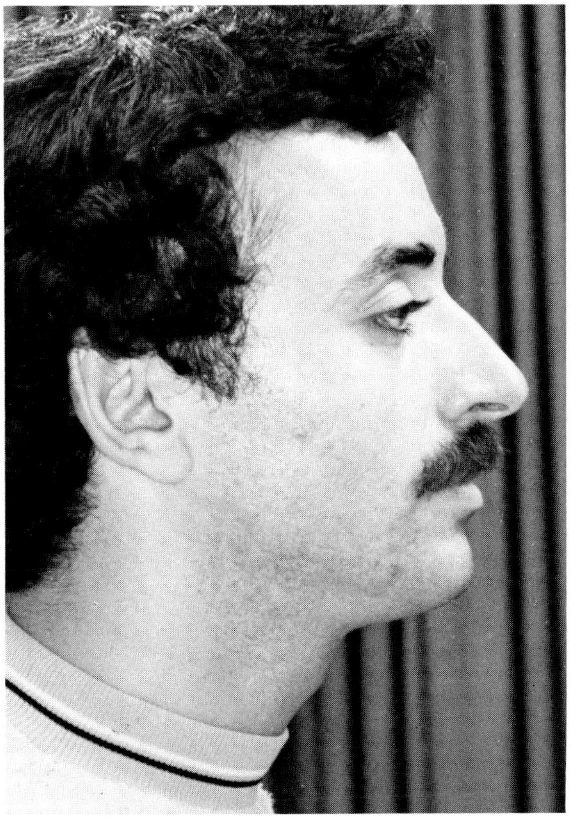

Case report 2: Reconstruction of dorsum using septal cartilage

This 28-year-old actor requested rhinoplasty because professionally it had become important that his nose appear straight in photographs from both the side and front. He was emphatic in his request that there be no change in appearance except for the straightening of his nose.

On lateral view, there is nothing to suggest the presence of a short nasal bone. The dorsum is slightly high, the tip is lower than the dorsum, and the nasolabial angle is 90 degrees. The nostril is notched, and the alar lobule inserts lower than the columella.

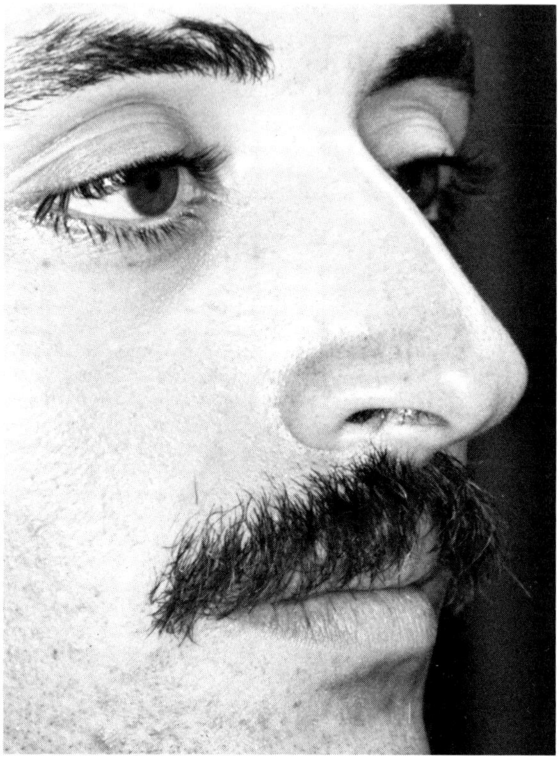

On right oblique view, the slight dorsal convexity is more visible. The tissues are fine and thin, and the tip cartilages appear to be well structured. There is a suspicious concavity in the entire middle third of the nose and a narrowness to the dorsum. Both features are characteristic of an absent or short bony pyramid. On this view, the left upper eyelid margin crosses behind the approximate level of the caudal end of the bony pyramid.

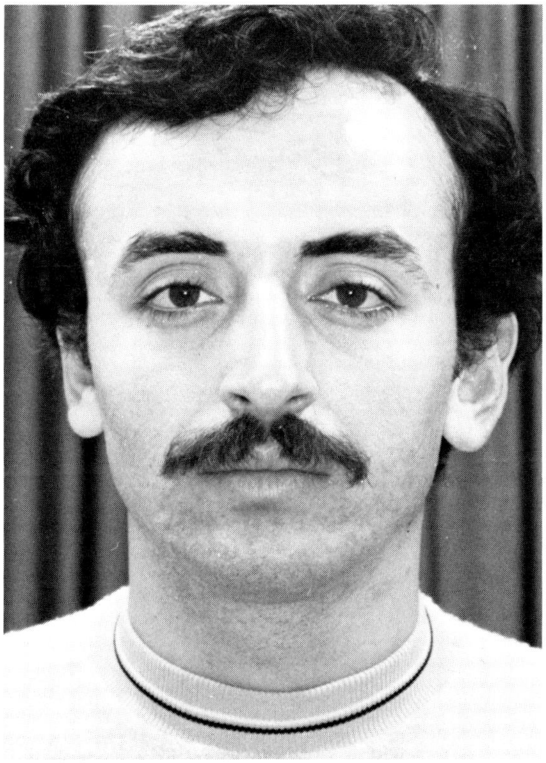

On front view, the middle third of the nose is disproportionately narrow. The edges of the frontal processes of the maxilla can be seen as faint light reflexes, which form brackets around the central nasal configuration. There is a marked septal deviation—a common finding in these cases because the nose with a short bony pyramid is especially vulnerable to injury.

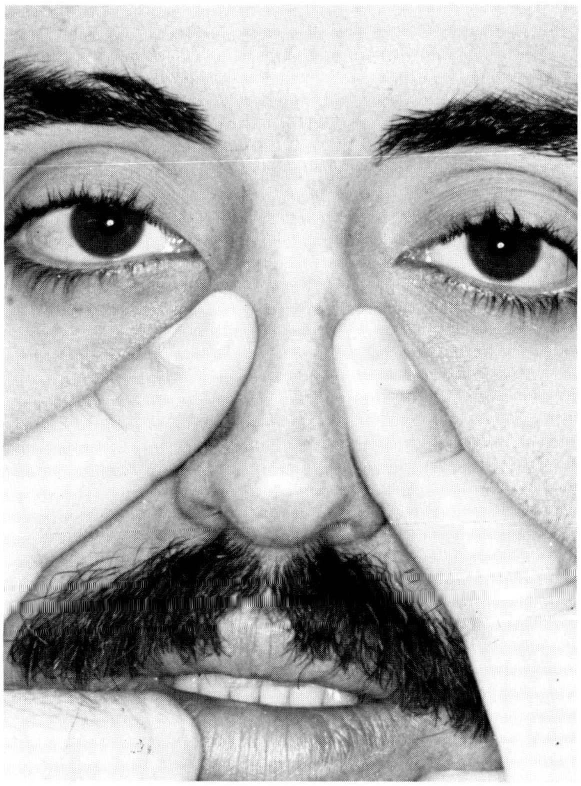

Palpation of the bony pyramid is the simplest and most certain method of assessment. The patient was asked to compress the central third of his nose, which makes the caudal borders of the bony vault visible. The bony pyramid is approximately one-fourth the distance from the radix to the angle of the septum.

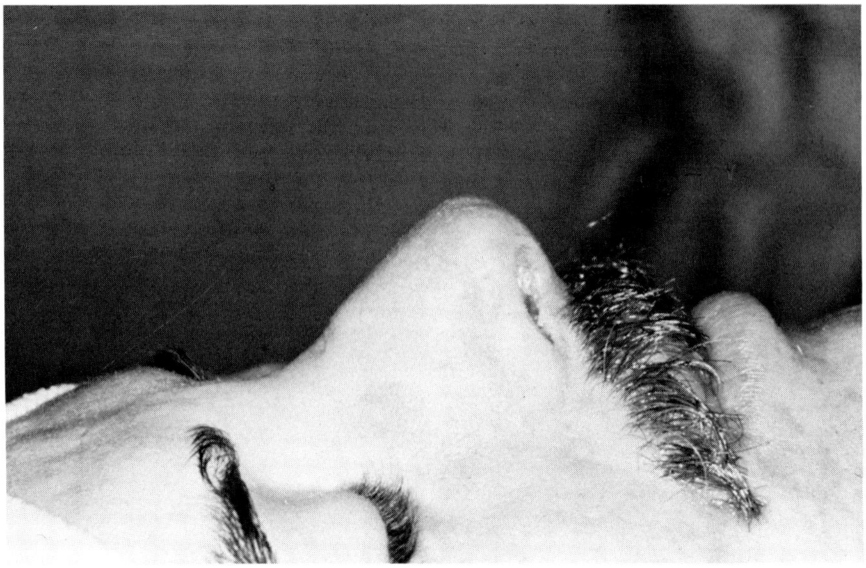

SURGICAL PROCEDURE

Following limited skeletonization over the upper cartilaginous and bony vaults, the bony dorsum was reduced slightly with a Foman rasp.

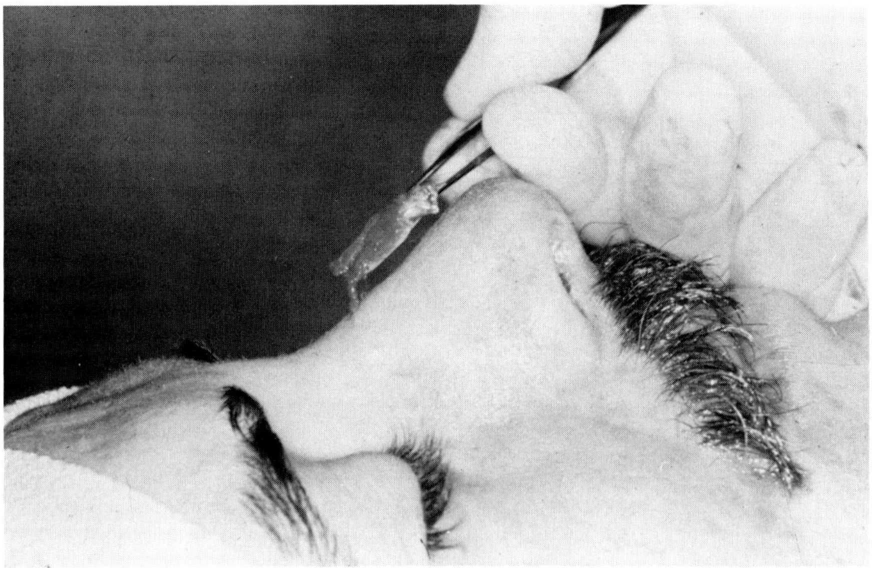

The dorsal segment of the upper cartilaginous vault is shown following resection. The resected portion was too small for use as a dorsal replacement.

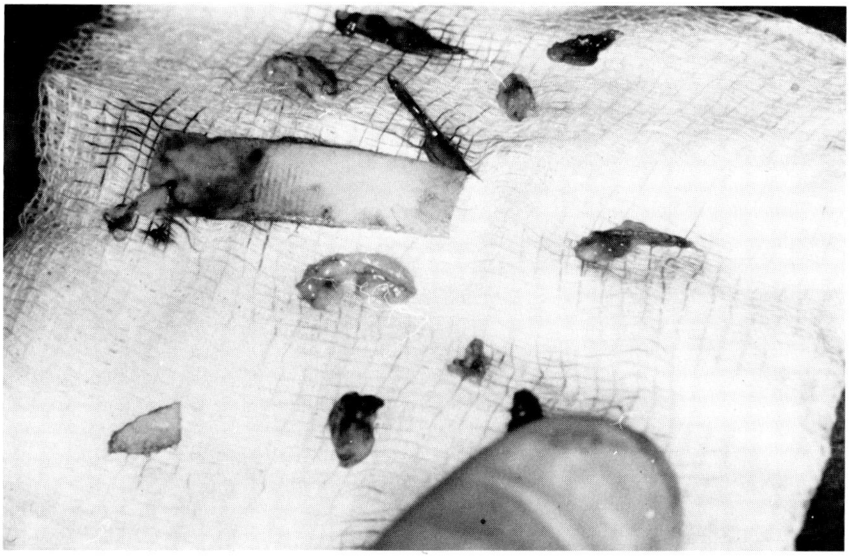

A septoplasty was done to relieve an obstruction on the left side of his nose. All unused pieces were trimmed and replaced in the septal pocket.

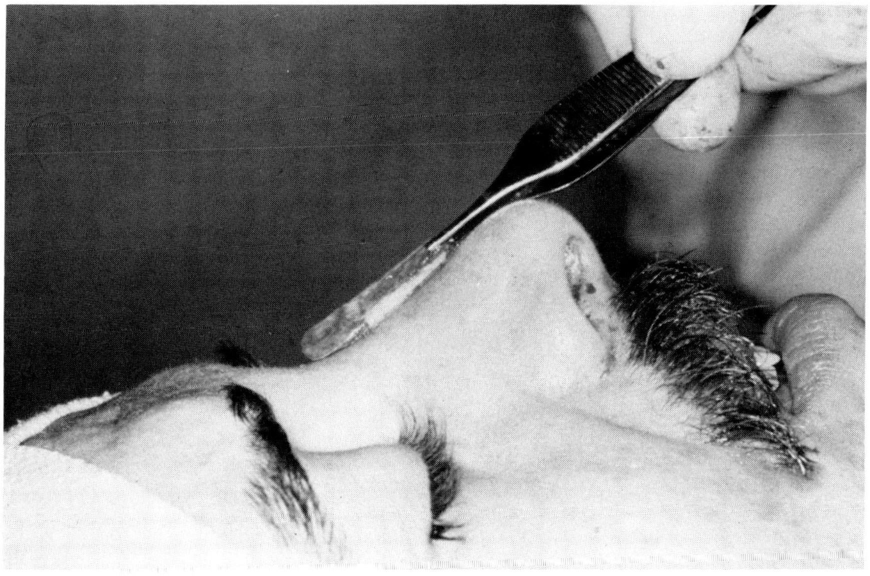

The cartilage, with attached perpendicular plate, was cut, and the sides were beveled to re-create the new dorsum. The thin ethmoid bone placed over the radix produces the least palpable evidence of a graft.

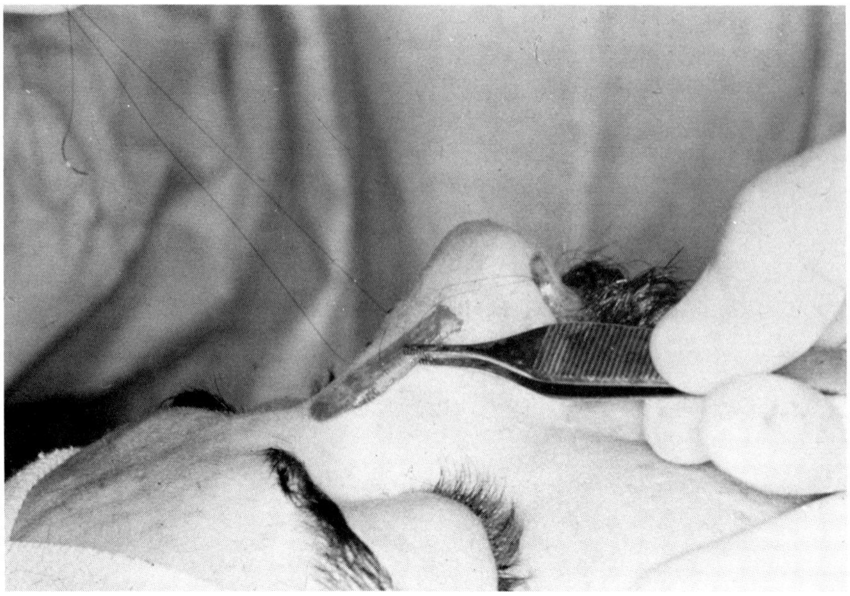

The graft was secured with a mattress suture of 6-0 nylon. (It is unnecessary to fix the graft in place with a percutaneous suture if the pocket for the graft is just large enough to accommodate it.)

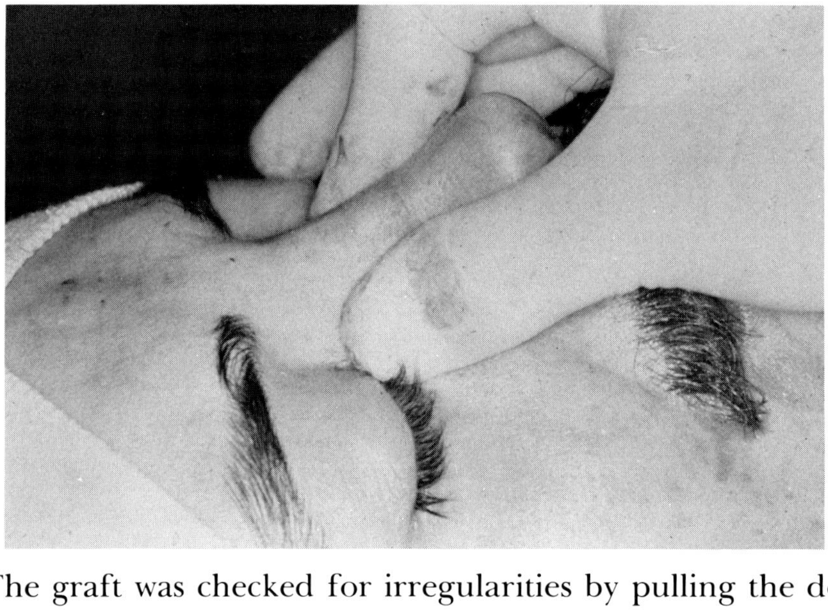

The graft was checked for irregularities by pulling the dorsal skin tightly over it.

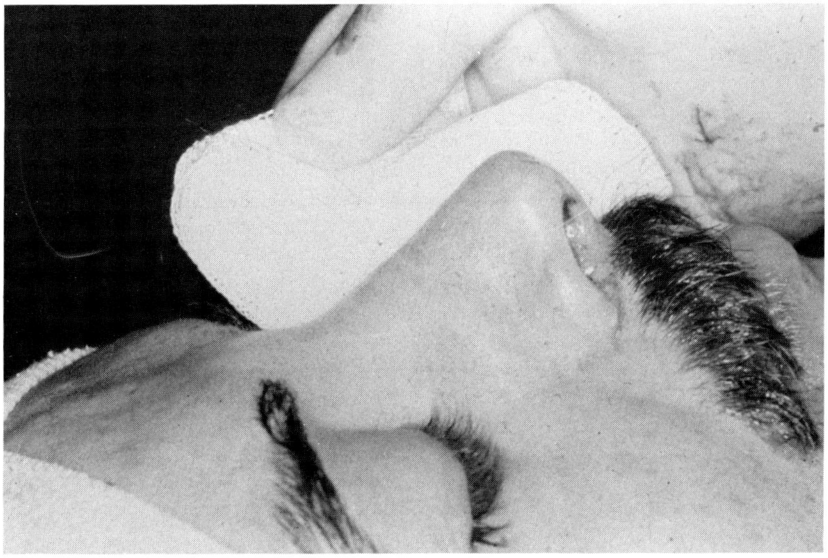

Final assessment of the dorsal contour was made.

Summary of surgical procedure

1. Limited skeletonization over the upper cartilaginous and bony vaults
2. Transfixion incision to the nasal spine
3. Trim of redundant membranous septum, but no excision of cartilage
4. Reduction of the bony dorsum by rasping
5. Scalpel trim of the roof of the upper cartilaginous vault
6. Major septoplasty
7. Delivery of the lower lateral cartilages through rim incisions
8. Trim of the cephalic portion of the lateral crura
9. Formation of a new dorsal roof by a septal cartilage graft

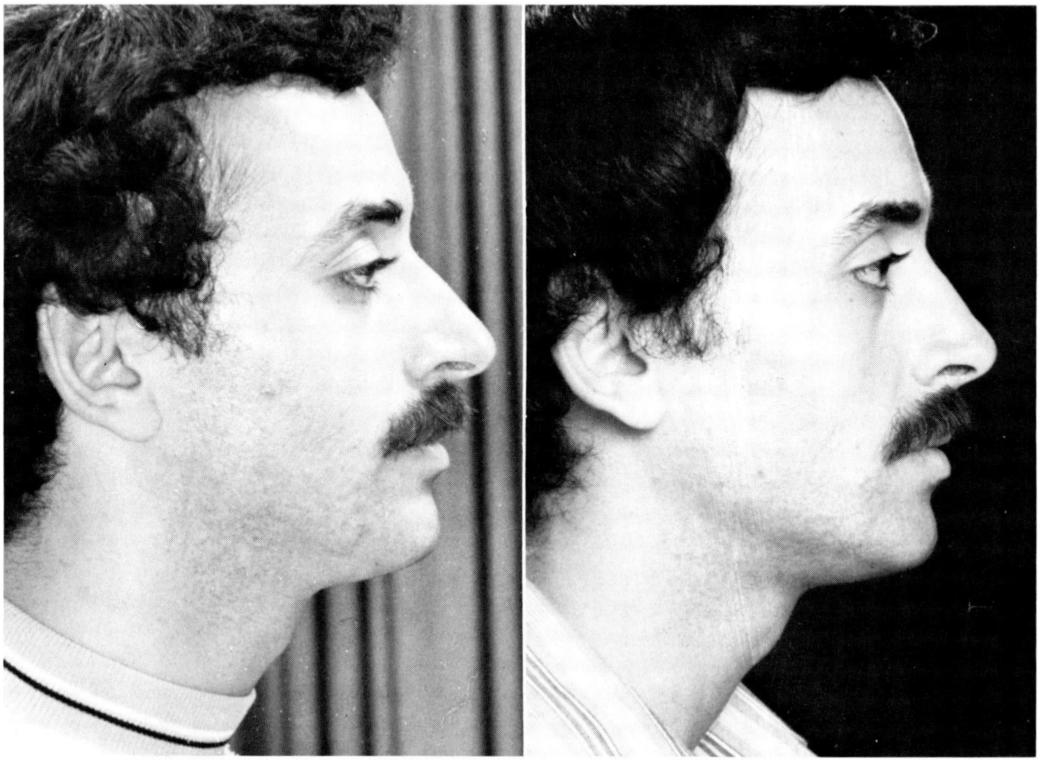

POSTOPERATIVE RESULTS

The postoperative photograph was taken 4 years after surgery. On lateral view, the slight dorsal convexity has been replaced by a straight dorsum with a natural dorsal irregularity. The tip is now the highest point in the dorsal line. The nasolabial angle is just slightly more open. The position of the alar lobule has been changed so that it is higher in relation to the insertion of the columella. The cephalic rotation of the tip was accomplished by resection of only a small segment of the membranous septum.

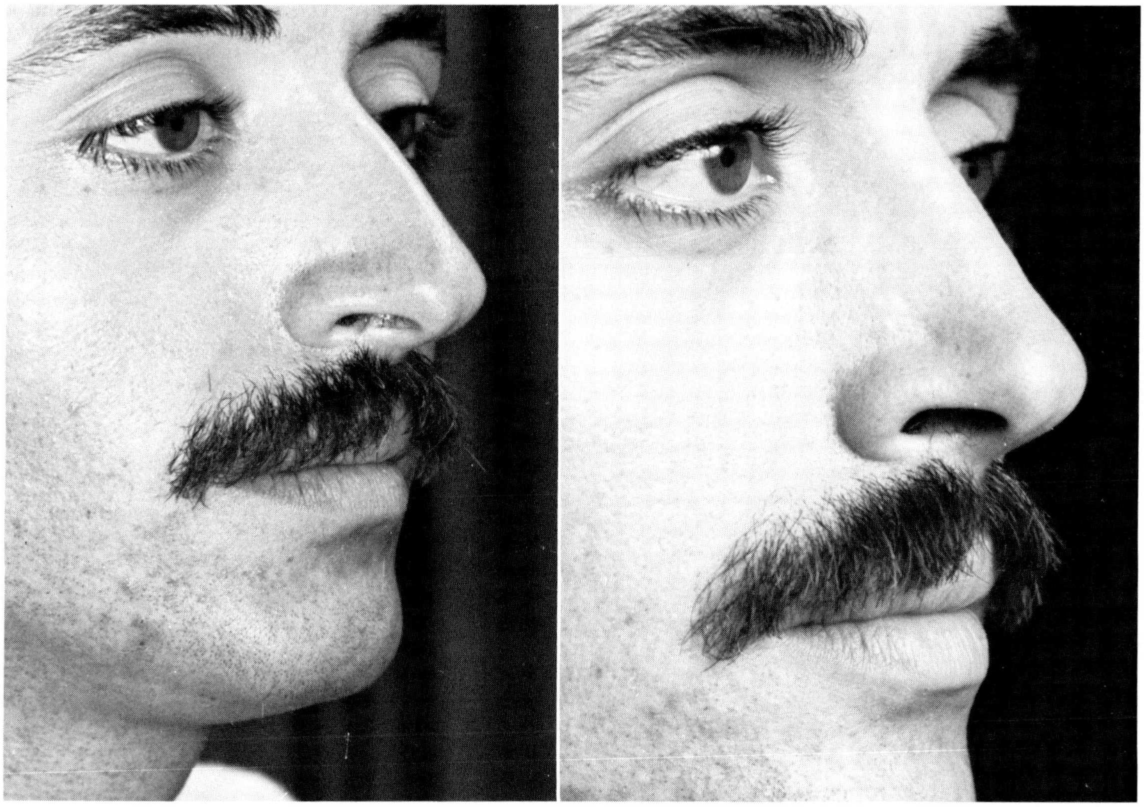

A dorsal graft forms a straight and broader dorsum, as seen on oblique view.

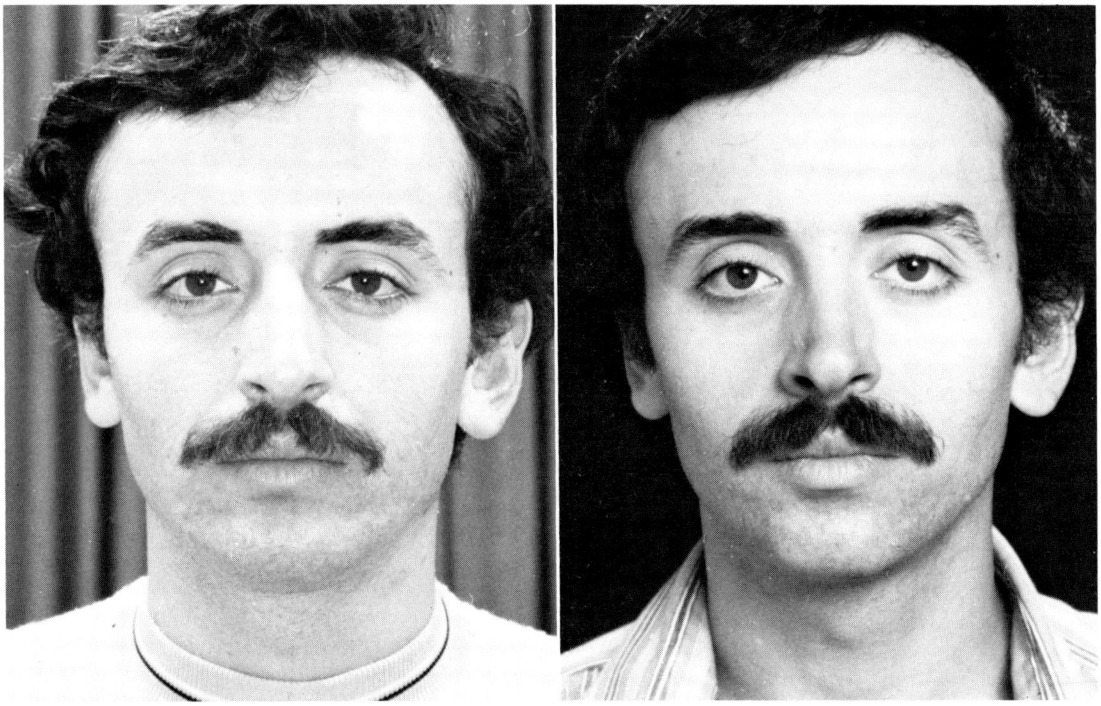

Postoperatively, the dorsal graft improves the nasal alignment and proportion. The light reflexes over the frontal processes of the maxilla form brackets around the central part of the nose in both photographs.

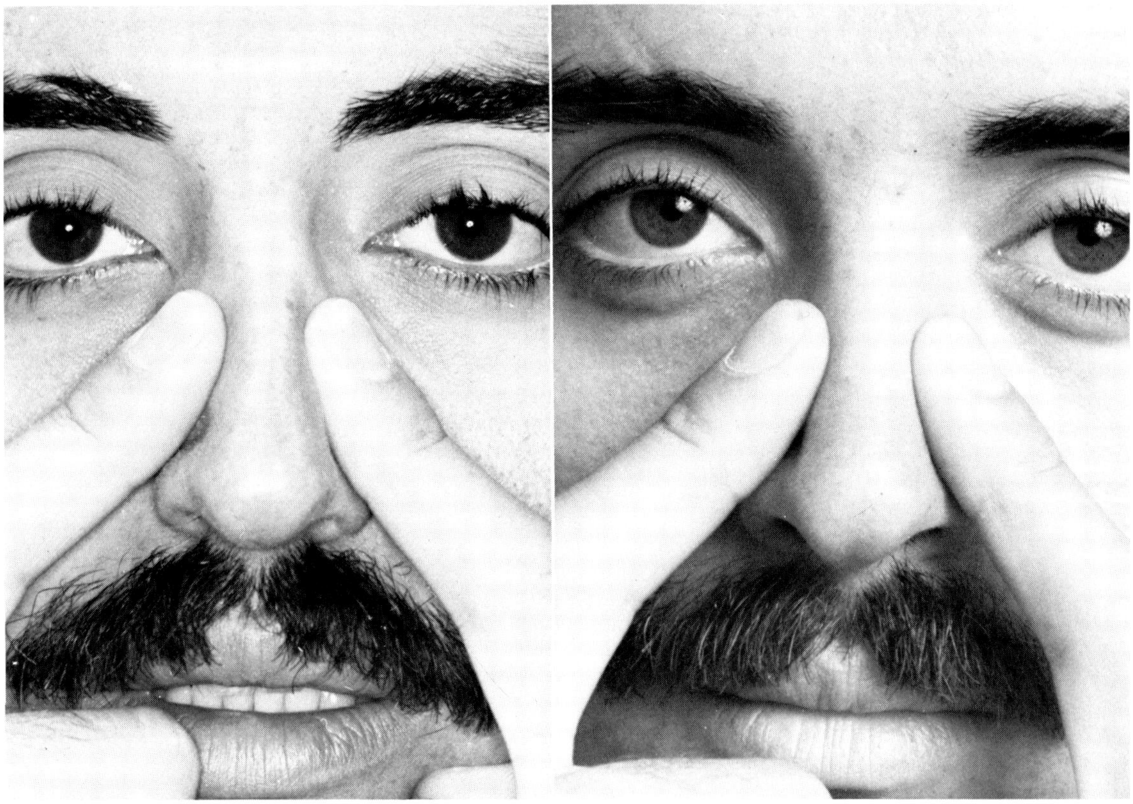

The discontinuity of the upper cartilaginous vault from the bony pyramid has been virtually eliminated by the dorsal graft.

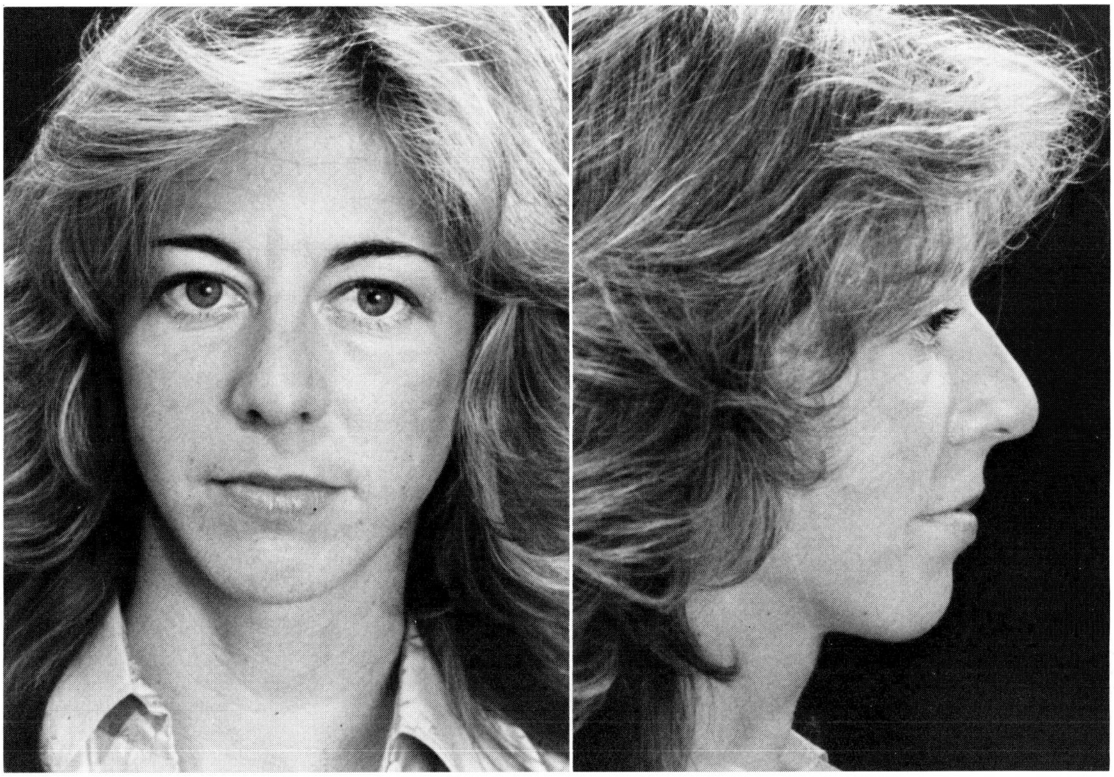

Case report 3: Lateral augmentation

Most patients with short nasal bones have a characteristic narrowness to the central third of the nasal contour because of a lack of bony support. However, this is not the case when the soft tissues are substantial enough to provide lateral fullness. This patient has a deceptively normal-appearing nasal configuration, seemingly well suited for a standard rhinoplasty.

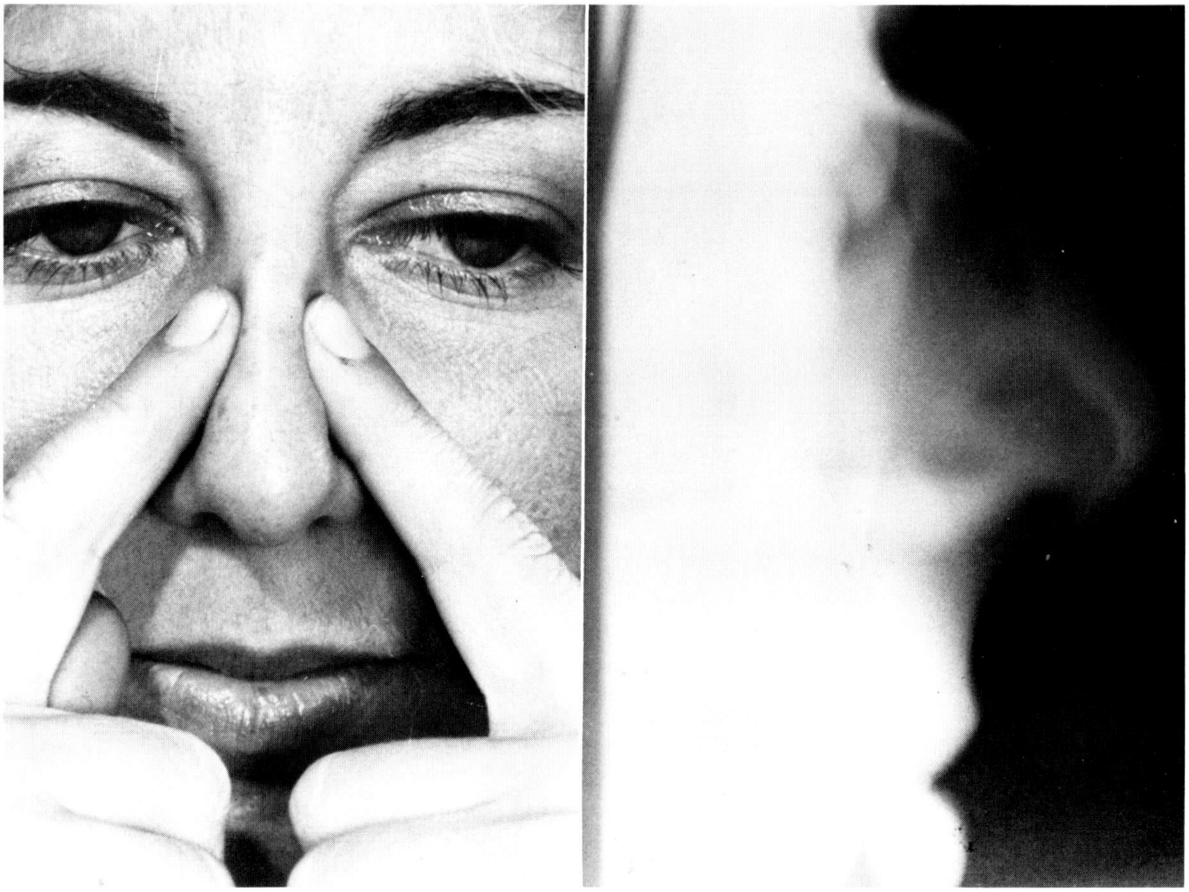

During examination it was determined that the nasal pyramid was short. The patient was asked to compress the sides of her nose to outline the caudal edge of the bony pyramid. X-ray film confirms the diagnosis.

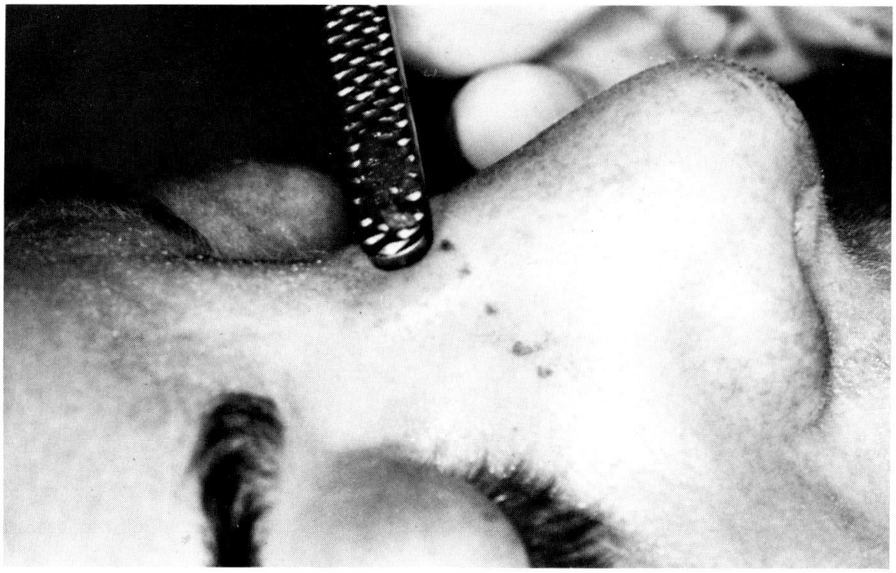

SURGICAL PROCEDURE

Following skeletonization, the bony dorsum was rasped down slightly.

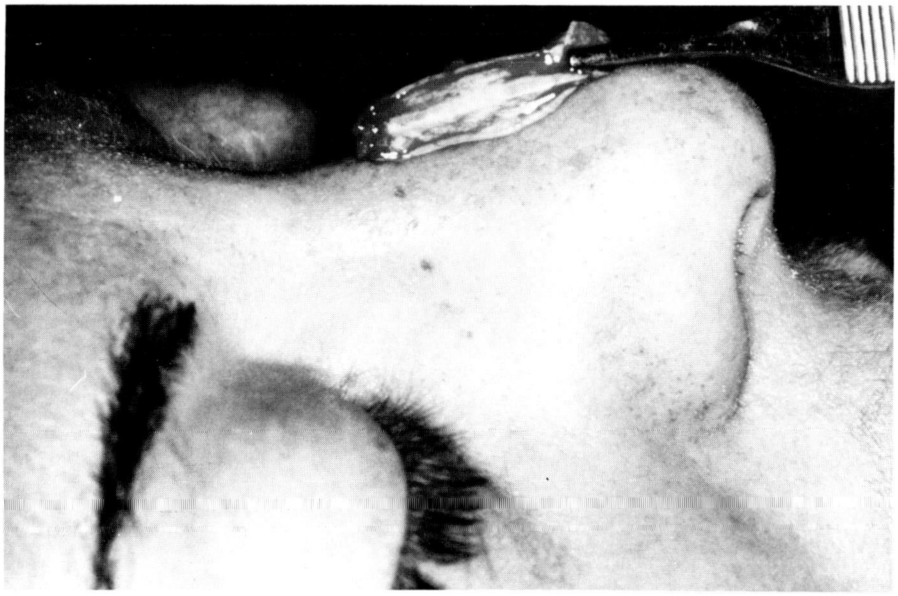

This was followed by a trim of the major portion of the cartilaginous dorsum using a knife. The resected specimen is shown.

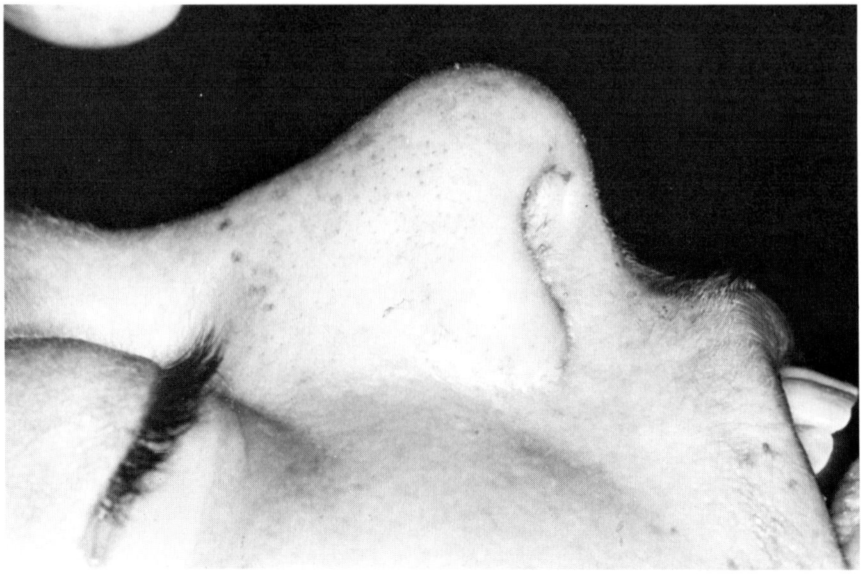

With reduction of the dorsum, the heaviness of the soft tissues is evident.

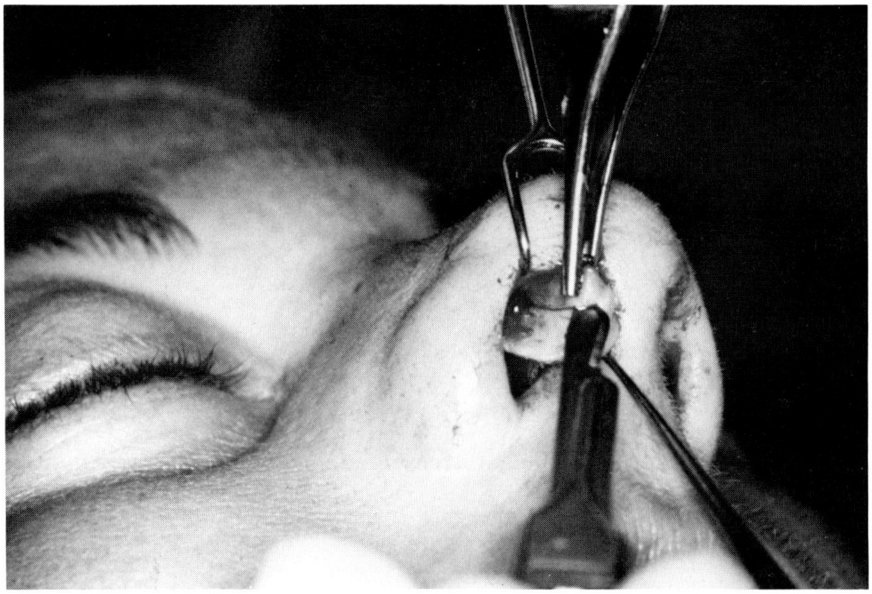

The tip cartilage is delivered through a rim incision and is found to be relatively thin. A preliminary cephalic trim is followed by attenuation of the dome in an attempt to obtain as much projection as possible.

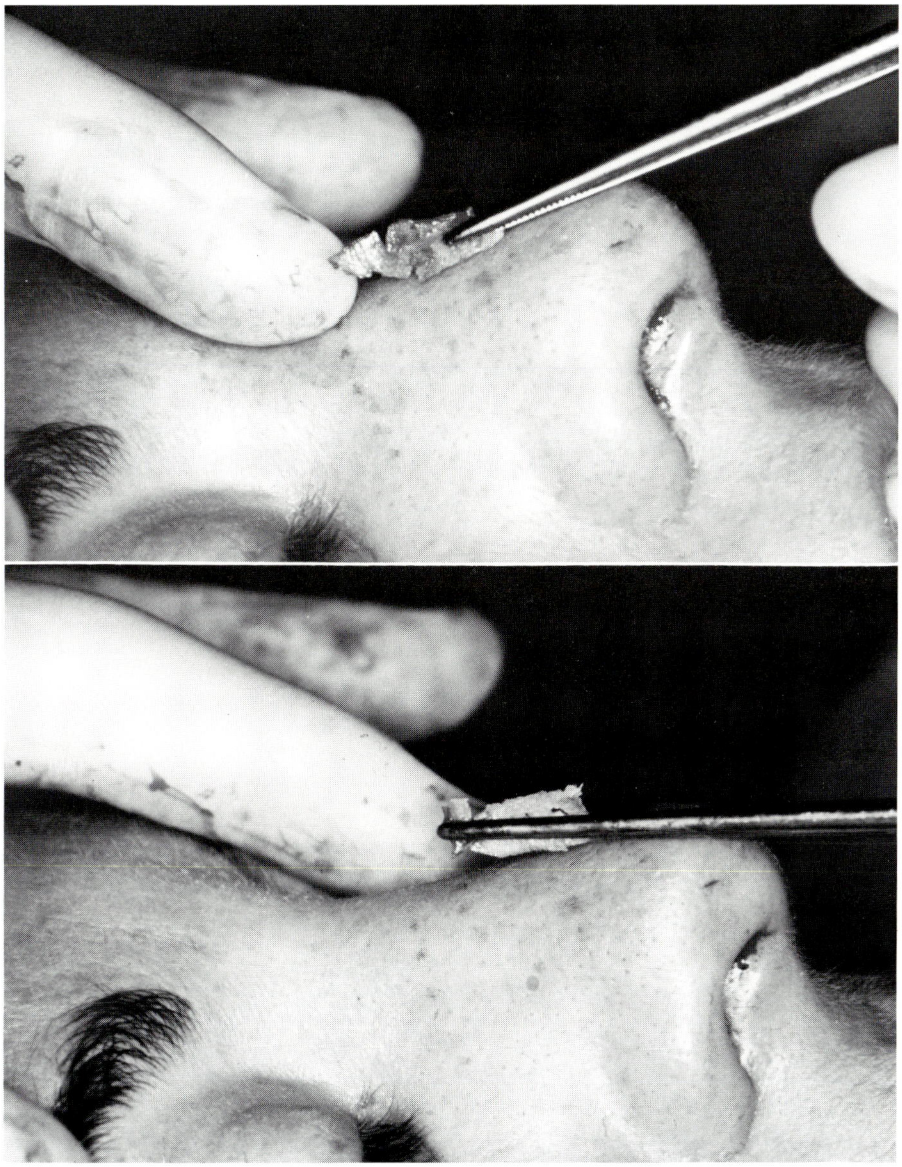

Because of the substance of the tissues, I thought that adequate contour could be provided by simply augmenting the lateral walls of the upper cartilaginous vault. Small crushed segments of cartilage were placed on both right and left sides.

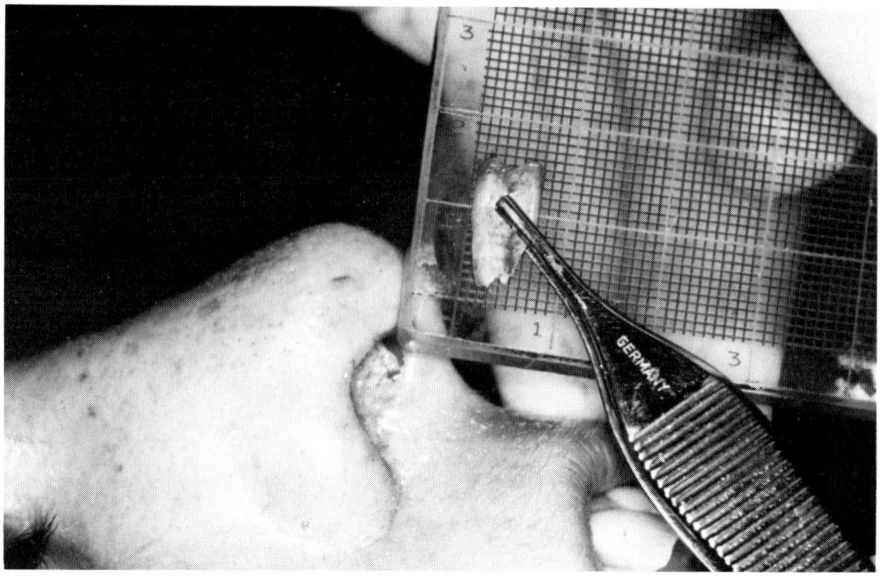

A tip graft was obtained from part of the resected dorsum.

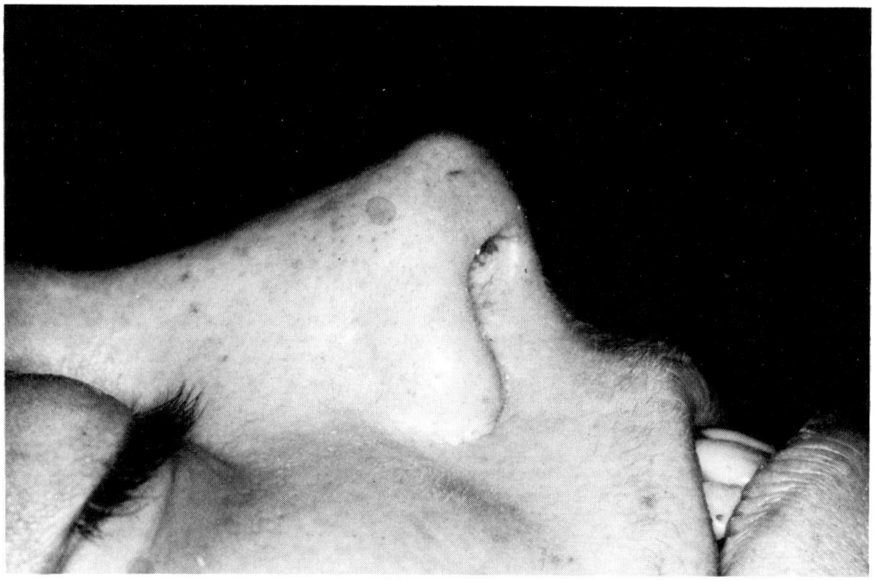

The added projection of the tip following placement of the tip graft can be seen.

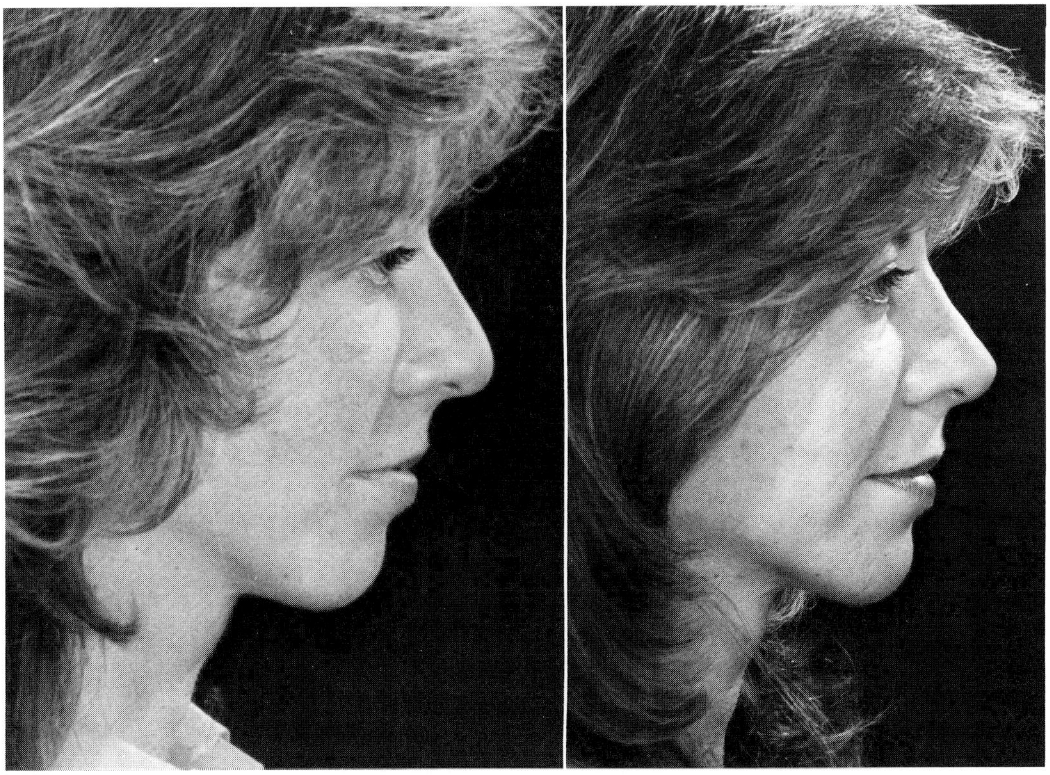

POSTOPERATIVE RESULTS

Postoperatively, an irregularity at the dorsal line occurs just caudal to the bony vault. The basal configuration and tip projection are improved.

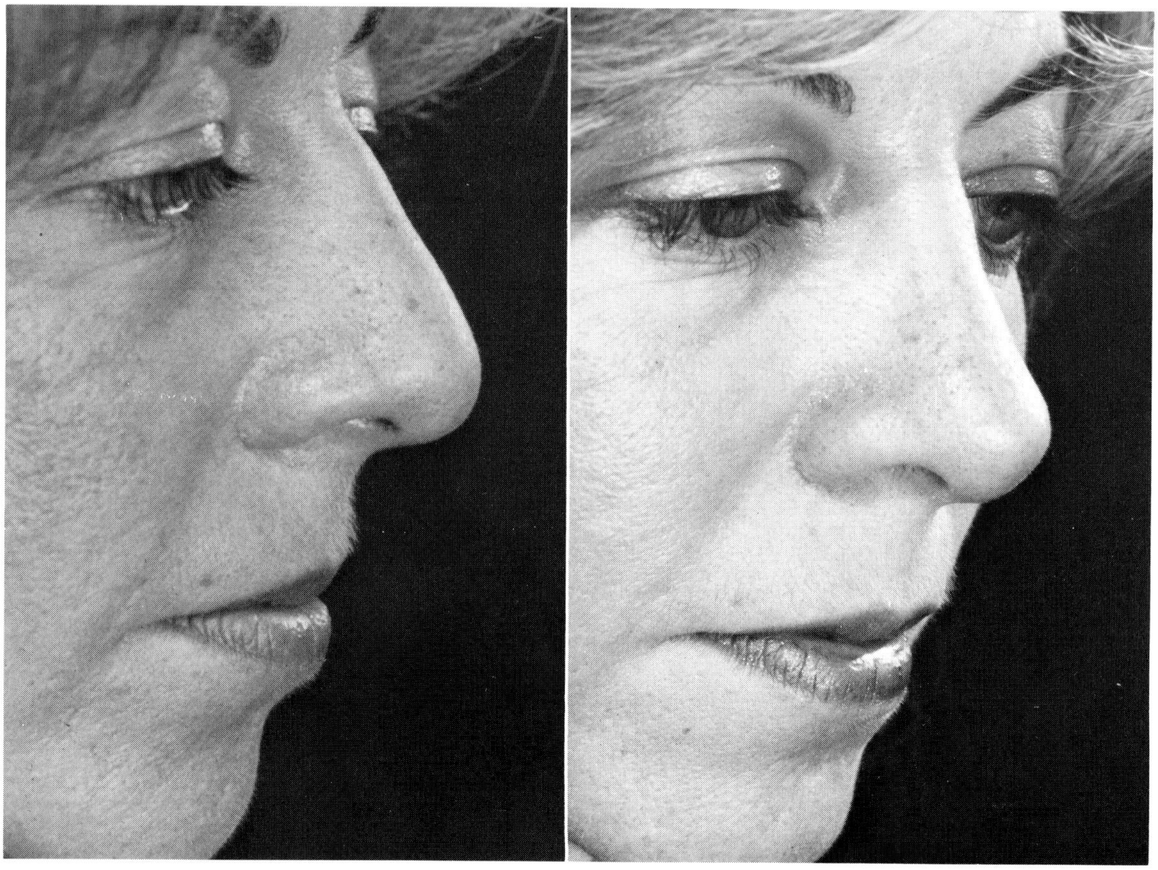

On right oblique view, there is an irregularity in the dorsal line at the edge of the short nasal bone despite the attempt to mask it by lateral augmentation. The central narrowness would have been greater without the lateral grafts. However, a better dorsal contour could have been obtained by full dorsal replacement.

Summary

To avoid the functional and aesthetic postsurgical problems that are likely to occur with short nasal bones, the following directives are recommended:

1. *Make the diagnosis.* The clinical significance of short nasal bones should not be underestimated. Palpation of the bony pyramid should be a part of the preoperative evaluation of every rhinoplasty patient.
2. *Consider no fracture of the nasal bones.* If short nasal bones are fractured following resection of the dorsal roof, the lateral nasal walls may collapse medially.
3. *Plan to reconstruct the dorsum.* The roof of the upper cartilaginous vault should be reconstructed. A well-prepared strip of septal cartilage makes an excellent roof. The Skoog technique of reinsertion of the resected dorsum is an effective alternative but requires some experience in making the initial cuts.

CROOKED NOSE

Historically, radical surgery has been advocated for correction of the crooked nose. A full-scale attack on the septum—incising, excising, scoring, morselizing, inner fixation, and swinging-door maneuvers—has been advocated for putting the nose in the midline. But such militancy for the sake of straightness is rarely necessary and always hazardous. The compulsion to place the septum in an absolute vertical plane is not based on normal anatomy, since most septums are not straight. Nor should midlining be the central surgical objective in the treatment of crooked noses. Clearly, the two main objectives are: (1) to produce a nose that appears straight and (2) to attain patent nasal airways. To these ends, a midline septum may be totally irrelevant.

Although radical surgery is sometimes indicated in extreme cases, most often the use of onlay grafts to create an illusion of straightness is sufficient. Portions of the obstructing septum should be carefully resected; then selected pieces can be placed onto the areas of concavity. Any remaining pieces can be crushed and replaced in the mucoperichondrial pocket. By this method, the nose appears straight and is functionally improved without jeopardy to its support.

Deviation of the bony pyramid is seen subsequent to trauma or following rhinoplasty when a high anterior septal deviation has prevented the nasal bones from being symmetrically mobilized. Deflection of the upper cartilaginous vault is most often caused by deviation of the septum but can also result from an avulsion or collapse of an upper lateral cartilage following rhinoplasty. The nasal tip can appear twisted because of a caudal dislocation and deviation of the septum or because of a unilateral deficit of lower lateral cartilage, usually following rhinoplasty. Whatever the cause of the crooked nose, camouflage techniques usually are successful.

Case report 1

This patient sustained a fracture of the bony pyramid during a basketball encounter. At the time of injury the nose was carefully packed and splinted. One year later, there was a slight deviation of the entire bony pyramid to the right and almost complete obstruction of the right nasal airway and narrowing of the left.

Although the need for functional correction was obvious, the patient's major concern was the aesthetic distortion. The profile was excellent, and he was specific and clear in his request that there be absolutely no aesthetic changes except to straighten the nose. This slight asymmetry was ideally suited for the onlay technique.

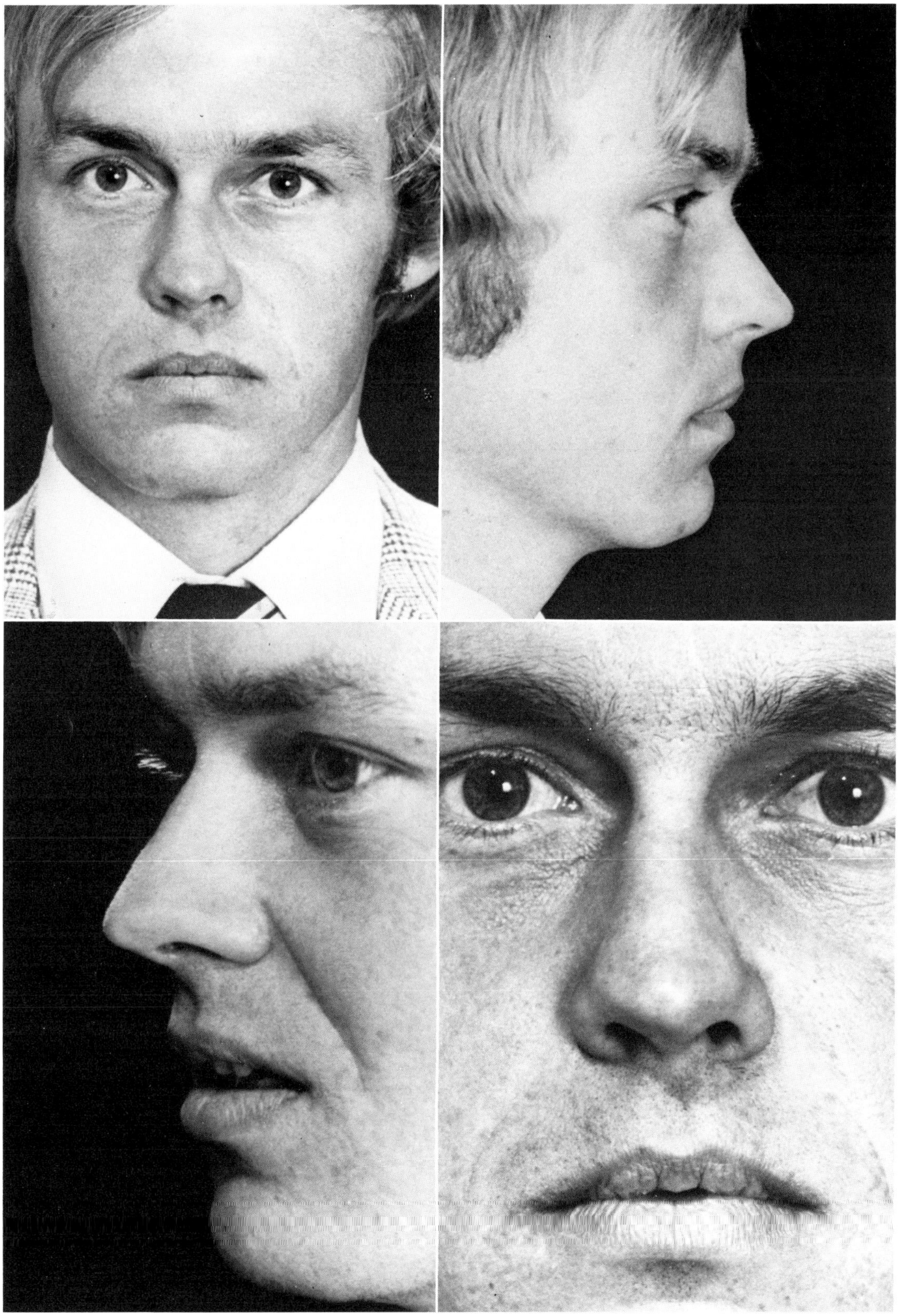

SURGICAL PROCEDURE

The surgical correction of the airway included resection of a major portion of the septum, part of the vomer, and the inferior borders of both turbinates. The distorted pieces of cartilage were crushed, and the entire mucoperichondrial pocket was relined with the crushed cartilage.

A piece of cartilage approximately the size of the wall of the left bony pyramid was prepared. An incision was made over the left upper lateral cartilage, and the dissection was carried to the root of the nose on the left side. The cartilage graft was placed over the depressed nasal bone, augmenting it just enough to give the appearance of symmetry. Following surgery, the airway is excellent and the nasal contour symmetrical.

Summary of surgical procedure

1. No skeletonization
2. Major septoplasty and partial vomerectomy
3. Replacement of crushed cartilage in the mucoperichondrial pocket
4. Bilateral partial inferior turbinectomy
5. Placement of septal cartilage graft over the left nasal concavity

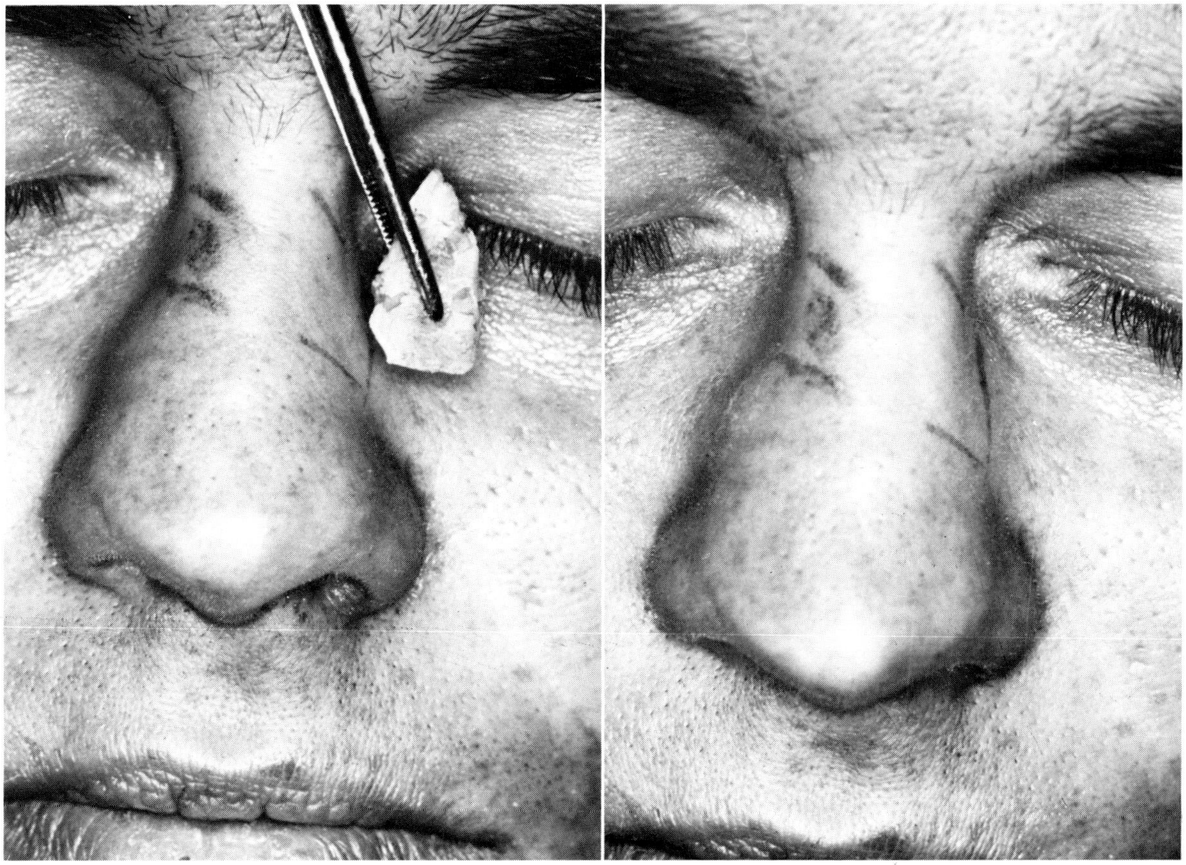

DISCUSSION

This man has a bony vault that is aesthetically too narrow for his nasal base. The injury that displaced the entire vault to the right actually moved the right nasal bone into better relationship with the base. This can be appreciated by covering the left half of the face so that only the right half of the nasal contour is seen.

The simple onlay graft technique has improved the relative positions of the upper and lower nasal vaults, corrected the asymmetry, and restored the nasal airways. These goals were achieved with virtually no postoperative morbidity—a fact that would certainly argue for the conservative approach to this crooked nose.

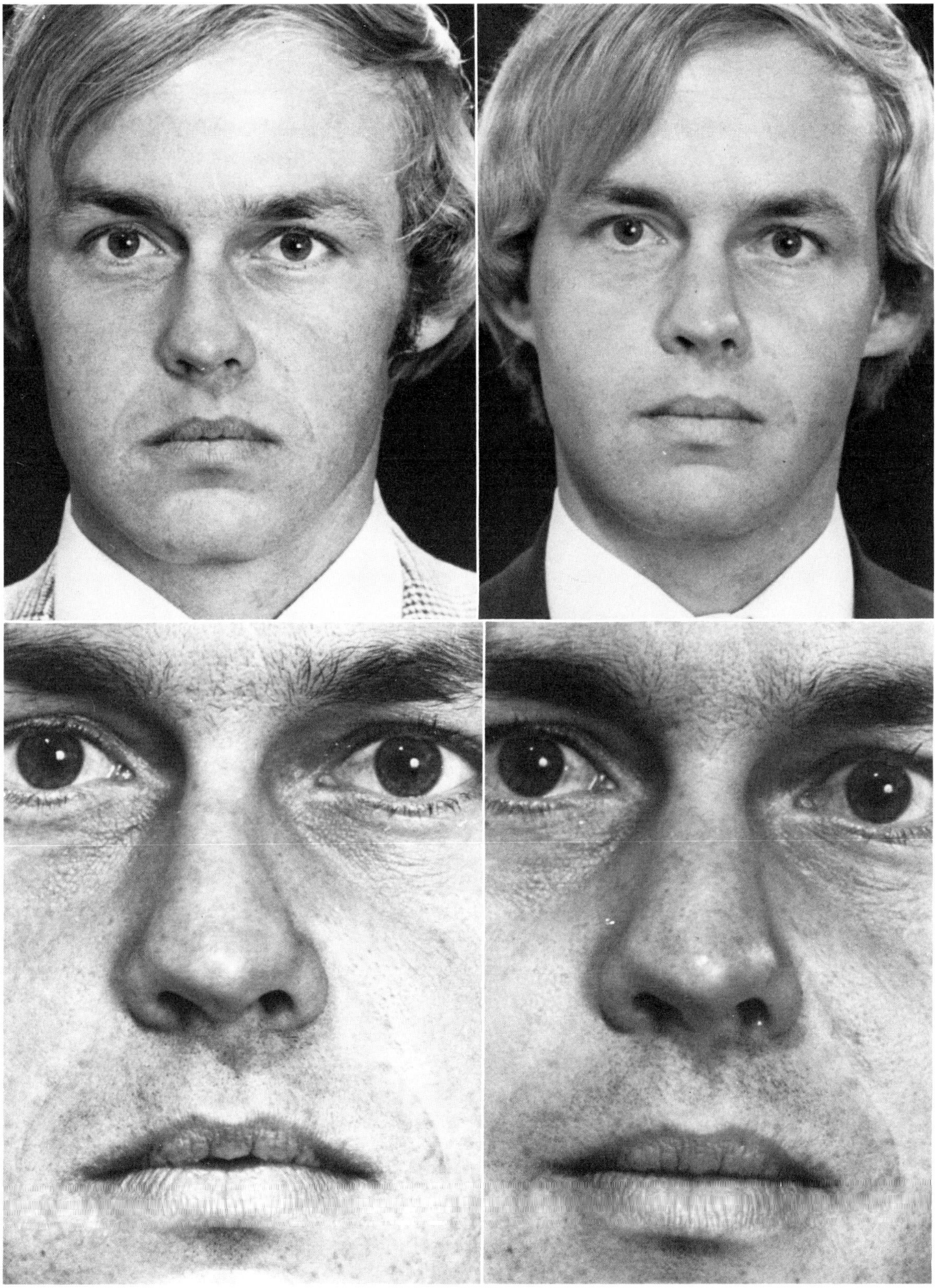

Case report 2

A primary rhinoplasty and submucous resection were performed 6 months following a traumatic nasal fracture. Initially, the surgery appeared to be successful, but within 6 weeks the airways were again obstructed, and the nose remained crooked. A second rhinoplasty was done 8 months later in an attempt to relieve the obstruction and straighten the nose, but to no avail. The patient was then referred to me for evaluation.

On examination the lateral view was unremarkable except for a retrusion of the subnasion. On front view, the entire pyramid is displaced laterally to the right. The oblique views are typical of this deformity, appearing retroussé on one side and having a dorsal hump on the opposite side. Internally, some of the caudal and central cartilaginous septum had been resected. However, there was a high angulation of the septum against the right nasal bone, which prevented its medial repositioning after osteotomy. The vomer and ethmoid contributed to the almost complete posterior obstruction.

Reconstruction was first directed to the septal/ethmoid/vomer deformity. The selective resection and replacement of septal cartilage and bone provided an adequate nasal airway. After the airway had been successfully treated, preserving the integrity of the dorsal caudal septum, a very careful osteotomy was done on the right side only. (Had there been a question about the integrity of the dorsal segment, no osteotomy would have been done.) The laterally displaced right nasal bone was adequately mobilized, whereas the support provided by the left medially displaced bone was not violated. Mobilization of the left side of the bony pyramid would have required fracture of the remaining dorsal ethmoid and cartilage, which, in combination with a fracture of the right nasal bone, could result in a saddle deformity. The left concavity was simply augmented by a cartilage graft overlay.

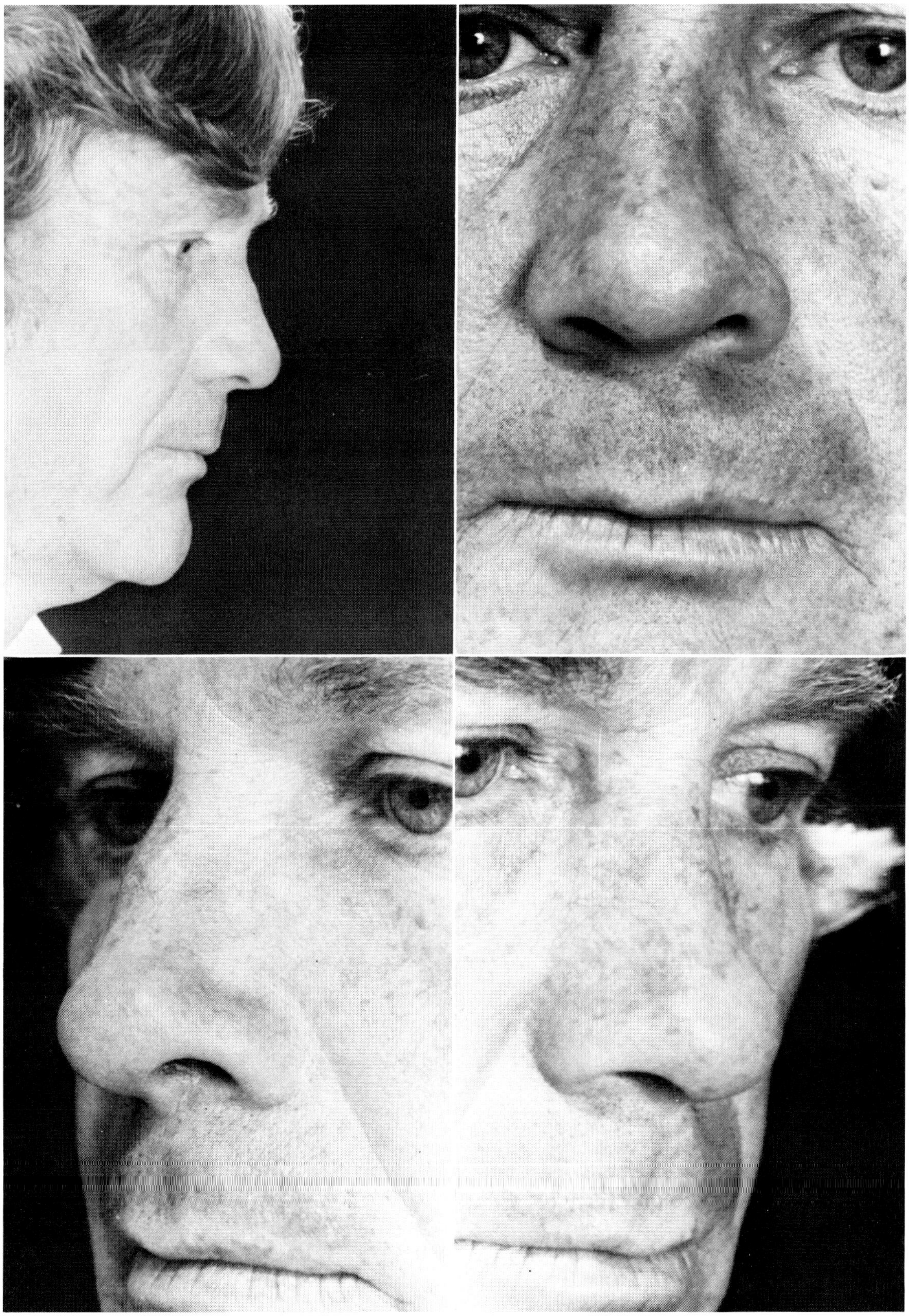

On postoperative lateral view, the dorsal line is straight, and the area of the subnasion has been improved by a small graft. The front view displays a nearly symmetrical nasal pyramid. The airways are patent 1 year following surgery.

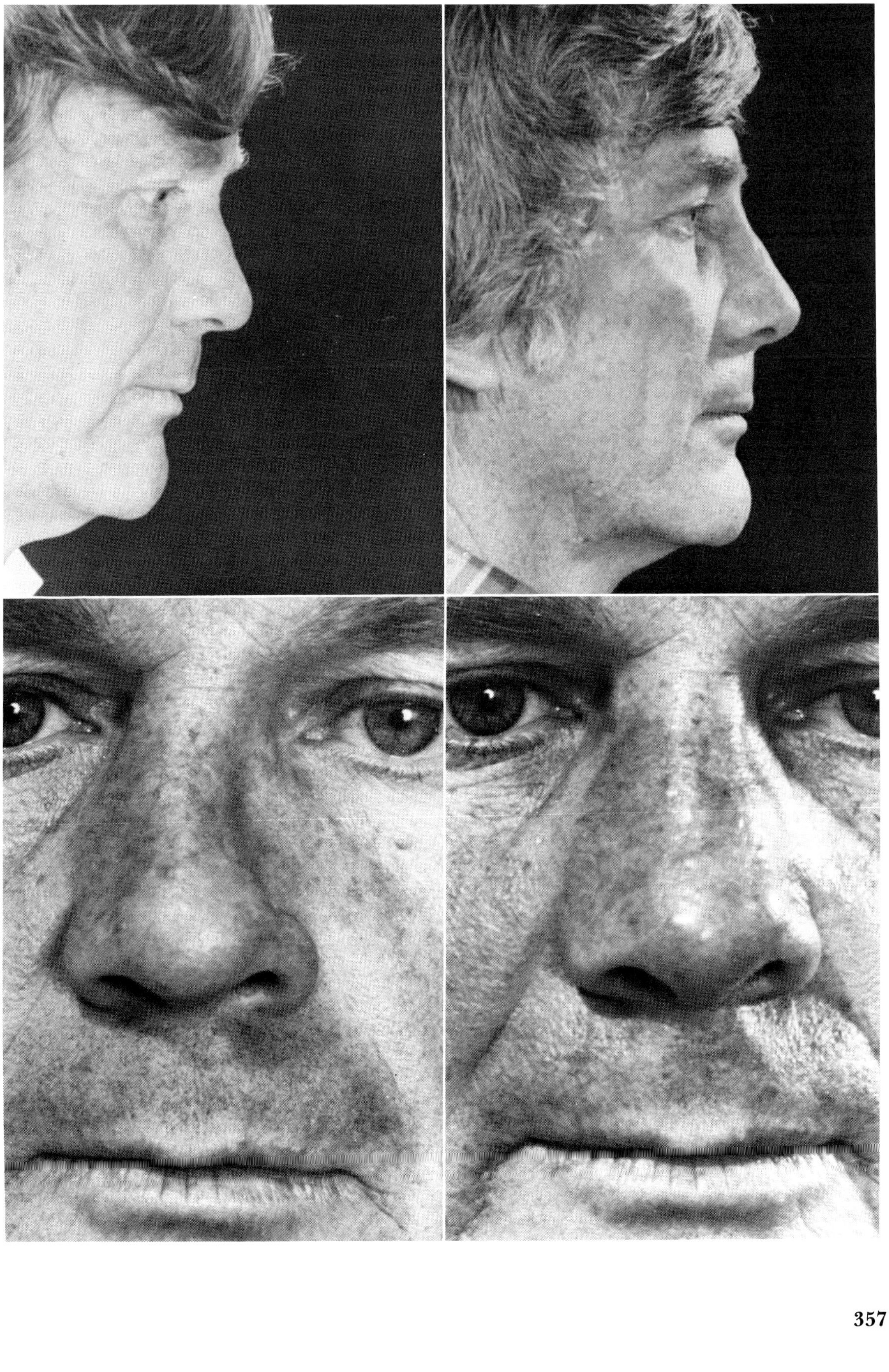

The oblique views are within the normal range of symmetry, though the augmented left is still more concave than the right. Greater medial placement of the right nasal bone would have been improbable without fracture of the dorsal attachment of the ethmoid.

Summary of surgical procedure

1. Limited skeletonization
2. Major septoplasty, with partial resection of ethmoid and vomer
3. Replacement of the cartilage surplus in the mucoperichondrial pocket
4. Right lateral osteotomy
5. Septal cartilage graft over the left nasal concavity
6. Small septal cartilage graft over the subnasion

DISCUSSION

The treatment of the crooked nose in the posttraumatic patient with a history of multiple surgical procedures is a particular problem. The potential for increasing functional difficulties and aesthetic deformity is greater as scar tissue increases and skeletal support decreases.

The two prior surgeries performed on this patient included a resection of the central portion of the quadrangular cartilage with scoring of the dorsal segment. Though this appeared to mobilize the skeletonized nose, it did not, in fact, remove the obstructing ethmoid and vomer; nor did it modify the high anterior deflection of the septum.

Because final correction necessitated more radical management of the septal obstruction, structural integrity was the first consideration in planning to straighten the nose. Onlay grafting was elected because it spares all the remaining support. The final result is a wider nose, but one that is more symmetrical and has functional airways.

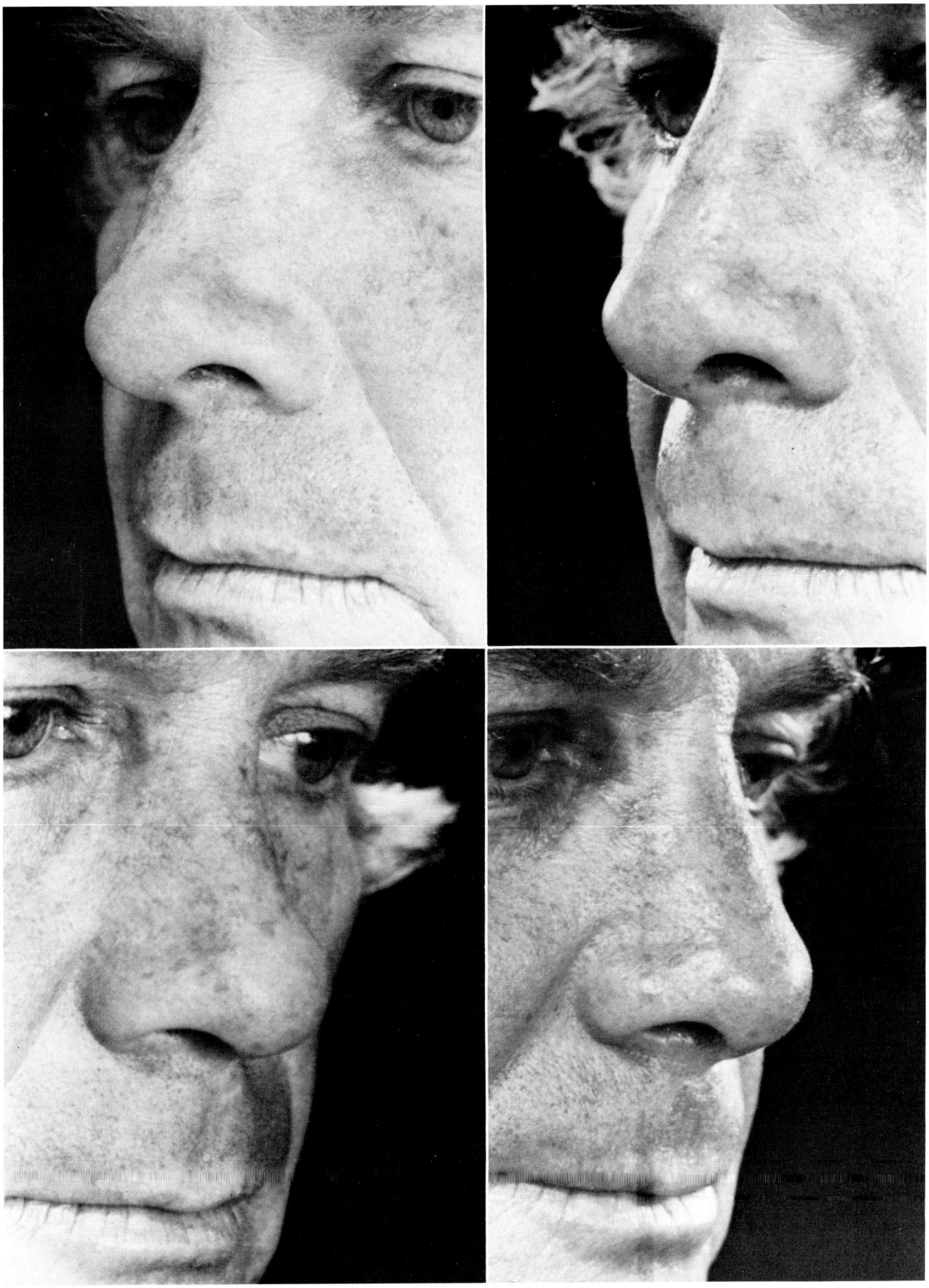

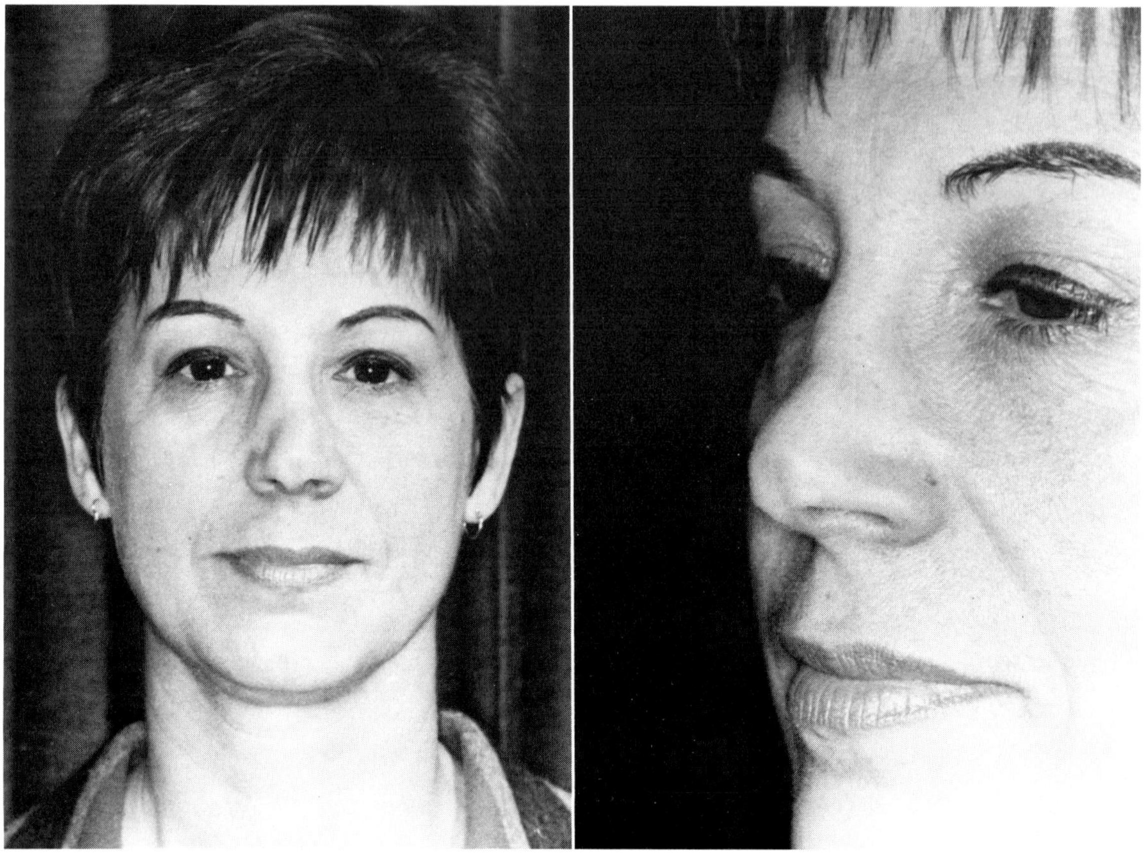

Case report 3

Rough handling of tissues can cause a separation of the upper lateral cartilages from the bony vault. This may result in a unilateral or, in this case, bilateral alteration in the nasal contour. This patient's deformity was accentuated by an irregular and overreduced dorsum.

The cleft in the center of the nasal lobule adds to the multiple irregularities seen on oblique view.

Summary of surgical procedure

1. Limited skeletonization
2. Septoplasty for onlay material
3. Osteotomies
4. Dorsal graft
5. Right lateral wall graft
6. Tip graft
7. Alar wedge resections

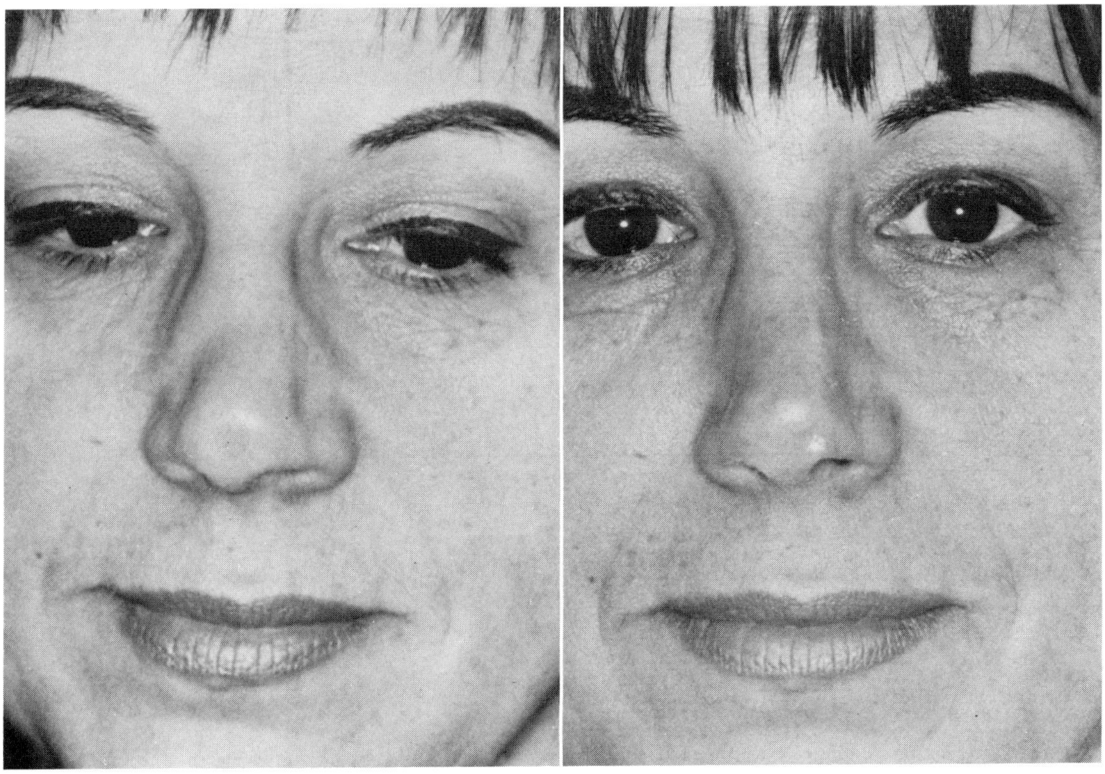

POSTOPERATIVE RESULTS

Following surgery, there is still some irregularity of the right nasal wall, but the striking discontinuity of the lateral nasal walls has been favorably modified.

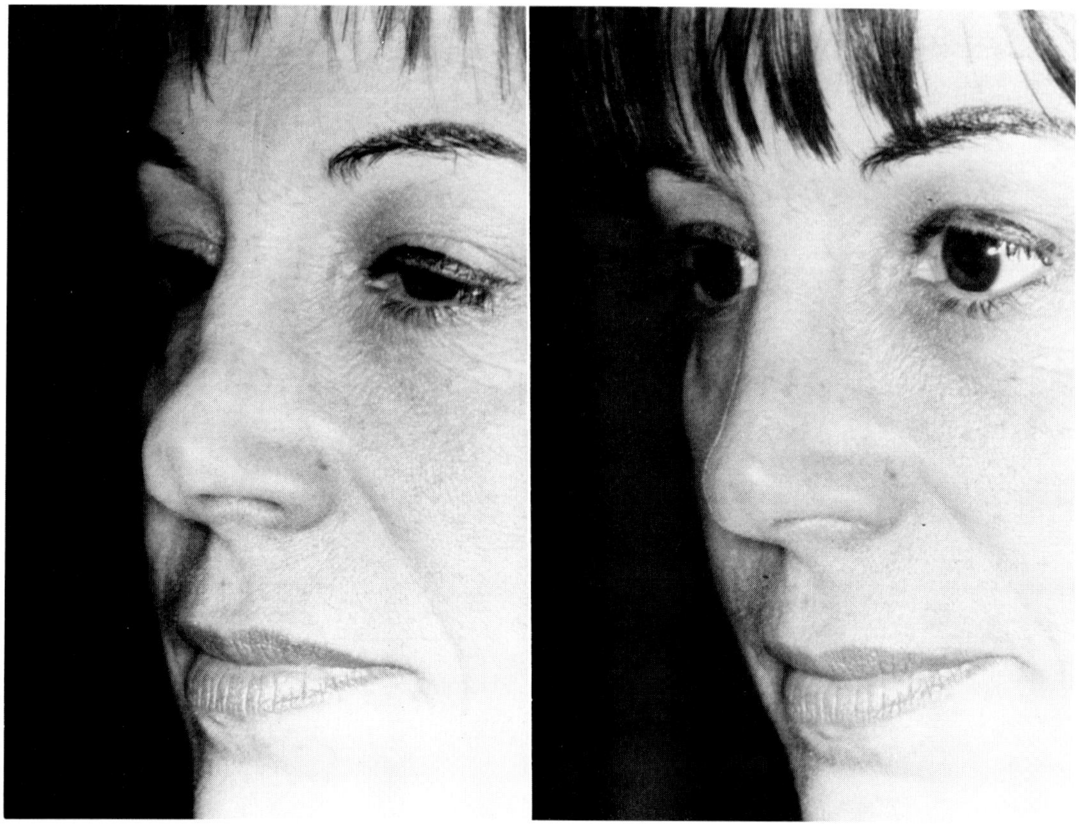

The superciliary ridge joins the radix and the lateral nasal wall to form a smooth, uninterrupted line to the slightly projecting tip. The cleft in the tip has been filled out by a cartilage tip graft.

DISCUSSION

When the upper lateral cartilage is detached from the nasal bone, the first priority is to obtain function. The placement of a dorsal graft in this patient served to provide some lateral distraction of the nasal walls to ensure function of the internal valve.

Realignment or reattachment of the upper lateral cartilage to the nasal bone on the right side was not feasible because of the presence of fibrous tissue between the articulating edges. This permanently displaces the cartilaginous attachment medially. This relationship is fixed regardless of the position of the nasal bone. Because the cuff of cartilage that normally attaches to the nasal bone is so short (2 to 3 mm), there is no practical way to dissect it out and reattach it. In this case, the use of onlay grafts was the best method of producing the illusion of alignment while maintaining good nasal function.

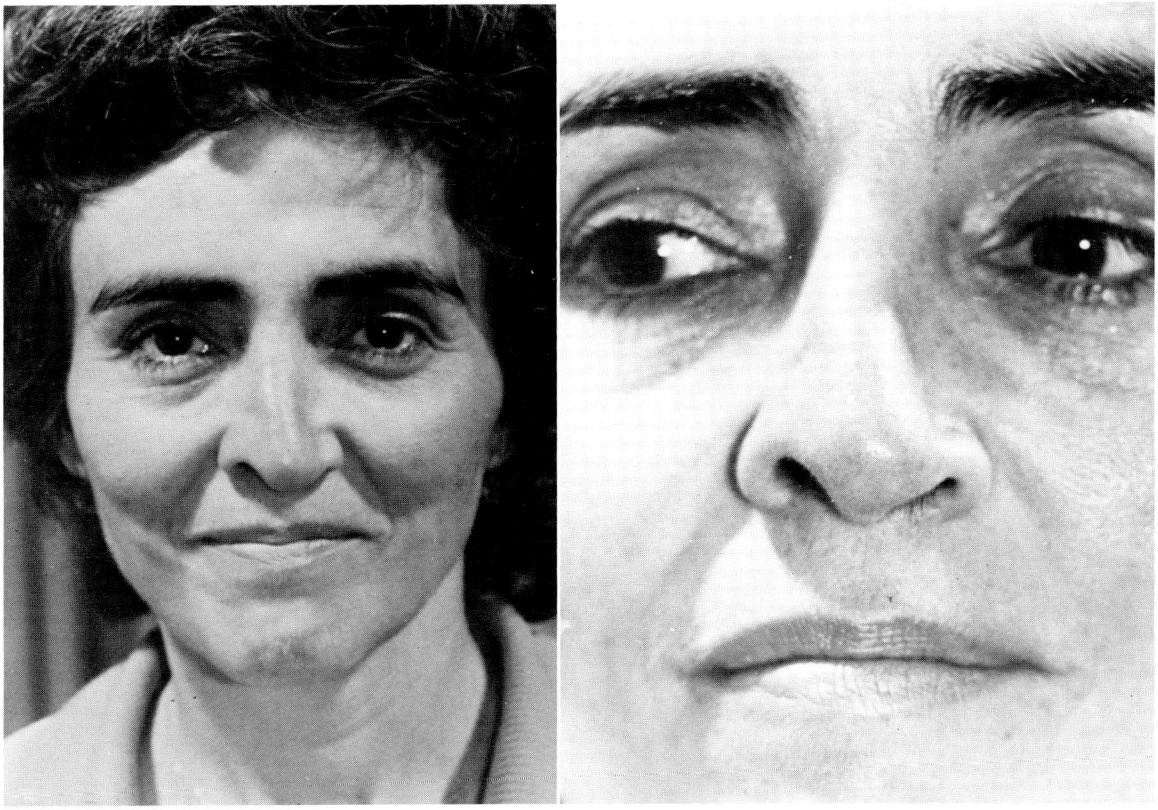

Case report 4

This 47-year-old patient with an undiagnosed high septal deviation was seen 18 months following a primary rhinoplasty. On front view, the tip deviates to the left. The overall impression is that of a crooked nose. The notched ala on the right adds to the twisted appearance of the tip. Just above the right alar lobule there is tissue atrophy caused by injections of a steroid that were given in an attempt to lower the alar rim. This depression on the right accentuates the concavity on the left.

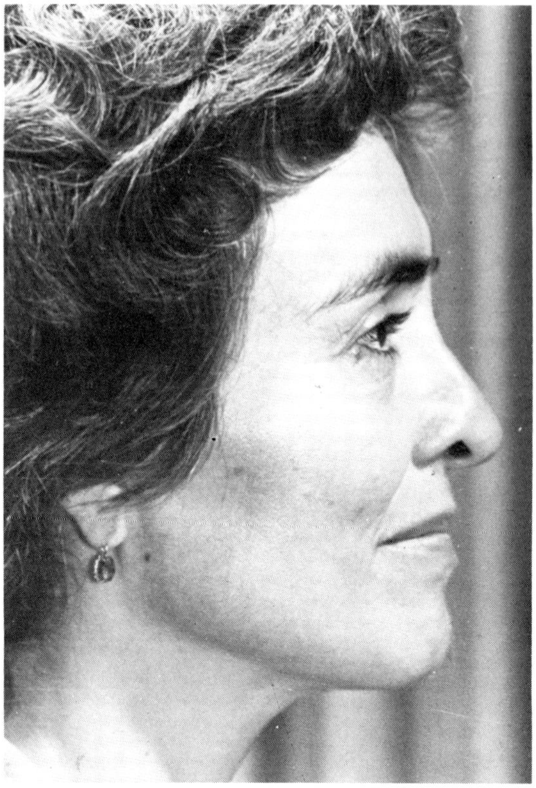

On lateral view, the dorsum appears high in relation to the tip. The right ala is notched. The nasolabial angle is acute, and the subnasion is retrusive. The relationship of the columella to the alar rim is poor.

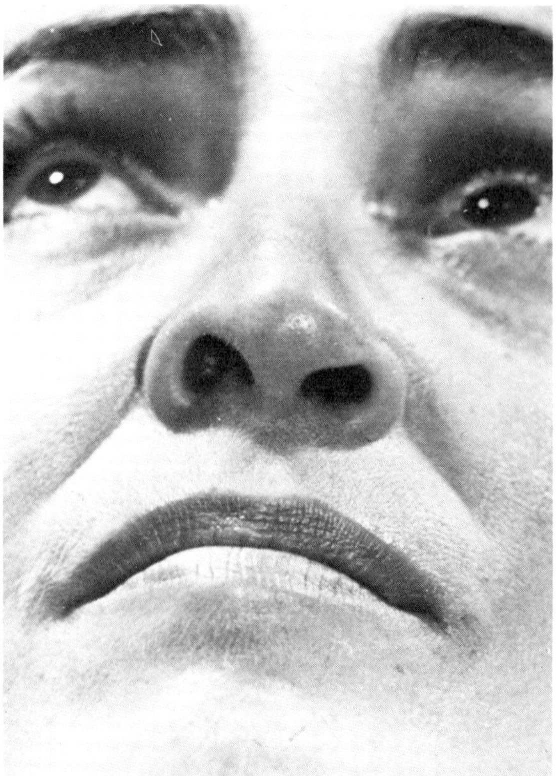

The basal outline has a horizontal axis, making it appear more rectangular than triangular. The nares are in disarray.

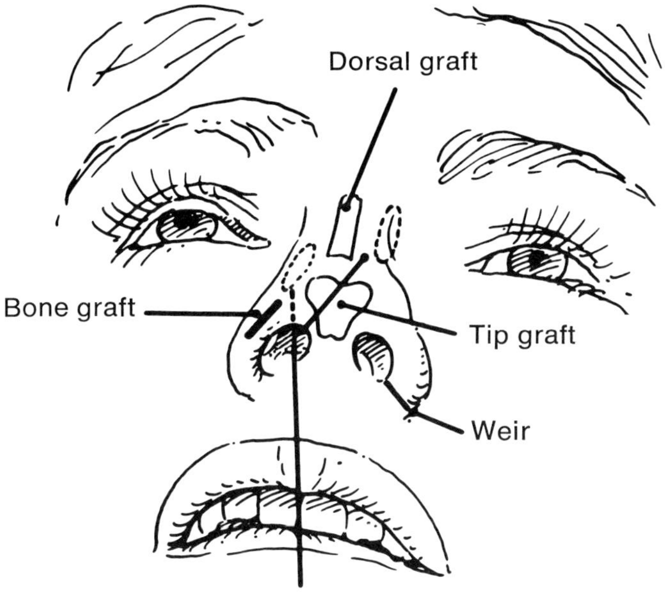

Summary of surgical procedure

1. Correction of functional problems
   a. Major submucous resection
   b. Partial perpendicular plate resection
   c. Partial vomer resection
   d. Bilateral partial inferior turbinectomy
2. Wide skeletonization, with cephalic rotation of the tip
3. Dorsal graft of septal cartilage
4. Onlay lateral graft over the left concavity
5. Small onlay graft over the depressed area on the right
6. Skin graft to release the scar on the right nostril
7. Ethmoid bone graft to the right alar rim
8. Septal cartilage tip graft
9. Bilateral alar wedge resections

POSTOPERATIVE RESULTS

The postoperative appearance is especially noteworthy, since there was no fracture of the nasal bones. Dorsal grafting in addition to bilateral nasal wall augmentation provided the illusion of symmetry.

Symmetry of the nasal tip was accomplished by (1) cephalic rotation, (2) release of the scar contracture by skin grafting the right vestibule, and (3) a small graft of ethmoid placed in the right alar rim.

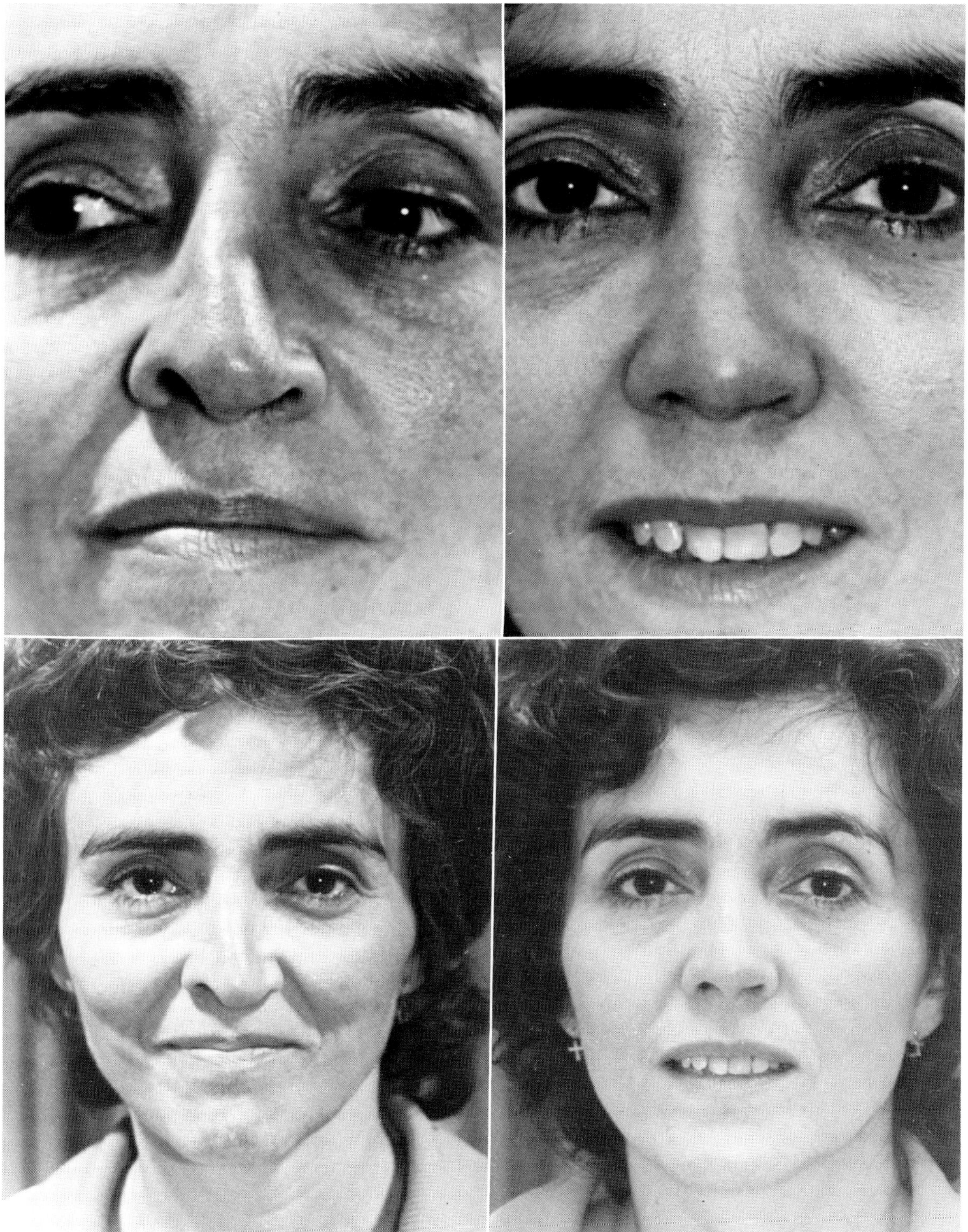

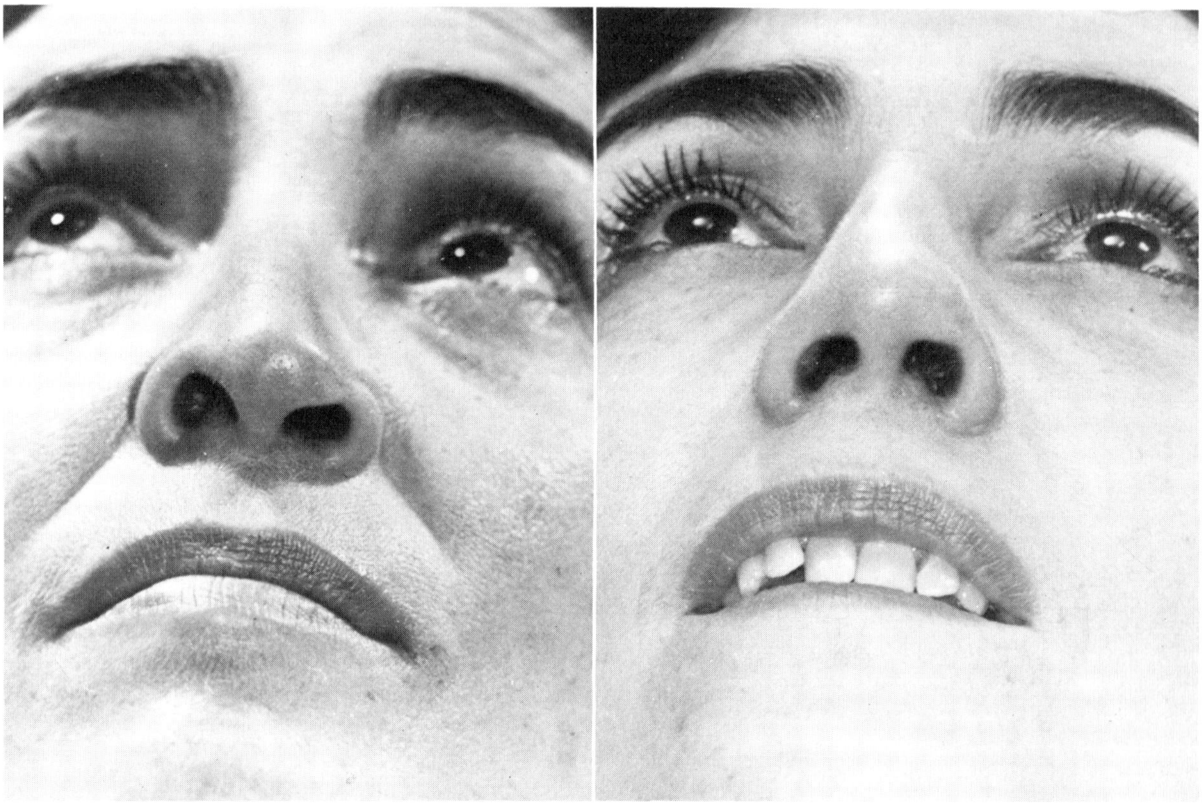

On basal view, the shift in the nostrils from a horizontal plane to a more vertical one is in part caused by the elevation of the dorsum by a cartilage graft. The nasal base was further improved by a tip graft of septal cartilage and bilateral alar wedge resections.

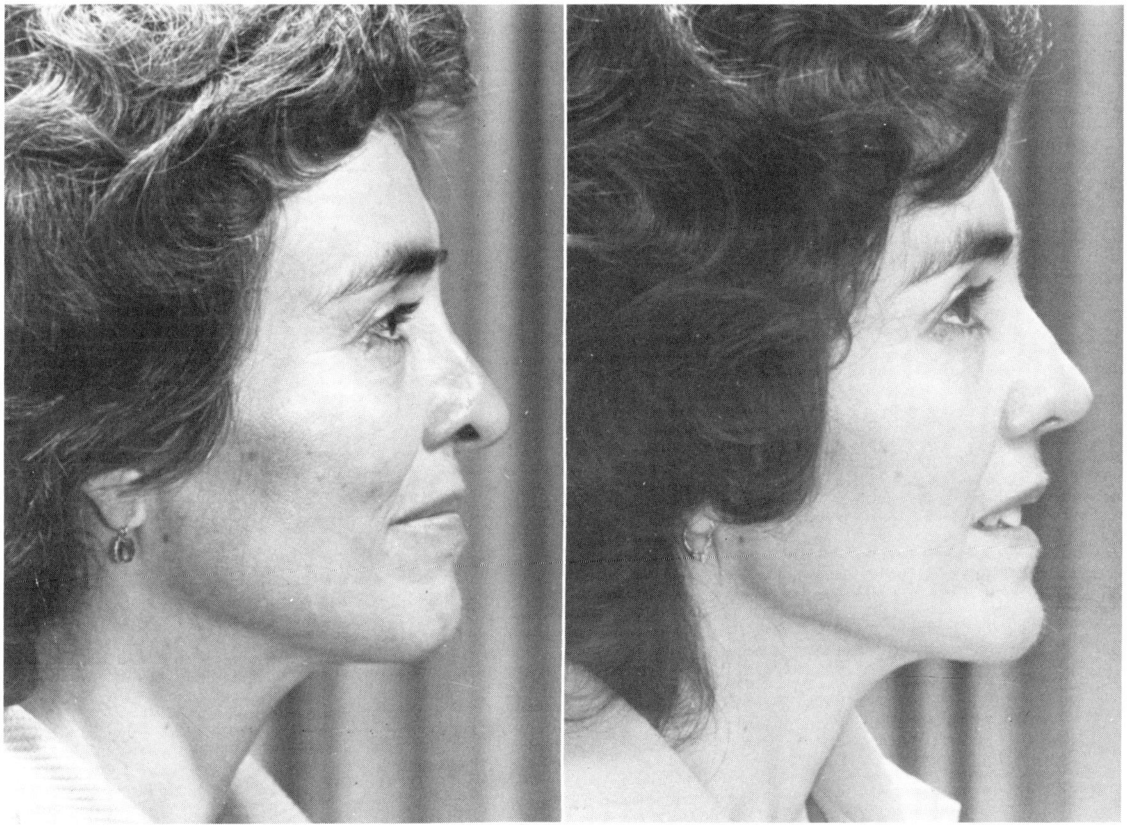

In the absence of a single strip of usable cartilage, two rectangles of cartilage were used for augmentation. Consequently, on lateral view the dorsum appears irregular. The increase in height of the dorsum at the radix was approximately 3 mm. The nasal tip graft is not visible because of the heavy tissues of the tip, but it has served to elevate the tip just above the dorsal line. The bone graft to the right alar rim, release of the scar contracture with skin grafting, and alar wedge resections improved the alar-columellar relationship.

DISCUSSION

A more conventional approach to this patient's crooked nose would have been difficult if not impossible because of her thick, calcified, and distorted septum.

Artistic conceptualizations of methods in surgery are frequently too simplistic and do not consider the pathologic changes that occur following injury. Attempts to score or morselize this septum to the midline would have been impossible. Moreover, the thickness and calcification of cartilage near the dorsum would not allow the unfolding that artists' drawings depict.

Radical procedures were unnecessary because the onlay graft technique provided a satisfactory result with minimum risk.

TIP WITH INADEQUATE PROJECTION

The tip with inadequate projection (TIP) is defined as any nasal tip that cannot be raised above the dorsal line by any alteration of tissues in or adjacent to it. The diagnosis of the TIP is primarily visual. Although it occurs with many combinations of tissues, there is a common, identifying feature; that is, the tip seems to be pulled in toward the nasal spine. This is caused by a short columella, an inadequate arch of lower lateral cartilage, or a combination of the two. Also characteristic is a downward inclination of the nasal tip despite an open nasolabial angle. These characteristics are not exclusively found in poorly projecting tips, but their presence is a diagnostic aid as well as a caution sign.

Frequently, patients with high dorsal lines appear to have adequate tip projection because of the upward distraction of the tip by the high dorsum, which is misleading. To determine the actual tip height, the lip should be brought forward to counteract all stresses on the tip. The distance from the base of the columella to the domes of the tip cartilages is the actual tip height. If this is insufficient to project to or above the estimated line of the new dorsum, tip grafting is indicated.

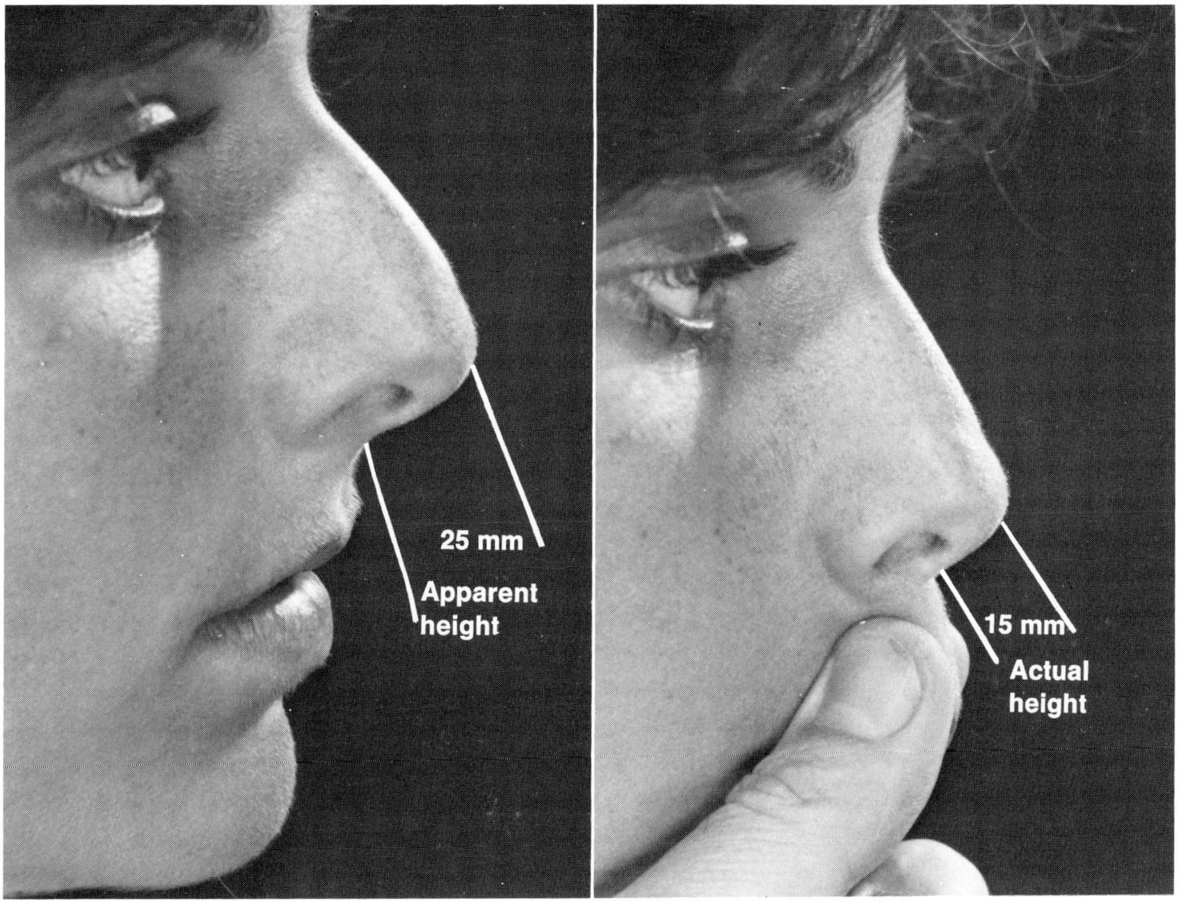

If a TIP is unrecognized or untreated, projection of the tip above the dorsal line cannot be accomplished. Furthermore, if the dorsum is overresected in an attempt to achieve this effect, a supratip deformity may result because of the inability of the tissues in the supratip area to contract to the reduced skeleton (see p. 384).

The solution to the TIP must begin with an understanding of the nature of the problem preoperatively. The projection potential of the nasal tip is limited by the size and construction of its parts. Since it is counterproductive to try to reduce other nasal tissues to match a retrusive tip, one must think in terms of conservative resection of tissues and augmentation of the tip in order to achieve correct proportions. I have had consistently good results with the use of a tip graft of septal cartilage, as described in Chapter 4.

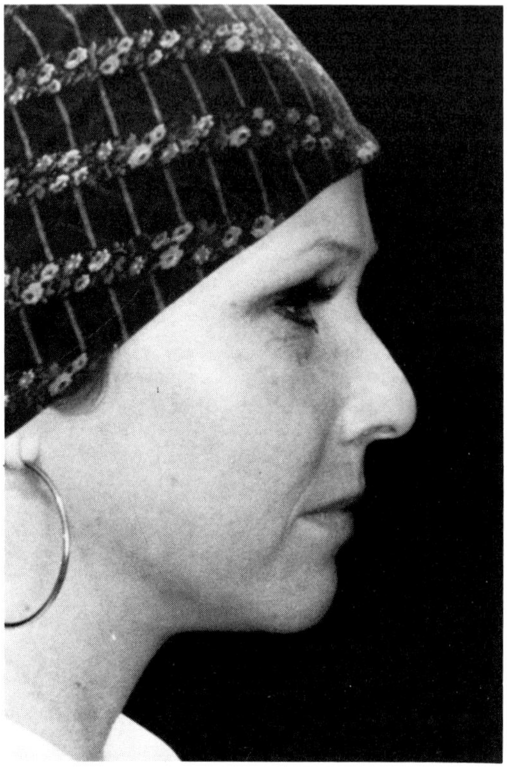

Case report 1

The appearance of a patient with a TIP is often deceptive. On lateral view, the initial impression is that of a prominent nose with a large dorsal hump. However, on closer examination it can be seen that the hump appears to be large because of a low radix and an inadequately projecting tip. If the radix were raised 2 mm, the hump would be virtually eliminated.

The nasolabial angle and the relationships of the basal parts are excellent. The columellar-alar complex is within normal limits, yet the tip appears to be flattened. The nose seems to incline downward despite the open nasolabial angle, which is characteristic of a TIP.

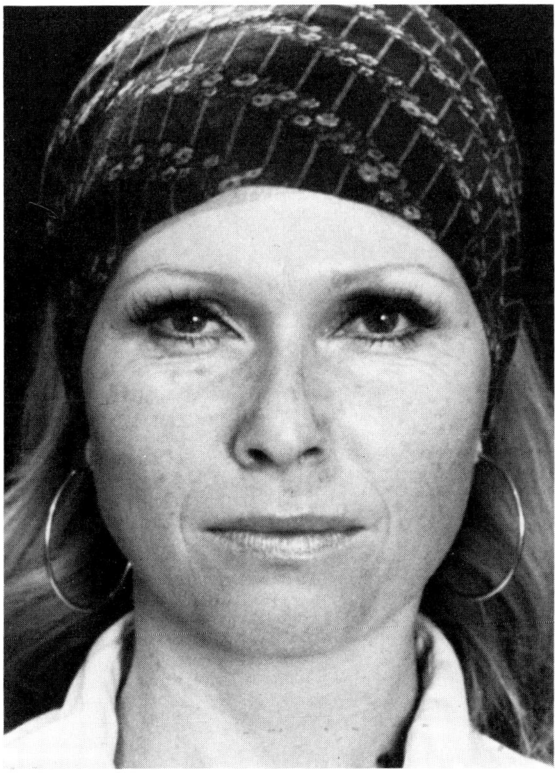

On front view, the bony pyramid is already narrow for the broad base. Osteotomies to further narrow it would compound the disproportion. In general, the nasal contour is good, but the tip is flat and broad. The only feature of her front view that should be changed is the nasal tip.

Summary of surgical procedure

1. Minimal skeletonization, with a transfixion incision to the middle third of the membranous septum
2. No resection of the caudal septum or nasal spine
3. Rasp of the bony dorsum 1 mm
4. Reduction of the cartilaginous dorsum 1 to 2 mm
5. Delivery of the tip cartilages through rim incisions
6. Trim of the cephalic parts (leaving 5- to 6-mm wide lateral crura) and attenuation of the dome areas with scoring cuts
7. No osteotomies
8. Tip graft of septal cartilage

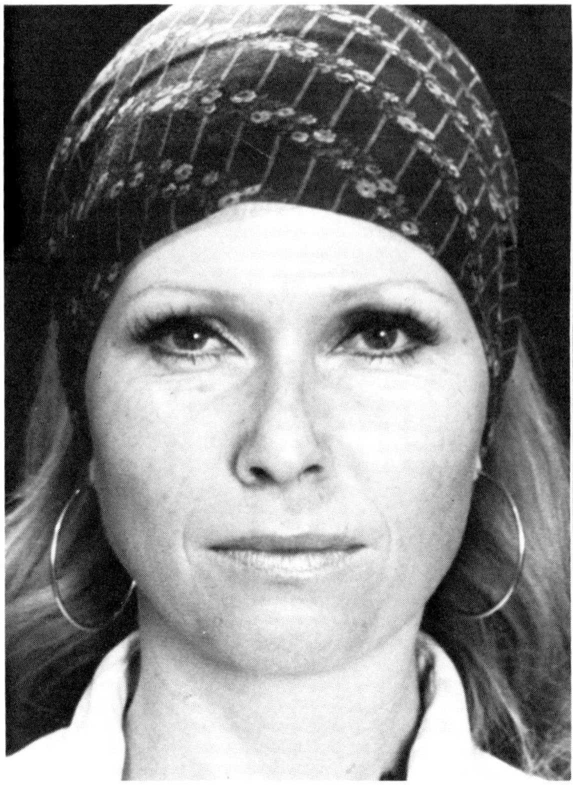

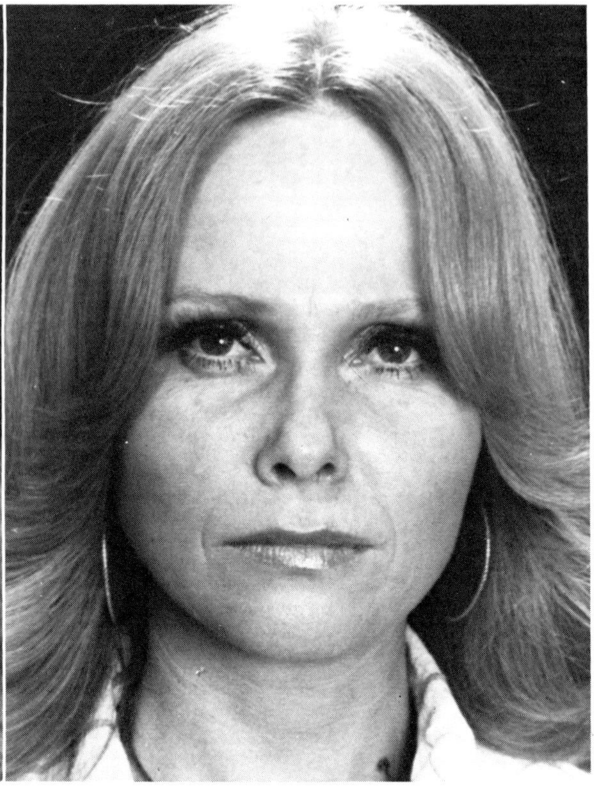

On front view, reduction of the dorsum by 1 to 2 mm has not created a problem with continuity but has produced a slightly broader-appearing dorsum. This has improved the overall balance of the nose.

Preoperatively, a diffuse light reflex is seen over the nasal tip. Postoperatively, the light reflects from the elevated tip as a central highlight, and the nasal base appears narrower and more projecting.

Postoperative right lateral and left close-up lateral views illustrate the effectiveness of elevating the tip and preserving the dorsal height. The good basal relationships are undisturbed. Tip projection has been obtained with the use of a tip graft of septal cartilage.

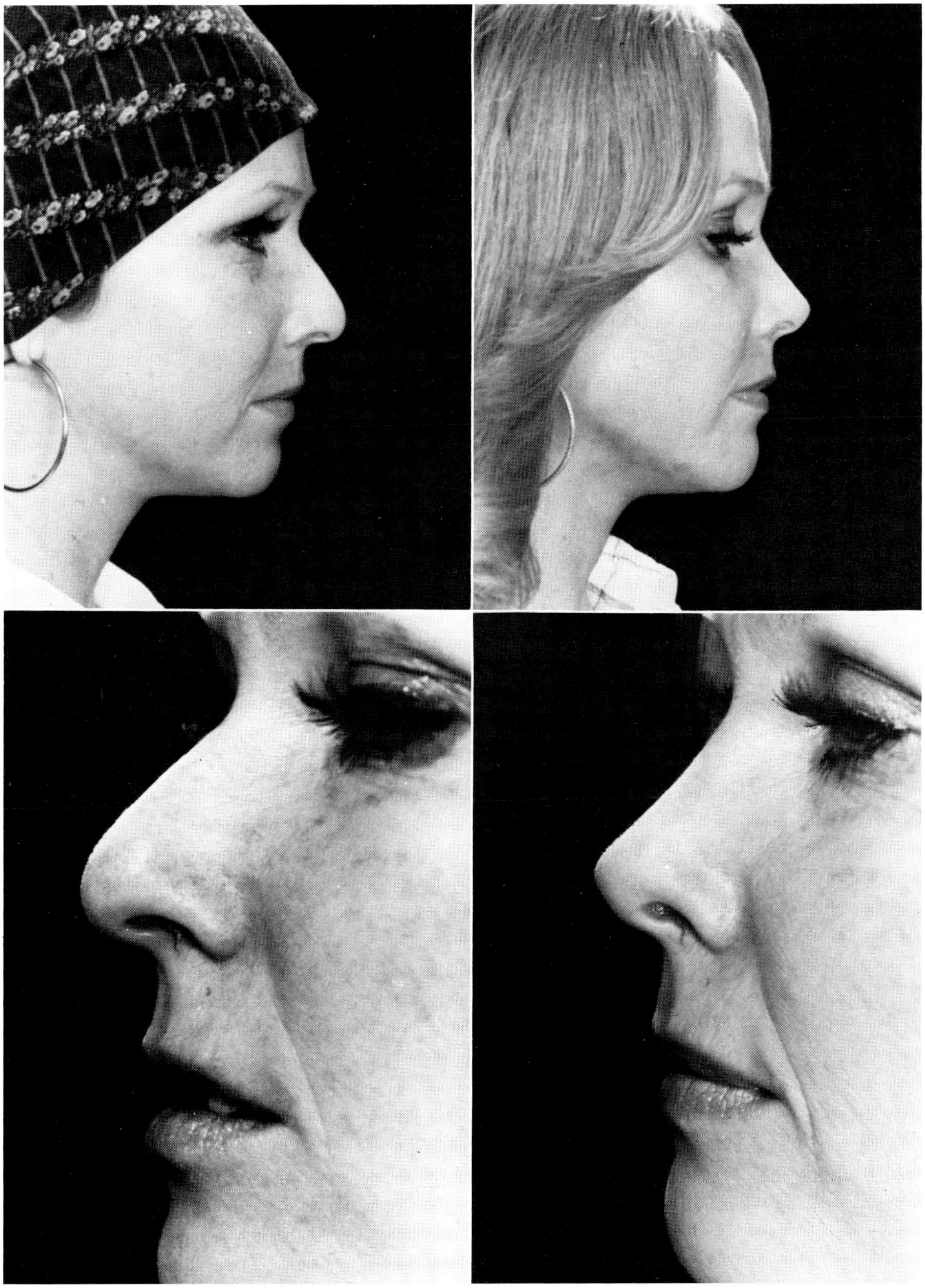

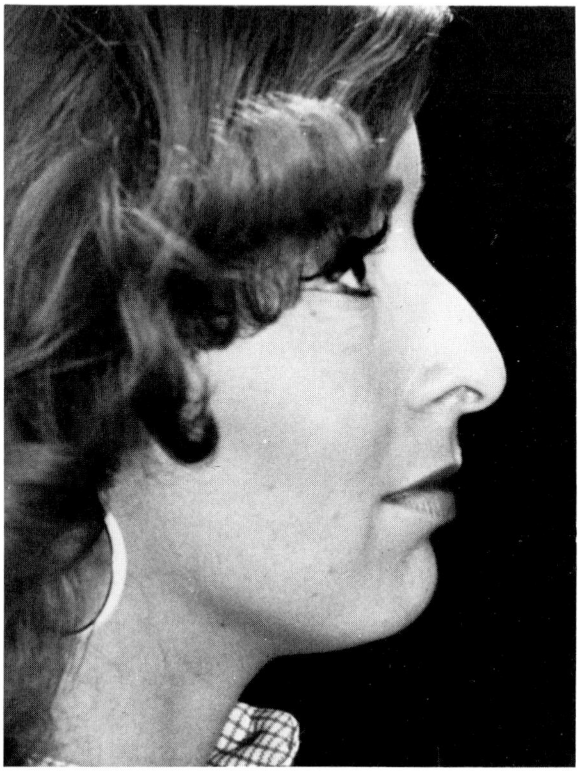

Case report 2

This patient's nose has a marked resemblance to the patient's nose shown on p. 372. Similar nasal configurations can be seen in patients with a TIP.

On lateral view, the dorsum seems high in relation to the low radix and low tip profile. If a finger is placed over the tip, the need for only slight dorsal resection becomes apparent. The columella is low for the slightly arching alae. The central notch in the ala is indicative of a fragile and vulnerable alar rim. Preservation of as much lower lateral cartilage as possible is imperative.

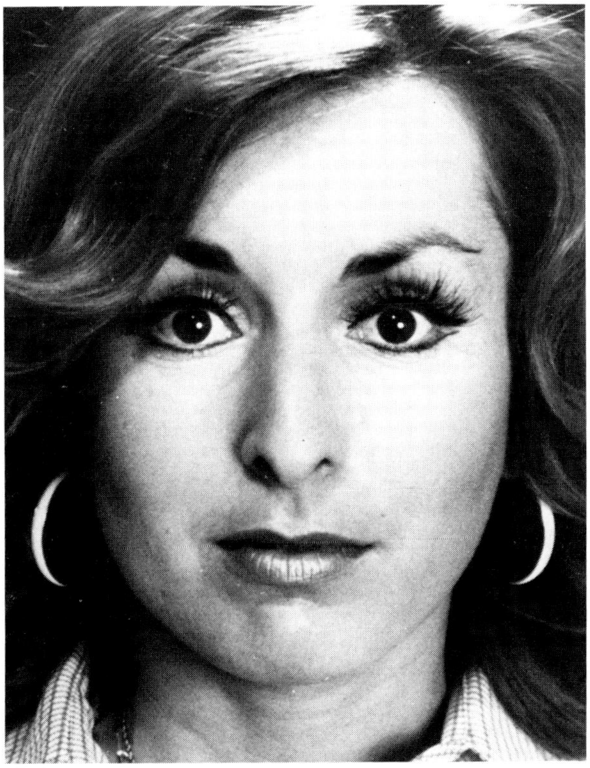

On front view, the bony pyramid is broad, and the nasal base is misproportioned because of the high-arching alae and the low-hanging columella.

Summary of surgical procedure

1. Limited skeletonization
2. Transfixion incision to the nasal spine
3. Reduction of the nasal spine with bone rongeur
4. Reduction of the caudal septum 3 mm
5. Reduction of the dorsum approximately 3 mm
6. Delivery of the tip cartilages through rim incisions
7. Trim of cephalic parts (leaving 6-mm wide lateral crura) and attenuation of the dome areas by scoring
8. Osteotomies
9. Placement of a septal cartilage tip graft

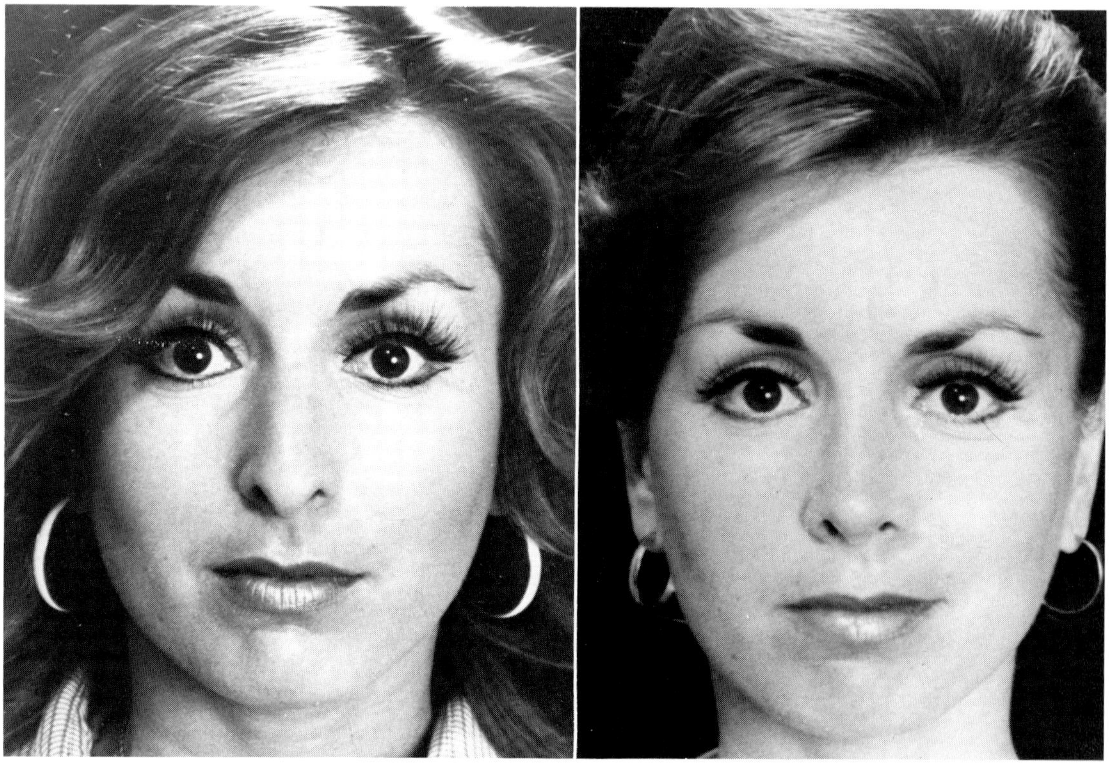

Postoperatively, the narrower bony pyramid is in good continuity with the superior orbital rims. The lateral nasal lines are slightly divergent, ending in a tip that reflects a central pattern of light. The improvement in the columellar-alar relationship has benefited the appearance of the high-arching alae.

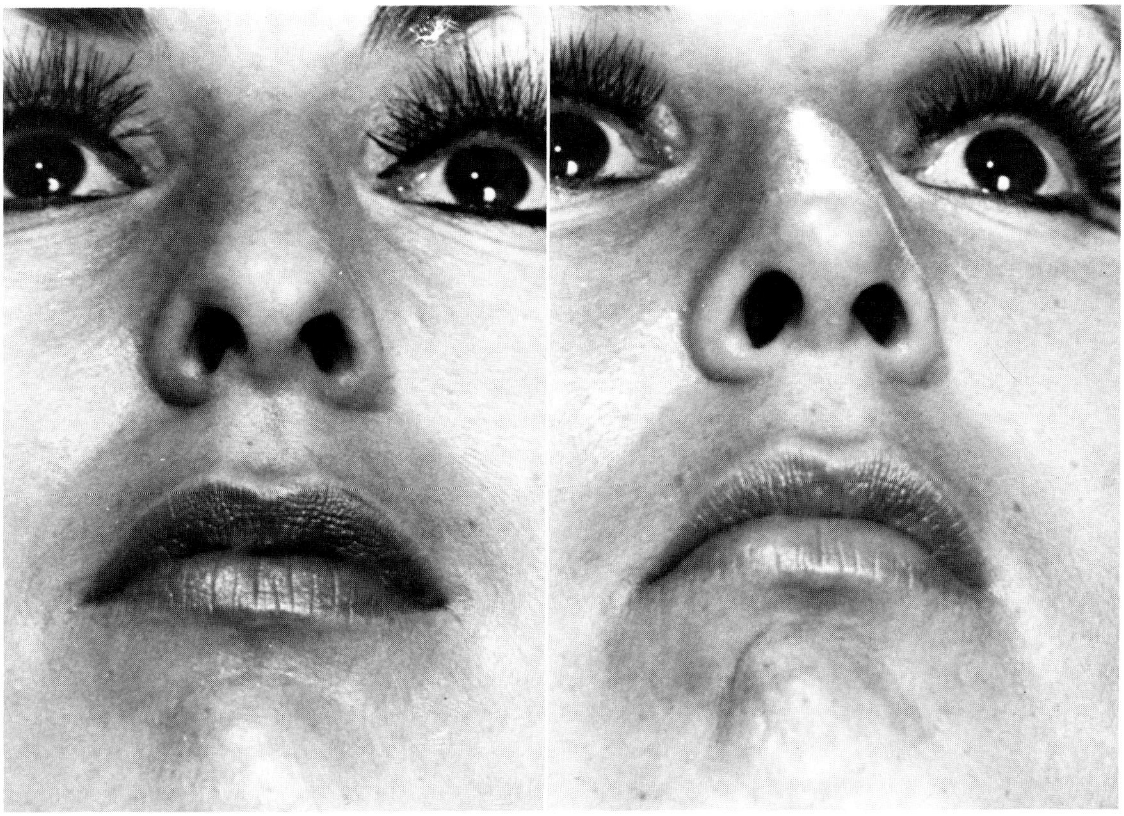

On basal view, the squat appearance of the nasal base has been altered by projection of the tip graft.

The right lateral and left close-up oblique views illustrate the dramatic effect of minimal dorsal reduction and tip augmentation in the patient with a TIP.

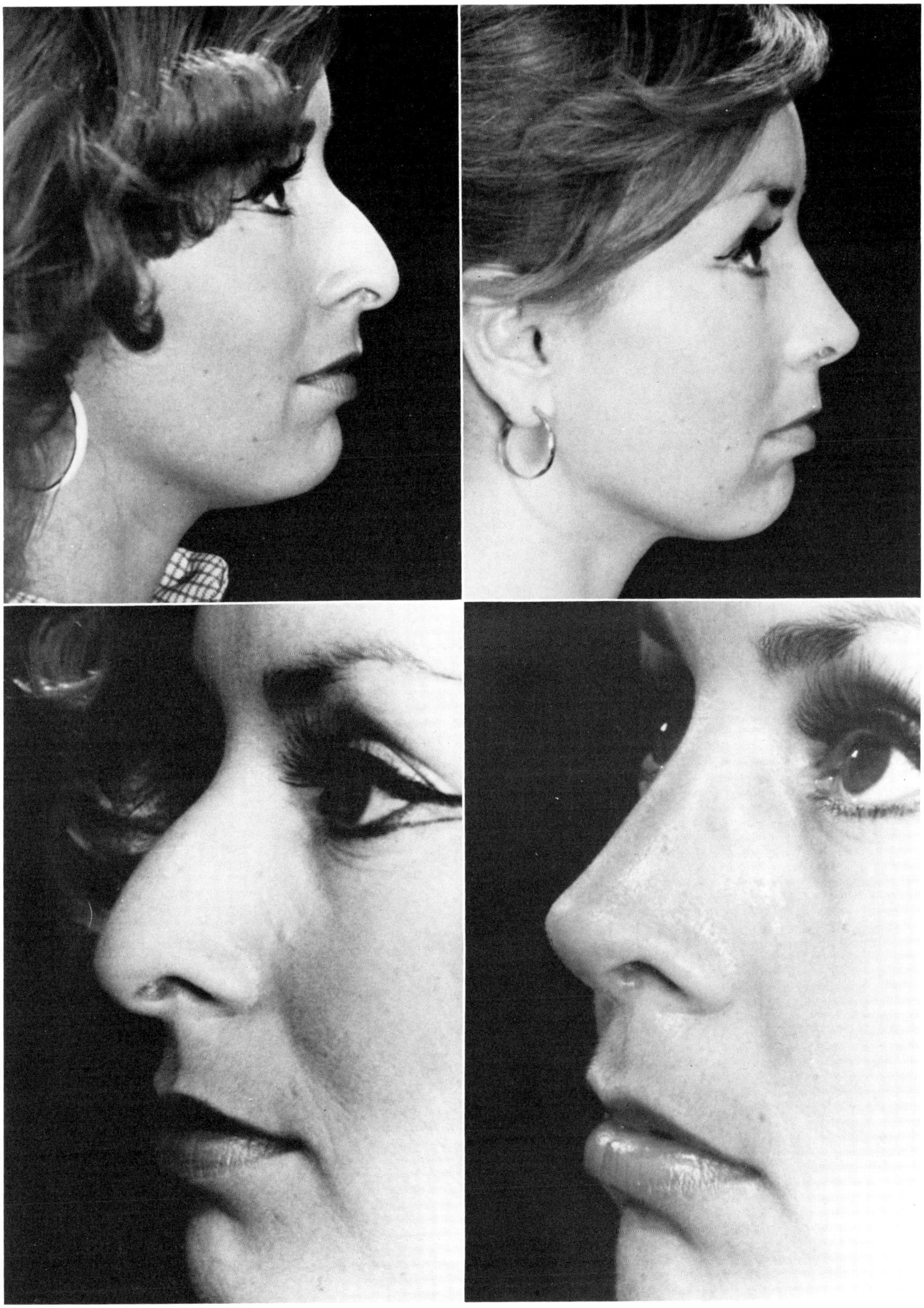

Case report 3

The combination of thick tissues, a high dorsum, and a TIP is a formidable surgical problem. Without elevation of the tip, even a modestly successful result is not possible.

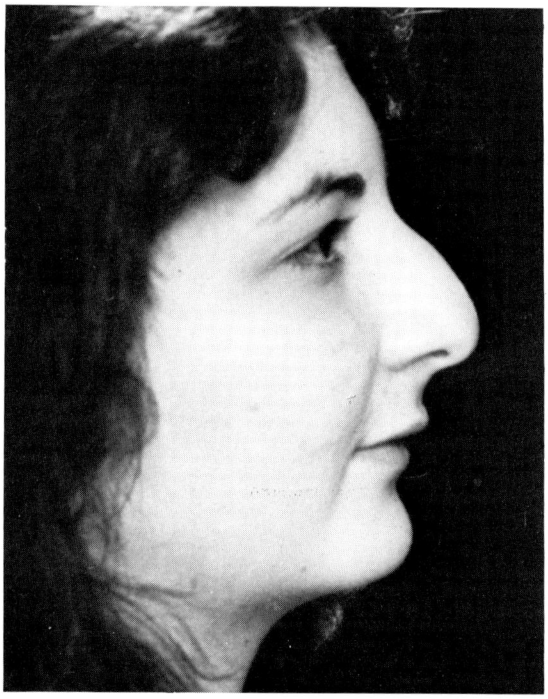

On lateral view, this patient appears to have a nasal configuration that would respond well to standard rhinoplasty except for the heavy tissues.

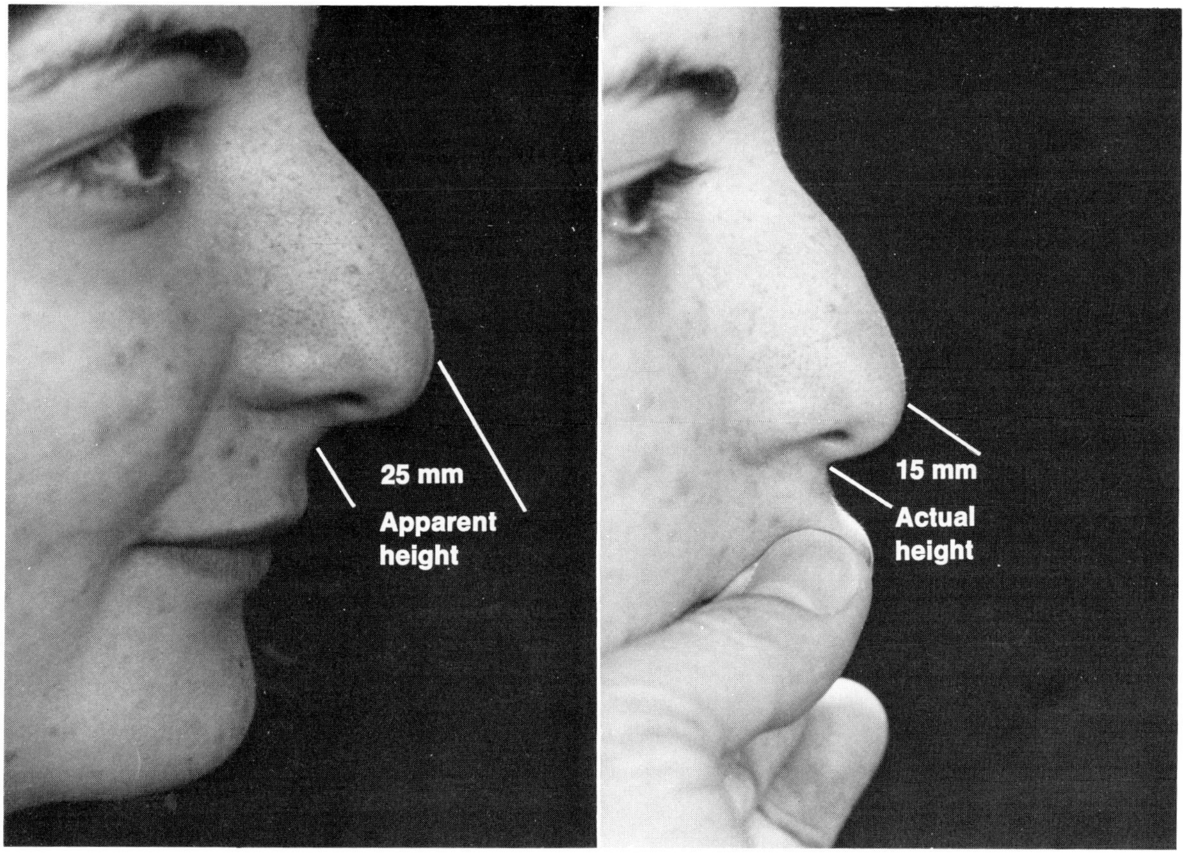

On testing for actual tip projection, one can see that there is not enough tip height to elevate it into a proper aesthetic relationship with the dorsum following reduction. Moderate reduction of the dorsum alone would not be sufficient for an adequate result.

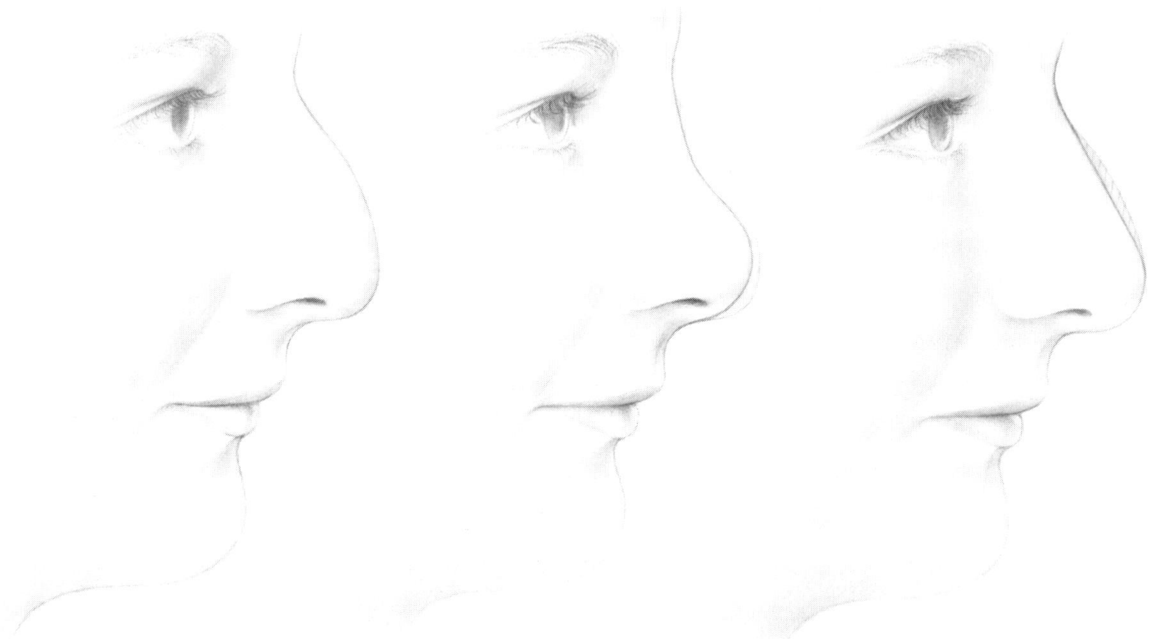

A drawing of the patient preoperatively is shown on the left. The center drawing of the patient portrays the theoretical result following moderate reduction of the dorsum. The thinner tissues near the radix contract well to the lowered skeleton, whereas the thicker tissues of the nasal base contract poorly. The resultant supratip fullness, which is one of the most common evidences of rhinoplasty, is inevitable with patients who have the compound problem of thick tissues and a retrusive tip. The drawing on the right shows that even if conservative resection of the dorsum were done, the lack of adequate tip projection would produce a disappointing result.

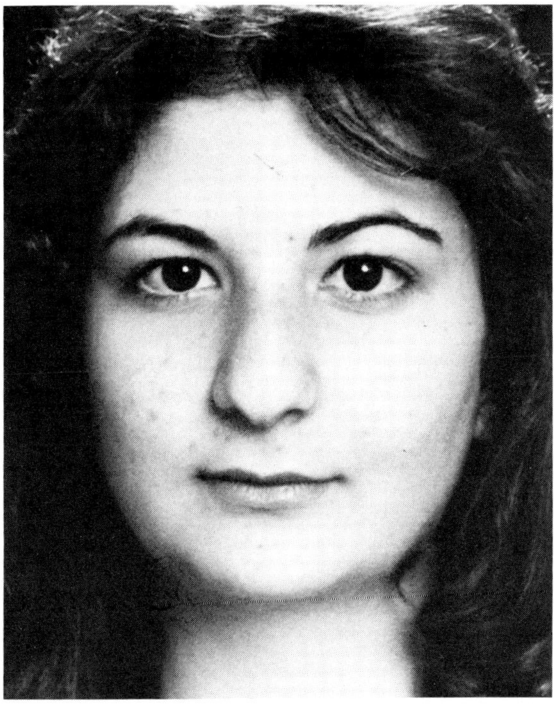

When confronted with an extremely broad radix, one is tempted to make it much narrower. All parts of this patient's nose are broad and large. In addition, the tissues are thick. If much narrowing of the bony vault were accomplished, disharmony of nasal parts would result.

Summary of surgical procedure

1. Limited skeletonization, including the membranous septum to the nasal spine
2. Reduction of the nasal spine and posterior caudal septum
3. Reduction of the bony dorsum 2 to 3 mm
4. Trim of the roof of the upper cartilaginous vault approximately 2 mm
5. Delivery of the tip cartilages through rim incisions
6. Trim of the cephalic parts and attenuation of the domes
7. Lateral osteotomies
8. Tip graft of septal cartilage

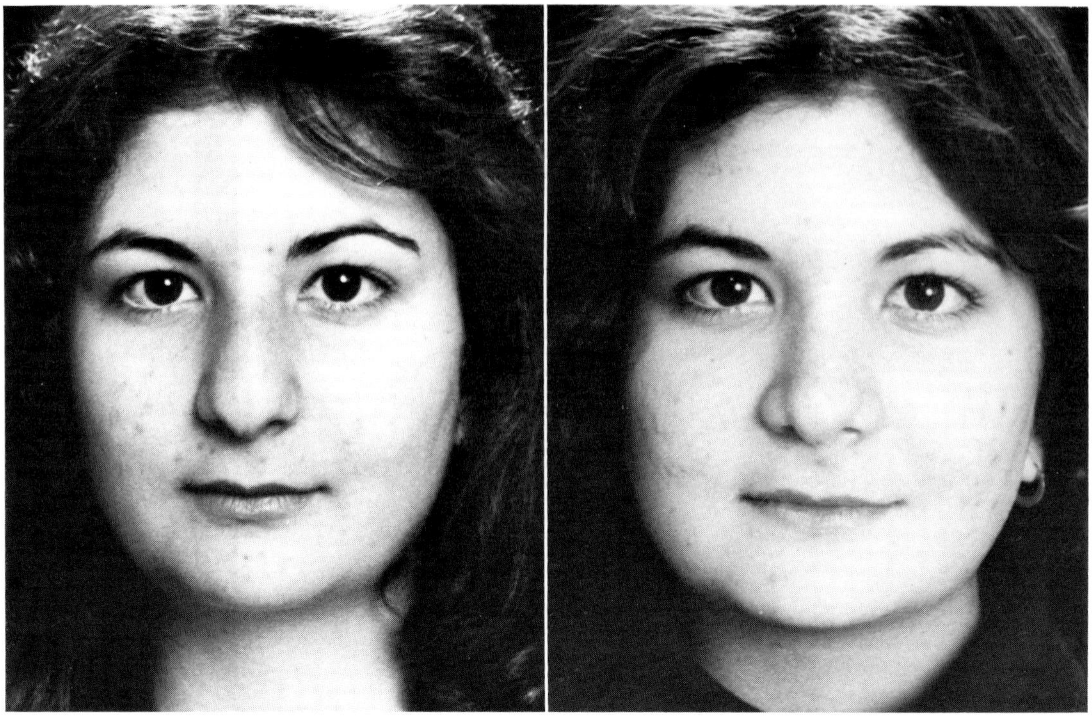

On postoperative front view, the nasal tip is better delineated, but the nose is still large.

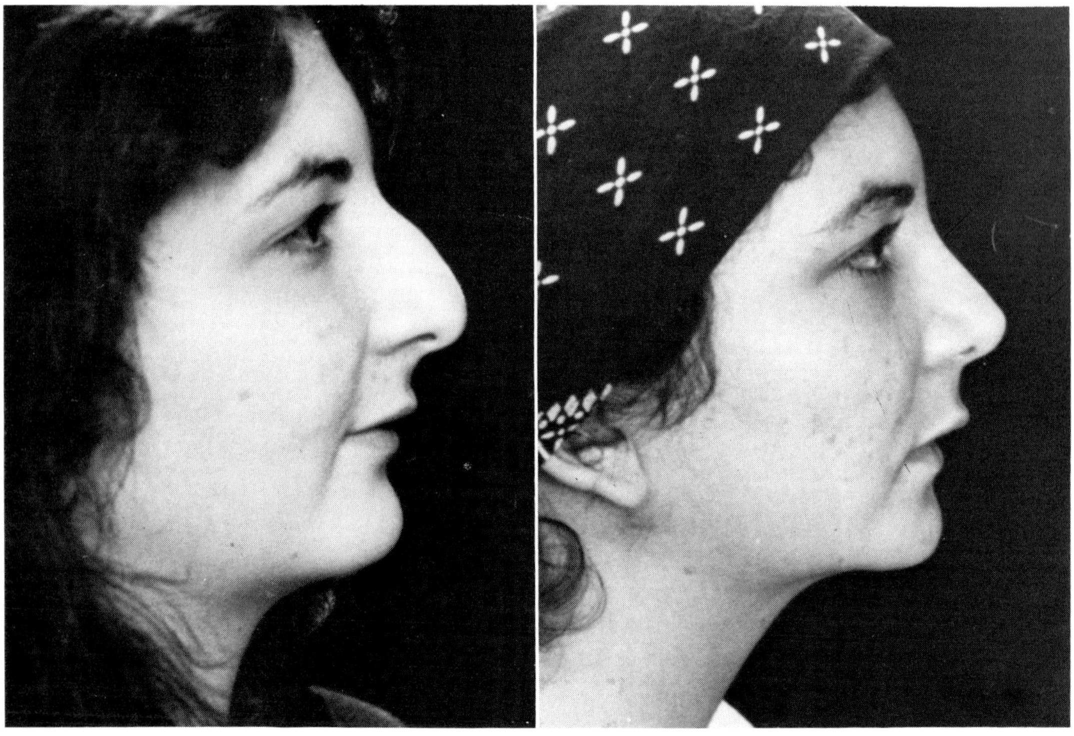

On lateral view, the dorsum is straight, and the tip has been elevated to the dorsal line. A conservative resection of the dorsum has maintained the necessary height to support the heavy tissues of the lower third of the nose.

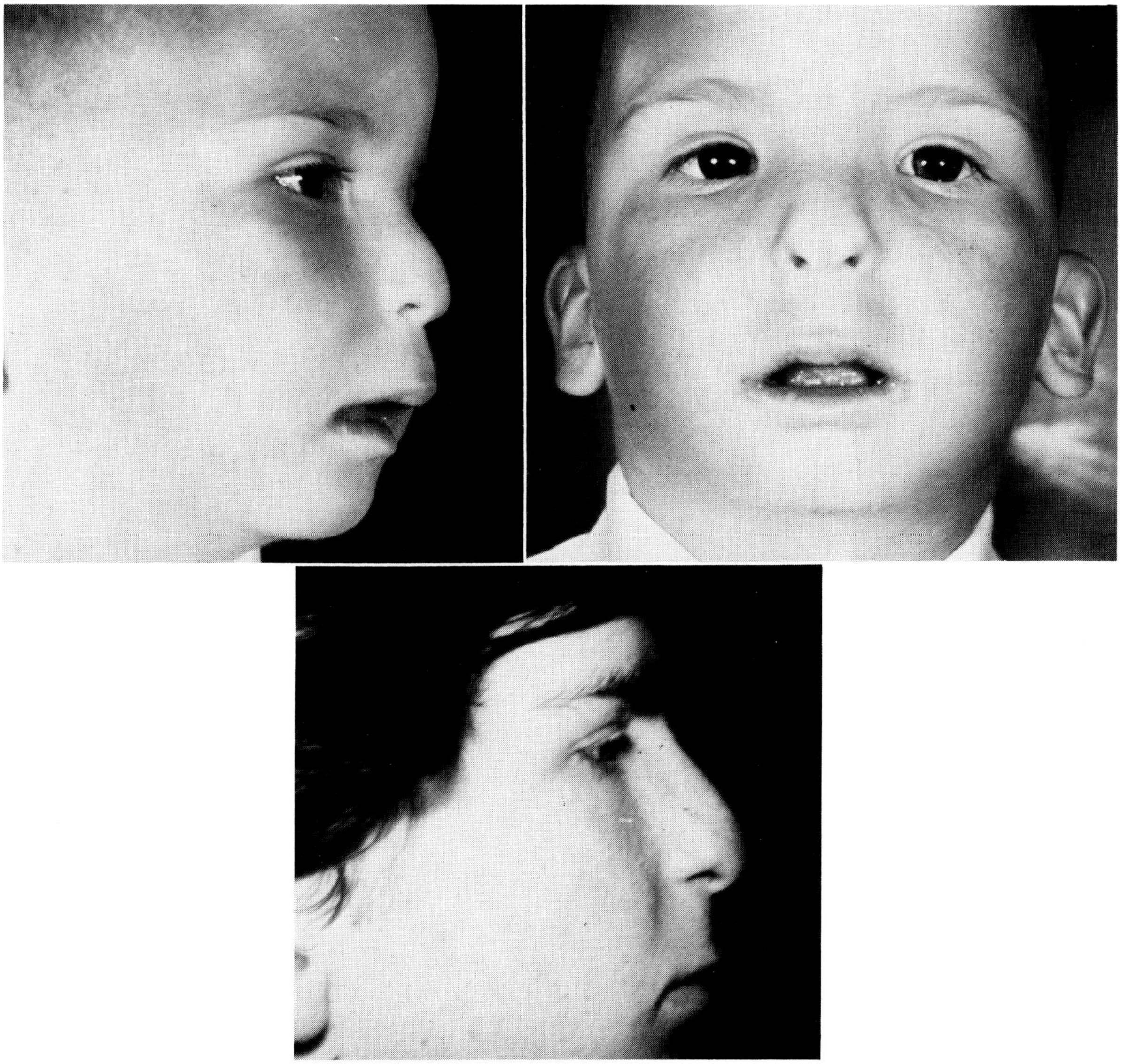

Case report 4

This patient is shown at 5 years and 16 years. The flat tip and short columella are characteristic of the TIP.

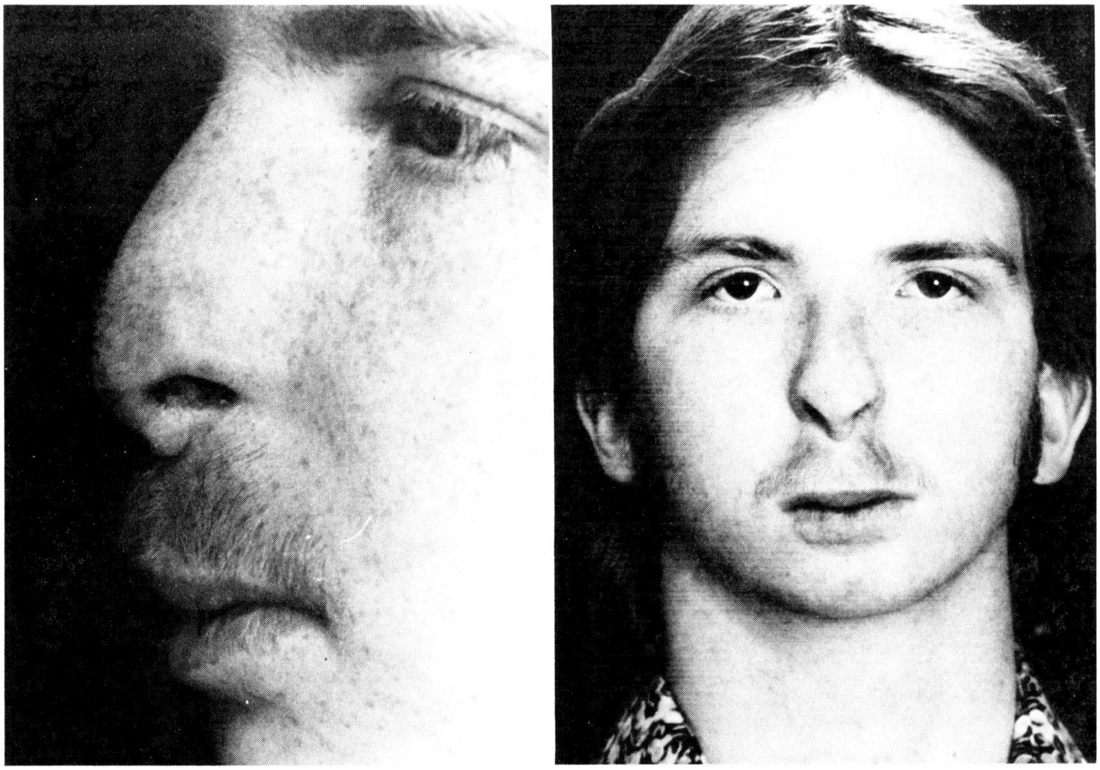

A primary surgical attempt to lengthen the columella by use of a composite ear graft failed to achieve the desired aesthetic result. Though the columella has been lengthened by the 6-mm graft, the problem of lack of tip projection persists.

The nasal tip is broad and flat. The poor alar-columellar relationship was worsened by the composite graft, which displaced the columella inferiorly.

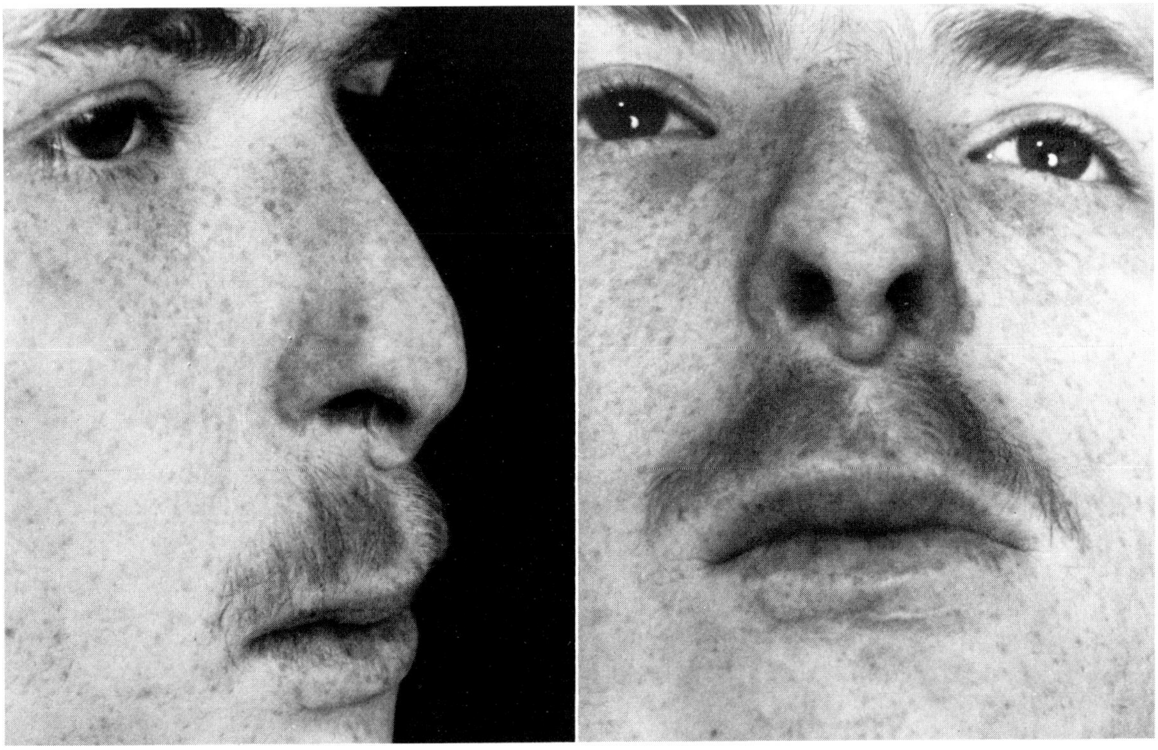

On right close-up oblique view, the effect of the composite graft is more visible. The primary aesthetic problem is a lack of tip projection.

The basal perimeter is almost square. Because of the extreme flatness of the tip, the anterior part of the perimeter is obscure.

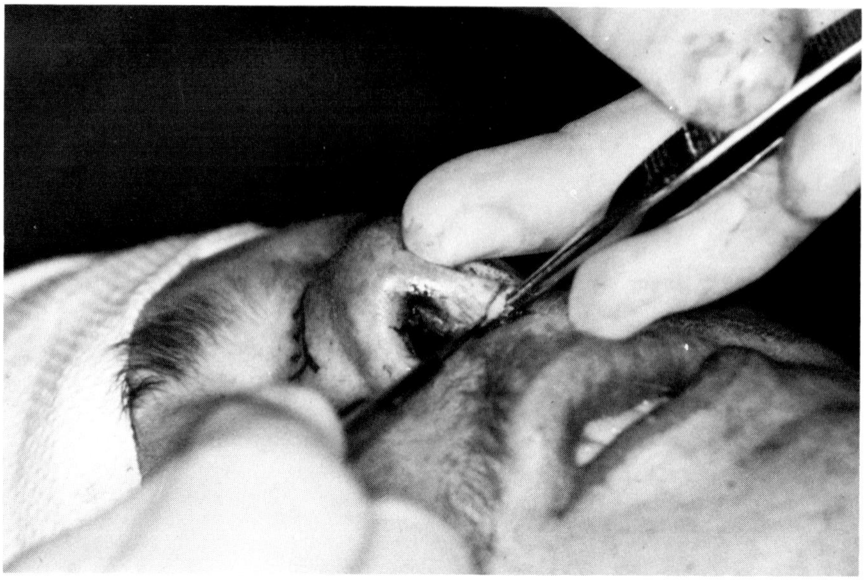

SURGICAL PROCEDURE

The redundant portion of the old composite graft was resected, allowing access to the columella.

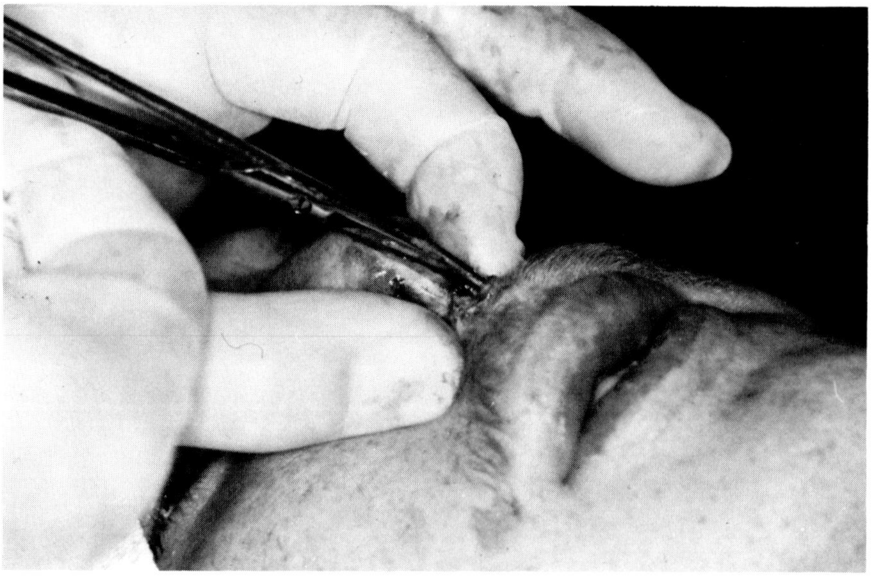

A pair of Joseph scissors was used to dissect a pocket into the columella, toward the spine, for placement of a supportive graft.

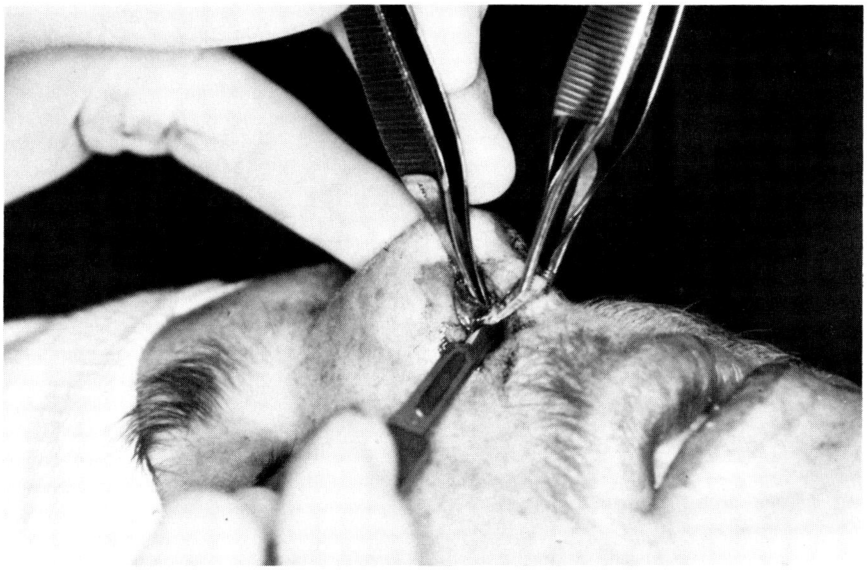

Initial skeletonization was followed by preliminary trim of the caudal septum.

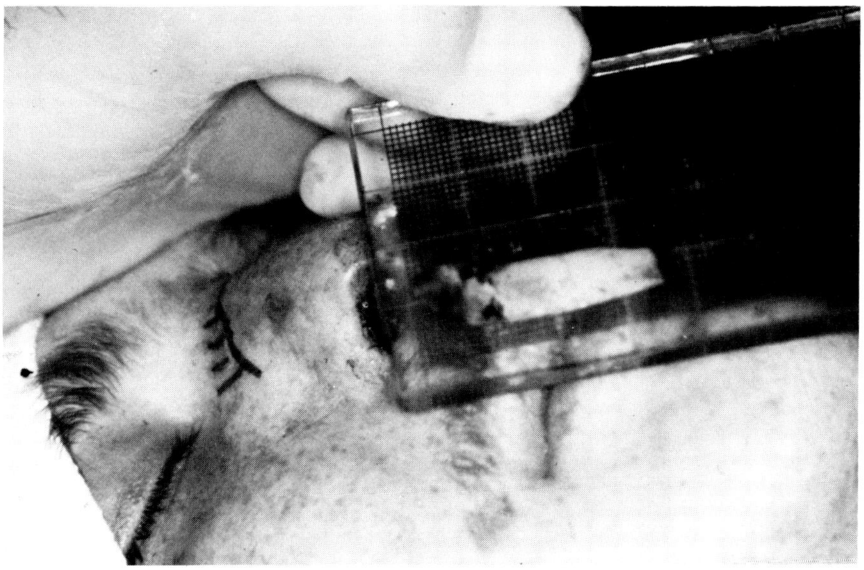

A submucous resection provided material for the planned reconstruction of the base of the nose.

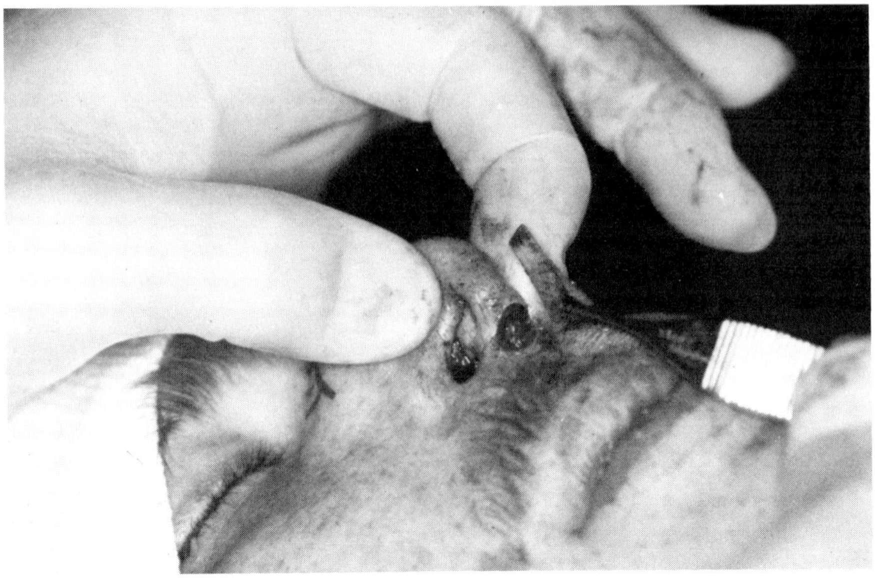

The 12 × 3 mm piece of cartilage was shaped.

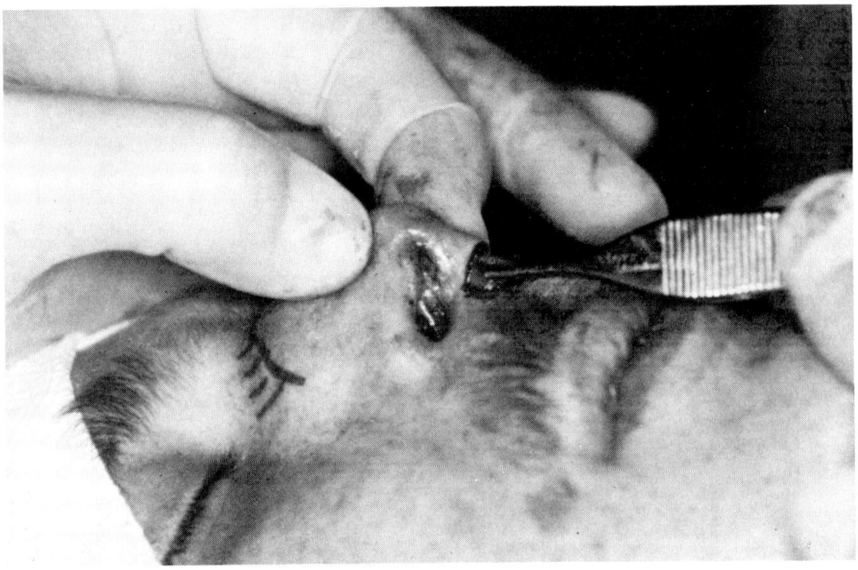

It was placed into the columella, with the larger end seated over the area of the nasal spine.

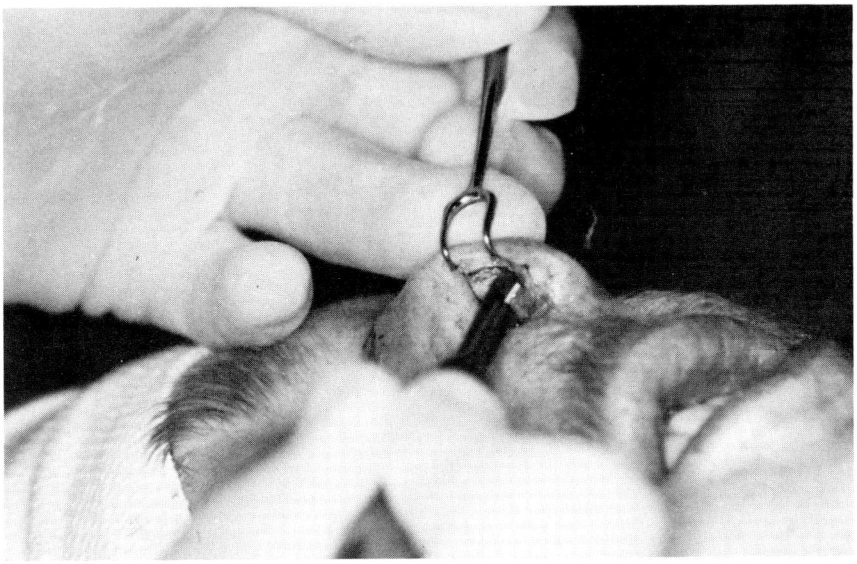

An incision was made into the tip lobule.

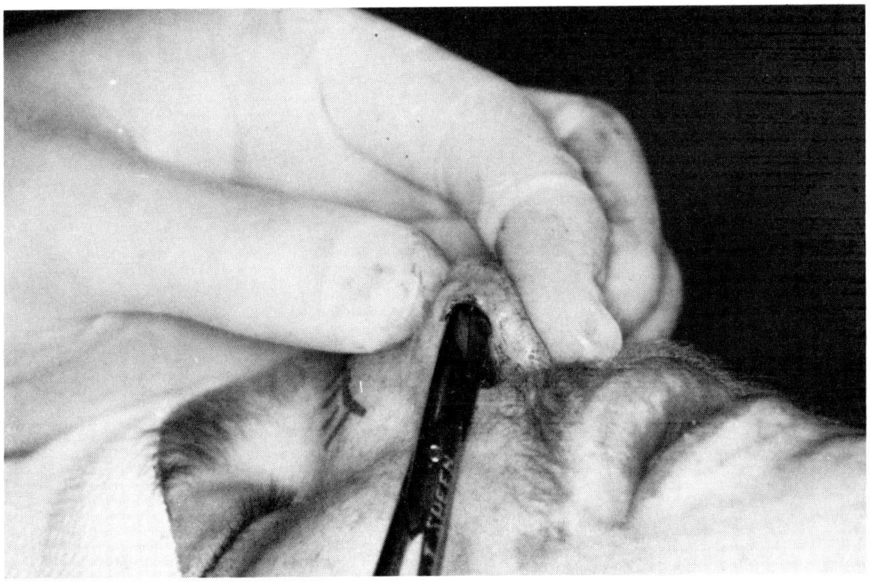

A pocket was dissected with Joseph scissors.

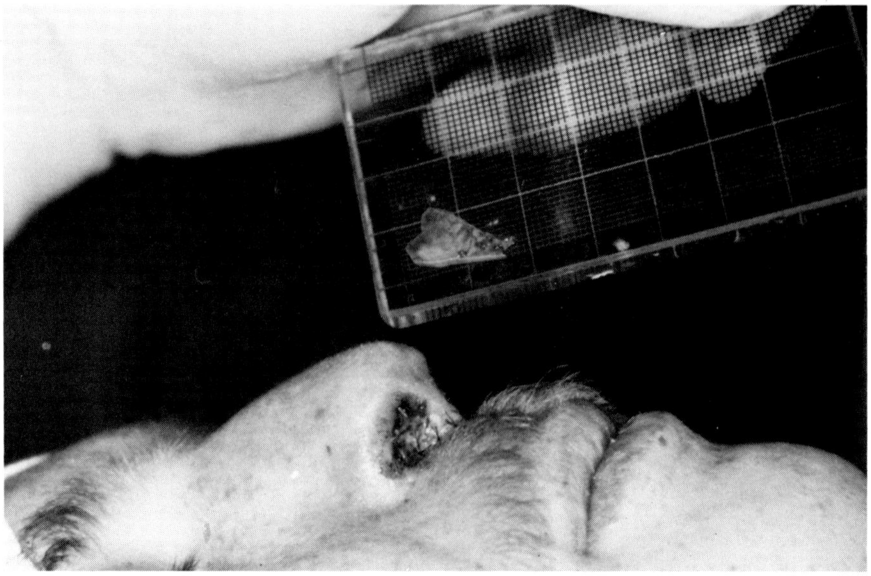

A large tip graft was fashioned.

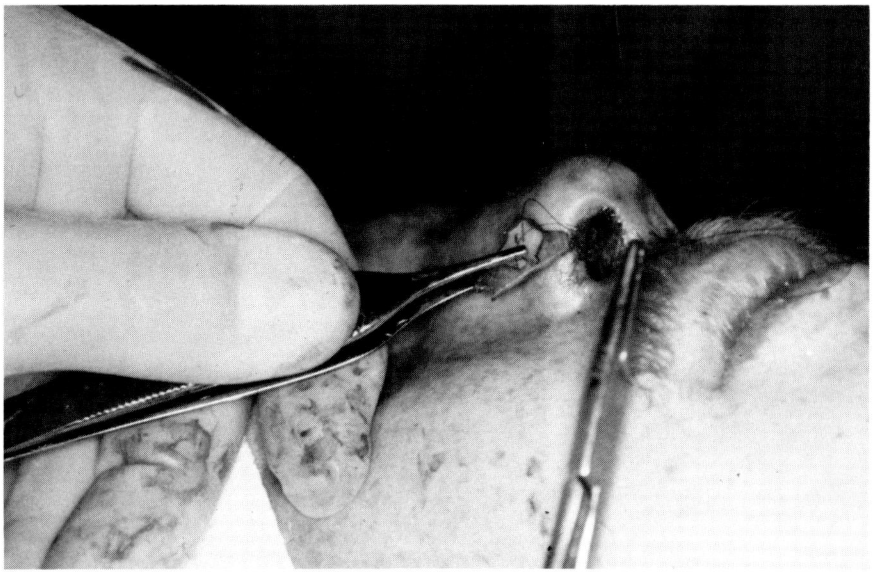

A small rectangle of cartilage was sutured to the anterior surface of the graft, which was fixed into position with a percutaneous mattress suture of 6-0 nylon.

Summary of surgical procedure

1. Limited skeletonization
2. Transfixion incision to the nasal spine
3. Resection of the nasal spine and posterior caudal septum 3 mm
4. Septoplasty to obtain graft material
5. Delivery of the lower lateral cartilages through rim incisions
6. Resection of approximately one half of the existing composite graft
7. Placement of a cartilage graft as a columellar strut
8. Tip graft of septal cartilage

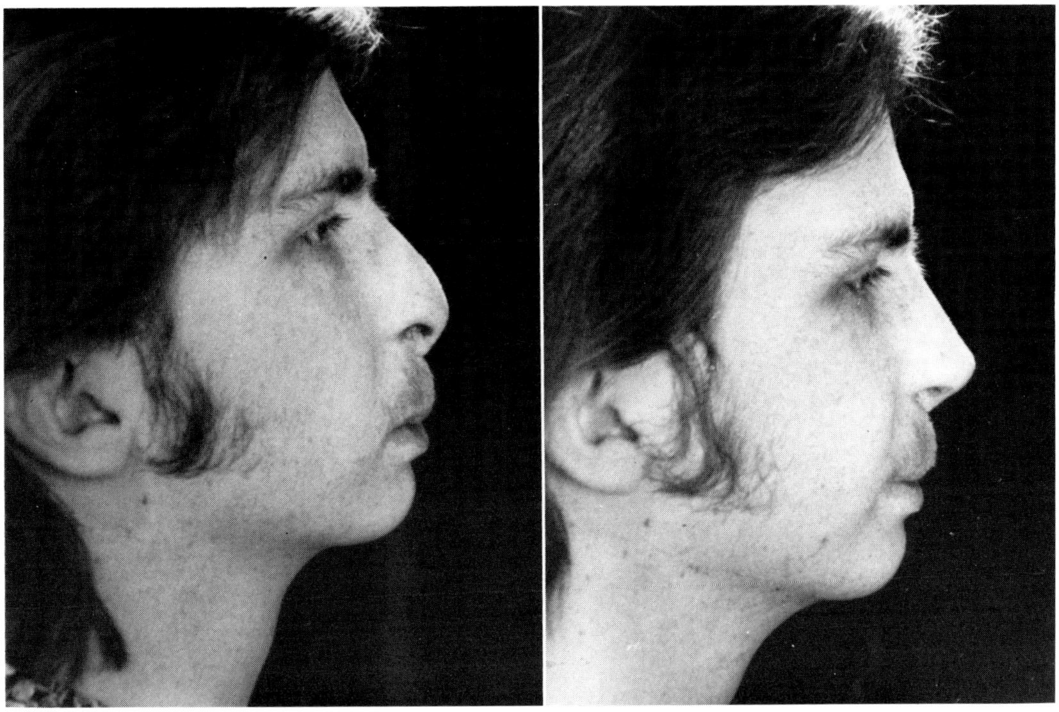

POSTOPERATIVE RESULTS

The most significant change on profile is the elevation of the tip above the dorsal line. The line from the tip to the insertion of the columella lacks the break at the columellar junction because of the placement of a columellar strut as a foundation for the tip graft.

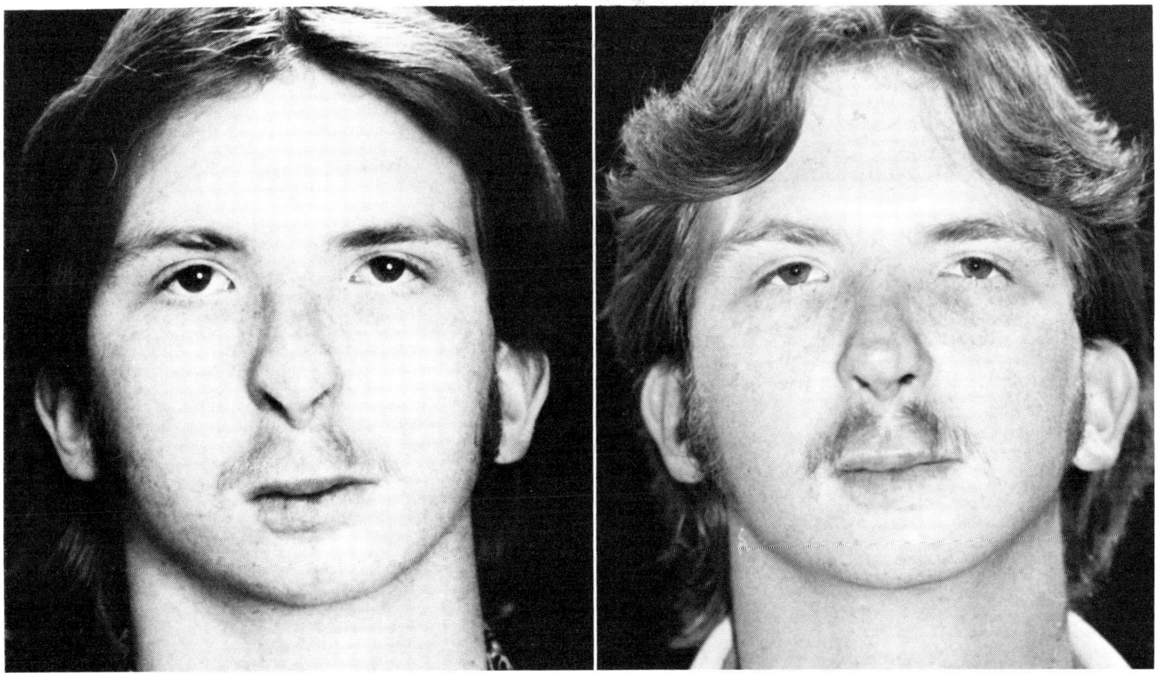

On front view, the projecting tip has altered the nasal contour favorably. The columella is in better position relative to the alar rims.

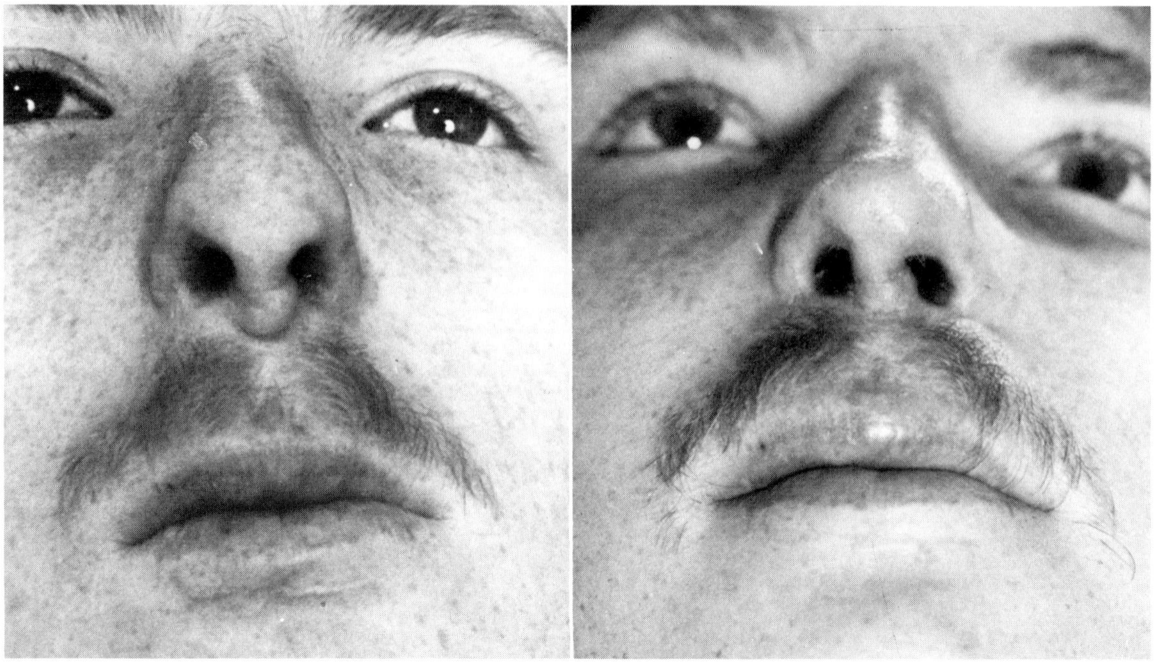

Extension of the tip by cartilage grafting produces a narrower and more delineated nasal base.

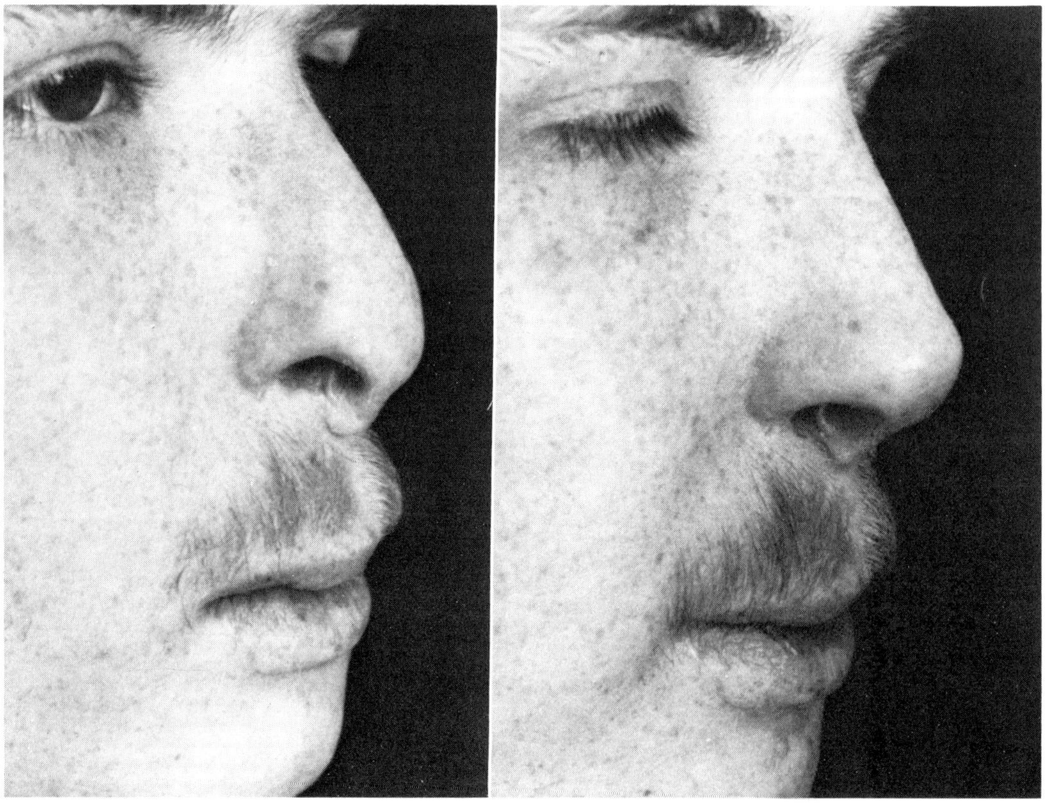

The columellar strut imparts an unnaturally stiff appearance to the base of the columella, but it provides excellent support to the columella and the tip graft.

ULTRAPROJECTING TIP

The ultraprojecting tip is a compound problem. It is not just a matter of large, gangling lower lateral cartilages, because all the parts of the nasal base are excessively long. In addition, one must contend with the towering tent of tissue overlying the large framework. To my knowledge there is no satisfactory method to significantly reduce the ultraprojecting nose. Therefore, the solution is to compromise.

The patient must understand preoperatively that surgery will modify tip projection but that the nose will still be large and projecting by the usual standards. The nostrils and columella will remain long, unless the surgeon resorts to external excisions.

Reduction of the ultraprojecting tip is limited by the amount and character of the soft tissue cover, which has a finite ability to contract. Moreover, when tissues contract, there is a concomitant loss of tip definition. Thus, inadequate framework results in a loss of definition or in frank distortion. Therefore, ample framework must be retained to ensure tissue draping.

The most common error in treating this problem is the attempt to produce a small nose, which invariably leads to overresection of skeletal parts. In the approach to surgery for the ultraprojecting tip, one should ask the question:Is it better to have a nose that is large and well contoured or a nose that is small and poorly contoured?

The surgical management of the ultraprojecting tip consists of: (1) conservative dorsal resection, (2) reduction of the nasal spine, and (3) reduction of the size of the arch of the lower lateral cartilage. The arch can be effectively reduced by conservative resection of the dome, but care must be taken that support of the tip is not jeopardized.

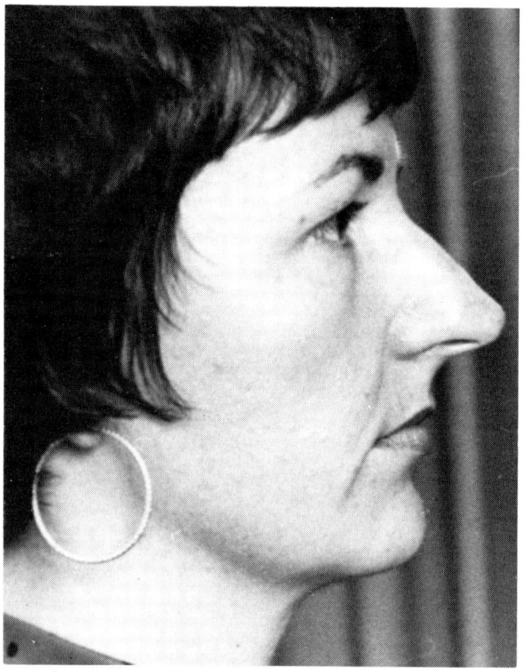

Case report 1

On profile, a well-contoured nose can be seen. All the requirements for an ideal nasal profile are present with one exception—the nasal tip is extremely projecting.

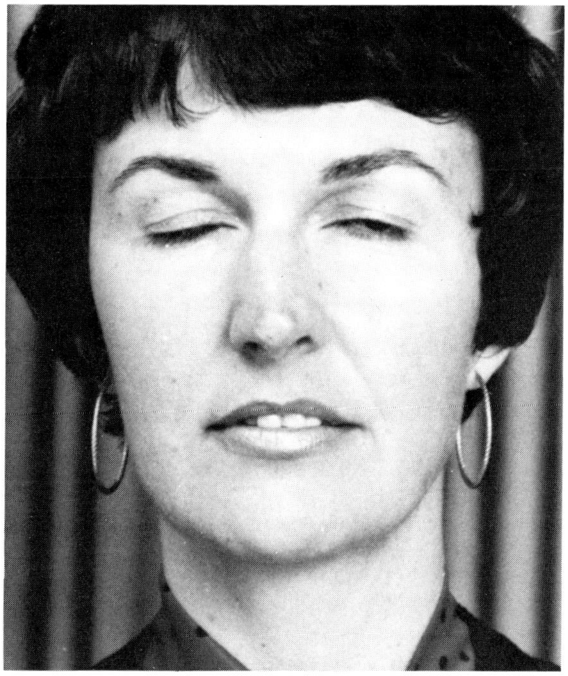

On front view, the bony pyramid is slightly broad for the base of the nose. The tip, which is narrow and sharp, blanches over the lower lateral cartilages. The projection of the tip cartilages is emphasized by concavities just lateral to the domes. The nose deviates to the right. The nostrils are visible, with the left nostril slightly higher than the right.

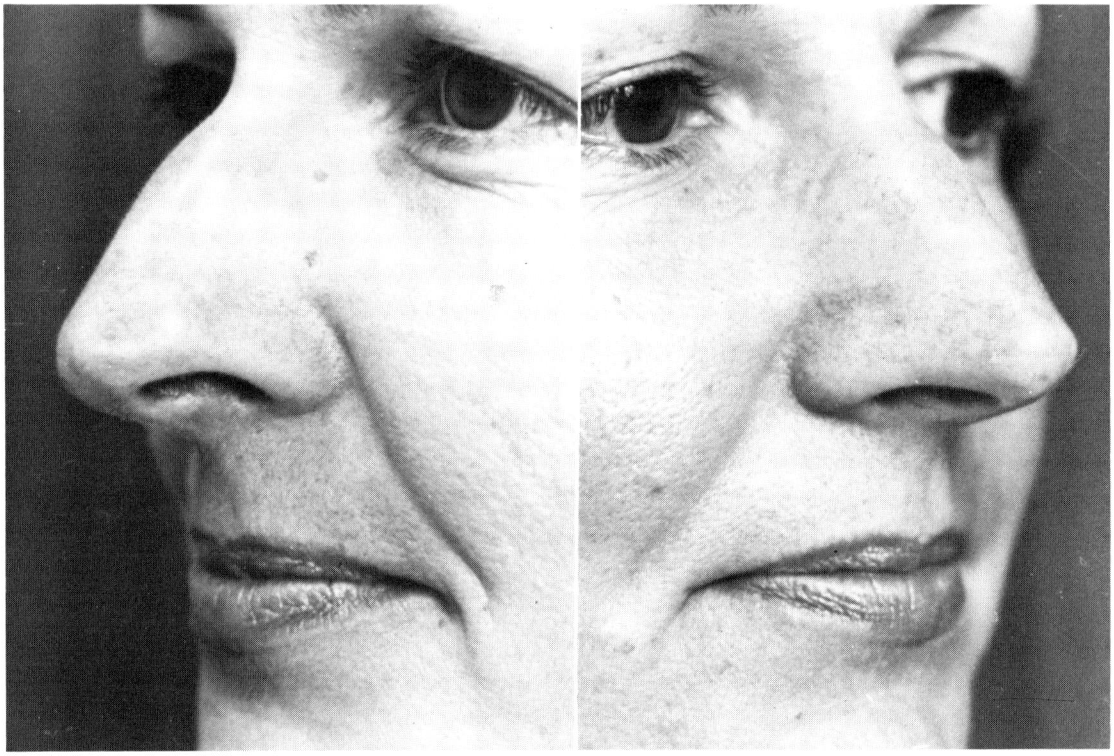

The right and left oblique views are different, with more dorsal irregularity on the left. Because of the slight dorsal prominence on the left oblique view, the tip appears to incline downward compared with the upward tilt on the right oblique view. The bony dorsum is broad and flat. By palpation, the nasal spine is found to be unusually prominent.

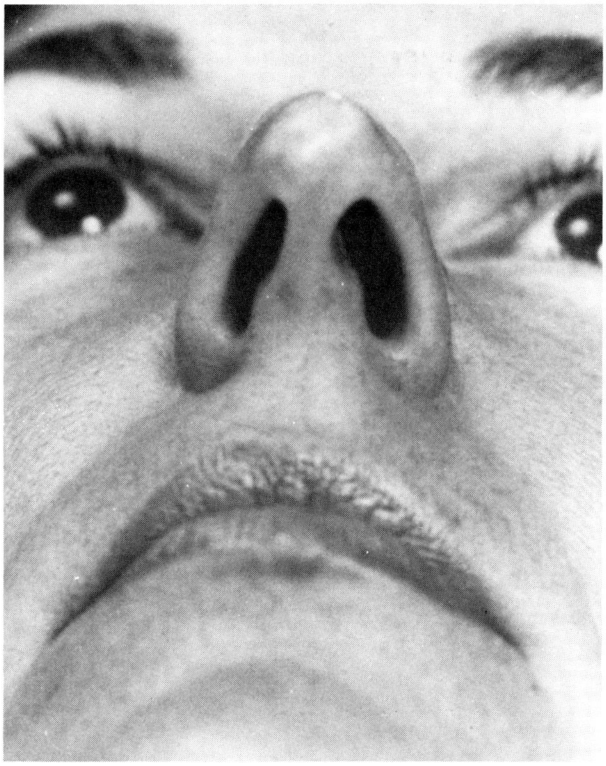

The basal configuration forms an isosceles triangle. The tip is narrow and overprojecting. The proximal two thirds of the columella is broad, causing some distortion of the nostrils. The right nostril is narrower than the left.

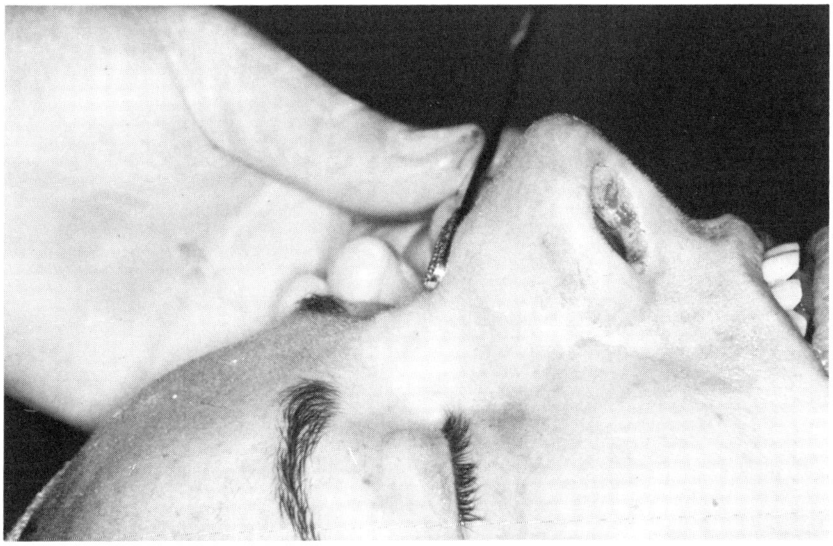

SURGICAL PROCEDURE

Following skeletonization, the bony dorsum is lowered with a Foman rasp. The rasp is shown at the junction of the lowered bony dorsum and the intact cartilaginous roof.

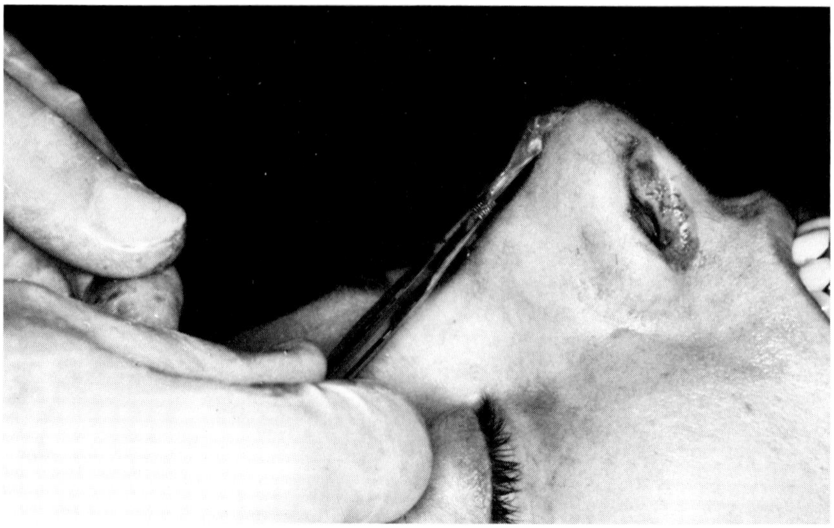

The roof of the upper cartilaginous vault is trimmed to the level of the bony vault. The resected roof is shown following its removal. The dorsal line is now well below the projecting tip.

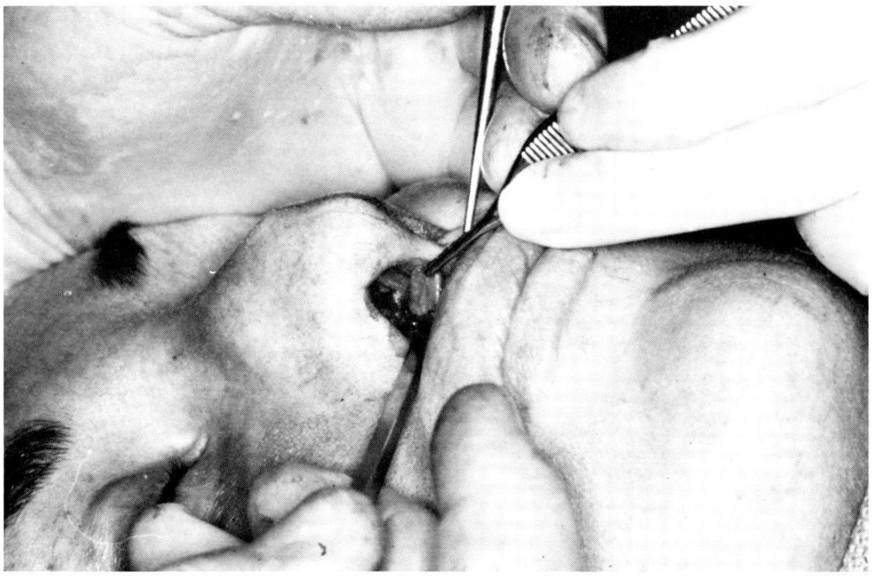

With the use of a 5-mm chisel, the nasal spine is reduced flush with the caudal septum and maxilla, producing a specimen of bone measuring 4 × 6 × 2 mm. This unusually large resection of nasal spine would normally cause lip retrusion. However, the bulk of tissues at the columellar base will provide adequate padding over the defect so that retrusion will not result. A segment of bone extending from the maxilla to the columella is resected as shown.

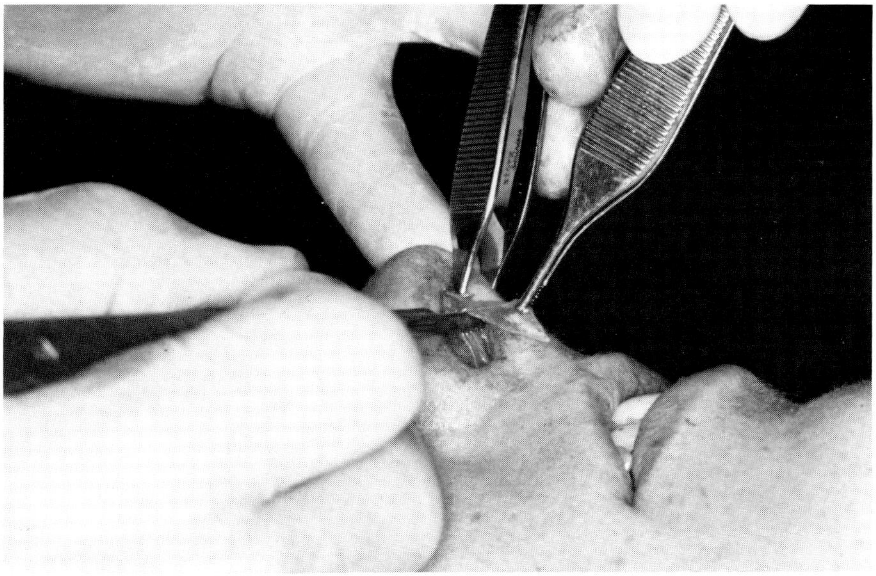

Because of the prominence of the caudal septum, a preliminary trim is done.

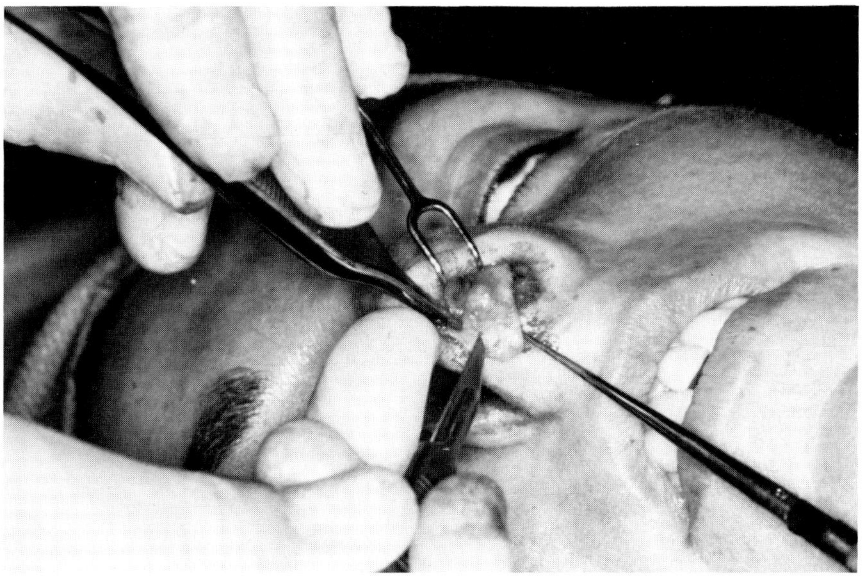

The lower lateral cartilage is exposed through a rim incision. The cartilage is found to be broad and substantial. The cephalic excess is trimmed, leaving behind a 6- to 7-mm wide lateral crus.

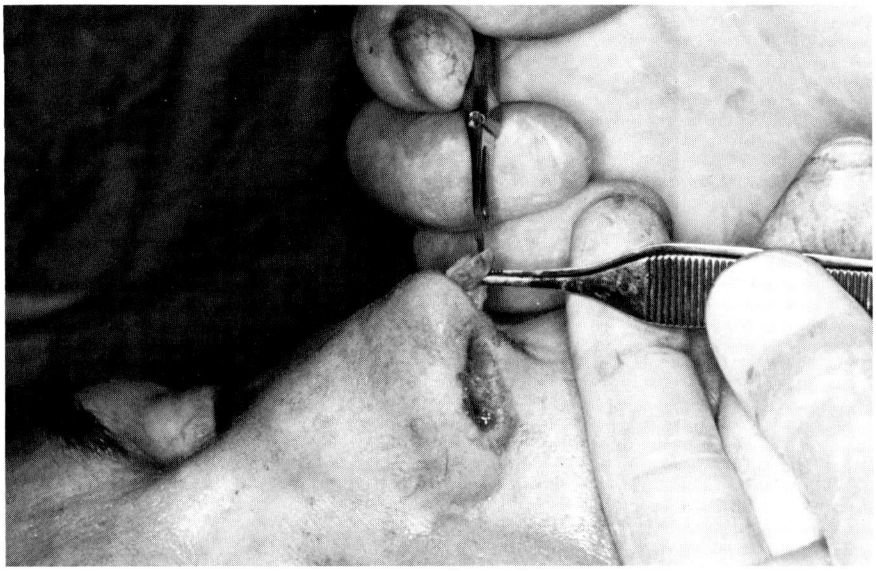

The highest point of the dome is marked mentally so that the central portion of the arch can be resected symmetrically. A 4-mm segment is excised.

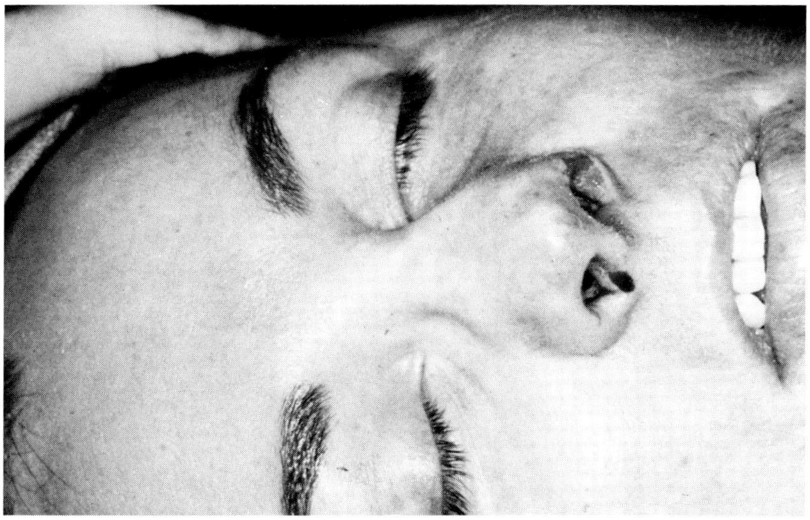

Following reduction of the dorsum, the breadth of the open roof is striking. Though the broad open roof has the ominous look of overreduction, I know that the height of the lateral nasal walls is sufficient to re-form the bony pyramid without difficulty.

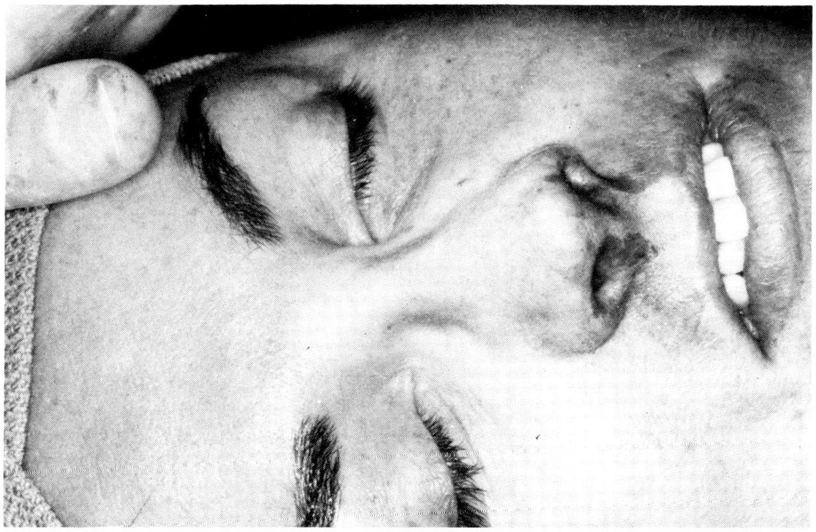

Following lateral osteotomies, slight digital pressure re-forms the pyramid without medial osteotomies.

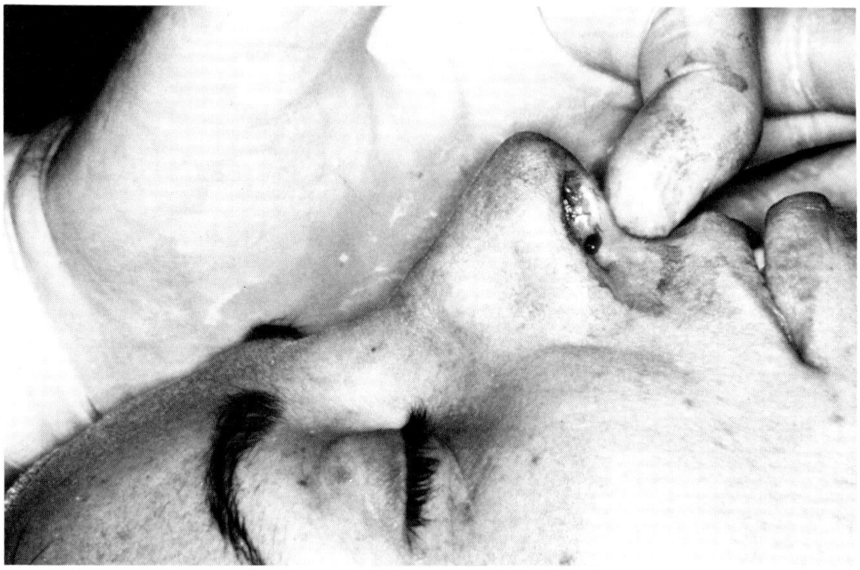

A final assessment is made. The slight fullness at the supratip indicates that the tissues will not contract to a smaller skeleton. Further reduction of the skeleton would likely result in a loss of definition.

Summary of surgical procedure

1. Wide skeletonization over the cartilaginous vault, modest skeletonization over the bony vault
2. Transfixion incision to the nasal spine
3. Trim of the caudal septum and the nasal spine
4. Reduction of the bony dorsum with a Foman rasp
5. Reduction of the roof of the upper cartilaginous vault
6. Delivery of the lower lateral cartilages through rim incisions
7. Trim of the cephalic part, with resection of 4 mm from the domes
8. Lateral osteotomies

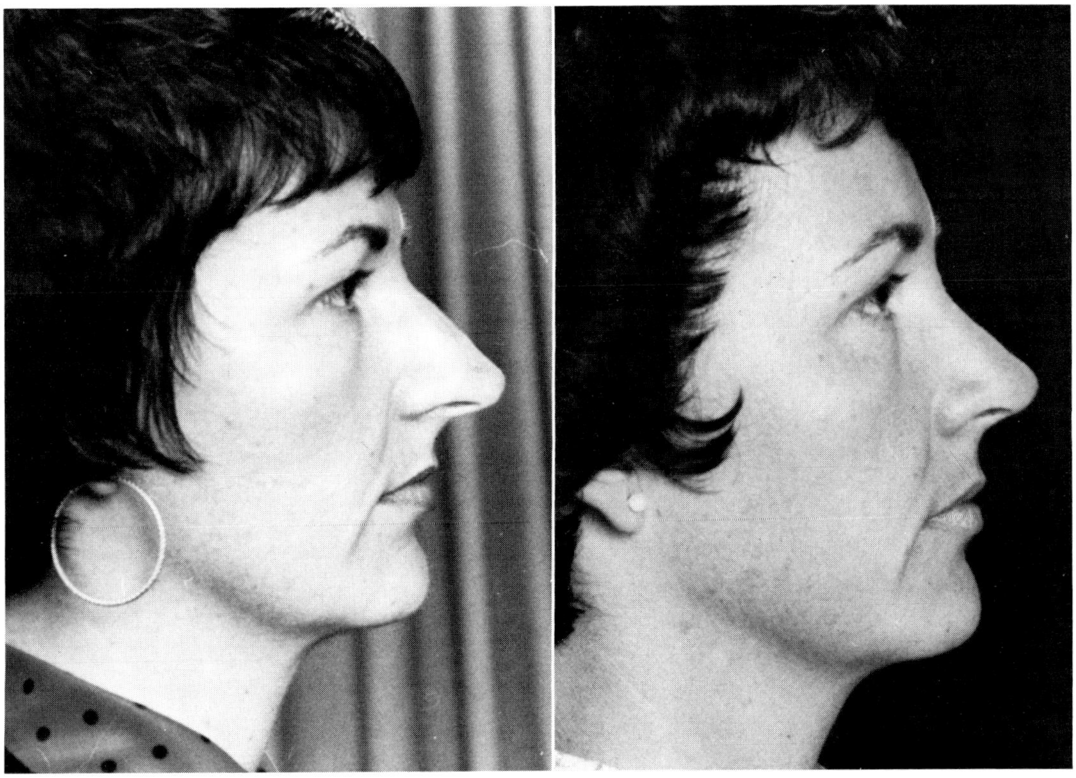

POSTOPERATIVE RESULTS

Postoperatively, there is a reduction in the projection of the middle third of the face although there is little discernible change in the identity of the nose. However, on critical examination, there is an obvious decrease in the height of the dorsum, a reduction in the projection of the nasal tip, and slight retrusion of the upper lip, which is well camouflaged by the fullness at the subnasion. Reduction of the nasal spine is an important step in the overall diminution of this nasal silhouette.

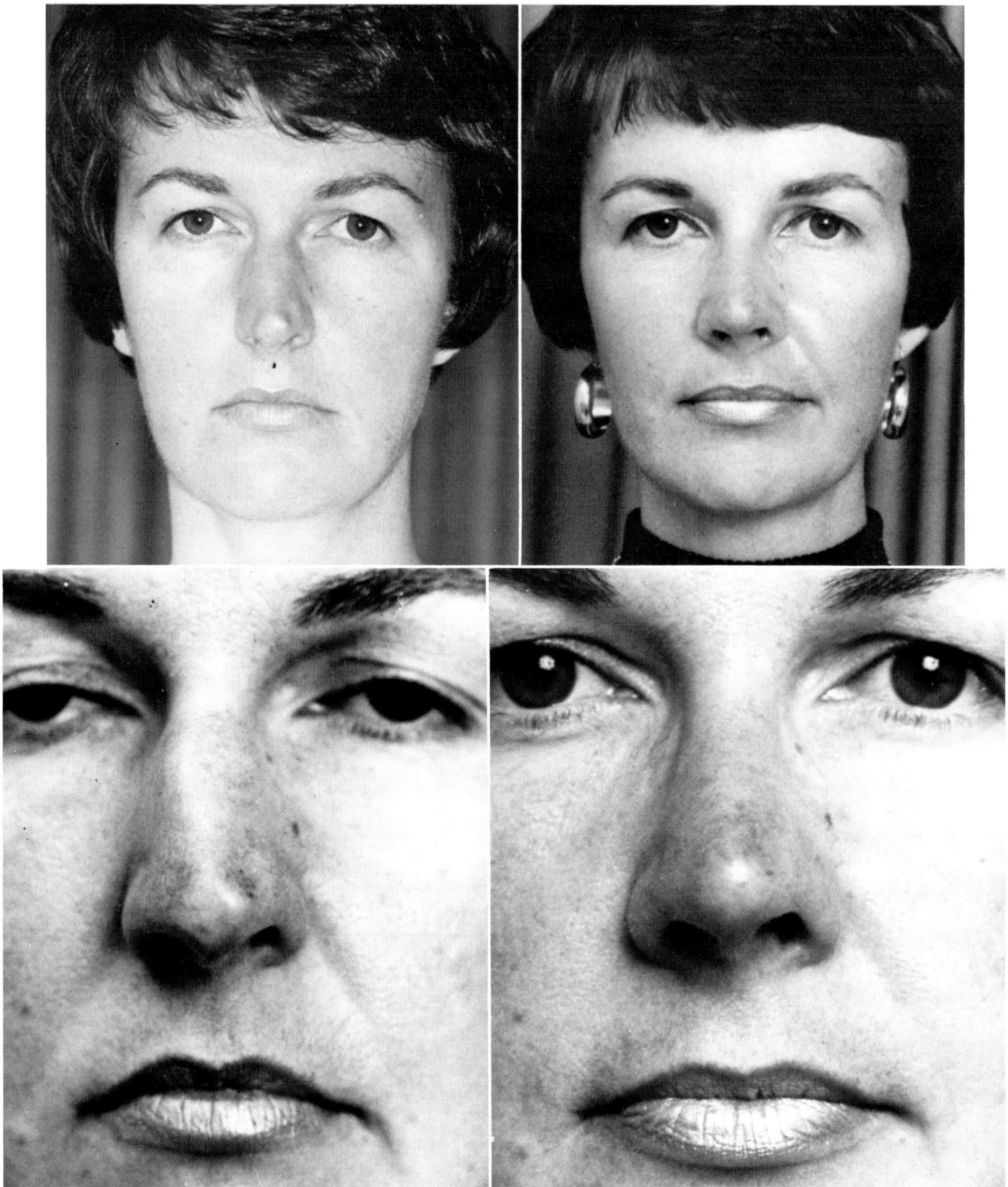

On front view, the nose appears shorter, and the nostrils are slightly more visible. The higher nostril on the left remains unchanged postoperatively. The nasal pyramid flows in smooth uninterrupted lines from the radix to the nasal base. The crooked appearance caused by the right dorsal irregularity of the bony vault has been corrected by a 2-mm reduction of the bony dorsum.

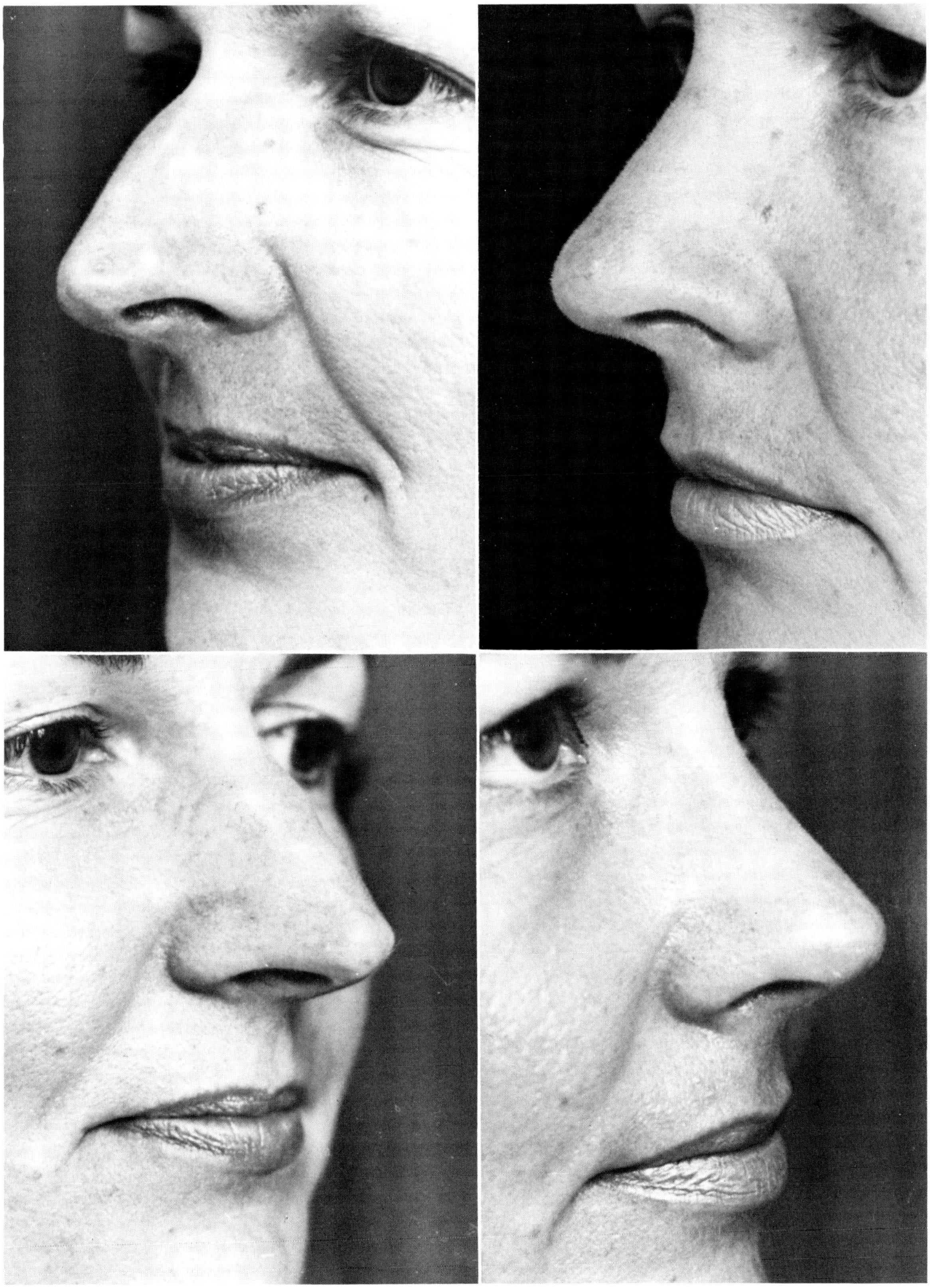

Postoperatively, the right and left oblique views are almost identical following correction of the dorsal irregularity. Though the nose remains large, the unusual characteristics that would designate it as ultraprojecting have been removed.

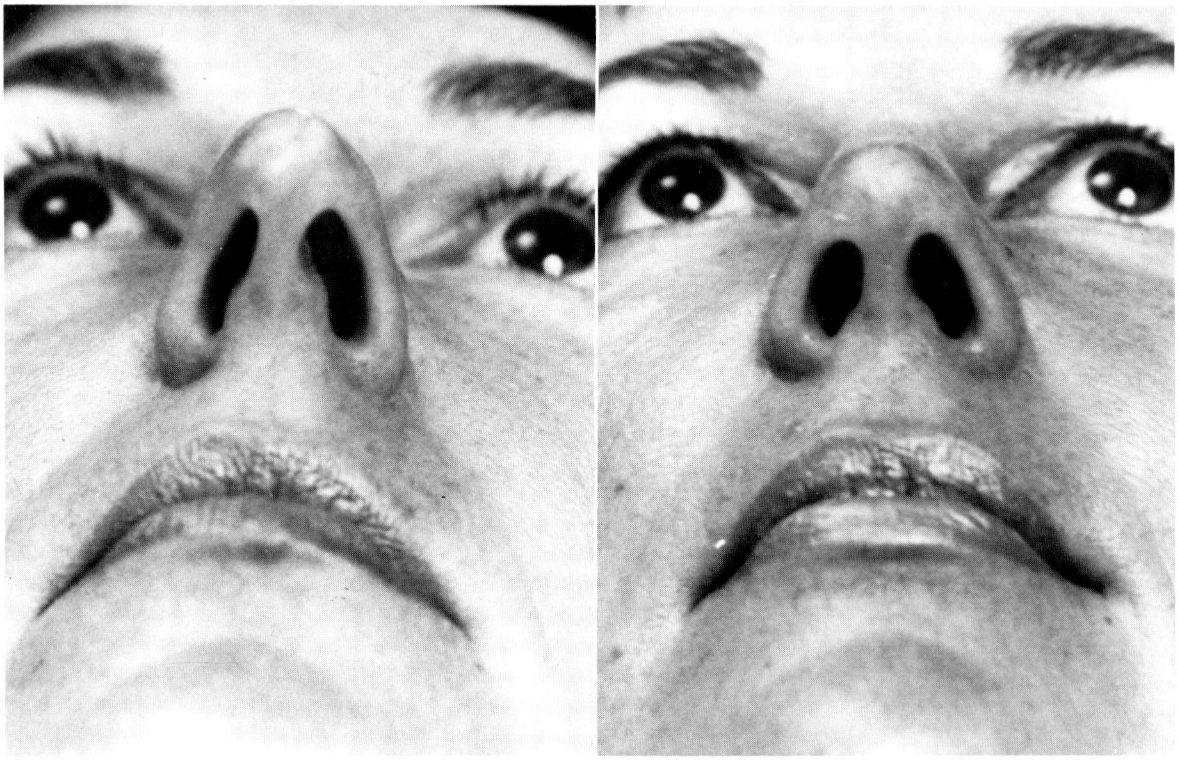

On basal view, the isosceles triangle has been changed to an equilateral one. The nostrils are slightly shorter and wider and are well supported by the 6- to 7-mm wide lateral crura.

Following partial resection of the nasal spine and caudal septum, there is less distortion at the base of the columella.

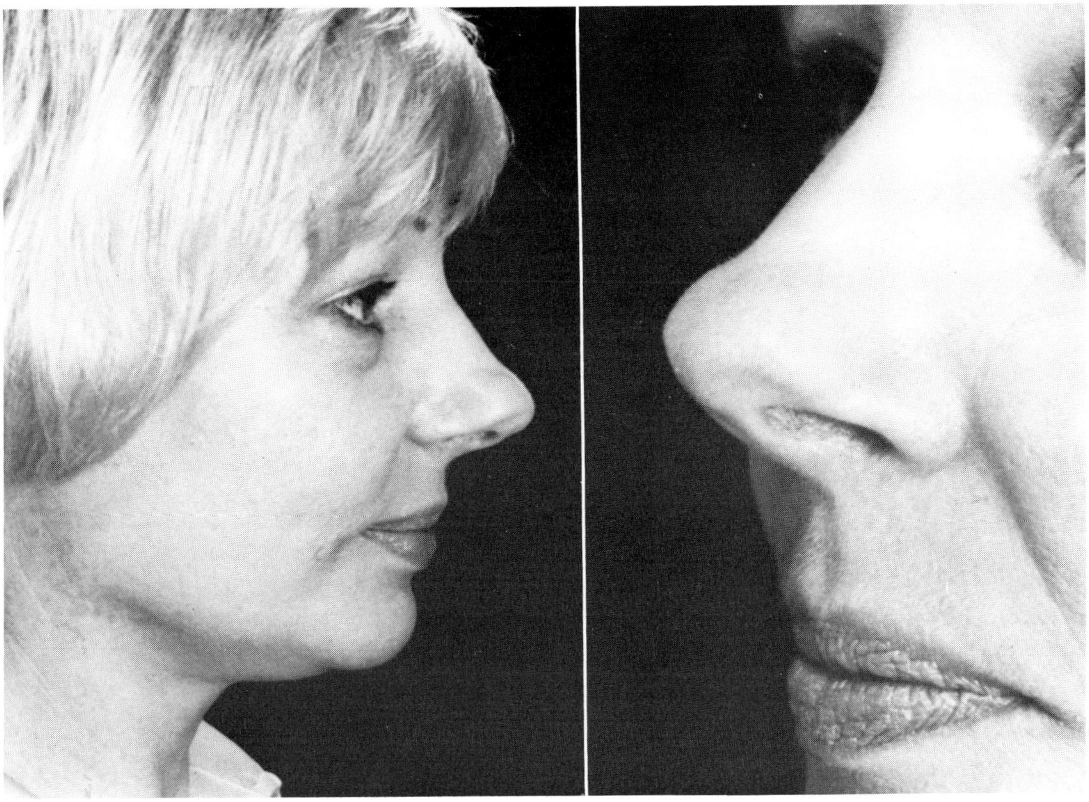

Case report 2

The lateral view of this patient displays a large, ultraprojecting but well-contoured nose.

On close-up oblique view, the massive basal configuration is evident. The facet over the soft triangle is exaggerated because of hypertrophy of the lateral crus of the lower lateral cartilage. The bony pyramid and upper cartilaginous vaults are in excellent alignment with each other.

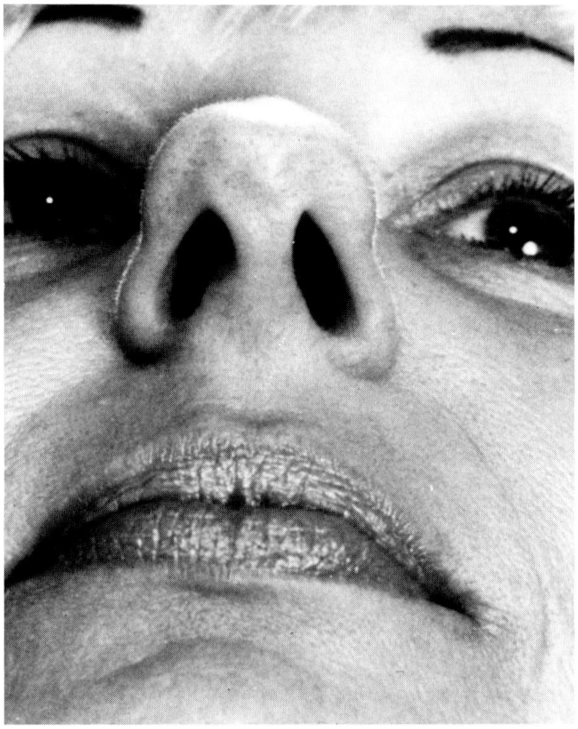

The basal perimeter is almost square. The columellar-alar complex is overwhelmed by the large nasal tip.

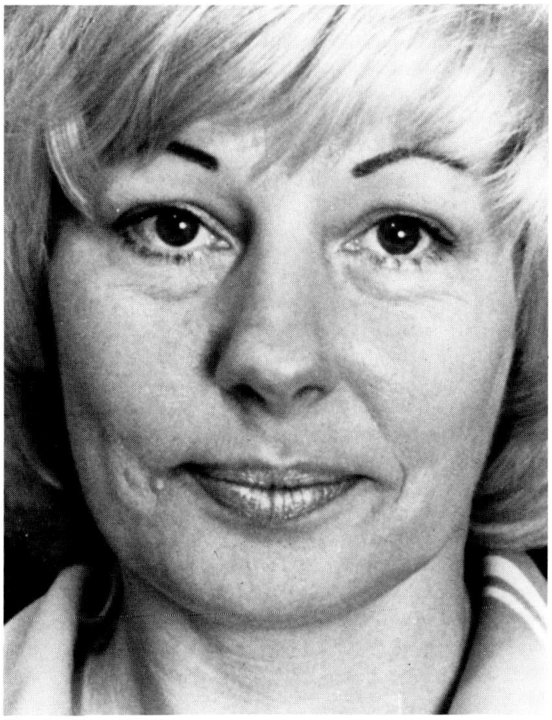

On front view, the nose does not appear inordinately large. Its length is in proportion to the face. Though the nose is slightly broad, it has nice lateral contours.

Summary of surgical procedure

1. Limited skeletonization over the bony and cartilaginous vaults
2. Transfixion incision to the base of the nasal spine
3. Conservative reduction of the nasal spine
4. Trim of the posterior two thirds of the caudal septum
5. Delivery of the lower lateral cartilages through rim incisions
6. Trim of the cephalic excess (leaving 5- to 6-mm wide lateral crura) and resection of 3 to 4 mm from each dome
7. Resection of 1 to 2 mm of medial crura
8. Bony dorsum reduced approximately 2 mm
9. Slight reduction of the cartilaginous dorsum
10. Lateral osteotomies

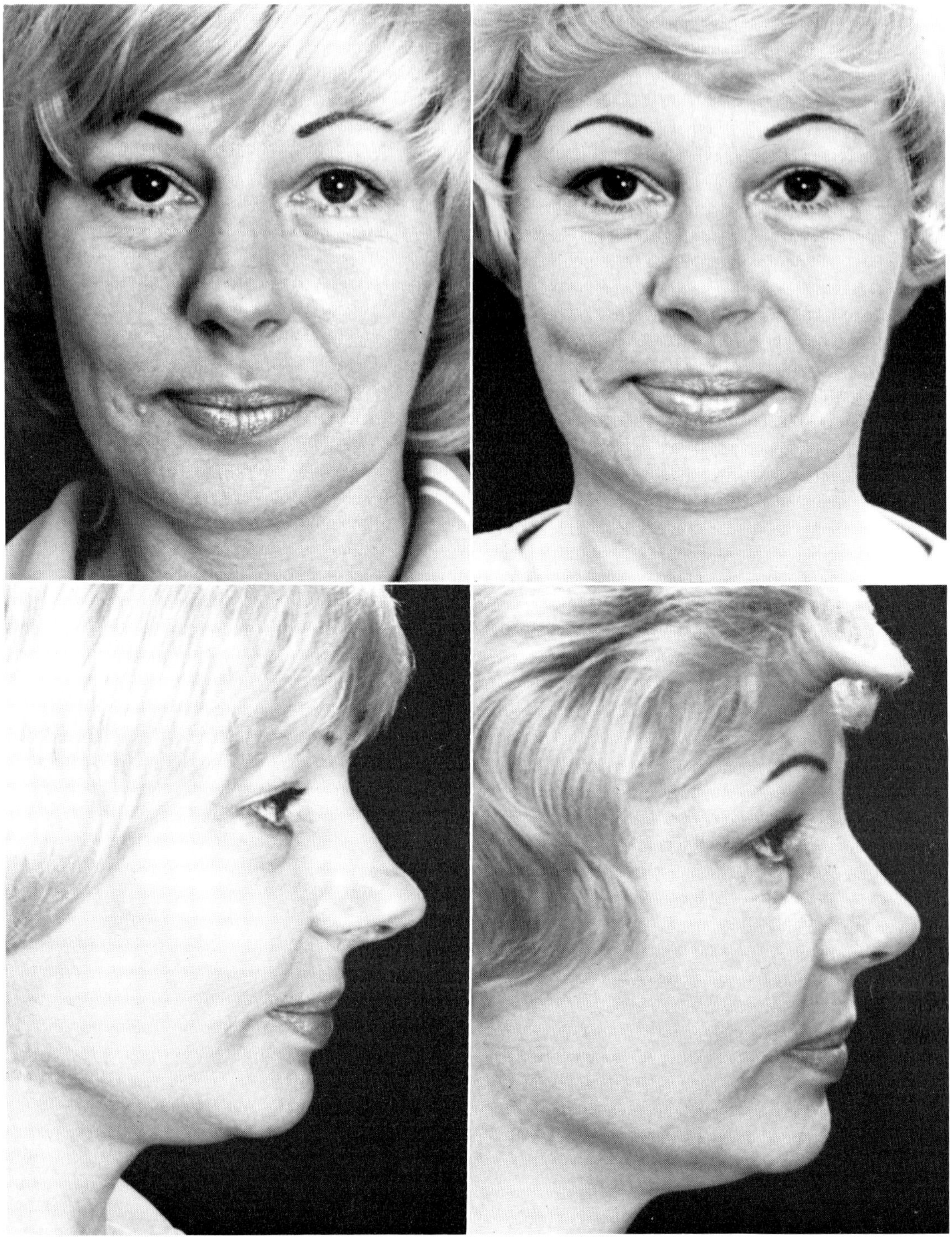

POSTOPERATIVE RESULTS

Postoperatively, there is virtually no change in the appearance of her nose viewed from the front. It is slightly narrower, and the tip is more refined. Laterally, the nose is still large, but the tip is less projecting. The dorsum is slightly lower. The nasal spine has been reduced, improving the columellar-alar relationship.

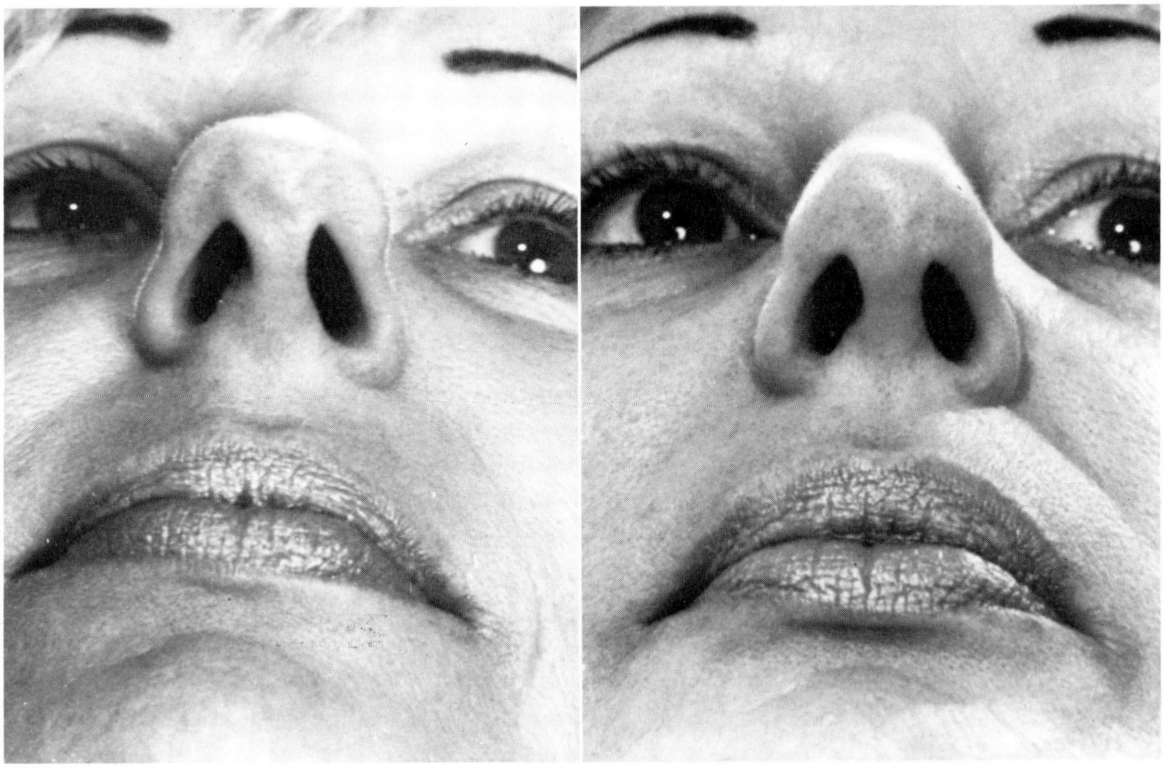

Postoperatively, the width of the nasal tip is decreased following a cephalic resection of the lower lateral cartilages, with a central, 4-mm resection of the arches of the domes. The tip has been reduced to its tissue limits without sacrificing aesthetic definition.

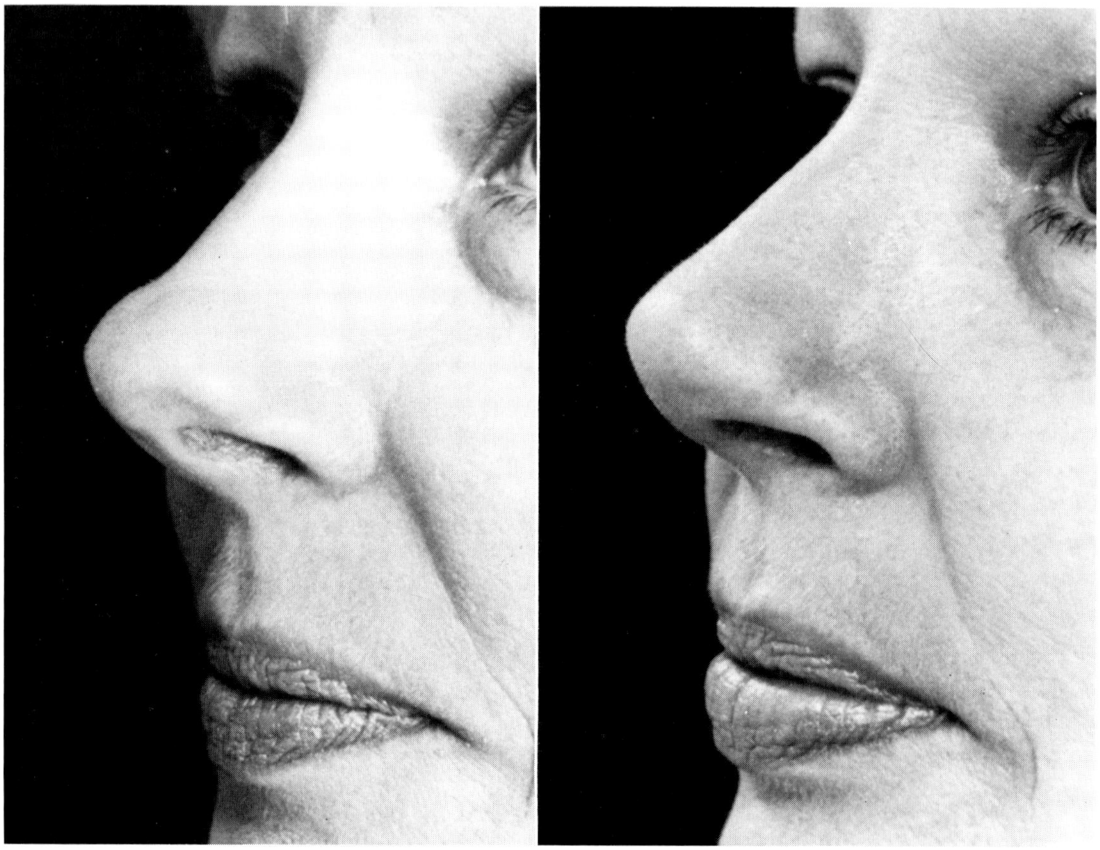

Because the lower lateral cartilages were not overresected, enough tip projection remains to provide a definite end point to the nasal contour on oblique view. The facet over the soft triangle has been softened, and the nostril appears shorter. The relationship of the tip to the columellar-alar complex has been improved.

Tissues become thicker as they contract to a reduced skeleton. If controlled, this can work in the surgeon's favor by hiding the edges of the transected medial and lateral crura.

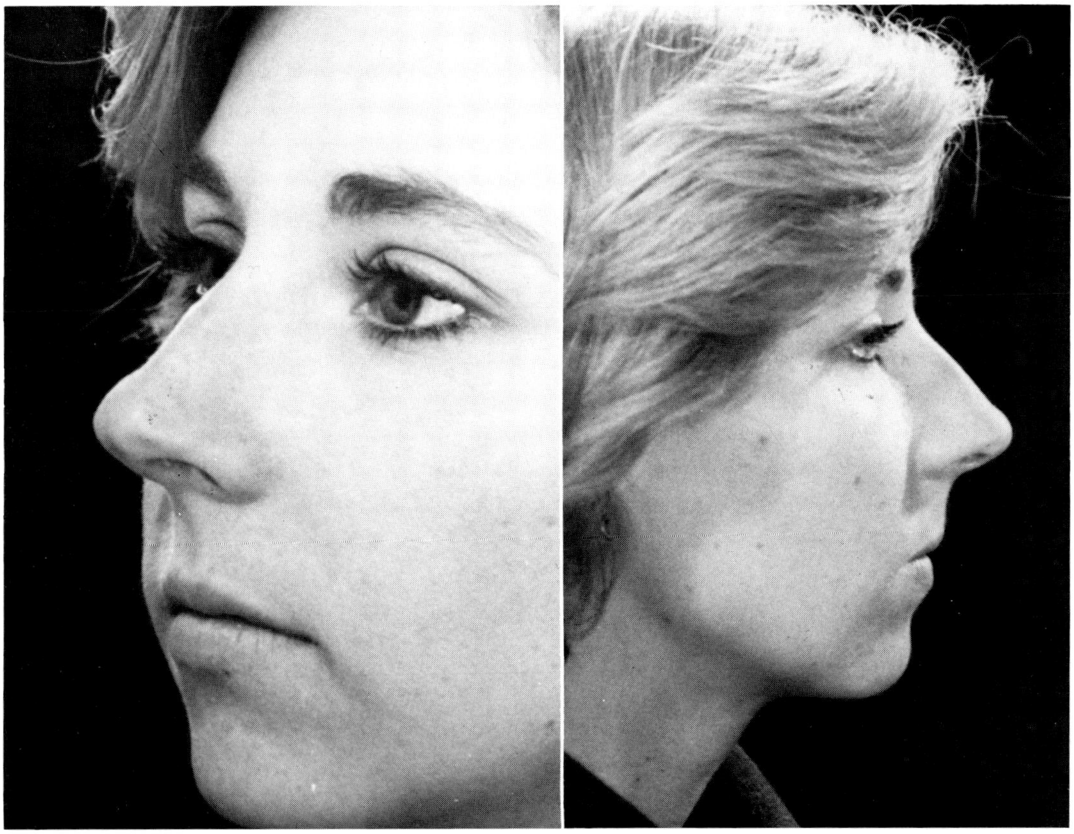

Case report 3

This patient requested a "softening" of the appearance of her nose, without identifiable change.

The overprojecting central third of her face is emphasized by a slightly retrusive chin. The nasal base is elevated from the face by the protrusion of the nasal spine and caudal septum. Although there is a slight dorsal hump, all parts of the nose are in good relation to each other. The tissues are well structured.

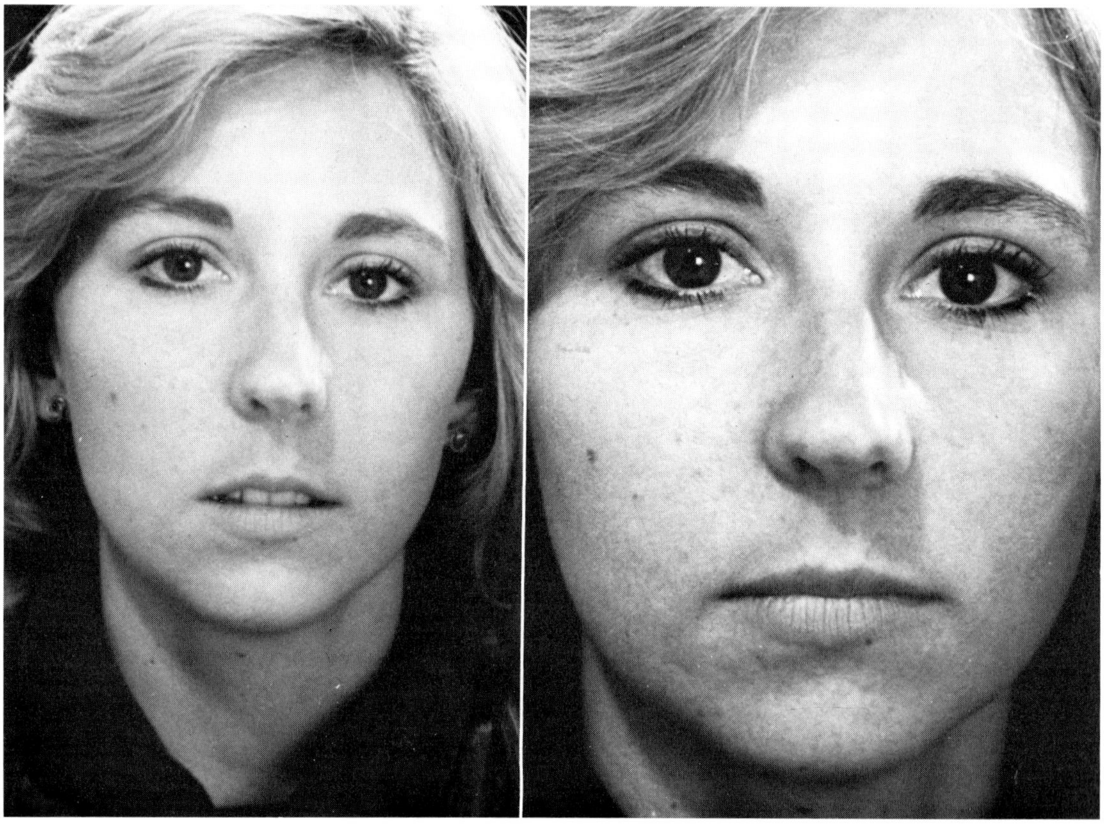

On front view, the size and shape of the nose are excellent except for a concavity on her right and a convexity on her left, giving the nose a crooked appearance.

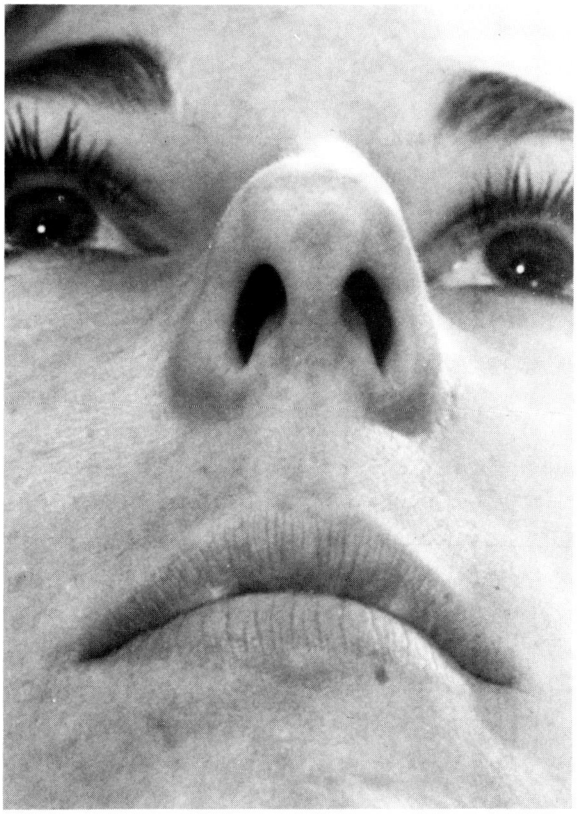

On basal view, the nose appears to be pushed away from the maxilla by the prominent nasal spine. The narrow nasal base is inconsonant with the overprojection of the nasal tip.

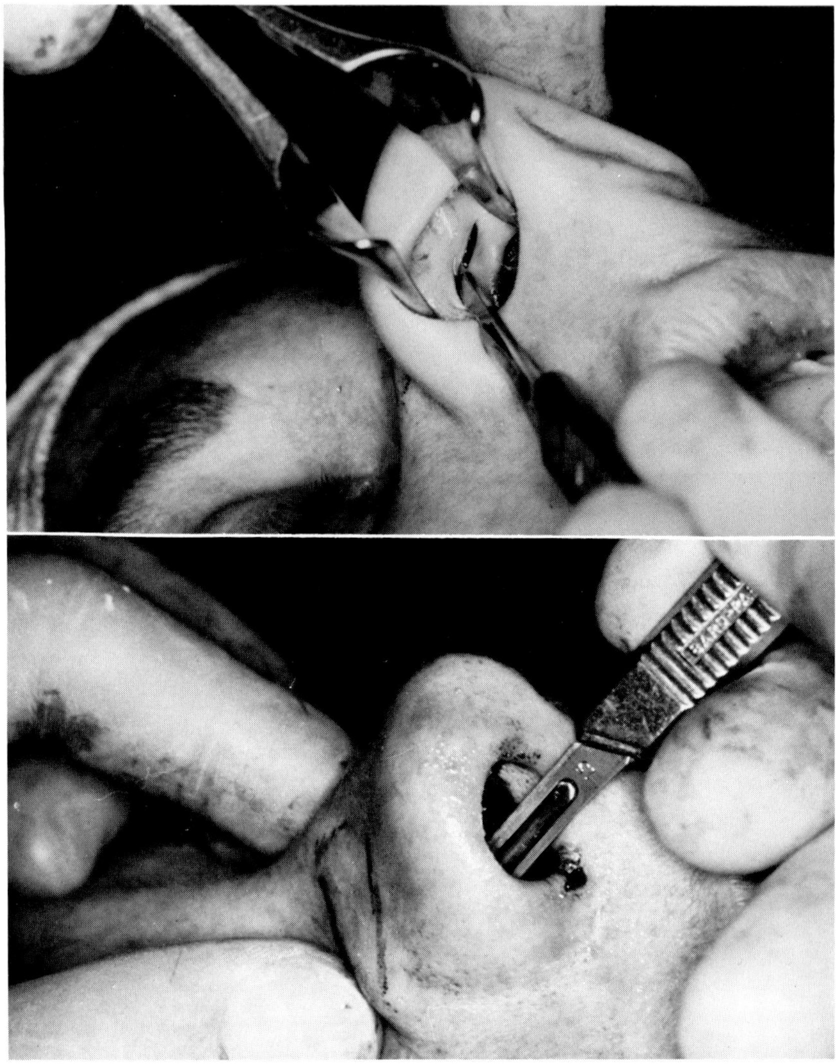

SURGICAL PROCEDURE

The usual intercartilaginous incision is made, but it is carried to the base of the pyriform aperture to allow as much redrape of the soft tissues as possible and to provide a pocket for grafting over the concavity on that side.

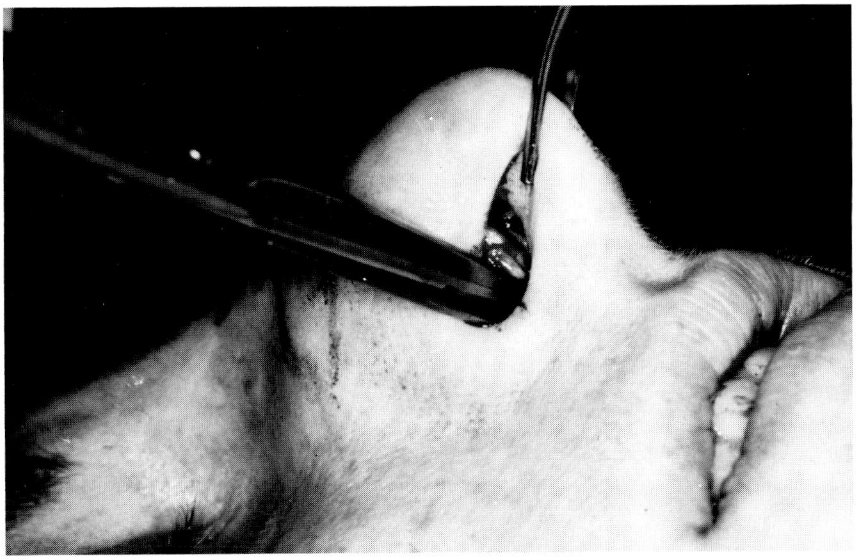

The membranous septum is incised with a Mayo scissors to the nasal spine in preparation for reducing the nasal spine and caudal septum.

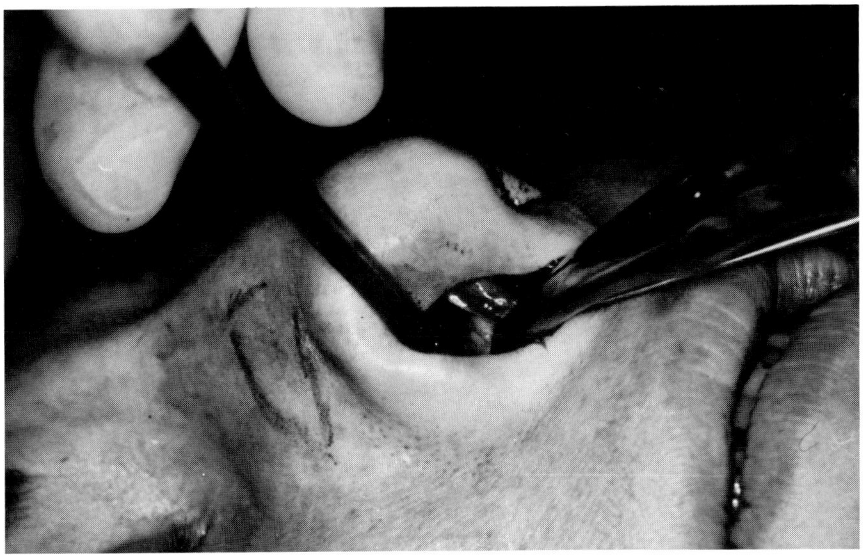

After the soft tissues are cleared away with a Joseph periosteal elevator, the nasal spine is reduced using a double-action rongeur.

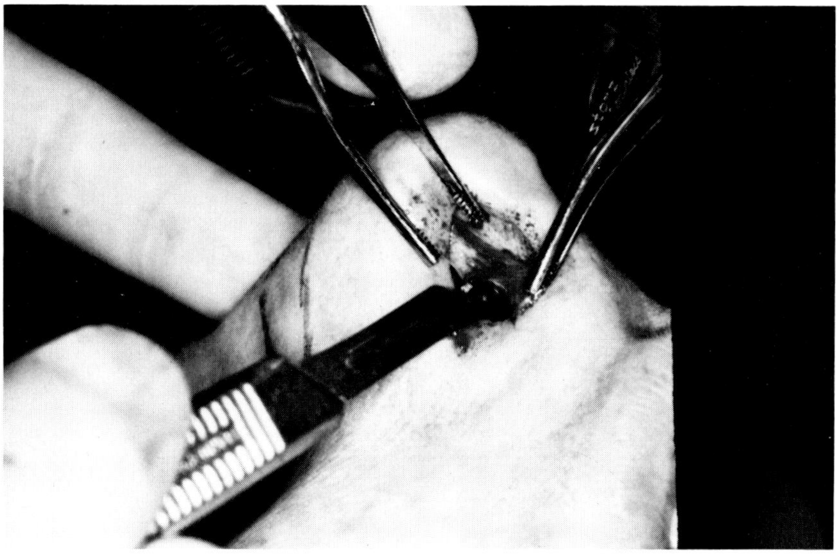

Approximately 4 mm of caudal septum is resected.

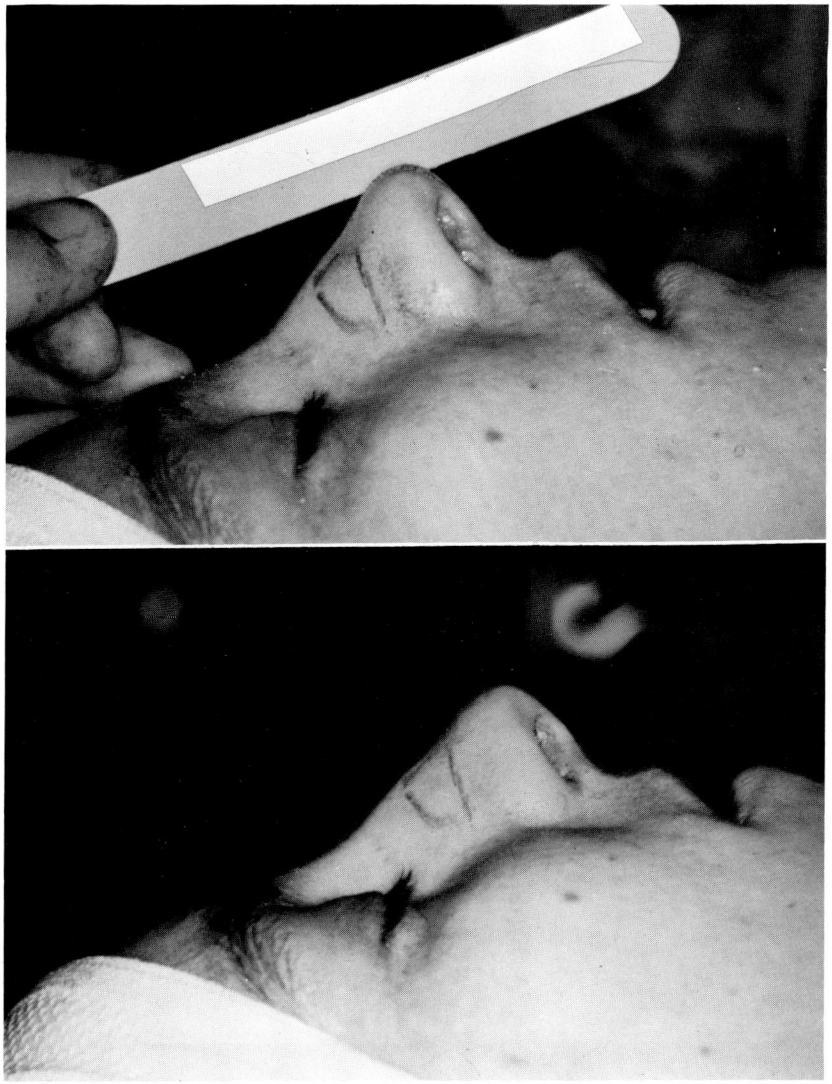

The effect of the nasal spine and caudal septum on the elevation of the tip can be seen in the comparative photographs of the patient before surgery and after partial resection of the caudal septum and nasal spine. There has been no other reduction of skeletal parts. The tip is now in line with the dorsum. At this point a judgment is made about the amount of dorsum to be reduced.

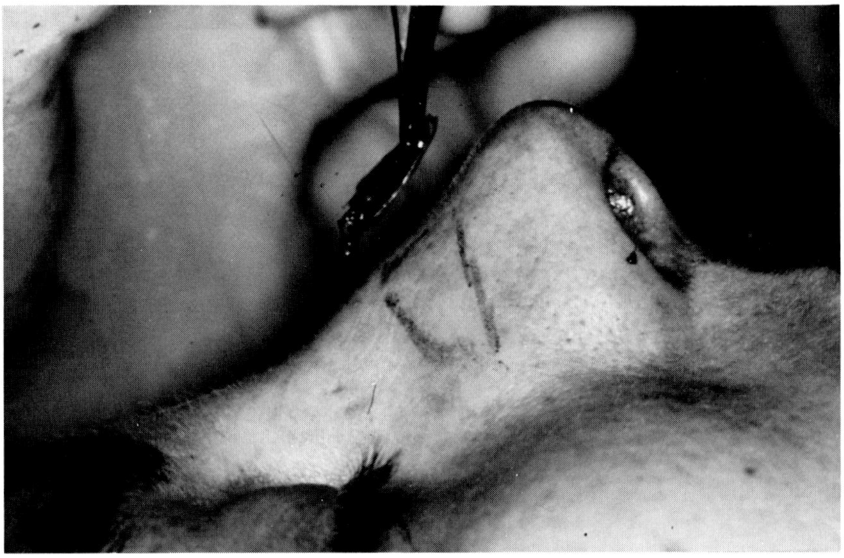

Following conservative reduction of the bony dorsum with a rasp, a portion of cartilaginous dorsum is resected.

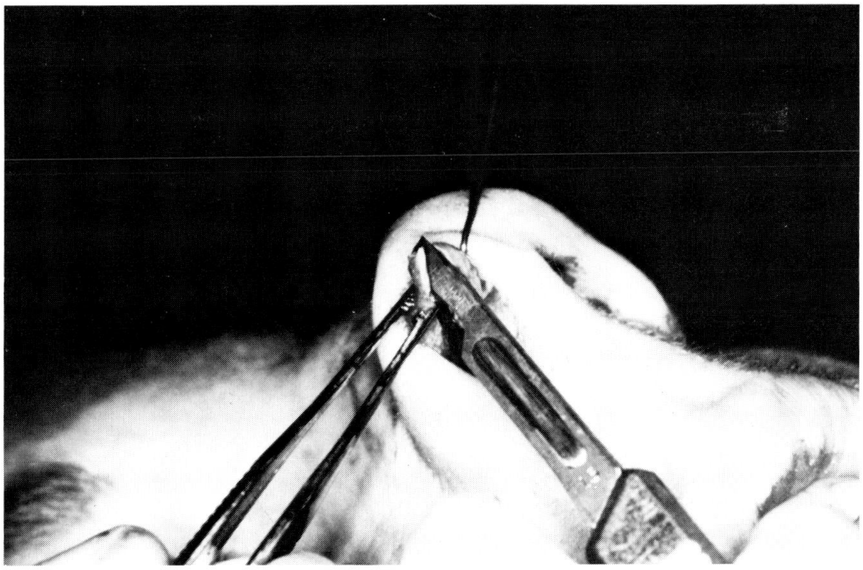

Tip reduction is accomplished by a 4-mm resection of the domes of the lower lateral cartilages. The first incision is made 2 mm medial to the central point of the dome.

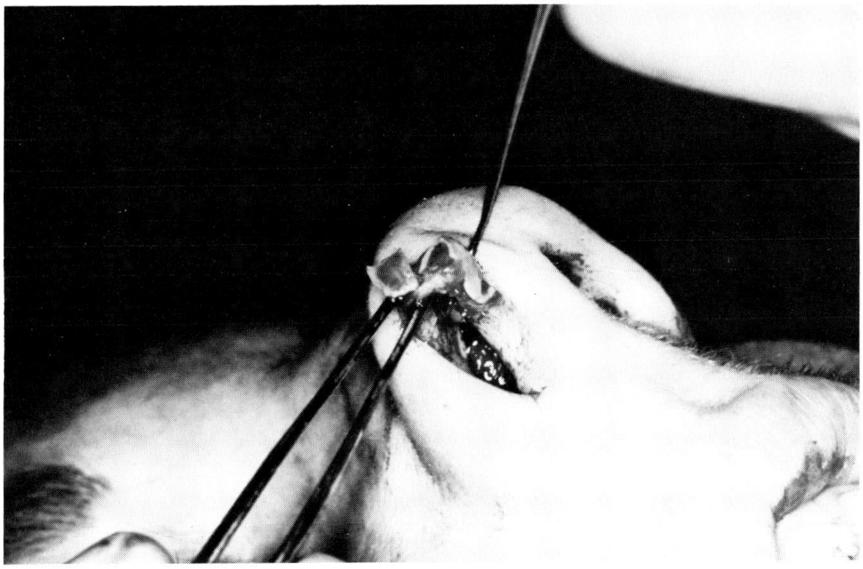

The second incision is made 2 mm lateral to the central point of the dome. The resulting sharp edges are carefully trimmed.

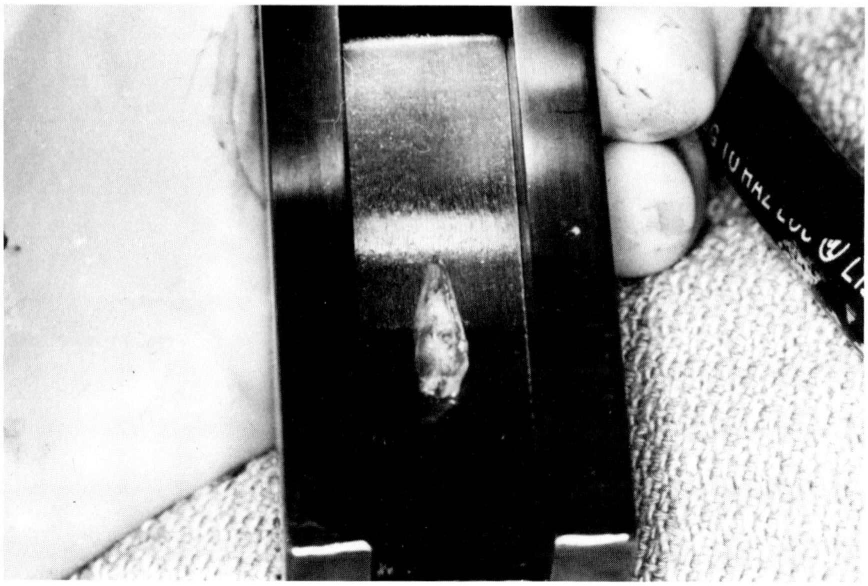

A small piece of cartilage is placed in the cartilage crusher.

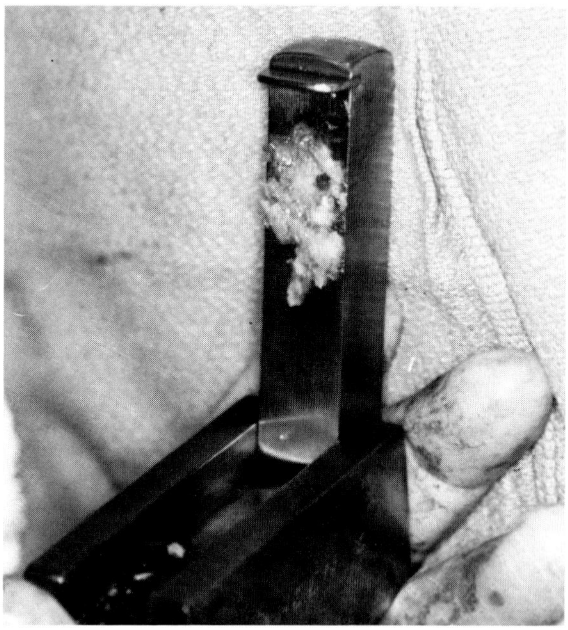

A light blow with a mallet renders a flat piece of cartilage for lateral wall augmentation.

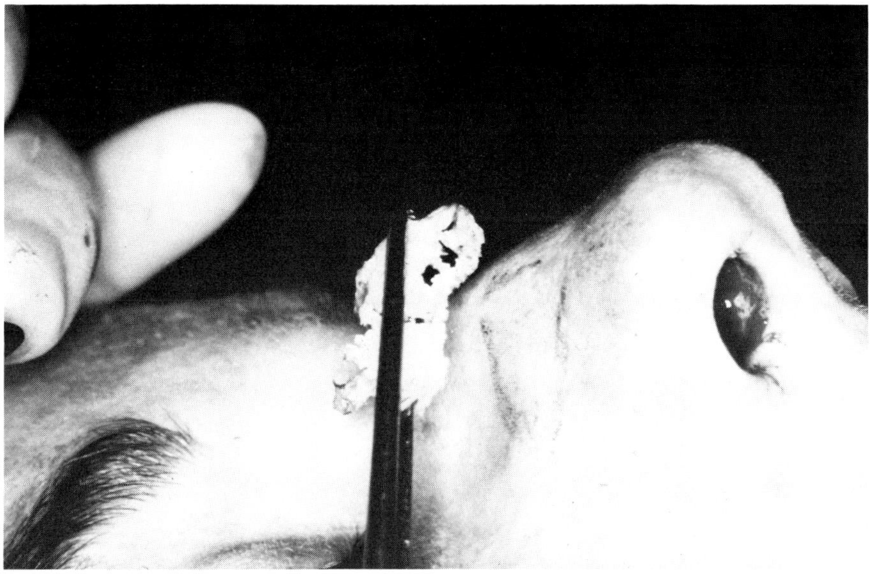

The graft is prepared for insertion over the right upper lateral cartilage.

Summary of surgical procedure

1. Wide skeletonization of the upper vault, limited skeletonization over the bony vault
2. Transfixion incision to the base of the nasal spine
3. Reduction of the nasal spine and caudal septum
4. Reduction of the bony roof
5. Reduction of the cartilaginous roof
6. Delivery of the tip cartilages through rim incisions
7. Cephalic trim and resection of 4 mm from the domes
8. Septoplasty for graft material
9. Onlay graft over the right upper lateral cartilage
10. Lateral osteotomies
11. Mentoplasty

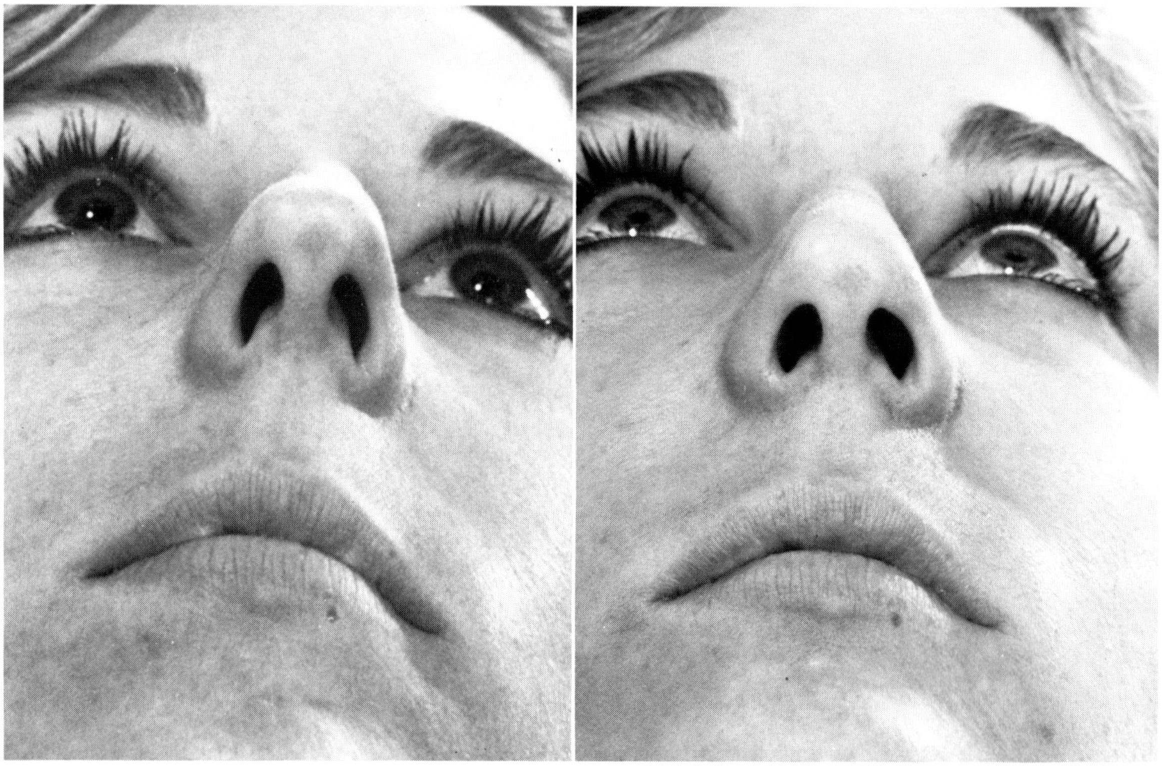

POSTOPERATIVE RESULTS

Postoperatively, there is a reduction of tip projection, with a more triangular basal configuration. The nostrils are shorter and broader as a result of the reduced projection of the tip.

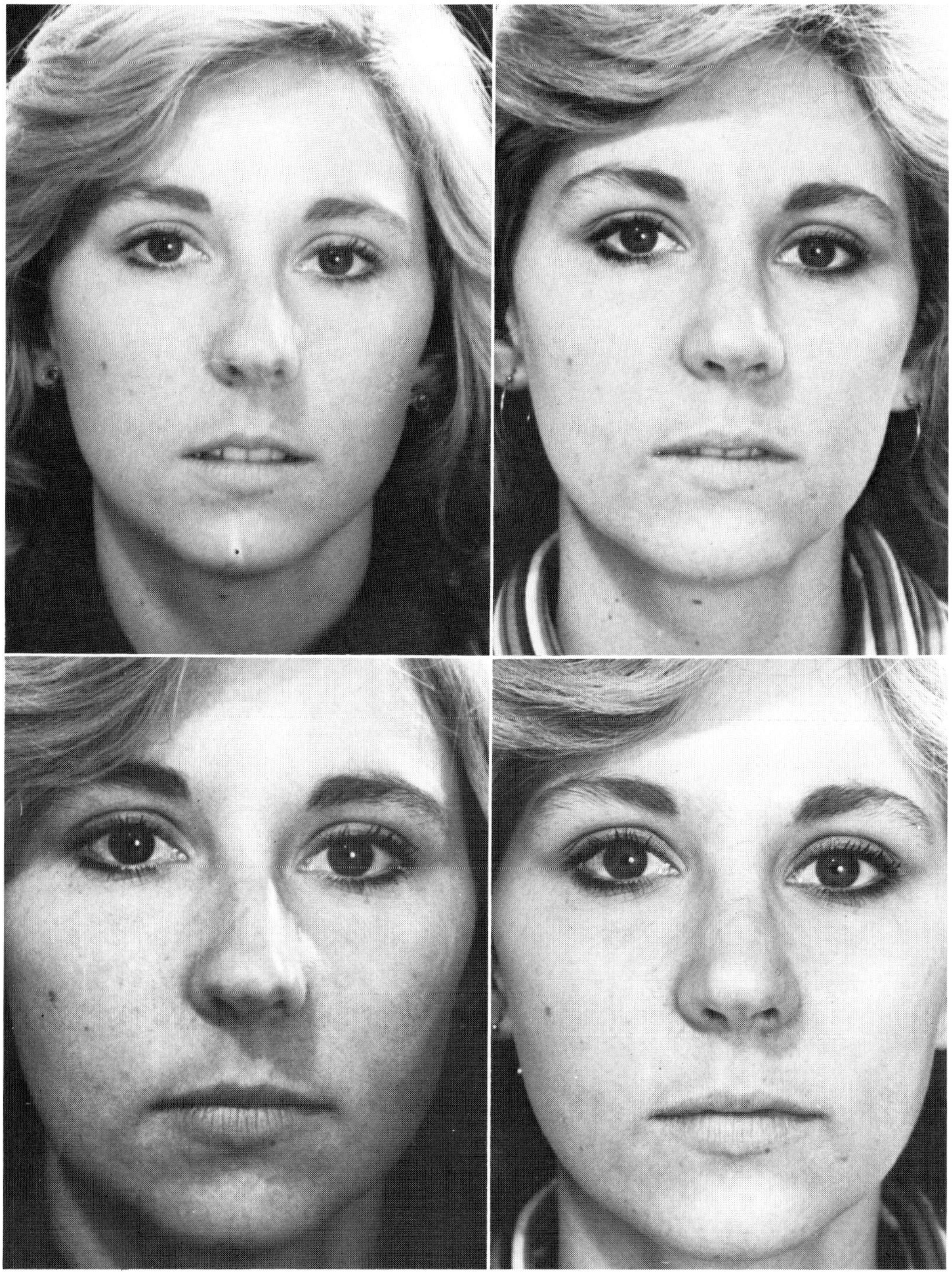

The curved appearance of the nose preoperatively has been corrected with the crushed cartilage graft over the upper lateral cartilage on her right.

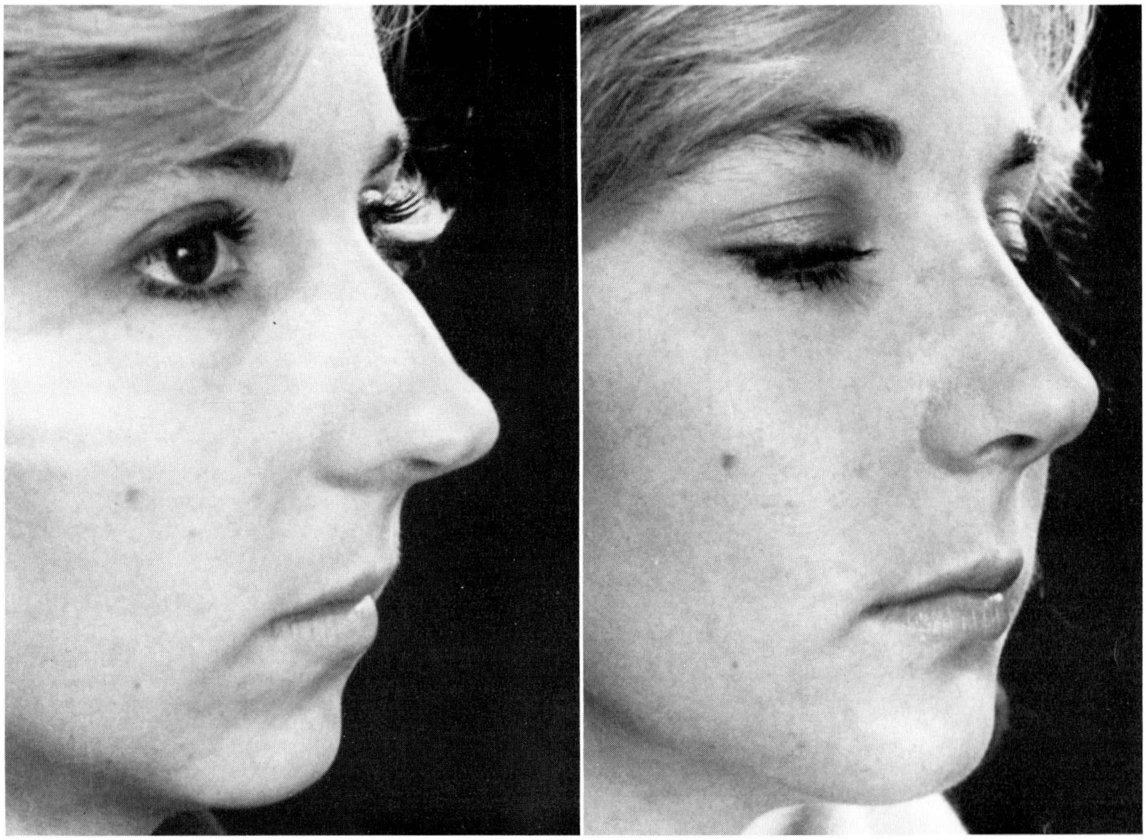

On oblique view, the preoperative dominance of the central third of her face has been modified by the decrease in nasal projection and by chin augmentation. The preoperative tip refinement has been retained in spite of the 4-mm reduction of the arches of the lower lateral cartilages.

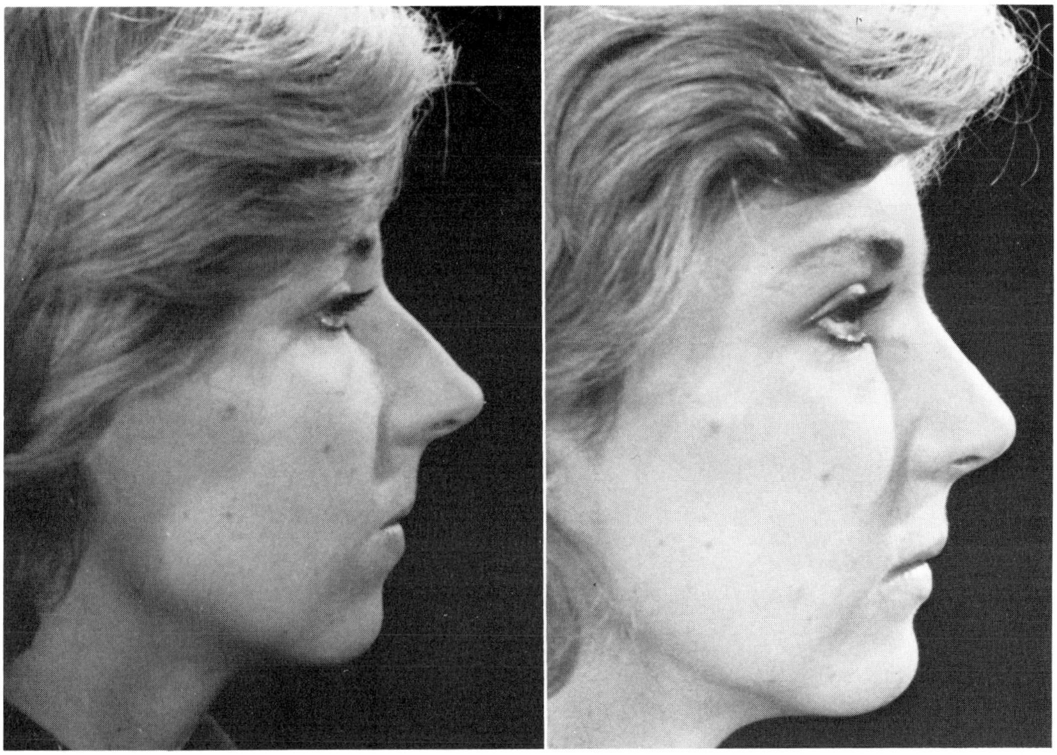

Reduction of the nasal spine has deepened the nasolabial angle and has produced a fuller, more attractive upper lip. The general appearance of her face is softer and better balanced. The tip no longer appears ultraprojecting, even though the surgical result is subtle.

MALPOSITION OF THE LOWER LATERAL CARTILAGES

Throughout the past I have been confounded by the occasional case when the nasal tip was not amenable to the usual contouring techniques. In these cases, in spite of normal columellar length and sufficient size and substance of the lower lateral cartilages, adequate tip projection and refinement could not be achieved. When it became apparent that the position of the cartilage might be responsible, these troublesome cases were reviewed, and interestingly, similarities were found—all were related to a malposition of the lower lateral cartilages. Since then I have recognized many cases of malposition, but only the more extreme cases have required special treatment. Relocation of the lateral crura or the placement of grafts into the alar walls has been the most effective means of treatment.

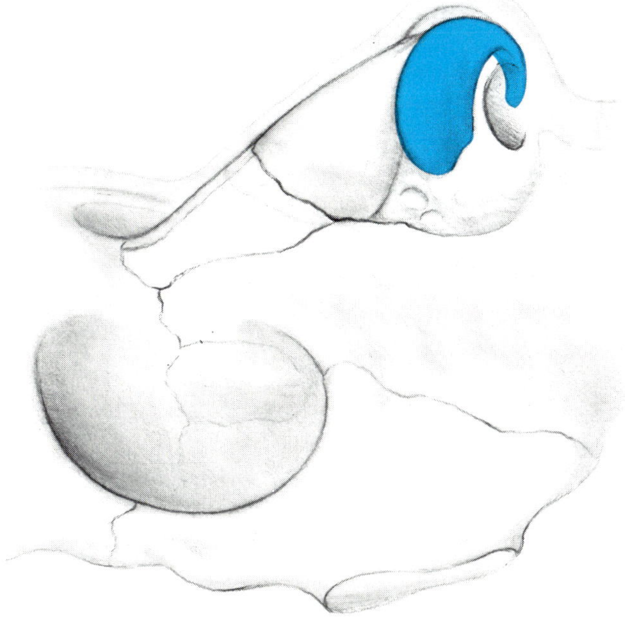

The normal relationship of lateral crus to alar rim

Since there are many variations in the position and contour of the lower lateral cartilages, it would be incorrect to state that there is a normal position or contour. However, most often the caudal edge of the lateral crus is parallel to the alar rim for half the length of the nostril. This position provides the lateral footing necessary to maintain tip projection when the lower lateral cartilages are rotated cephalad, visor fashion, during rhinoplasty.

Malposition of the lower lateral cartilages is defined as any displacement of the lateral crura from the usual parallel alignment with the nostril rims. This displacement is clinically significant when there is inadequate footing for support of the lateral crura.

Characteristic of the nose with malposition of the lower lateral cartilages is the combination of the following traits:

1. Vertical grooves forming a pair of parentheses around the tip, giving it a round appearance
2. Notches in the alar rims
3. Broad and flat nasal tip
4. Square basal perimeter

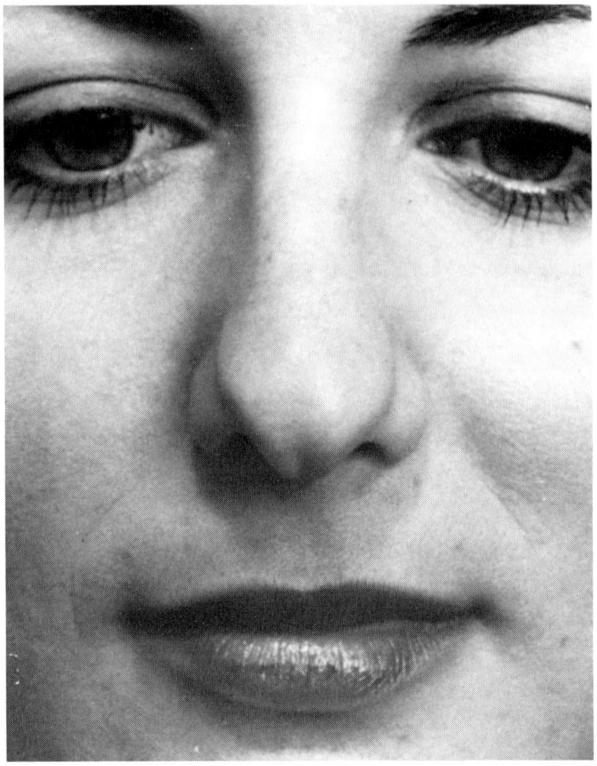

The parentheses around the tip are manifestations of the caudal borders of the lateral crura.

Notches in the alar rims are caused by lack of support to the lateral portions of the nostrils. Depending on the thickness of the skin, the position of the caudal borders of the crura is more or less visible.

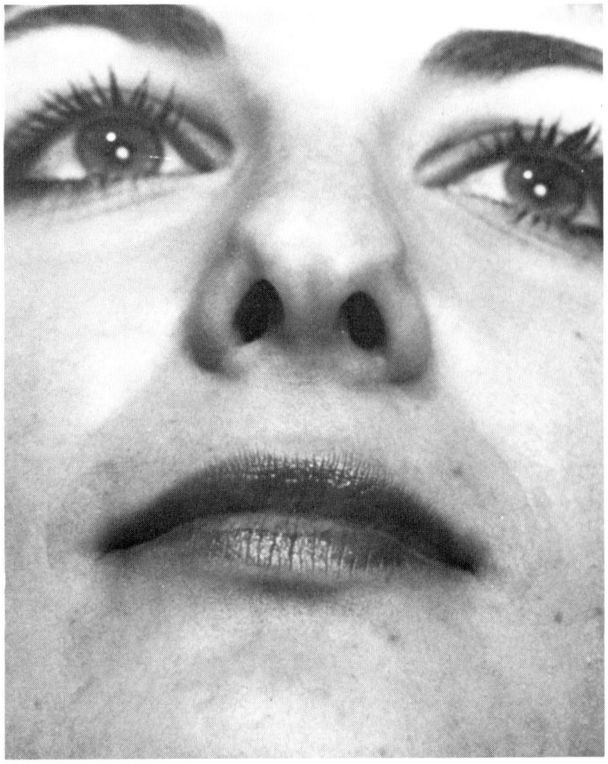

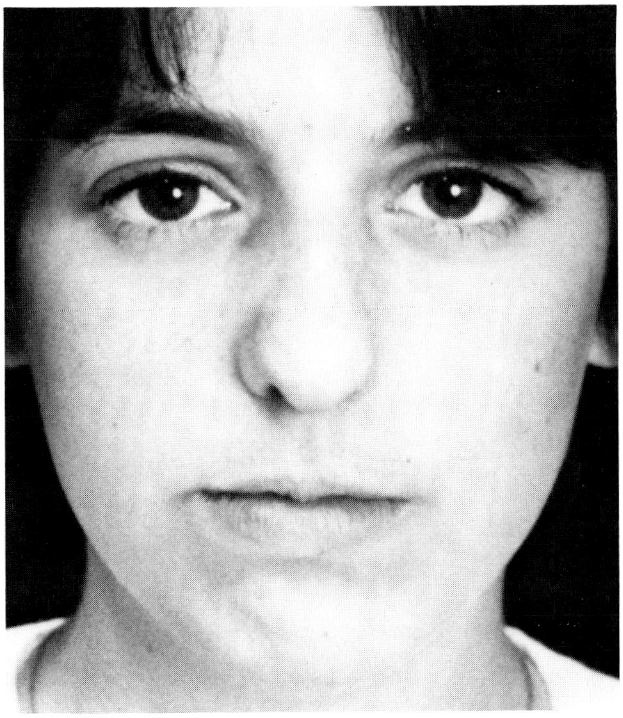

Placement of the lateral crura superiorly produces a large anterior mass of cartilage and decreases the projection of the domes. This results in a nasal tip that is broad and flat.

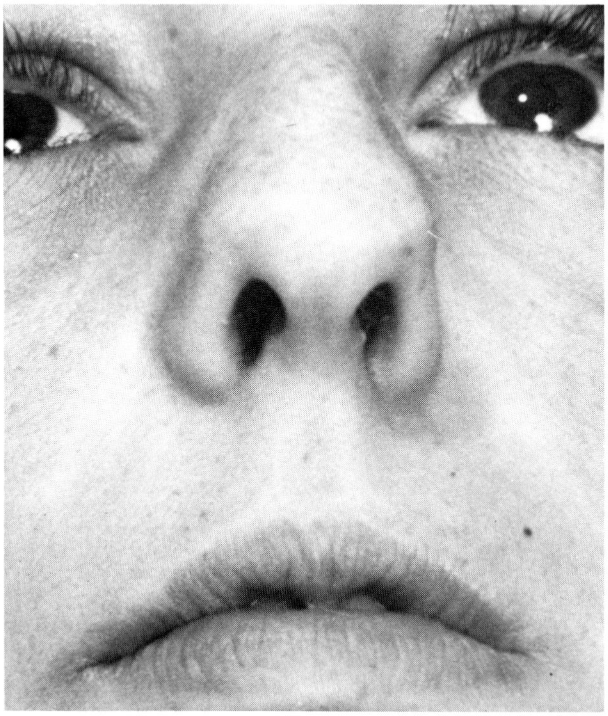

The ideal triangular base is possible only if the lower lateral cartilage forms an arch. With malposition, the footing of the lateral crus (lateral wall of the arch) has been displaced superiorly, which results in a lower, wider dome area, thus forming a square nasal base.

The use of a model demonstrates the mechanical basis for the visual effect of malposition of the lateral crura.

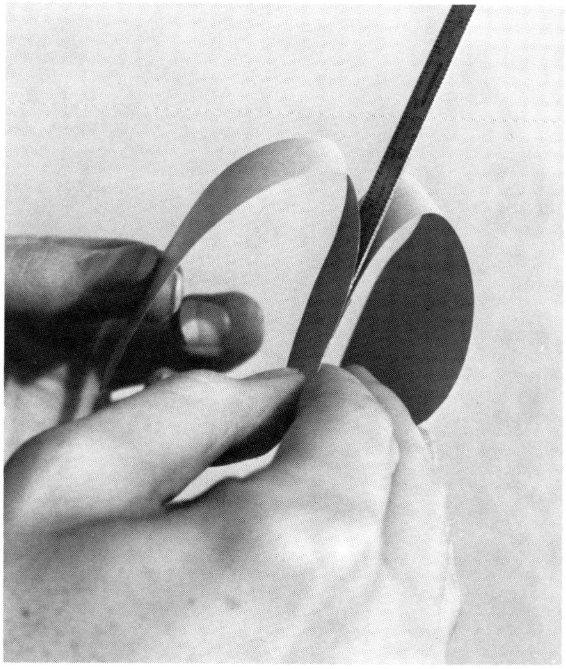

This basal view illustrates the usual contour and position of the lower lateral cartilages as they form double arches supporting the nasal tip.

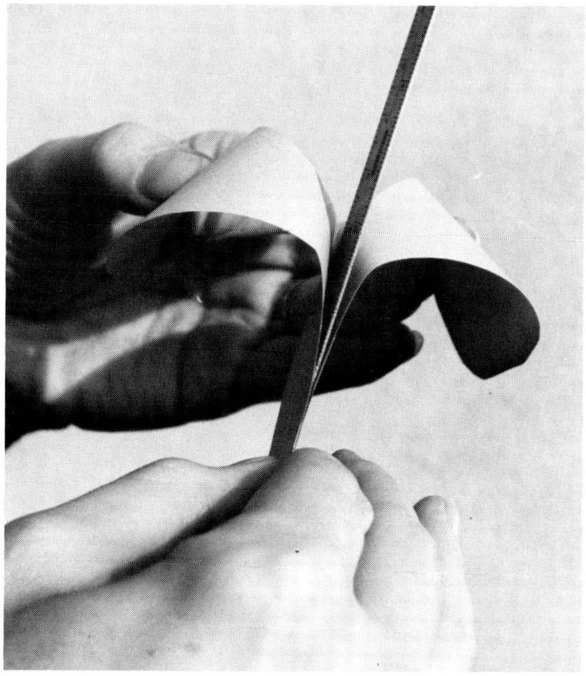

When the lateral crura are cephalically displaced, the domes widen as the lateral walls are moved superiorly.

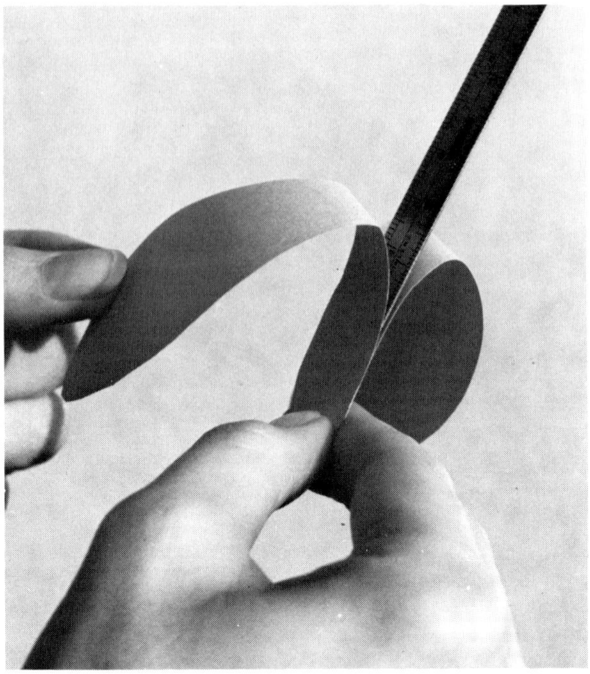

This is the usual position of the lateral crura viewed on oblique. The cephalic edge of the dome of the arch is seen at 43 mm on the ruler.

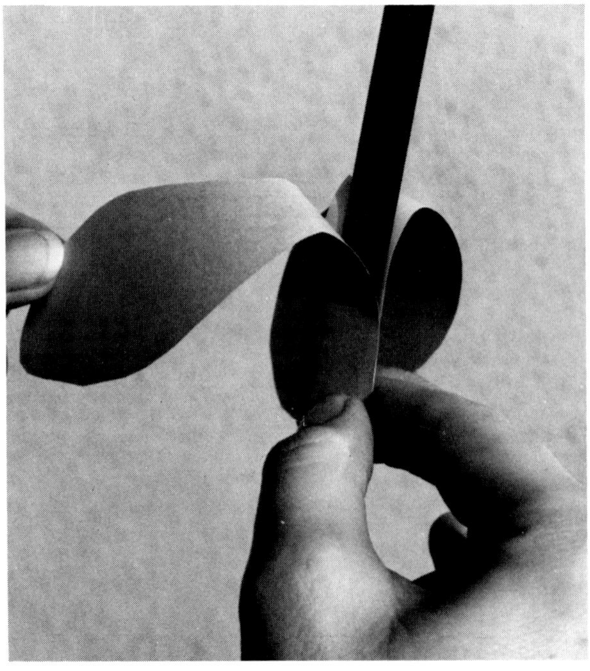

Following a slight upward rotation of the lateral crus, the dome broadens as it decreases in height to 36 mm on the ruler.

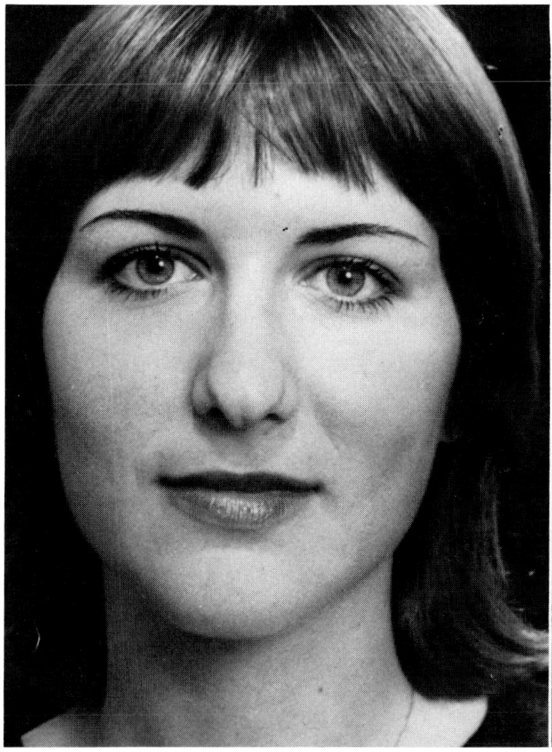
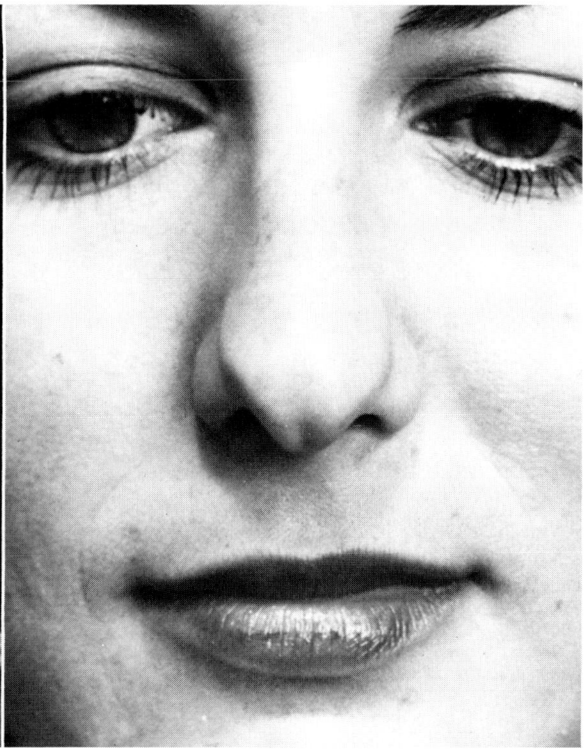

Case report 1: Malposition with relocation of lateral crura

This patient was diagnosed as having malposition of the lower lateral cartilages. On front view, the nose exhibits two characteristics of malposition:

1. Parentheses around the nasal tip
2. Broad and flat nasal tip

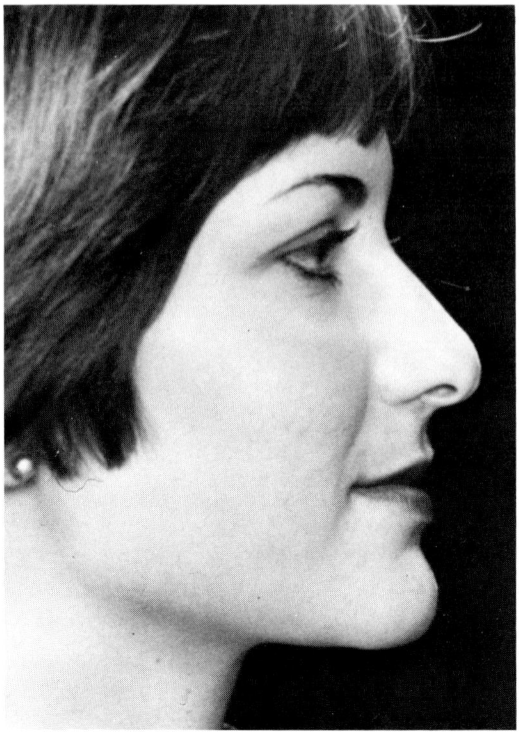

On lateral view, the tip seems well structured, but it is blunted because of a lack of projection of the lower lateral cartilages. In spite of the open nasolabial angle and a straight dorsum, the tip appears to be inclined downward (TIP).

On oblique view, the cephalic displacement of the lateral crus is demonstrated by light pressure on the lateral nasal wall. It also demonstrates the unsupported tissues lateral to the malpositioned cartilage.

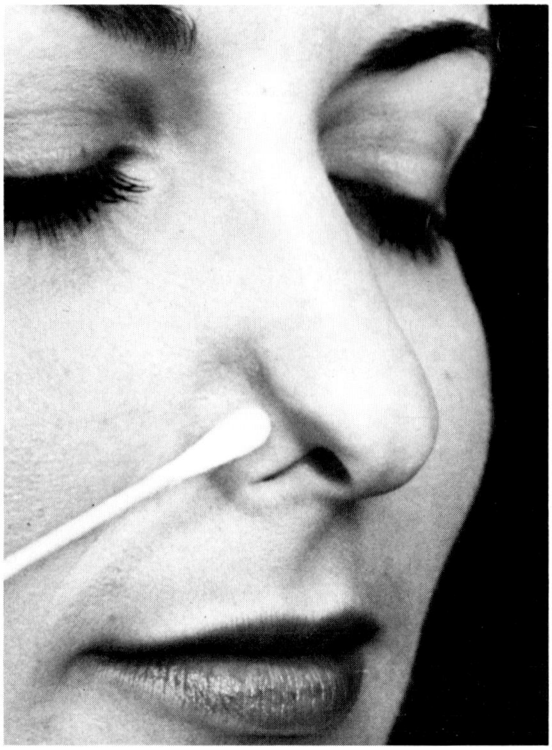

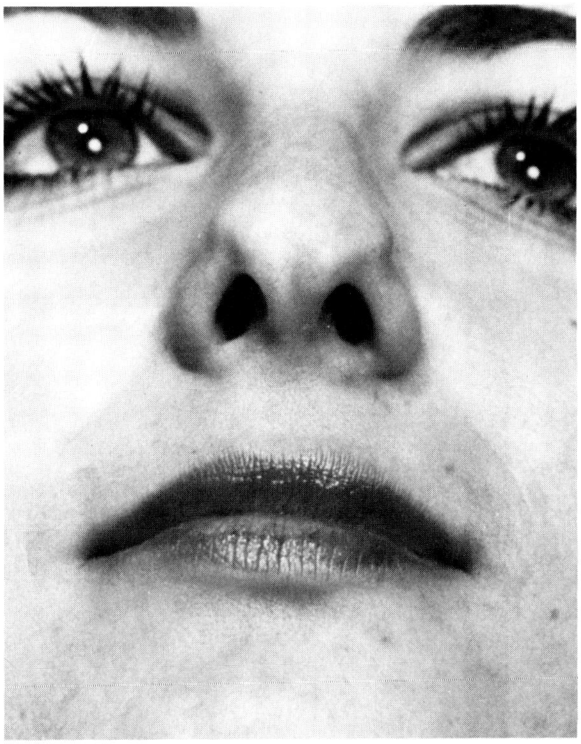

On basal view, the following characteristics of malposition can be seen:

1. Almost square perimeter
2. Notching of the alar rims at the caudal borders of the lateral crura

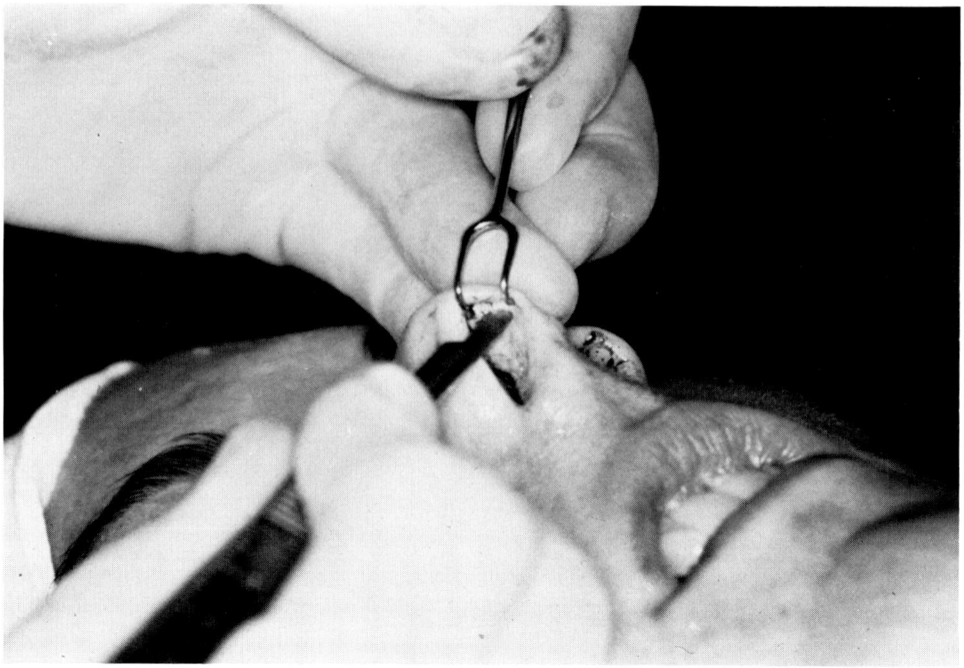

SURGICAL PROCEDURE

The rim incision begins medially at about the midpoint of the columella and then follows the caudal border of the medial crus to the area of the soft triangle.

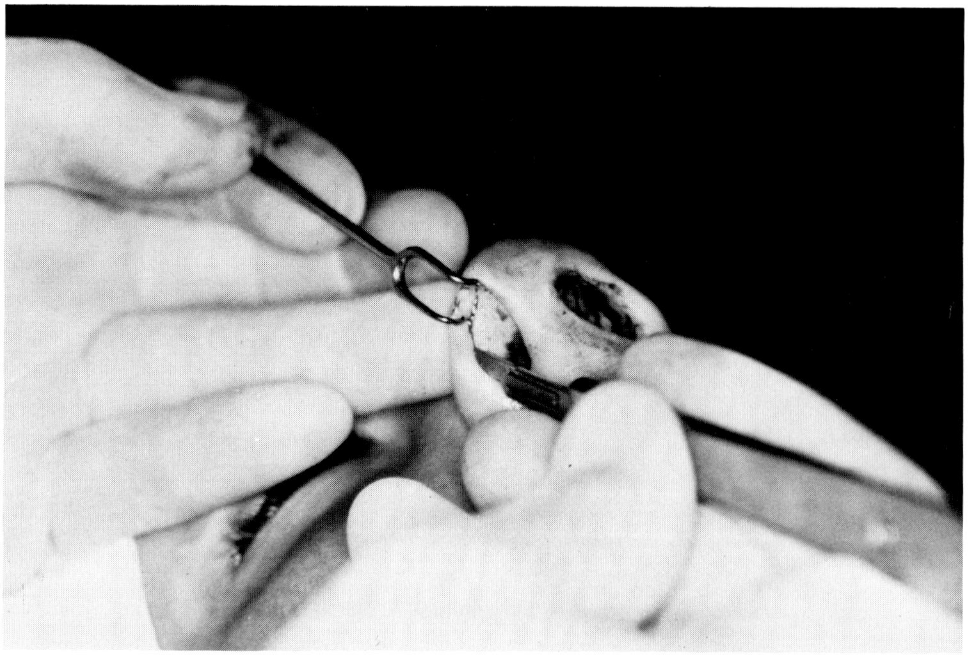

The incision is carried along the caudal border of the lower lateral cartilage past the area of the soft triangle. It then continues along a theoretical ideal placement of the lateral crus, or approximately 3 mm cephalad to the alar rim and parallel to it. The incision is carried as far laterally as necessary to accommodate the entire length of the lateral crus.

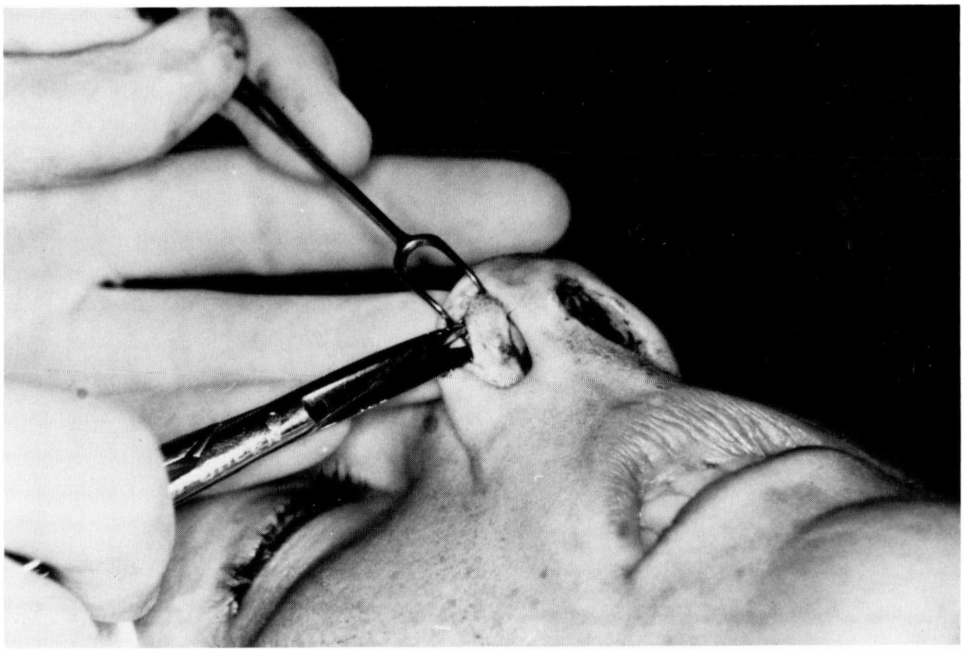

Dissection of the lateral crus begins near the dome where the caudal edge of the lateral crus can easily be found.

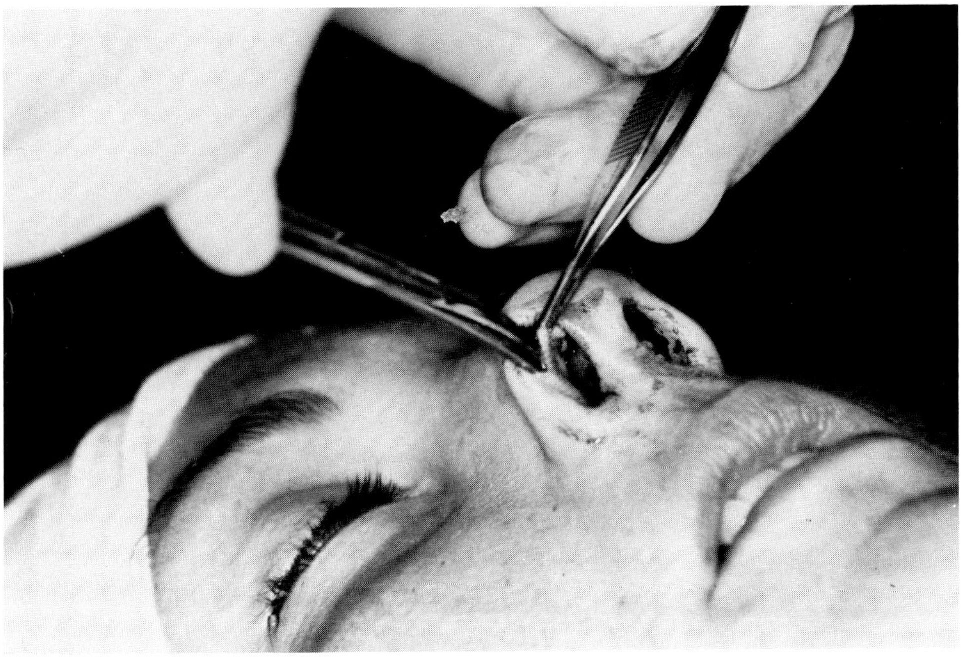

The dissection is carried laterally along the incision parallel with the alar rim. This progresses cephalad to the inferior border of the lateral crus.

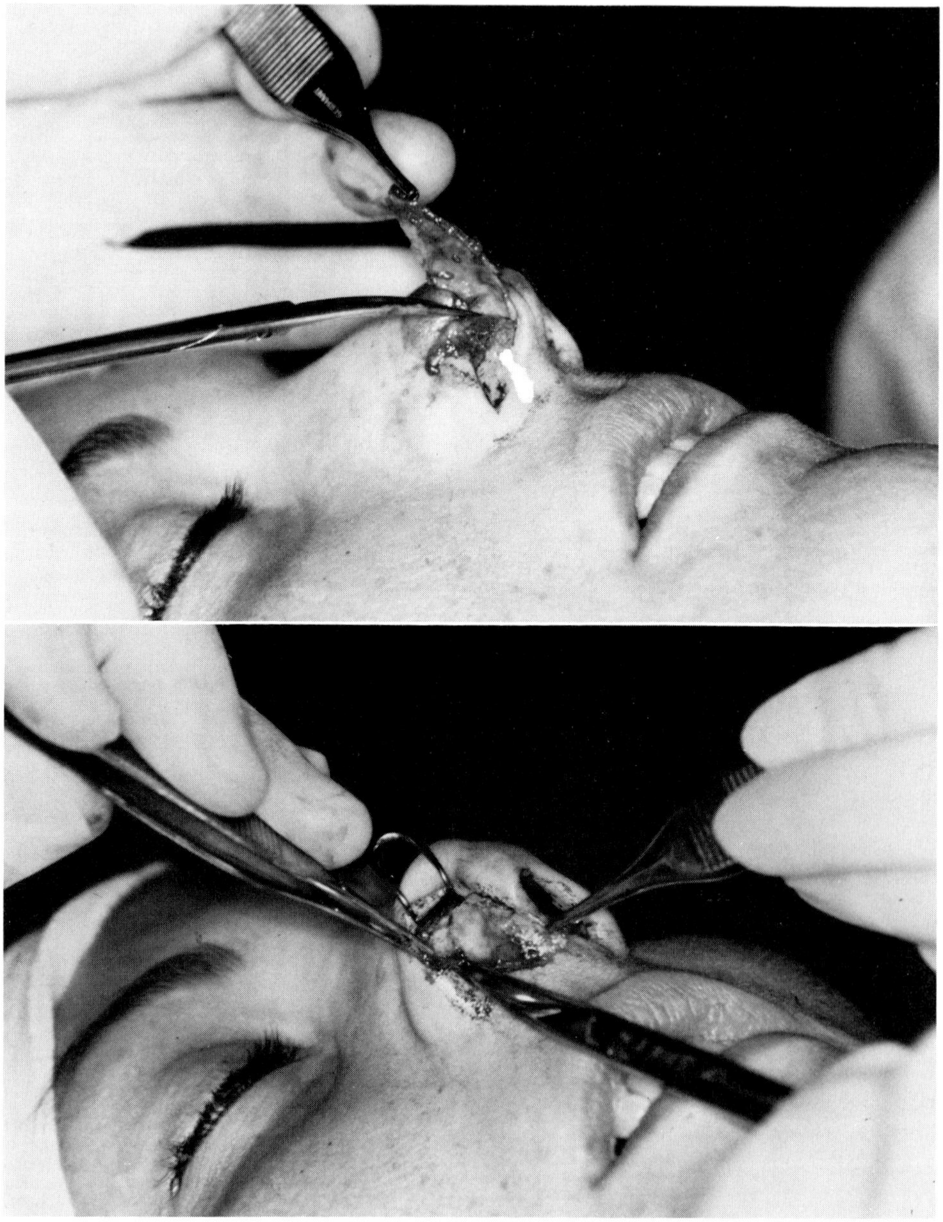

The lateral crus is completely separated from all soft tissue anteriorly and posteriorly as the dissection approaches the medial crus.

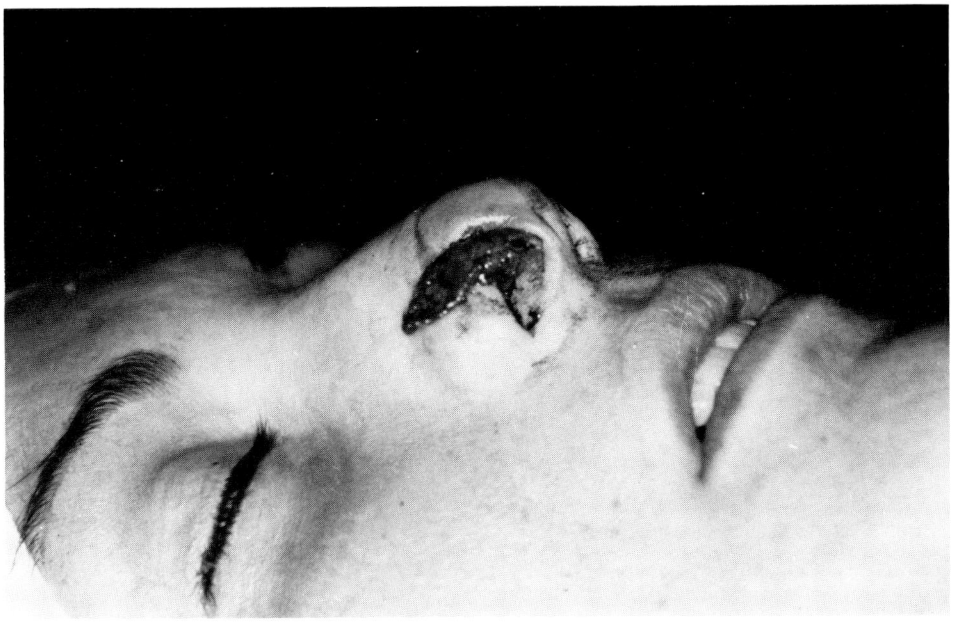

The malposition of the cartilage is obvious when the lateral crus is exposed. The cartilage is almost perpendicular to the alar rim rather than parallel to it.

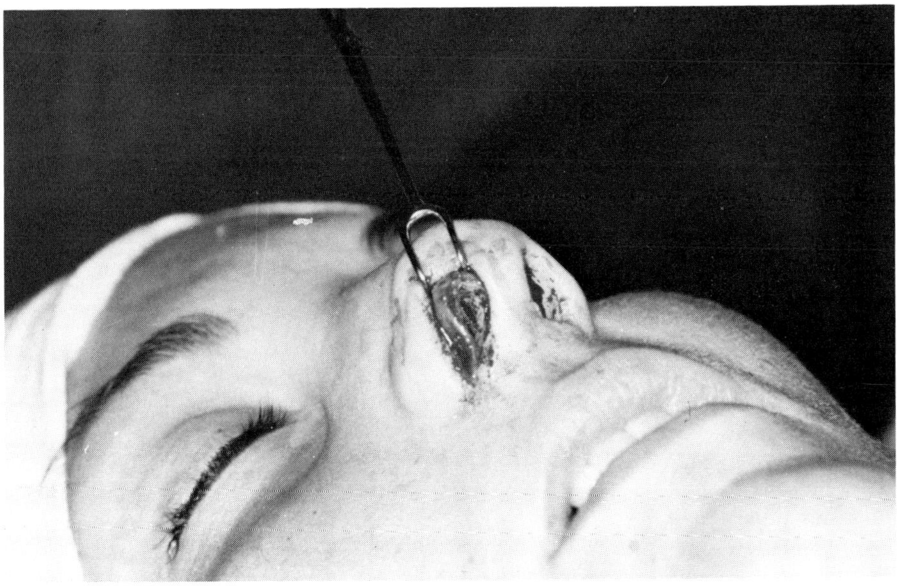

When placed in its correct position along the rim of the nostril, the lateral crus extends into the alar lobule.

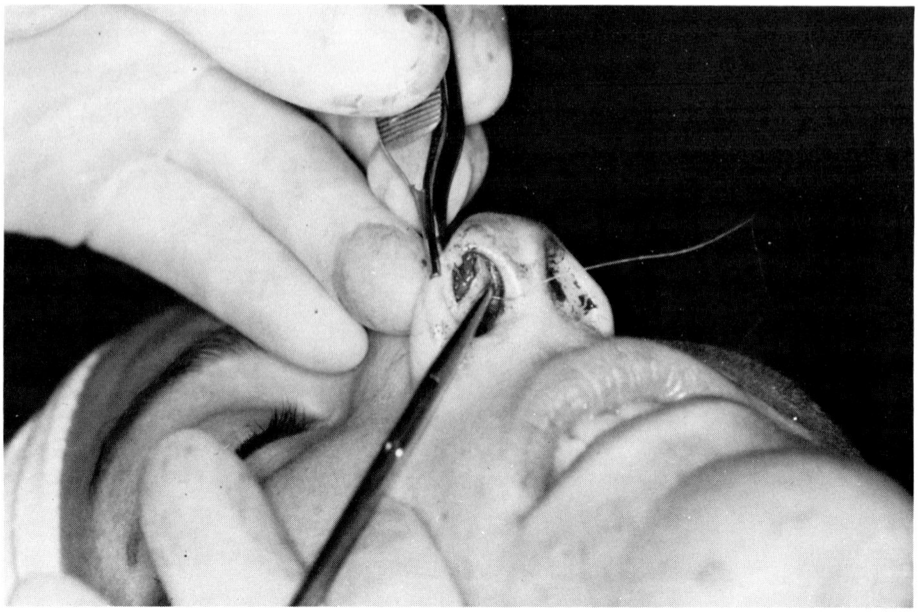

Three interrupted sutures of 5-0 plain catgut fix the lateral crus into its new position along the alar rim. Since attempts to gain more tip projection by advancing the crus caused distortion rather than projection, the cartilage was repositioned without stress.

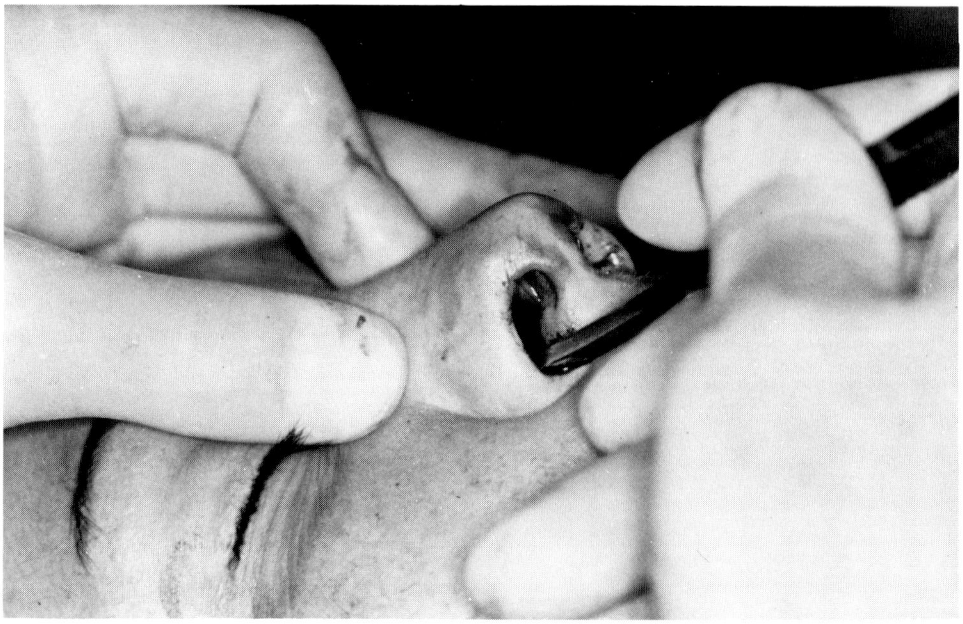

Lateral osteotomies begin low in the pyriform aperture and end high toward the radix.

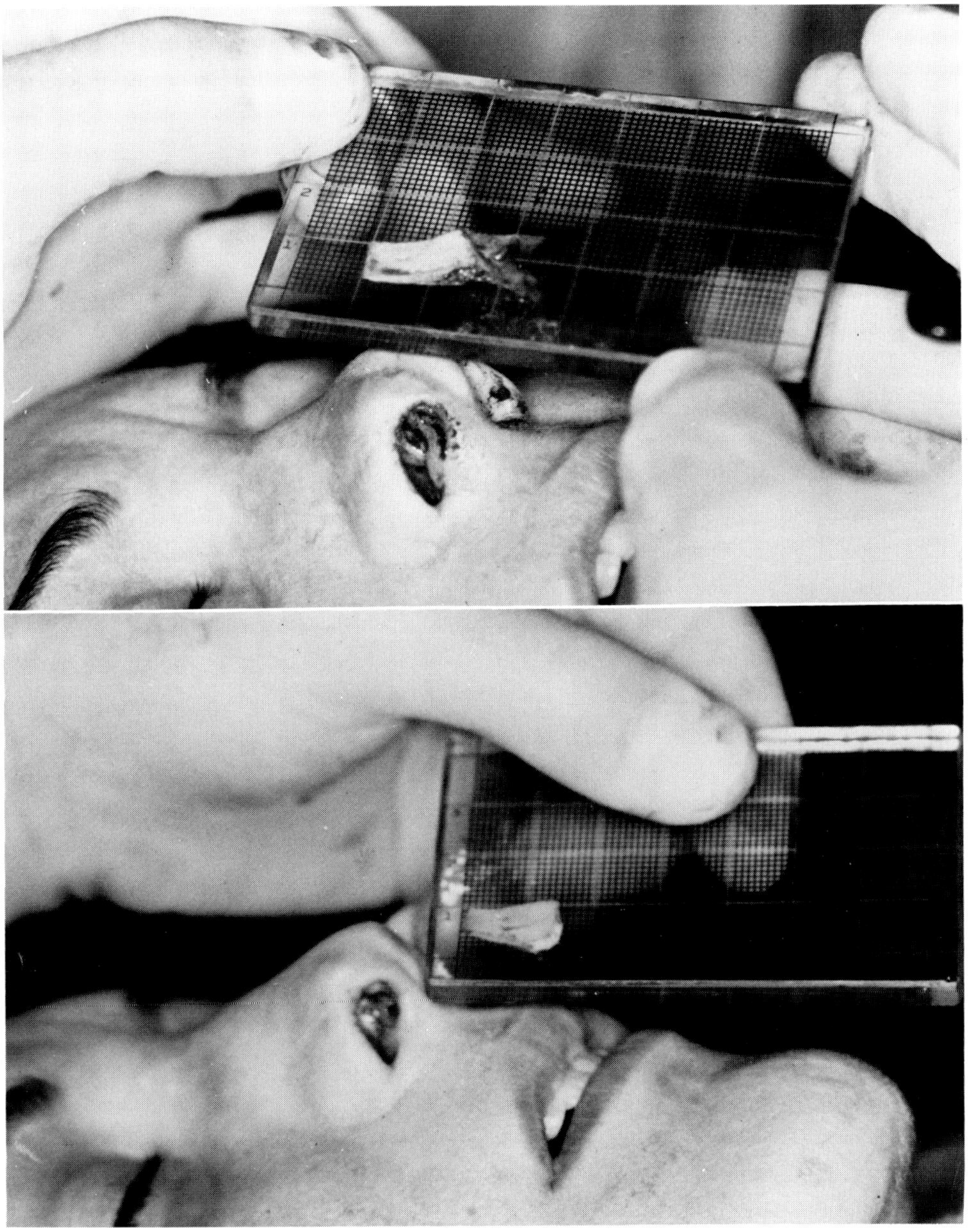

Because of persisting flatness of the nasal tip, a tip graft is fashioned from septal cartilage.

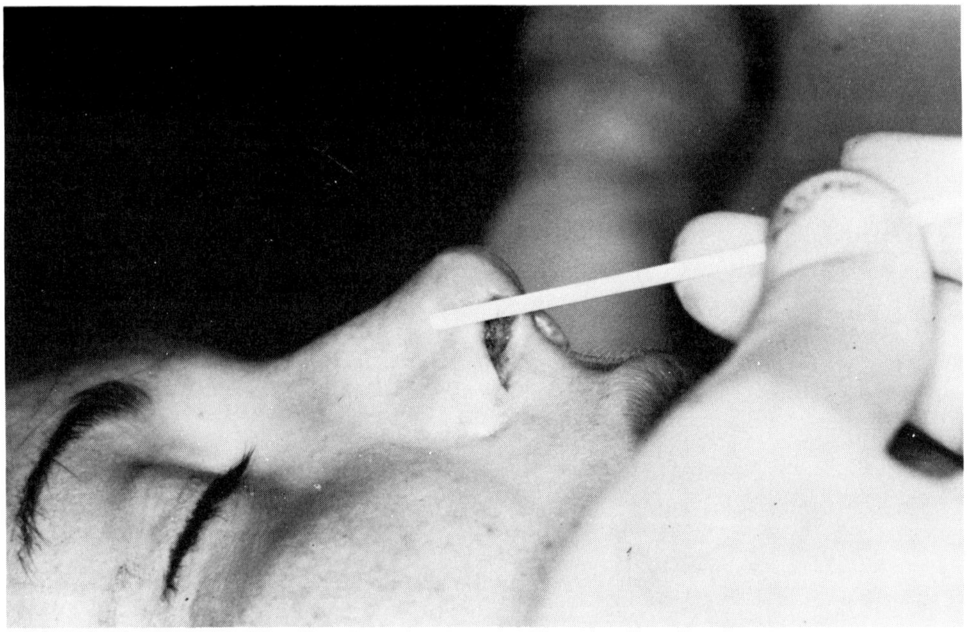

Following placement of the tip graft and repositioning of the lateral crura, the tip projects above the dorsal line, and the nostril rims are well supported.

Summary of surgical procedure

1. Limited skeletonization to the nasal spine
2. Reduction of the nasal spine
3. Reduction of the dorsum 2 mm
4. Delivery of the entire lateral crura of the lower lateral cartilages
5. Reposition of the lateral crura
6. Submucous resection for graft material
7. Lateral osteotomies
8. Tip graft of septal cartilage

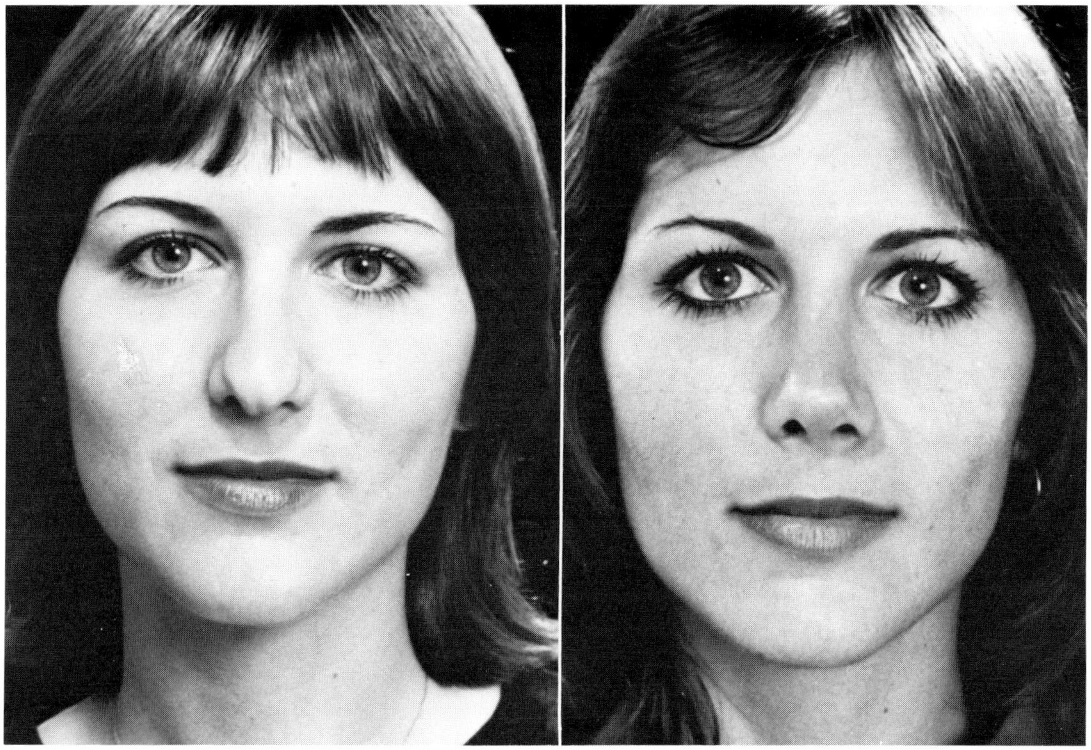

POSTOPERATIVE RESULTS

Postoperatively, the nose appears shorter because of the projection of the nasal tip, even though the actual length was retained. The parentheses, which are pathognomonic of malposition of the lateral crura, have been ablated.

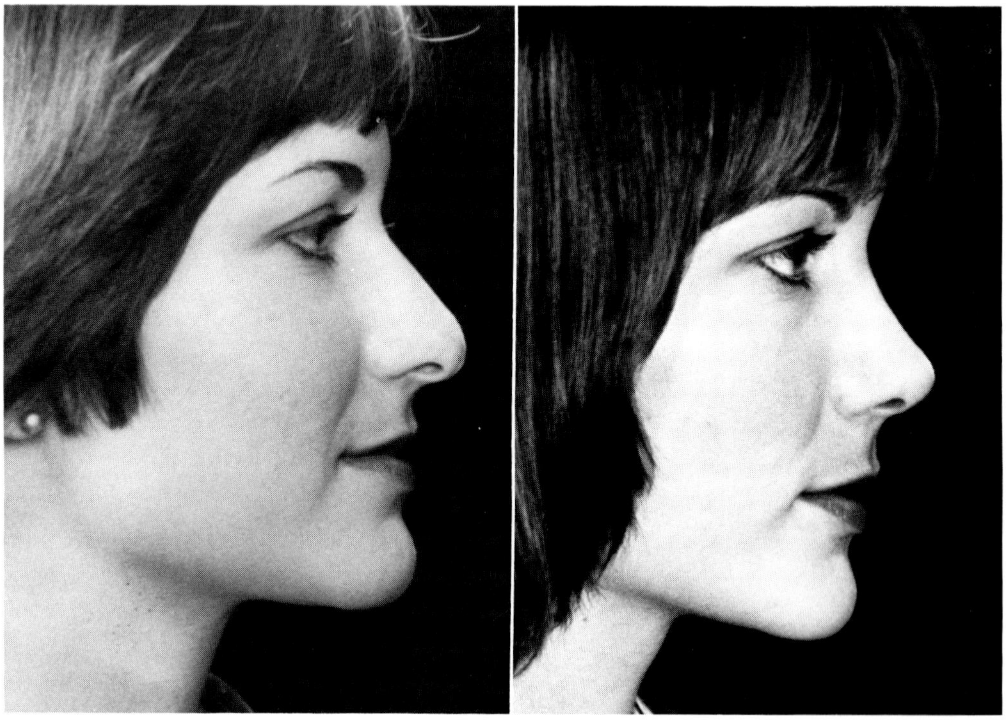

On lateral view postoperatively, the most important change in the nasal profile is the tip definition obtained by the tip graft. A minimal reduction of the dorsum has preserved the well-proportioned size of her nose. Slight reduction of the nasal spine without resection of the caudal septum has maintained the length of her nose but deepened the nasolabial angle, producing a slightly longer lip and better separation of lip from columella.

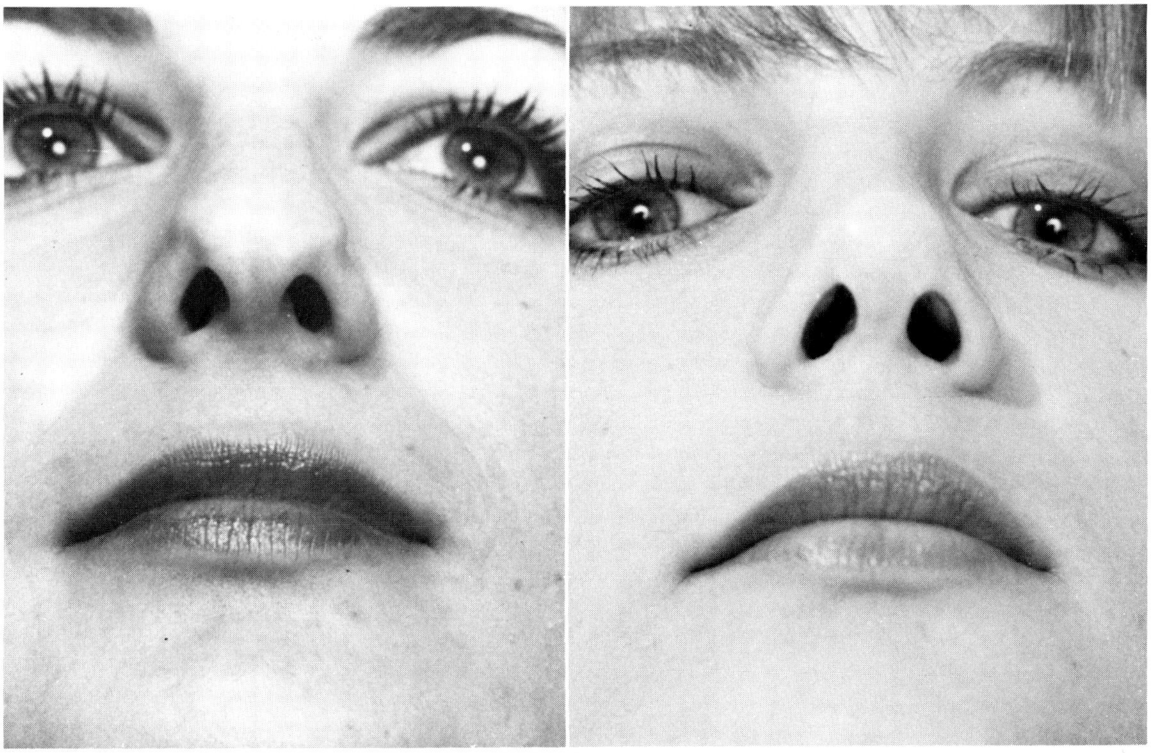

On postoperative basal view, relocation of the lateral crura has eliminated the notches in the alar rims. The basal perimeter has been changed from square to triangular.

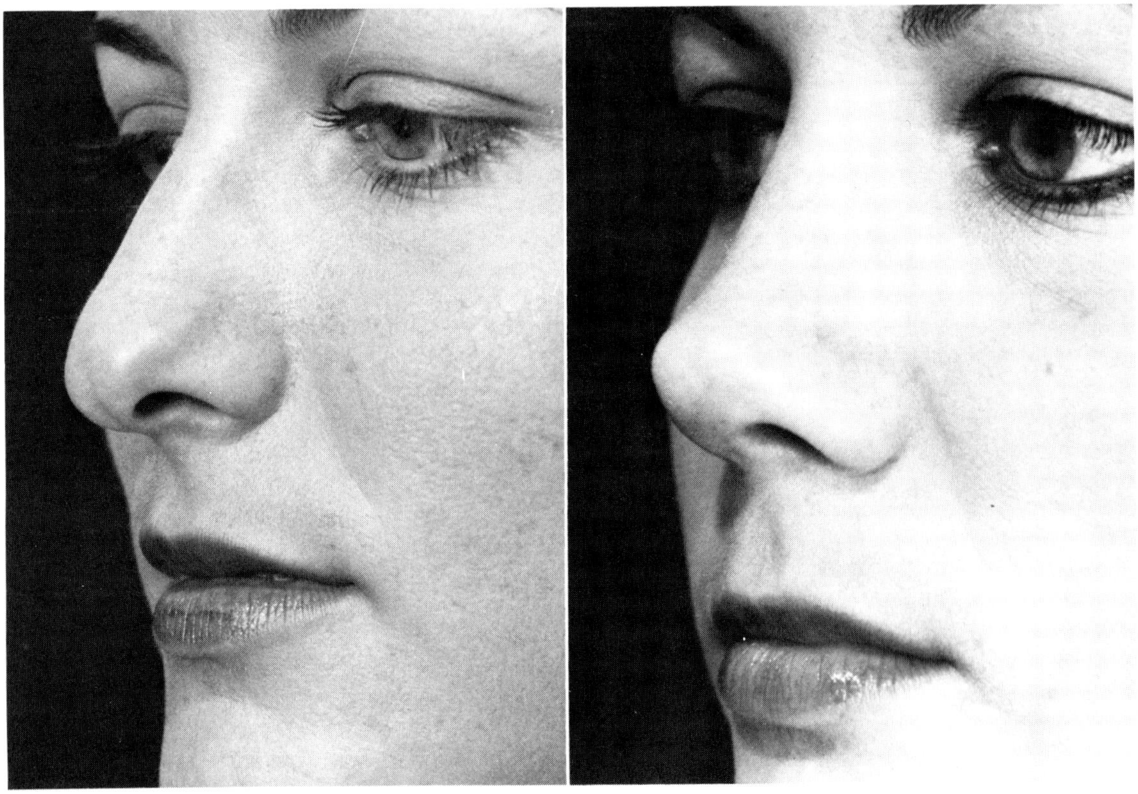

Postoperatively, the change in location of the lateral crus has provided visual continuity of the alar rim.

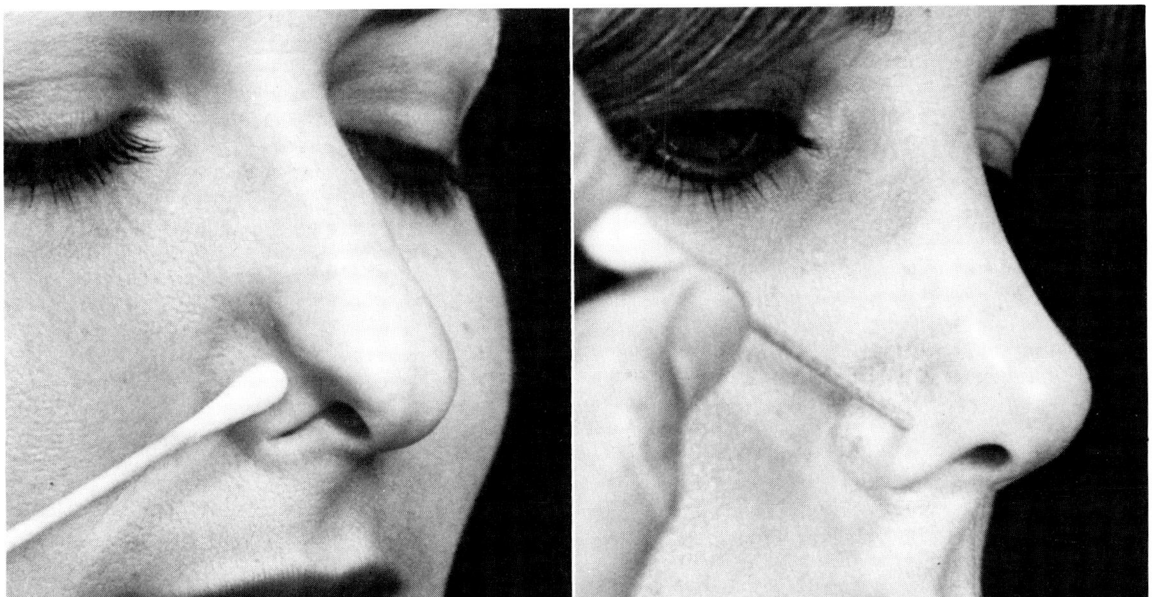

Pressure on the lateral nasal wall with an applicator demonstrates the excellent support supplied by the repositioned alar cartilage.

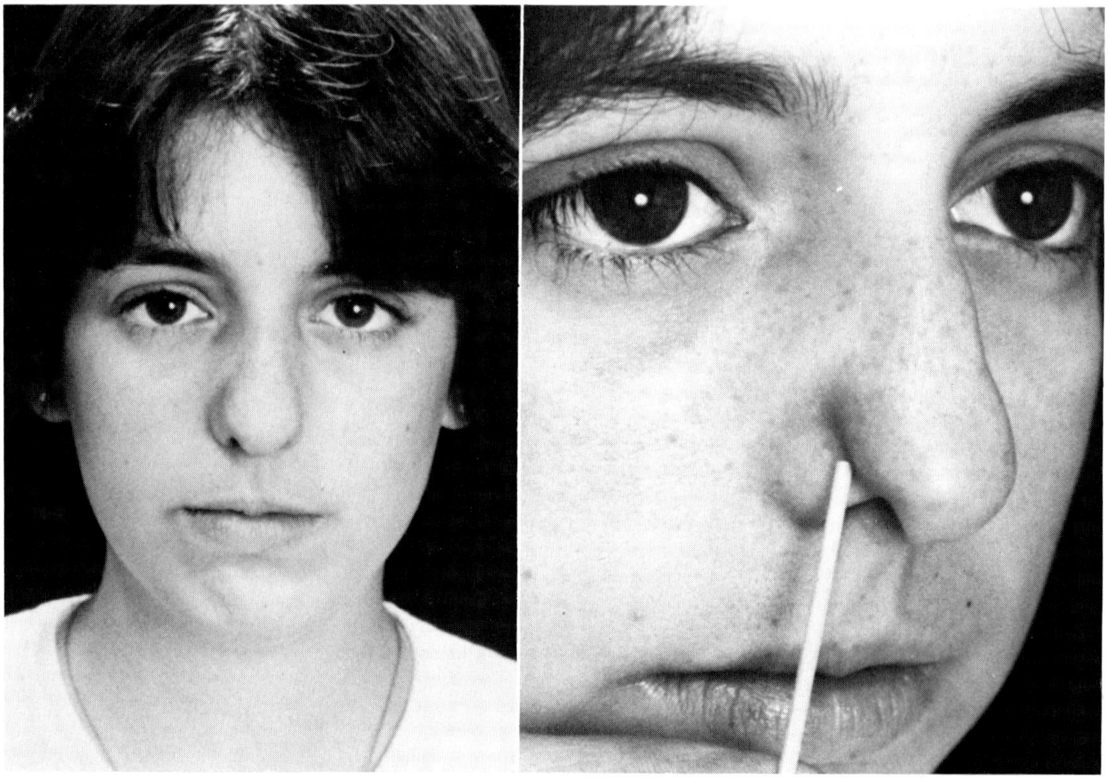

Case report 2: Malposition without relocation of lateral crura

Malposition of the lower lateral cartilages does not require relocation of the footing of the lateral crus if the footing provides the necessary support for projection of the cartilaginous arch.

This patient on front view has the typical round, flat tip bordered by parentheses. The nasal contour is pear shaped.

The right oblique view illustrates the test for the lateral limits of the tip cartilage.

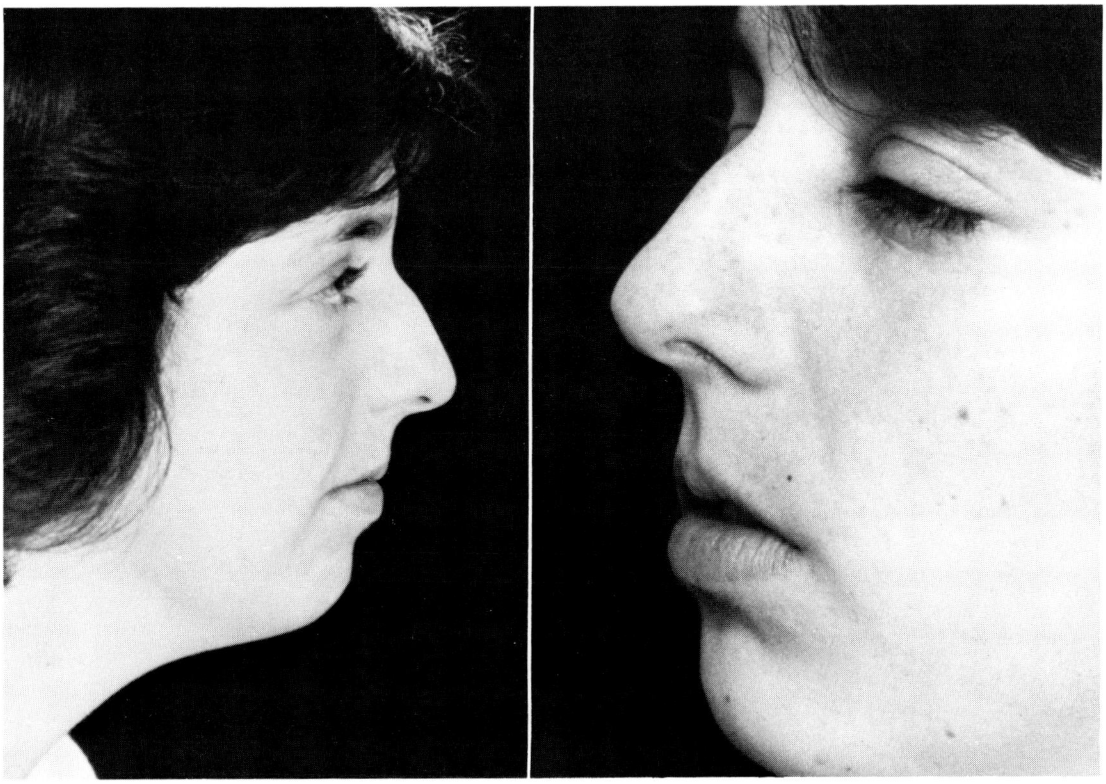

On lateral and left oblique views, the nose appears longer and more refined than it does on front view. There is a slight dorsal hump, but the relationships of the base are excellent.

Since the tip projects above the dorsal line, relocation of the lateral crus is contraindicated because projection could be diminished if the lateral crus were dissected from its attachments.

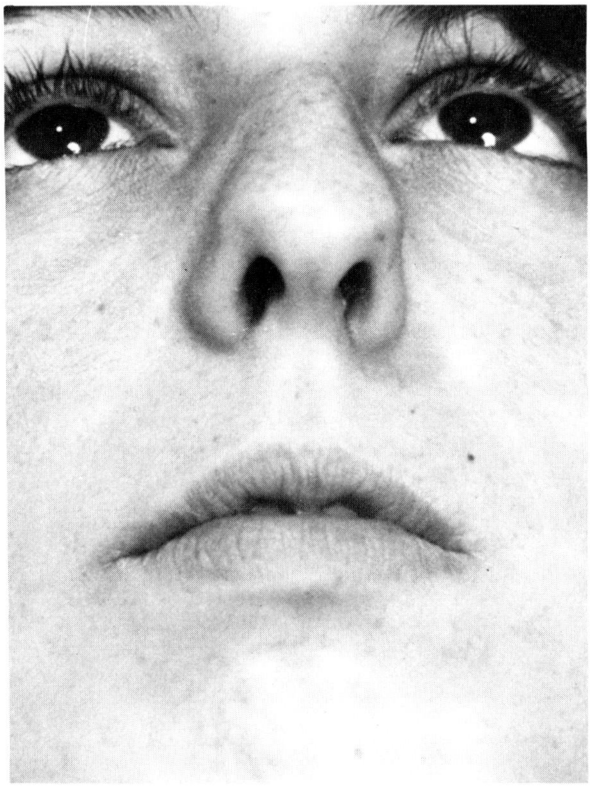

On basal view, the following characteristics of malposition can be seen:

1. Square basal contour
2. Notching of the nostrils at the lateral crura

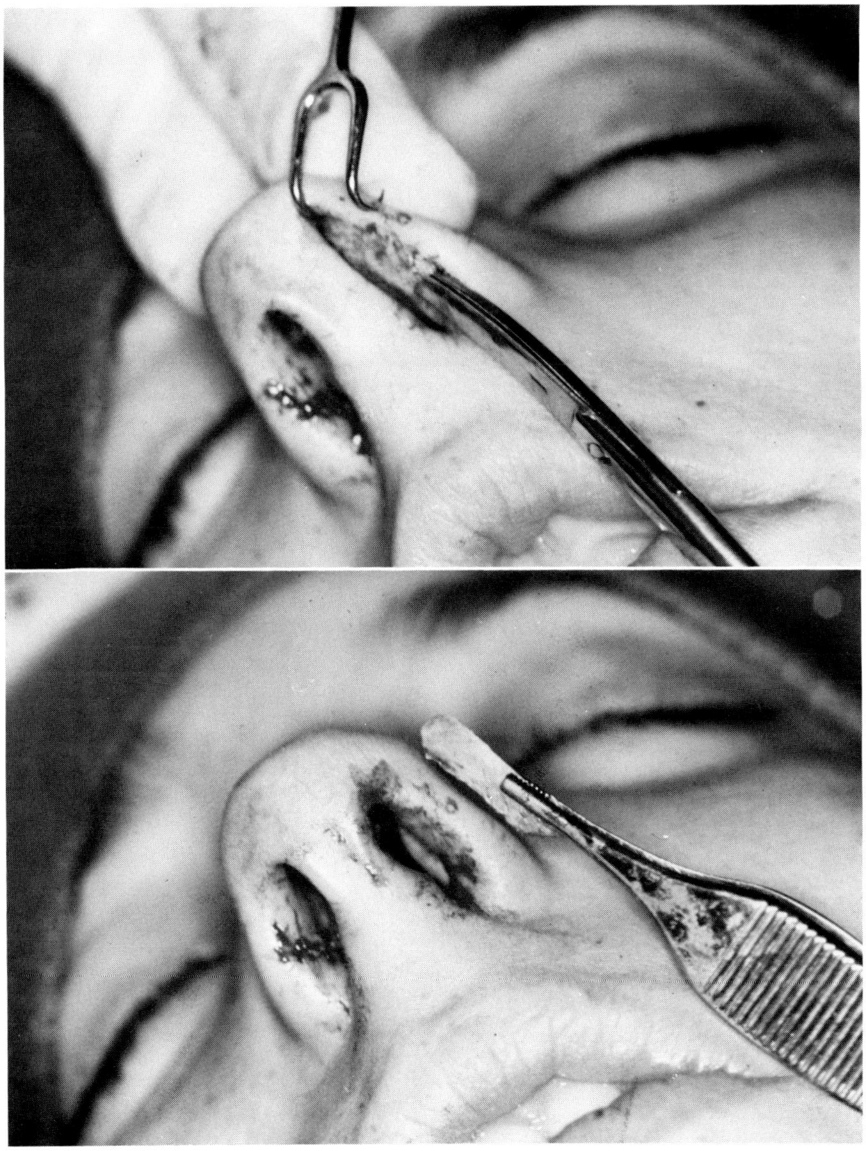

SURGICAL PROCEDURE

An ethmoid bone graft is placed along each alar rim to provide support to the area that would ordinarily be supported by the lateral crus of the lower lateral cartilage.

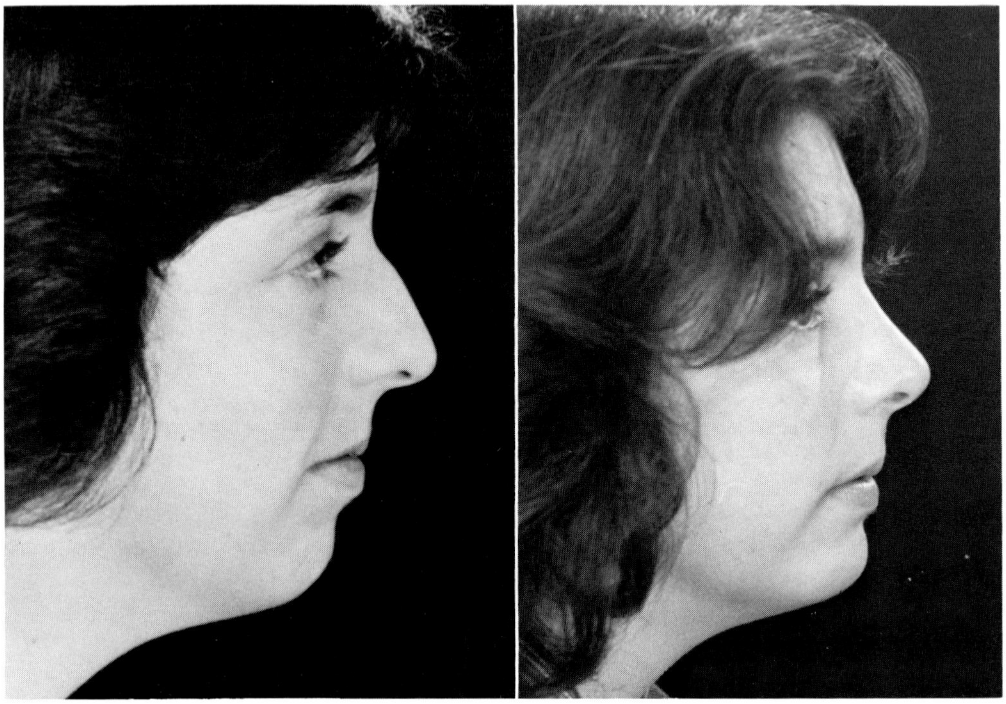

On right lateral view postoperatively, there is a straight dorsum with a tip that projects above the dorsal line. The relationship of tip to dorsum provides the illusion of an upward tilt to the nose even though the nasolabial angle has not been changed.

Summary of surgical procedure

1. Limited skeletonization to the angle of the septum
2. Reduction of the dorsum 2 mm
3. Delivery of the lower lateral cartilages through rim incisions
4. Cephalic trim and attenuation of the domes
5. Submucous resection to obtain perpendicular plate of the ethmoid
6. Lateral osteotomies
7. Ethmoid bone grafts placed in the lateral nasal walls

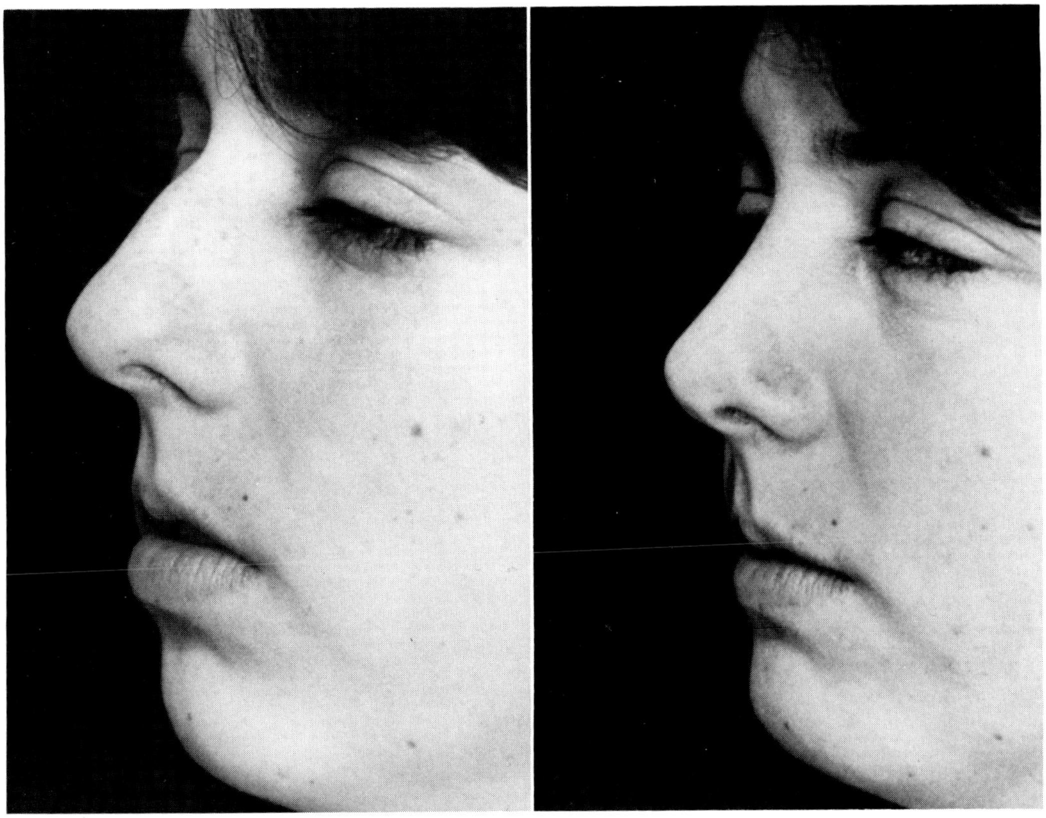

POSTOPERATIVE RESULTS

Postoperatively, the oblique dorsal line is straight and flows in continuity with the superciliary ridge and the nasal tip.

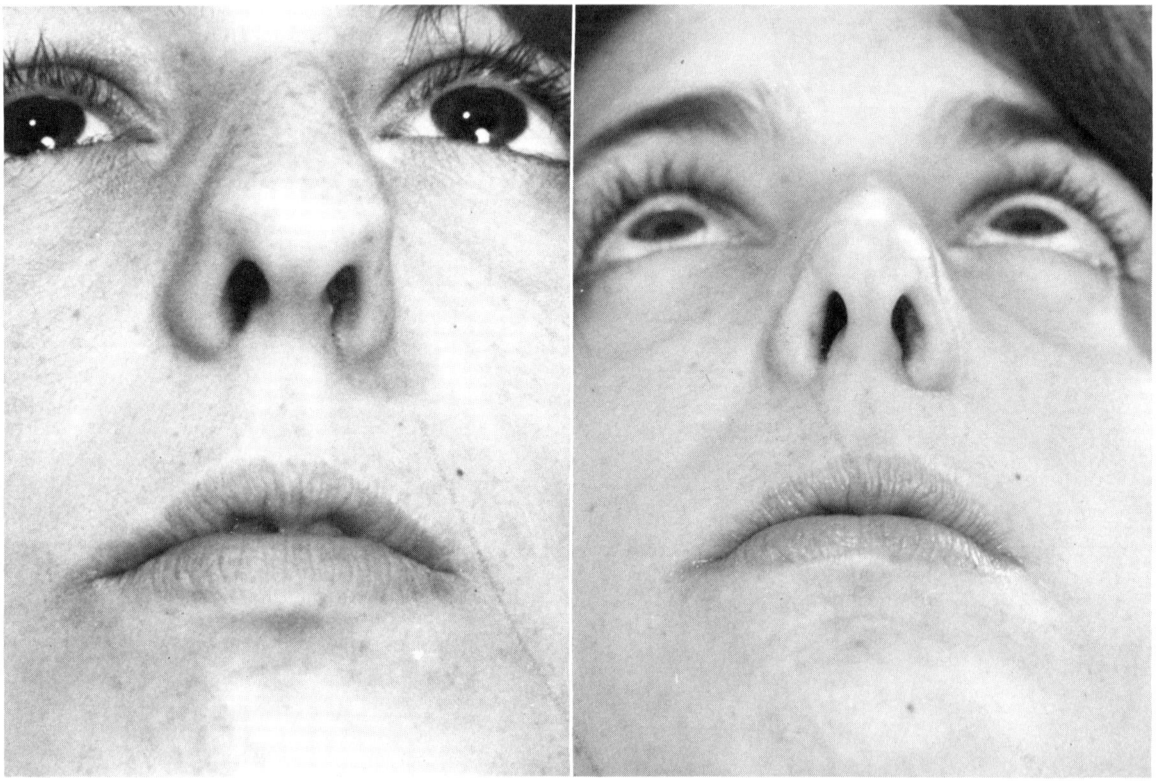

On basal view, the square basal configuration has been modified. The notches in the lateral nasal walls have been filled by the ethmoid bone grafts.

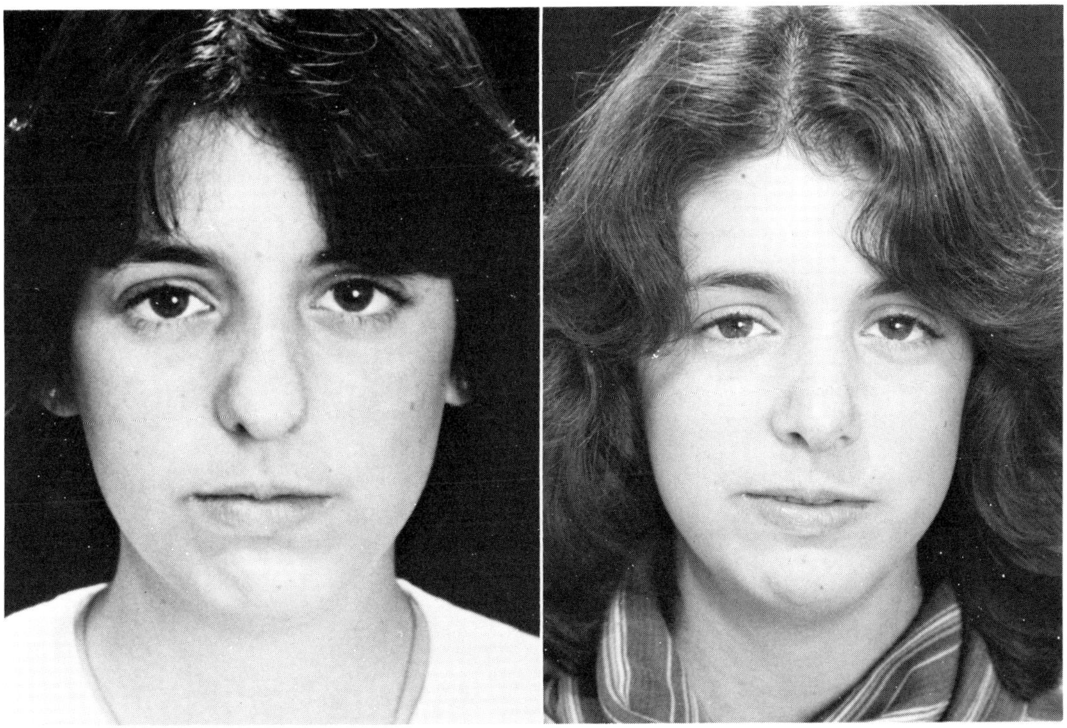

On front view, the nose appears longer even though it remains unchanged in length. The tip is more refined, and the parentheses are almost completely ablated.

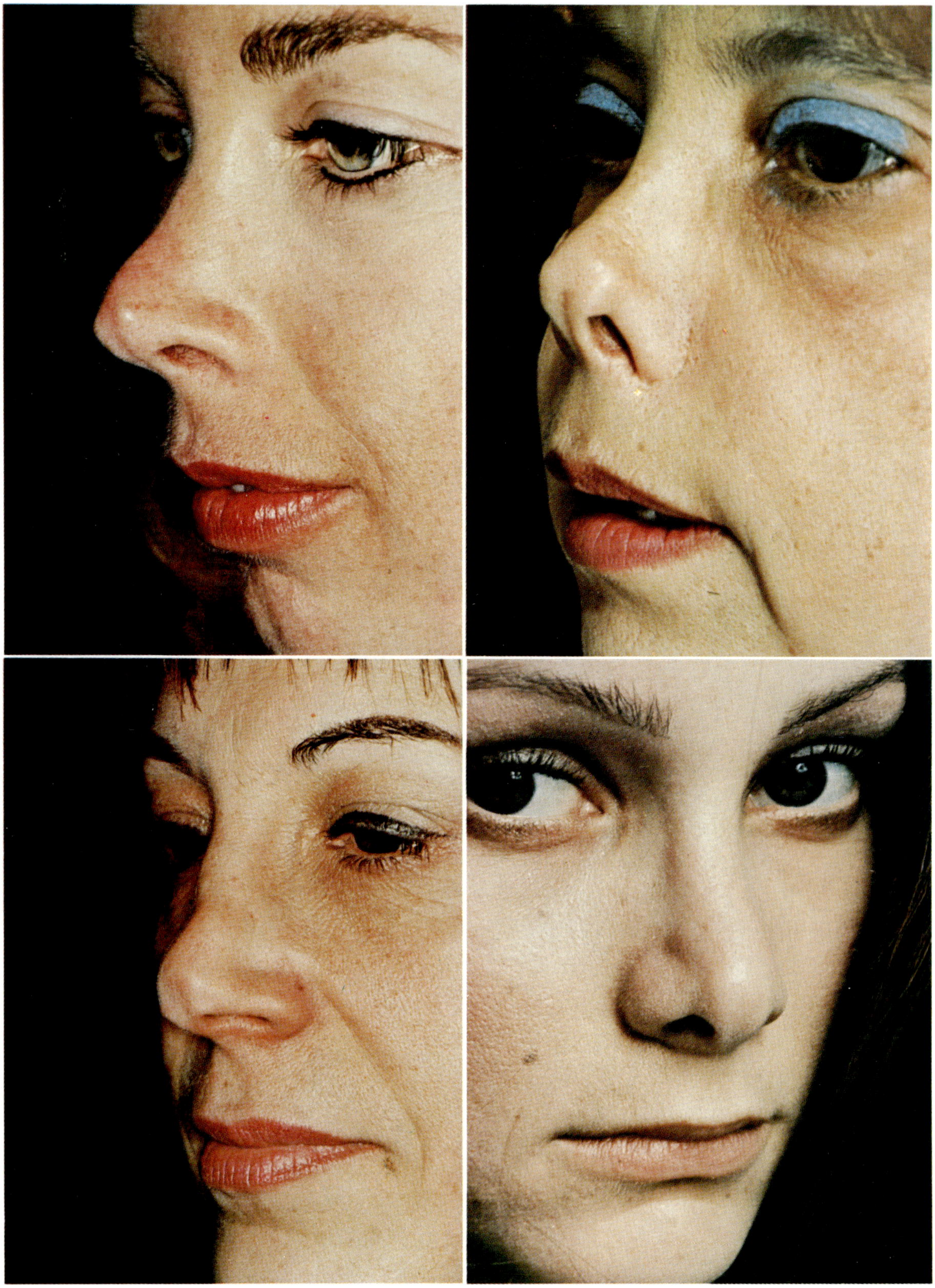

CHAPTER 7

Secondary rhinoplasty

Secondary rhinoplasty* is the "agony and the ecstasy" of nasal surgery. It is the agony because there are so many inherent handicaps and limitations—irrevocable tissue damage, tissue deficit, and scarring—that the surgeon can be caught in a quagmire of frustration and futility. The margin for error is painfully small, since each step is likely to be irreversible and may even make the deformity worse. If one does not operate, it is hard to tell a patient that there is little or nothing that can be done for an iatrogenic disfigurement. If one does operate and fails, it is harder still, for both the surgeon and the patient, to bear the consequences of that failure.

On the other hand, secondary rhinoplasty when successful is the ecstasy of nasal surgery because of the deep satisfaction that comes from performing well a complex and hazardous task. And for the patient it is truly ecstasy when a distorted, postsurgical nose is restored to near normalcy. Even those patients for whom little improvement is possible feel great joy and relief when a striking deformity is lessened or when a nonfunctional airway is corrected. Whether agony or ecstasy, it is only a transient moment for the surgeon. For the patient who must live with the results, it is an experience that lasts.

The small percentage of minor revisions that are inevitable in everyone's practice can be well taken care of by the primary surgeon. But if one surgeon performs two or more unsuccessful procedures, expert consultation is advisable. Regretably, patients are frequently returned to the primary surgeon, either for economic or medicolegal reasons, or because the next surgeon may not want to inherit someone else's problems. In my opinion this is a dangerous practice because the next surgical procedure may be the patient's last chance for a satisfactory result. The patient must be spared the irreversible, catastrophic consequences of repeated surgical procedures; thus great care must be taken when deciding *whether or not, when,* and *by whom.*

Little is written about secondary rhinoplasty as a distinct surgical entity. Unfortunately, this informational void does not reflect a lack of necessity, since the need for postoperative reconstruction is inordinately great. The presumption may be that secondary revi-

*Used to designate any rhinoplasty subsequent to a primary.

sion is a kind of "try it again" rhinoplasty. But it is not. Many aspects of approach and technique distinguish it from primary rhinoplasty, and these must be understood by the surgeon who undertakes secondary correction.

In general, these cases require a reverse approach to primary rhinoplasty. The surgical plan is based on retrospection because secondary repair frequently involves the reversal of what has been done, or overdone, in the preceding operation(s). In a primary rhinoplasty, normal anatomy and tissues can be expected. In secondary rhinoplasty the anatomy is distorted, the tissues are scarred, and the vascularity is diminished. These general findings one can be sure of; the particulars are sometimes impossible to anticipate.

The number and variety of problems encountered in secondary rhinoplasty prevent the use of a standardized approach. For this reason, one's own experience and the methodical analysis of case reports are the most valuable means of understanding this complex surgery. However, there are ground rules that can be generally applied and that must be followed for a favorable result.

GROUND RULES

The following ground rules have proved invaluable in the management of postsurgical nasal deformities:

1. Defer surgery until there is final resolution of the tissues.
2. Have a well-defined aesthetic concept.
3. Make a proper diagnosis.
4. Limit the dissection.
5. Use only autogenous material.

Deferring surgery

The necessary time lapse for complete wound resolution is approximately 1 year. In cases of multiple procedures or extraordinary scarring, tissue changes can occur up to 2 years. Serial photographs and examinations aid in the determination of the stability of the tissues in terms of edema, induration, vascularity, and contracture. There are minor revisions, requiring minimal dissection, that can be performed safely in 6 months, but as a rule, secondary rhinoplasty should not be undertaken for a minimum of 1 year following the last procedure.

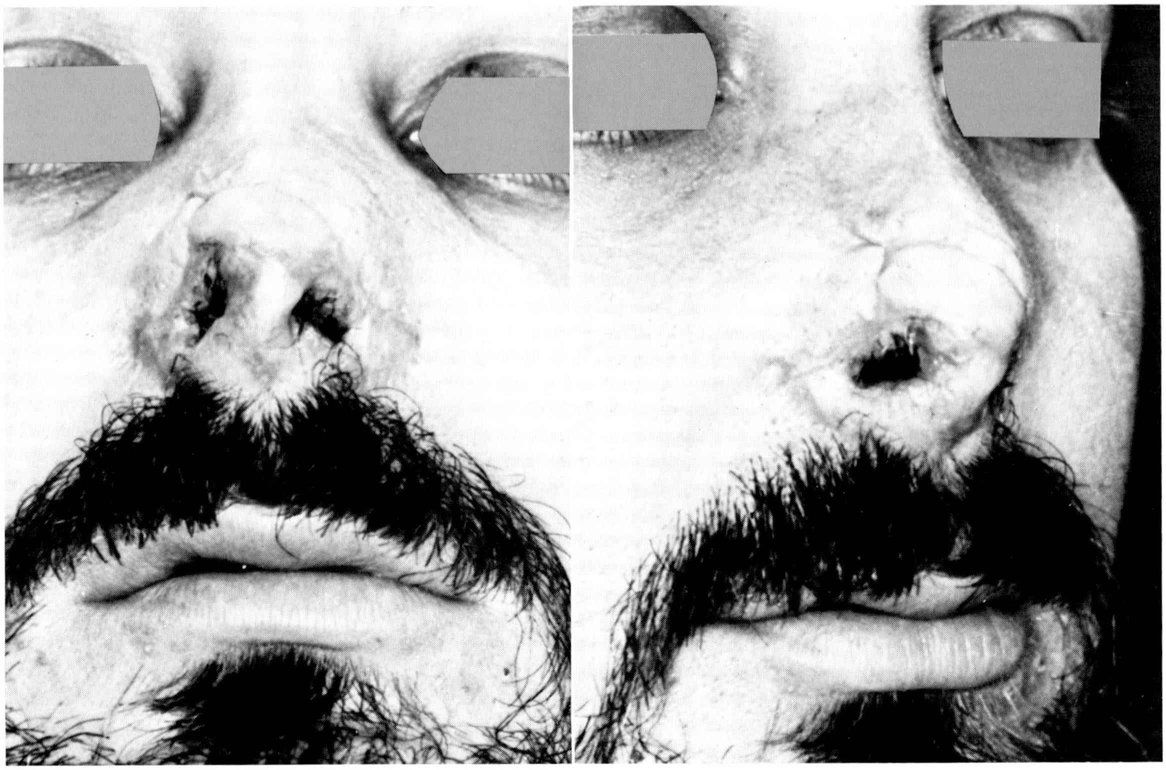

This patient demonstrates the effects of an aesthetic rhinoplasty followed by three revisional procedures that were performed within a 1-year period. The consequent vascular compromise, tissue loss, and scarring have resulted in tragedy for this 28-year-old man.

Having a well-defined aesthetic concept

This should not be a vague generalization, but rather a set of clearly defined relationships that integrate all the anatomic parts of the nose into a balanced whole. A well-defined aesthetic concept is particularly important in secondary rhinoplasty because in the absence of normal anatomy it is often quite difficult to determine exactly what is aesthetically awry. And obviously, revisional surgery should not be performed without definite aesthetic goals clearly in mind. For a detailed discussion of aesthetic concepts, please refer to Chapter 2.

Making a proper diagnosis

Diagnosis begins with the surgical history of the patient. In addition to the patient's subjective account of the prior operation(s), it is valuable to review preoperative photographs and any sequential postoperative photographs that can be provided. This will give the surgeon an idea of the problems presented by the original nose and of the surgical progression that produced the nose at hand. Although a review of operative records can be enlightening, experience has shown that operative reports are sometimes irrelevant since they may be merely a rote dictation of standard technique. Nevertheless, they should be reviewed if possible.

A thorough examination of all nasal parts provides the most reliable information for making a diagnosis. For internal examination, a headlight is mandatory. Using a headlight, one can evaluate the internal valve by tipping the patient's head back, and then, without touching the nose, observing whether or not the valve narrows (but not collapses) on inspiration. The condition of the turbinates and the structure and substance of the septum should also be evaluated. Since the septum is the primary source of reconstructive material, the surgeon must determine if it is of sufficient quantity and quality for reconstructive use.

Following a light application of 5% cocaine solution to the septal mucosa, an assessment of the septal cartilage can be carried out by transillumination of the septum and by palpation with a cotton applicator along the mucosa. Meanwhile, if one looks in the opposite nostril, the tip of the applicator can be seen to push out the mucosa where the septum is absent. One can be misled if the septal cartilage is very thin or if there is scarring or mucosal hyperplasia in the absence of septum, though usually an accurate assessment of the septum can be made.

On external examination, the overall nasal contour and specific nasofacial and intranasal relationships should be analyzed. It is especially important to note the condition of the tissues because this, more than anything else, will determine the nature and extent of the proposed reconstruction. An essential part of the preoperative diagnosis is the recognition of tissue limitations.

Case report 1: Combination of minor discrepancies

This patient is seen following a conservatively performed rhinoplasty. There is no major distortion. Many aesthetic aspects are satisfactory, yet the overall impression of the nose is poor. Examination of the nasal airways revealed no functional impairment of either side.

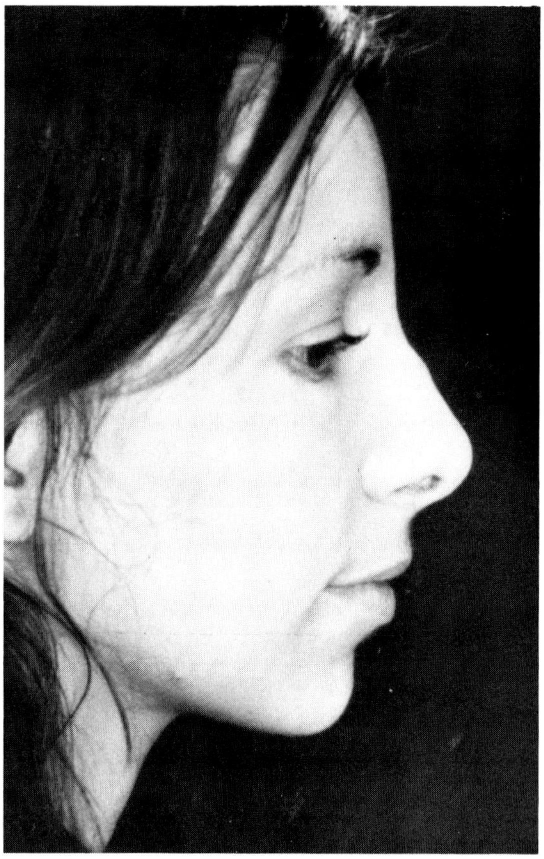

On lateral view, the dorsum begins at the radix and is almost straight, ending in a tip that is at the dorsal line. The tip is blunt and has no visible end point. The nasolabial angle is good, and the subnasion is full. The columella is in poor position relative to the alae.

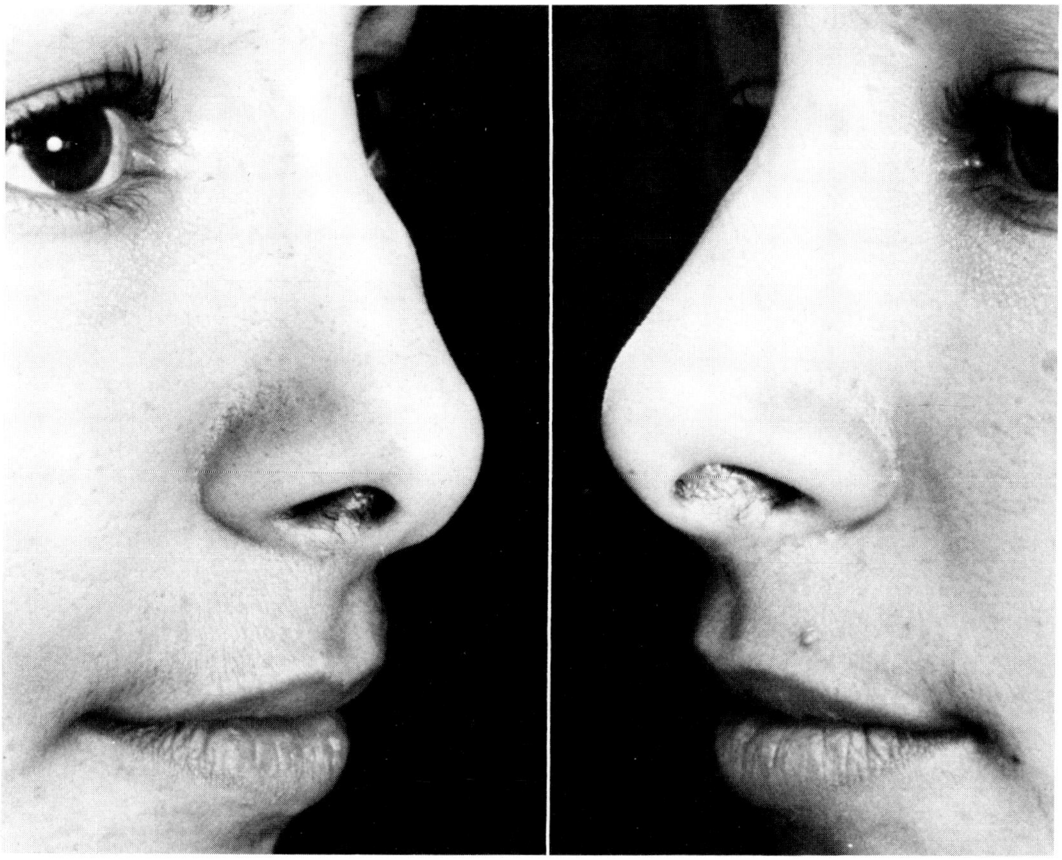

The dorsal irregularity on right oblique view compared with the relatively smooth dorsum on left oblique view indicates that the dorsal hump is left of the midline at the osteochondral junction. Both views illustrate a poor columellar-alar relationship and an unattractive show of vibrissae. The lack of tip delineation is largely responsible for the heavy appearance of the nose.

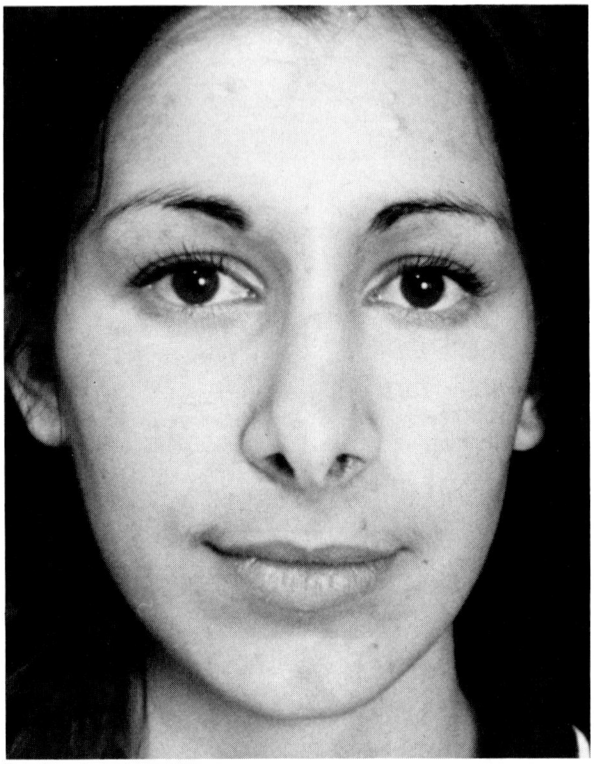

On front view, the lateral lines of the upper two thirds of the nose flow in continuity with the superior orbital rims. At the lower third, the lines join with parentheses around the nasal tip, then converge on the columella, which becomes their end point.

The lower third of the nose is the most objectionable aesthetic feature on front view. The alar flare is exaggerated by the parentheses, which separate the alar lobules from the tip. The lines that extend downward from the alar-facial grooves to the insertion of the columella are caused by the prominence of the nasal sills. The low columella distracts the sills inferiorly, exposing the nasal vestibule.

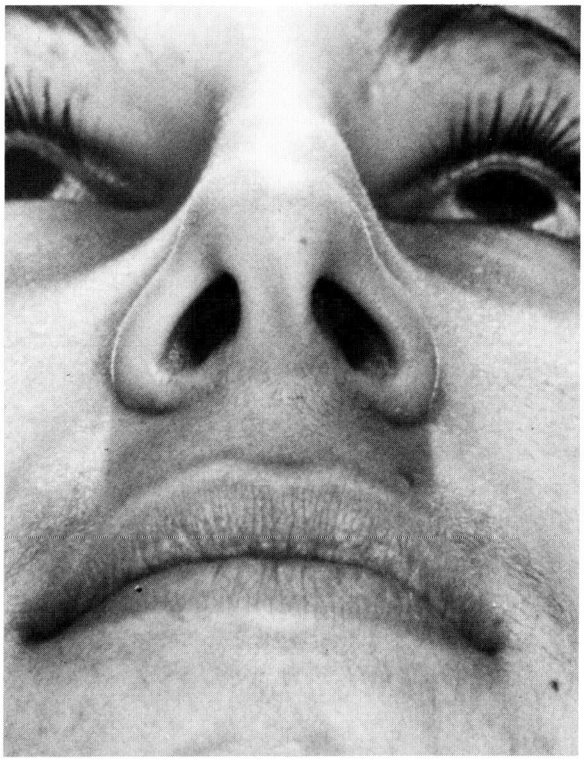

On basal view, the position of the dorsal bump is apparent. The nostrils are in good position and are well proportioned. The alar lobules are slightly redundant.

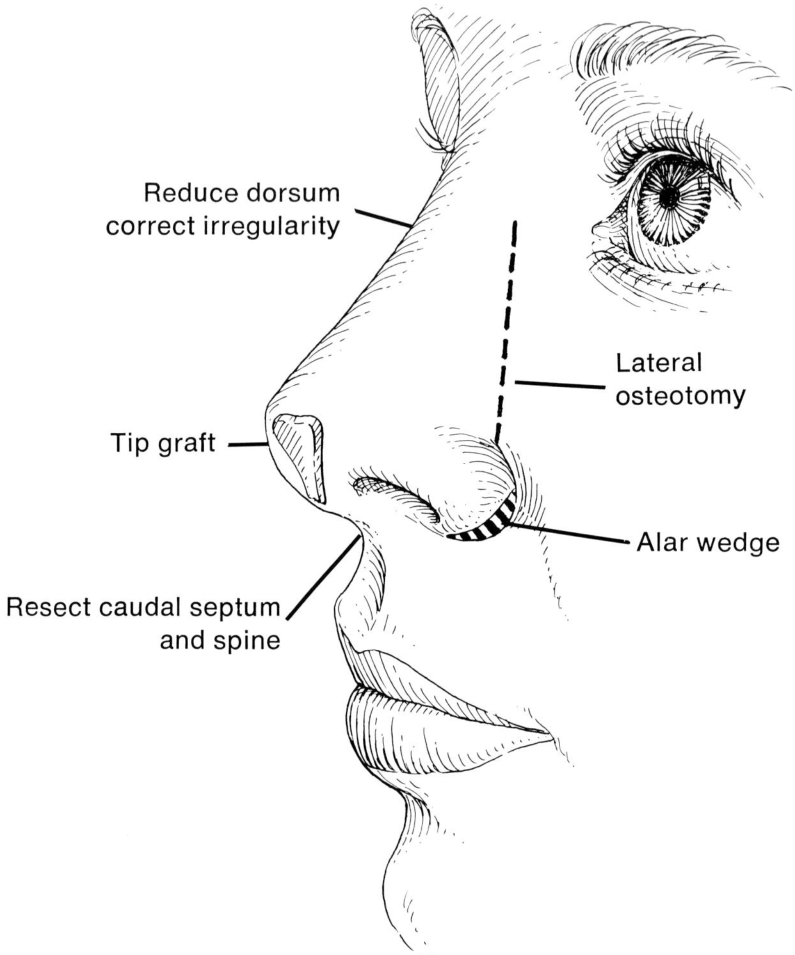

Summary of surgical procedure

1. Limited skeletonization over the cartilaginous and bony vaults
2. Reduction of the nasal spine 2 mm
3. Reduction of the entire caudal septum 3 mm
4. Reduction of the height of the dorsum 1 to 2 mm
5. Septal cartilage obtained for the tip graft
6. Placement of the tip graft
7. Lateral osteotomies
8. Bilateral alar wedge resections

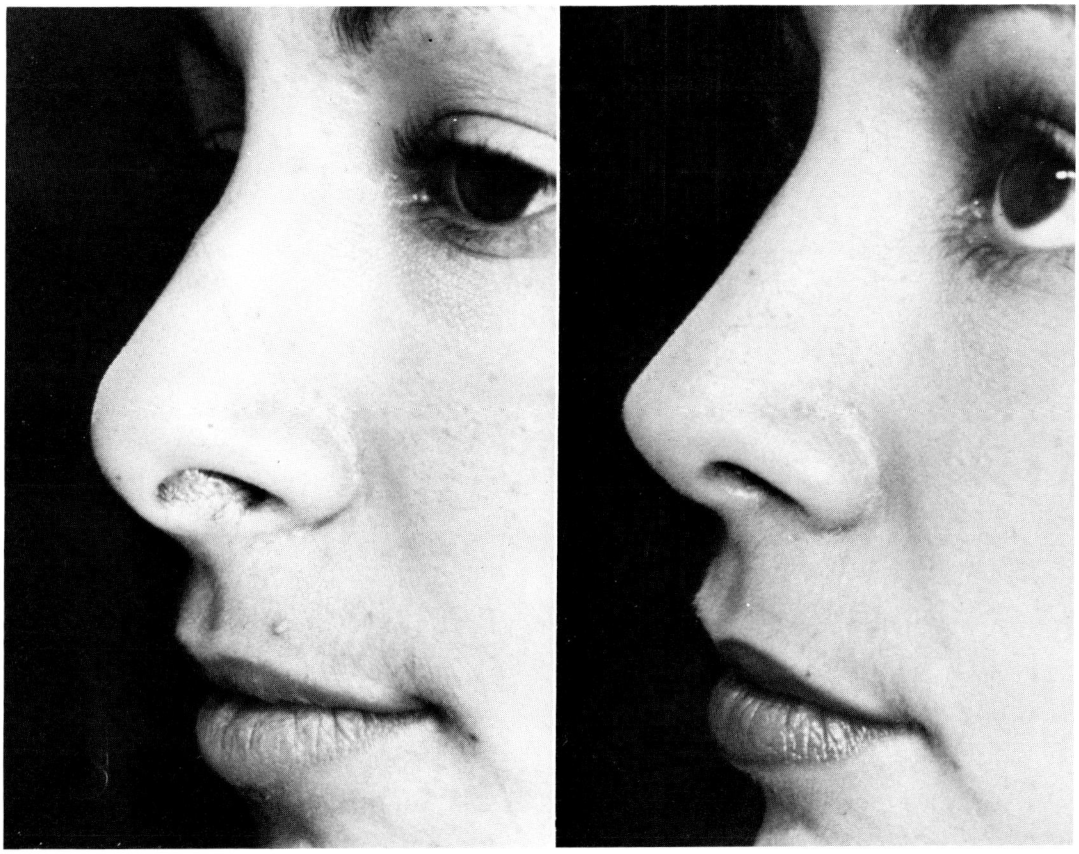

POSTOPERATIVE RESULTS

Postoperatively, the dorsum is straight, the tip has a definitive end point, and the relationship of the columella to the alae is improved.

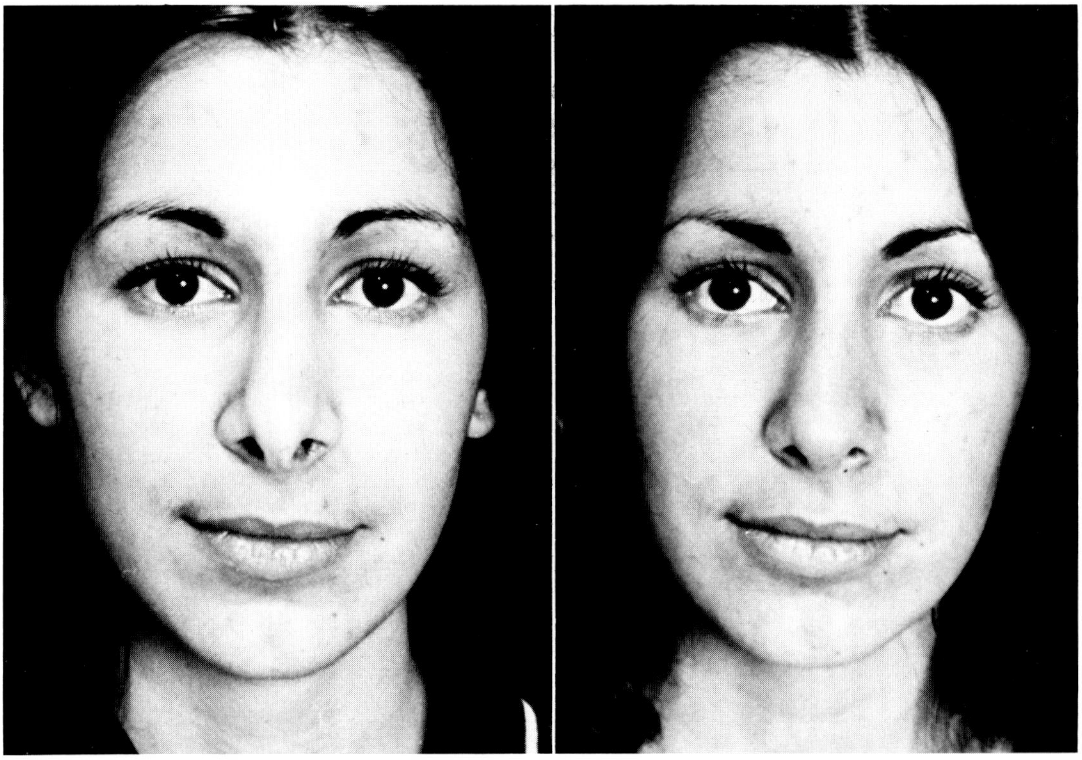

Preoperatively, the lateral nasal walls are seen to be almost parallel from the radix to the alar lobules. Following narrowing of the bony pyramid, the lateral nasal walls flow in divergent lines to the base. Elevation of the columella and reduction of the width of the alae have a favorable effect on the basal configuration.

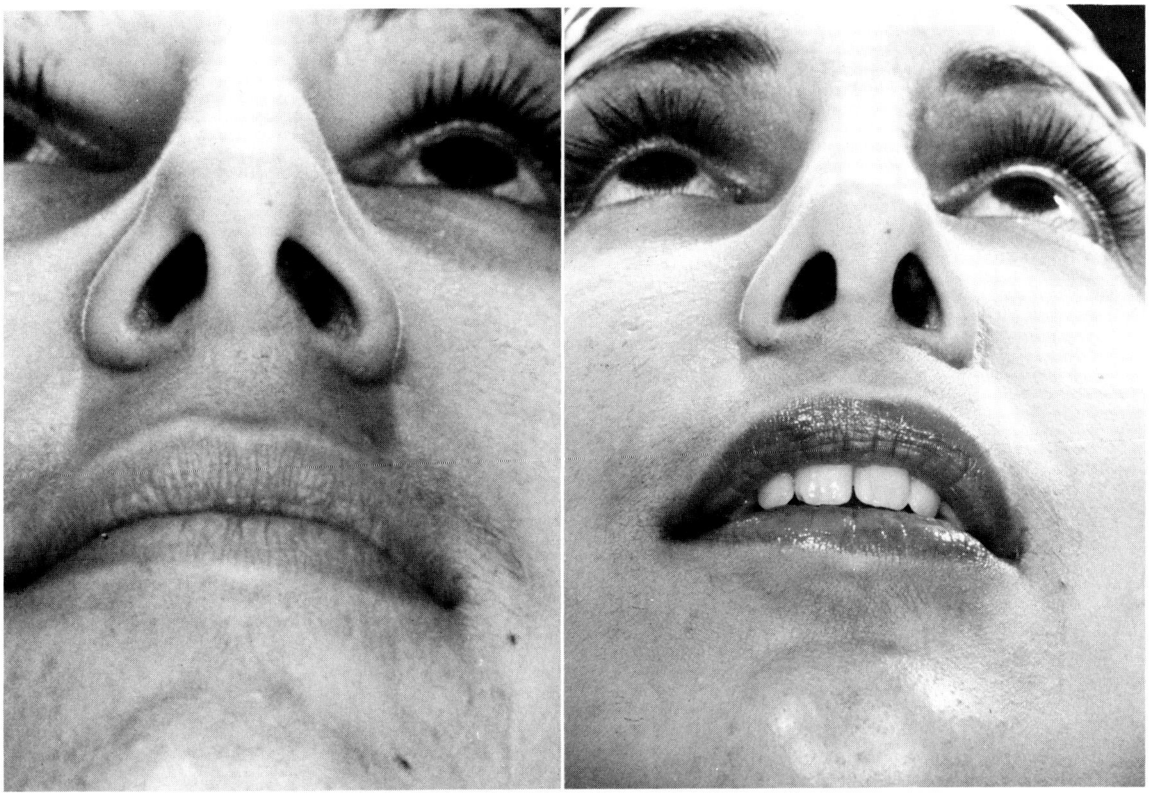

The slight excess of alar lobule has been reduced. The tip graft has narrowed and delineated the tip while re-creating the normal appearance of the domes of the lower lateral cartilages.

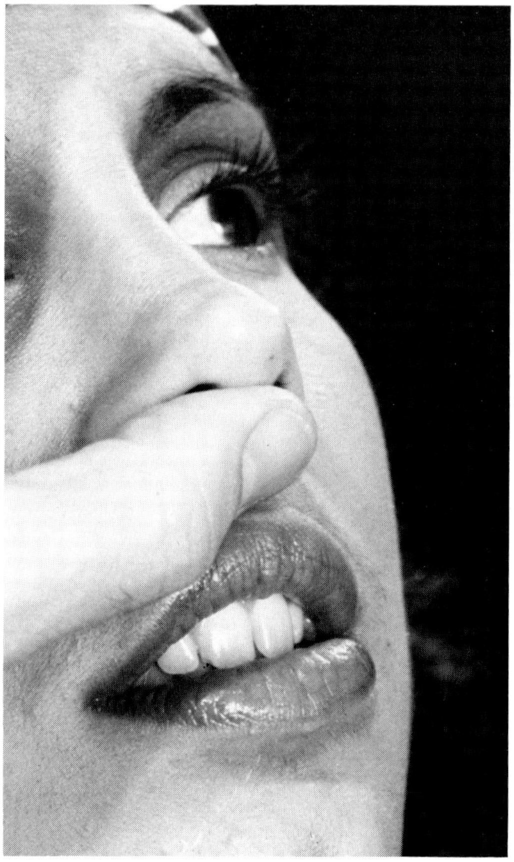

One year postoperatively the contour of the tip graft remains visible. With upward pressure on its base, the considerable width of the graft can be seen.

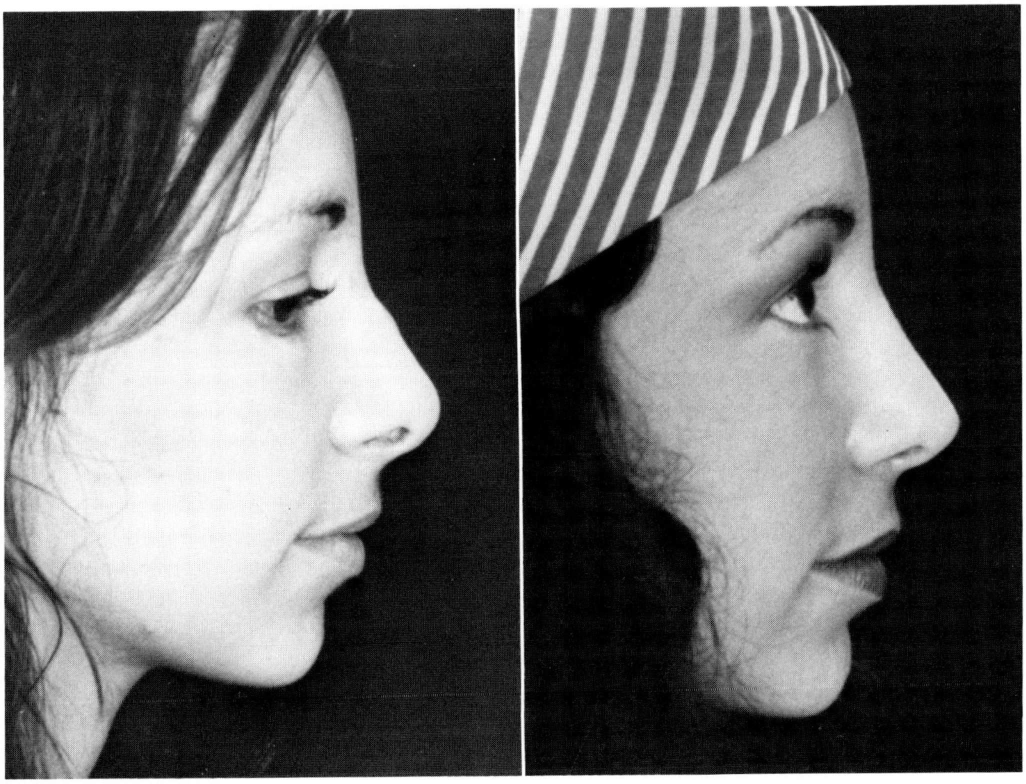

Postoperatively, all discrepant areas have been modified—dorsal irregularity, tip flatness, alar flare, prominent nasal spine, and caudal septum. Correction of the basal complex has added length to the lip.

DISCUSSION

This type of case requires finesse in diagnosis. In the absence of major deformity, attention to small details leads to the discovery of the offending parts or relationships. Because it is the sum of the discrepancies that made this nose unattractive, all of the discrepancies had to be corrected to achieve a total and attractive result. If only the dorsal irregularity were corrected, the overall appearance of the nose would not be significantly changed.

For a postsurgical nose, the condition of the tissues was exceptionally favorable. The skin was supple and fine, the framework was sufficient, and the septum was ample.

Because of the presence of many small nasal aberrations, this patient illustrates the need for a clear and specific aesthetic concept as well as for astute preoperative diagnosis.

Case report 2: Limitations of tissues

This 43-year-old man had a history of six operative procedures designed to thin out and reduce the nasal contour—all of which were unsuccessful. The patient was told that he formed scar tissue. This was reinforced in his mind because the result always looked better immediately following surgery. As time went on, the supratip area gradually raised above the level of the tip to form a classic "parrot's beak" deformity.

In addition to the obvious need for aesthetic correction, the nose was functionally impeded because of an ethmoid deformity that caused posterior narrowing and because of bilateral turbinate hypertrophy.

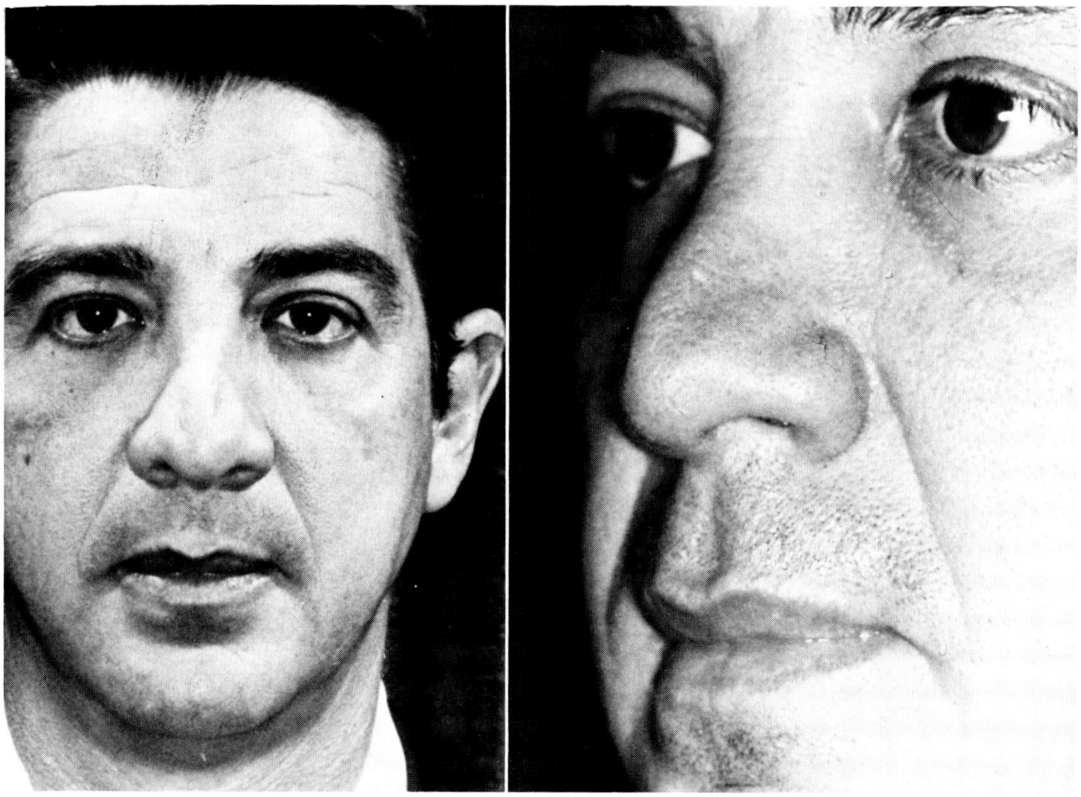

On front view, the deep vertical grooves accent a central ridge of tissues. The dorsum is low; the nasal base is massive. On oblique view, the heavy alar lobules and central ridge contribute to the cumbrous appearance of this nose.

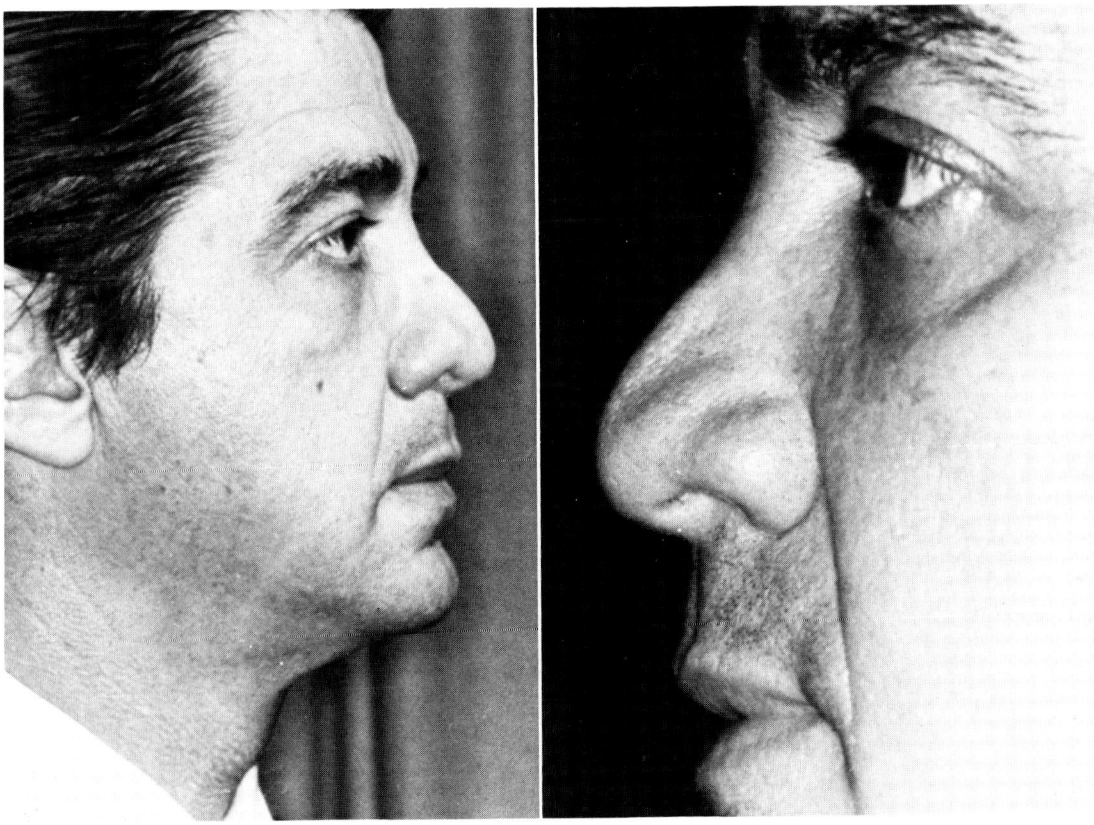

On lateral view, the dorsum is too low for the bulky lower third. Though the nasolabial angle is satisfactory, the nose has the appearance of downward inclination because of the high supratip area. The vertical grooves and the central ridge are evidences of repeated attempts to thin and reduce the dorsal tissues.

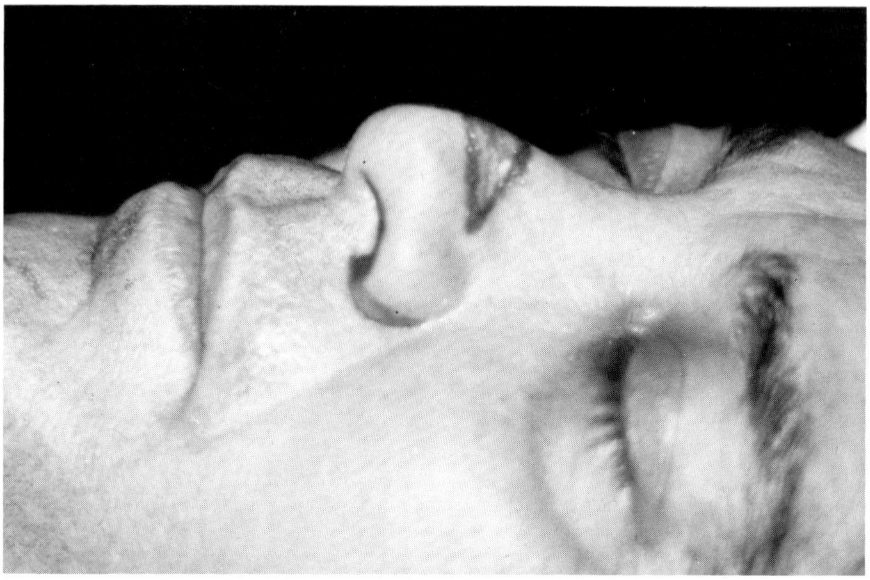

SURGICAL PROCEDURE

Preoperative markings show the generous horizontal excision, which measured 6 mm at its center.

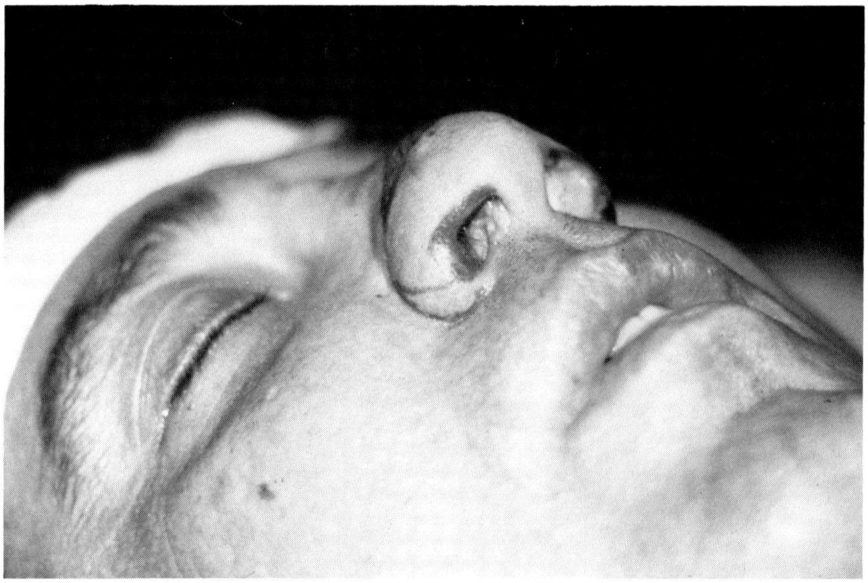

Markings on basal view show the extent of thinning of the alar walls in addition to reduction of the large alar lobules.

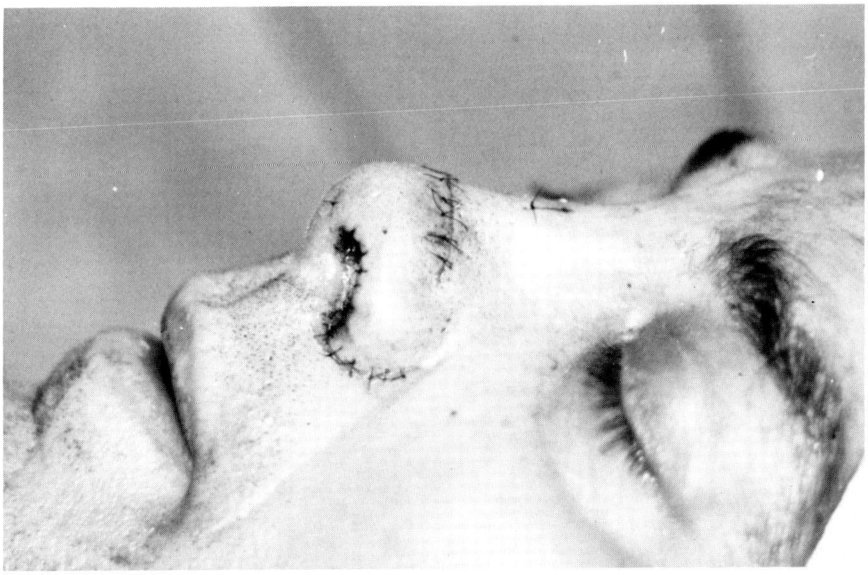

The dorsal graft of septal cartilage and the tip graft are secured with a single 6-0 nylon suture. Because the base of the nose was slightly dusky, the packing was kept to a minimum, and the dressing was placed without plaster and then removed in 24 hours.

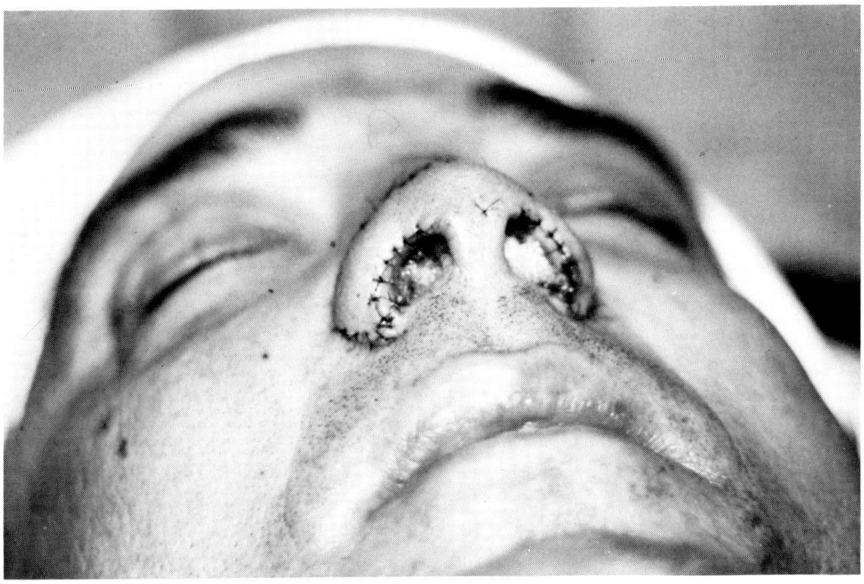

There is some reduction in the overall mass of the nasal base without narrowing the perimeter of the nostrils.

Summary of surgical procedure

1. Major septoplasty, with partial resection of vomer and ethmoid and partial inferior turbinectomy
2. Horizontal excision of soft tissues, not including mucosa
3. Three-layered cartilage graft to dorsum
4. Tip graft of septal cartilage
5. Sculpting resections of nostrils and alar lobules

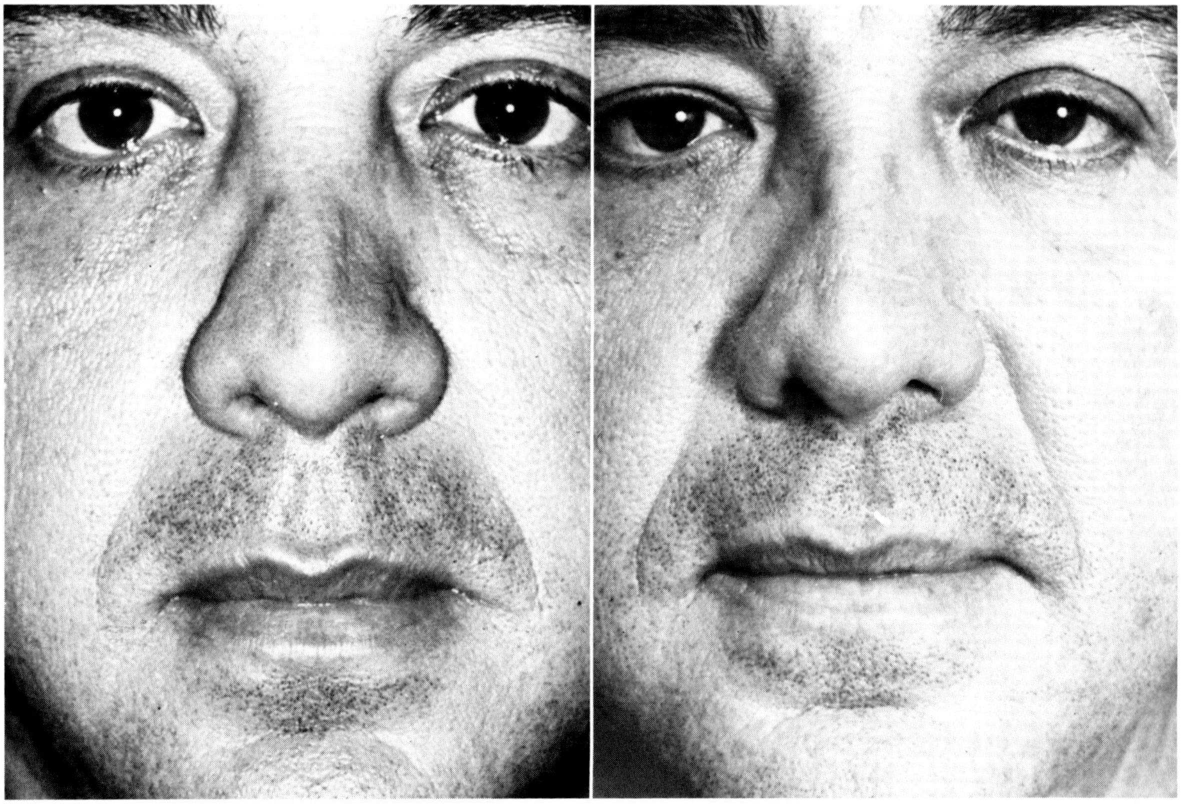

POSTOPERATIVE RESULTS

Seven years postoperatively, the nasal base, which has been narrowed by alar wedge resections, is still broad for the dorsal area. The horizontal scar is an acceptable exchange for the reduction of the ridged, redundant supratip skin. The elevation of the dorsum has added dimension to the central third of his face.

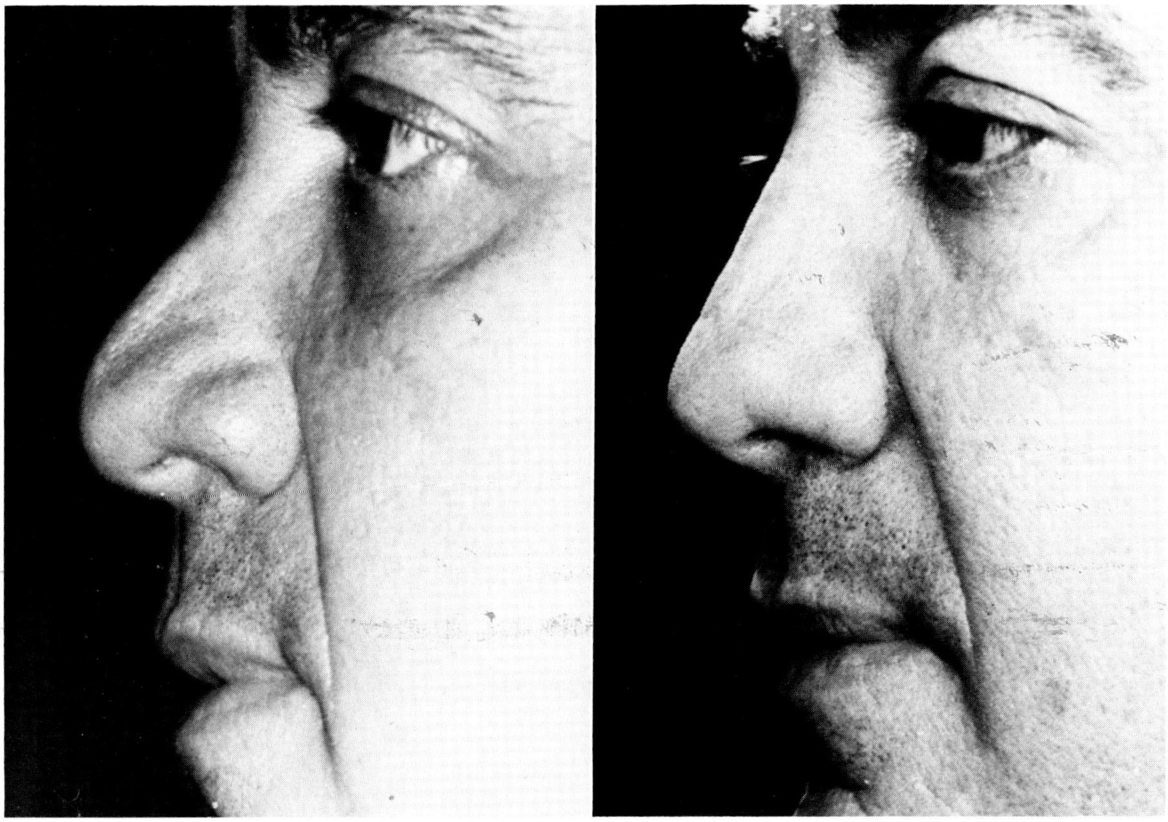

On lateral view, the dorsum is straight, the tip is almost in line with it, and the relationships of the nasal base are good. The scar is barely visible.

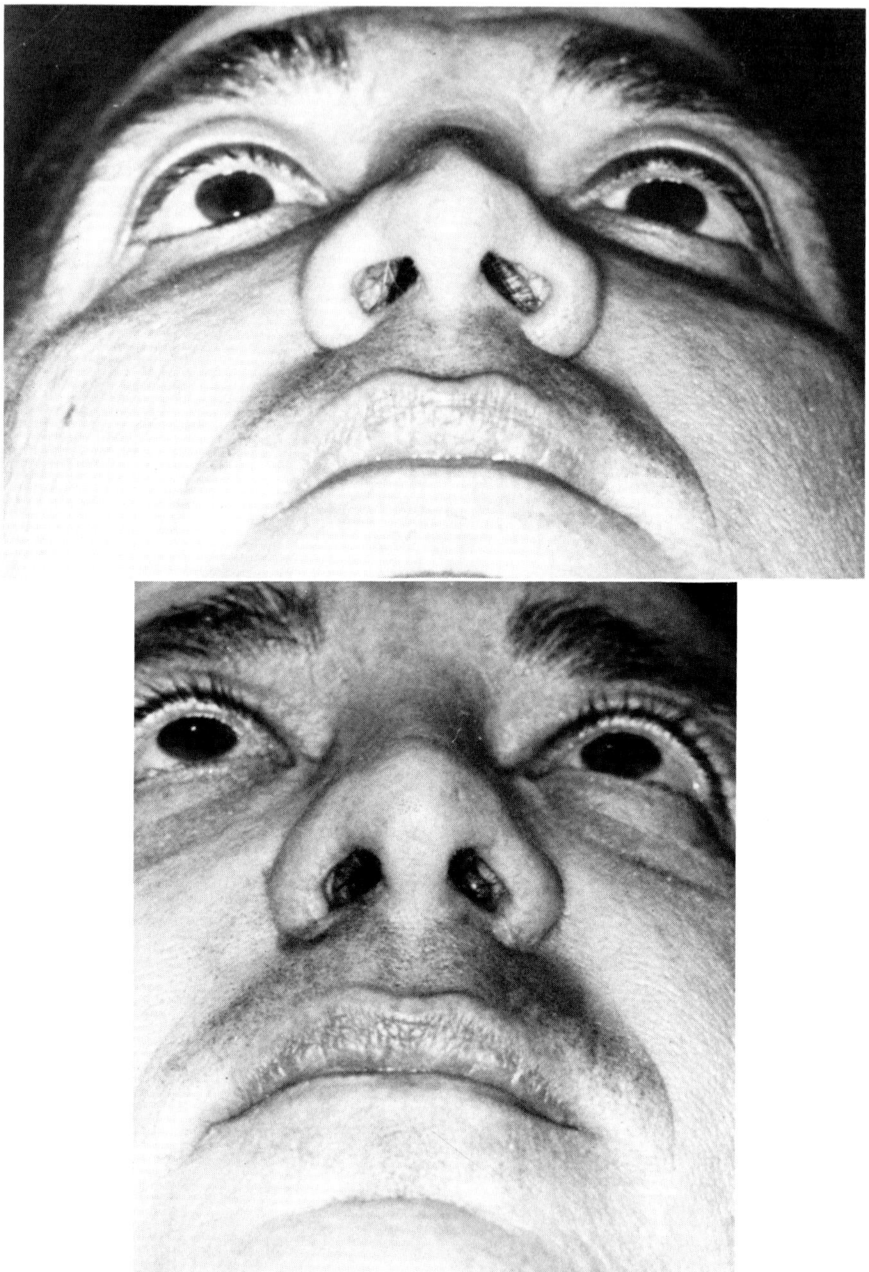

The nasal base is improved postoperatively but remains bulky. The perimeter of the small nostrils was not changed; however, their position was altered from horizontal to more vertical.

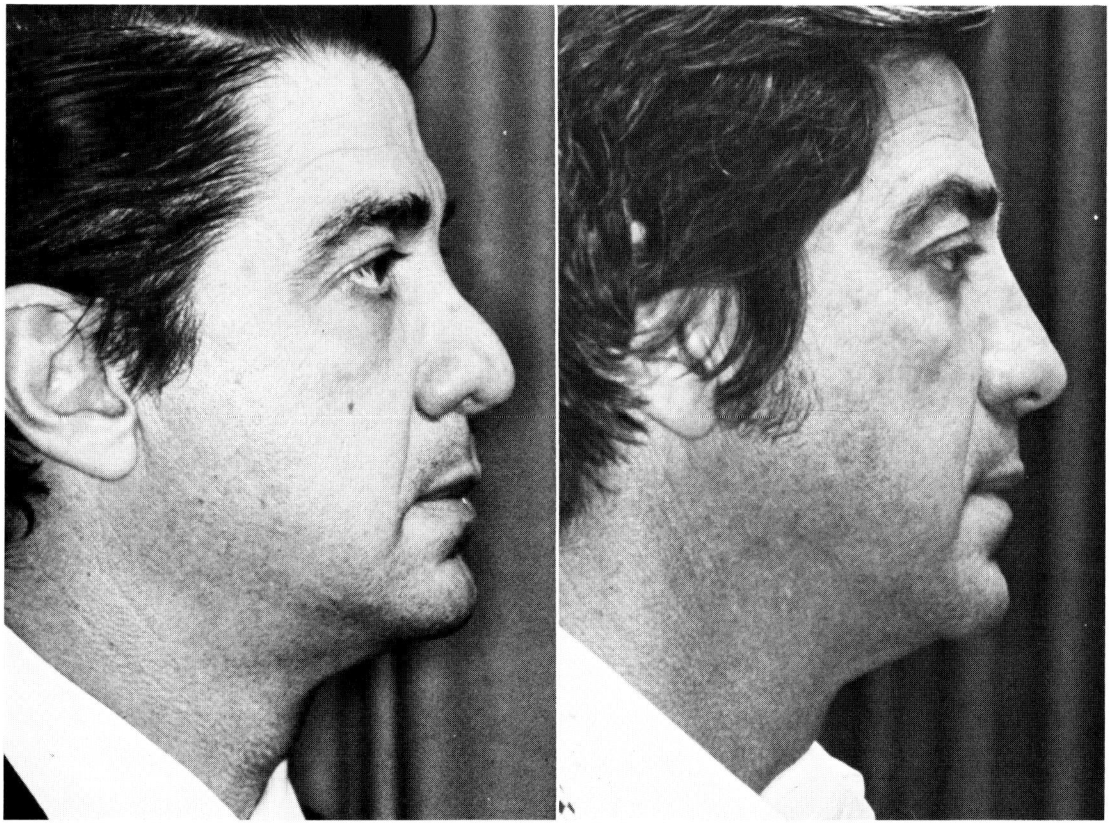

On right lateral view, the nasofacial proportion is improved. In spite of the scars across the dorsum and the base of his nose, the postoperative view appears less surgical than does the preoperative view.

DISCUSSION

The identification of the functional and aesthetic problems of a nose is only part of the diagnosis. Also important is a determination of the nature of those problems. Very often, one must point to the condition or limitations of the tissues as the source of postsurgical deformities. In this case, the prior surgeons recognized that the dorsal tissues were excessive, but they failed to recognize (six times) that these tissues would not contract down to the reduced skeleton.

An assessment of this patient's surgical history and his tissues would indicate that further subdermal dissection would not reduce the supratip fullness, since the tissues did not drape over the dorsal edge of the septum. The limits of tissue contractility had been reached.

Not only was this a problem of overreduced framework, but there was also an *actual* surplus (not relative, as in many secondary rhinoplasties) of soft tissues over the lower third of the nose. Therefore, the patient was advised that although dorsal augmentation would improve the nose, nothing short of external excisions of soft tissue would significantly change its appearance.

Following the patient's acceptance of the prospect of visible scars, a decision had to be made about the design and amount of excision. Excision of the long, vertical ridge of tissue was tempting, but if it were removed, the excision most likely would have been excessive. On the other hand, a transverse excision would eliminate some of the grooves and some of the ridge. Also, it would provide access to the dorsum for augmentation without disturbing tip circulation, and it would rotate the tip cephalad. The transverse excision had plain advantages.

The dorsal approach for augmentation ensured vascular continuity of all the tissues of the nasal base so that extensive alar wedge resections and a tip graft could be undertaken safely.

Limiting the dissection

A major difference in primary and secondary nasal surgery is the scarring and decreased vascularity usually present in the secondary patient. Because of this, patients who have had multiple procedures are in danger of tissue loss if routine rhinoplastic techniques are used. Extensive undermining is both unnecessary and hazardous. Every cut made in revisional rhinoplasty further compromises the remaining circulation. Therefore, the placement of every incision and the limits of dissection must be carefully planned preoperatively.

Although the nose is an extremely vascular organ that can withstand considerable surgery, it is not immune to unlimited assault. If, during the course of a revisional rhinoplasty, any or all of the following maneuvers are to be performed, consider the consequences to the blood supply:

1. Local anesthesia with epinephrine
2. Skeletonization
3. Supratip thinning
4. Transection of the membranous septum
5. Alar wedge resections
6. Tip exploration or tip graft of cartilage
7. Rigid splint over the nasal tissues

If excessive scarring is present, the danger should be obvious.

The following case presentation illustrates the development of a vascular problem subsequent to a revisional rhinoplasty that I performed.

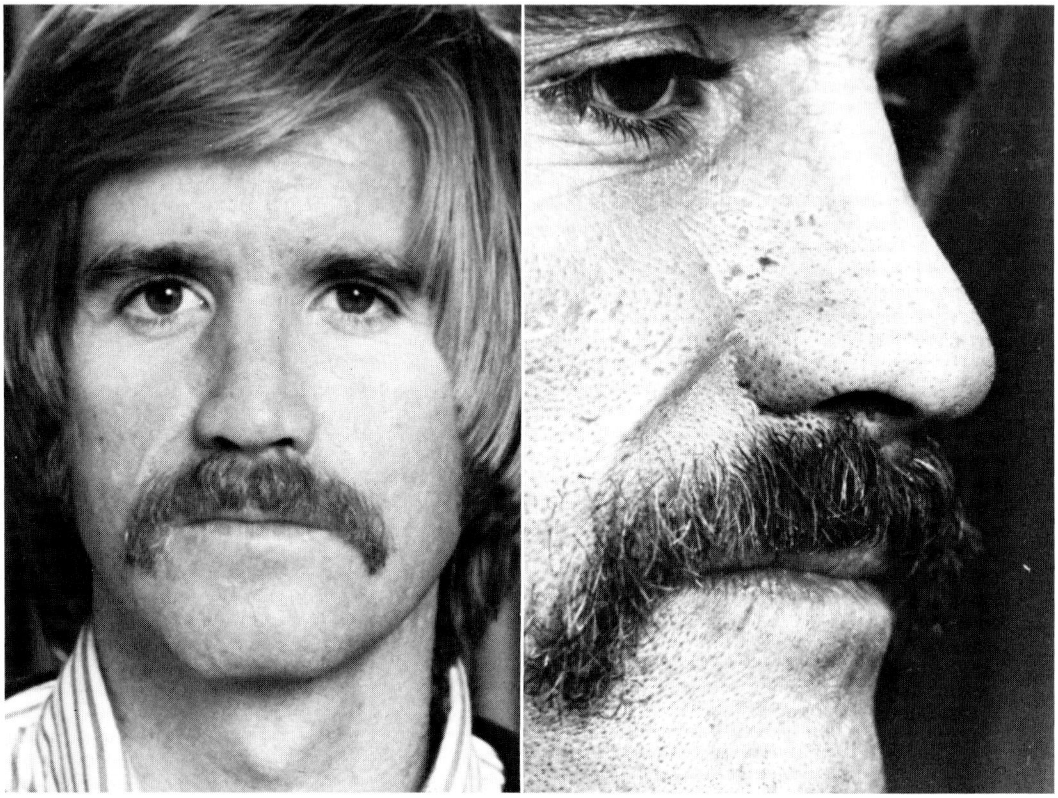

Case report

A 32-year-old patient is seen 14 months after the last of three rhinoplasties. The primary rhinoplasty was unsatisfactory because of supratip fullness. One year later a secondary procedure was done to thin out the supratip area and further reduce the skeleton. The result of the secondary was worse than the first; therefore, a third procedure was done to reduce the size of the nostrils and to place a silicone prosthesis over the dorsum.

The patient's primary complaints were related to the movable prosthesis, the lack of tip projection, and the relative supratip fullness.

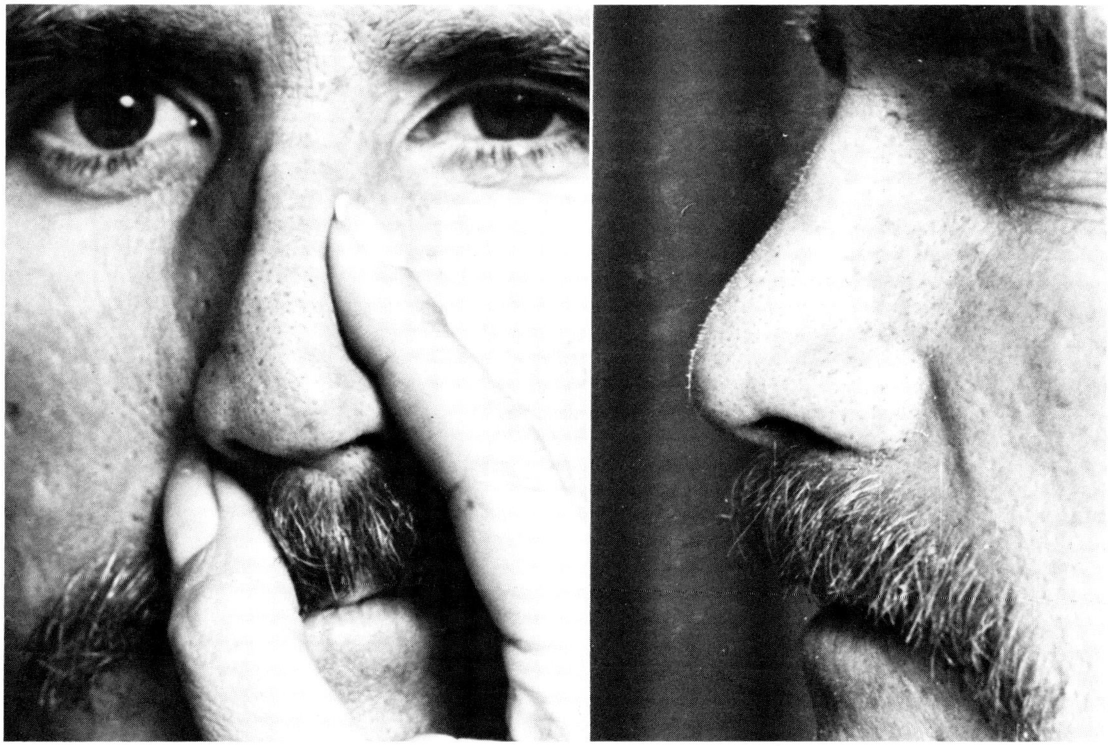

Examination confirmed a freely movable, firm prosthesis. On lateral examination, a well-healed surgical scar was found to extend over 75% of the alar-facial groove. The dorsum was straight, the supratip was slightly high, and the tip was flat. The nasolabial angle was 90 degrees.

Summary of surgical procedure

1. Bilateral intracartilaginous incisions
2. Dissection under the capsule of the prosthesis
3. Removal of the prosthesis
4. Resection of an ellipse of the membranous septum to the posterior third of the caudal septum
5. Submucous resection to obtain graft material
6. Dorsal graft inserted under the capsule
7. Tip graft inserted in a separate pocket

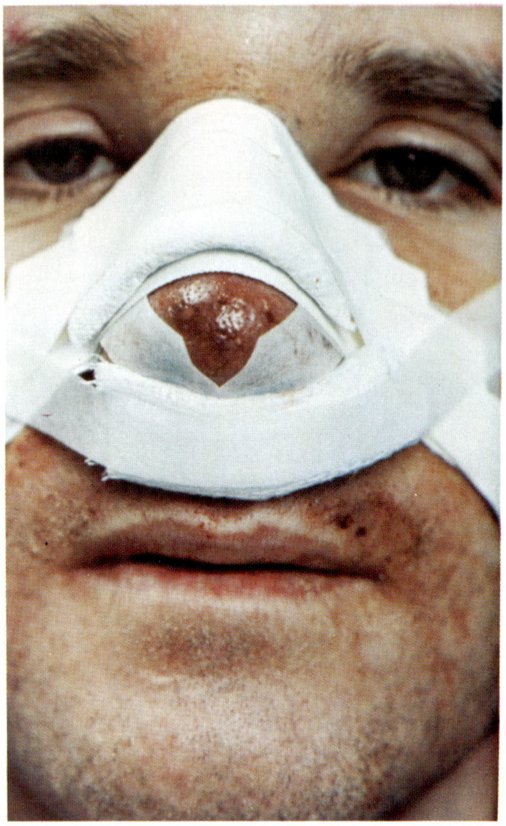

POSTOPERATIVE RESULTS

The patient is shown on the morning following surgery. The top packs of Adaptic gauze were removed from both sides. The plaster was removed, and the tape around the tip was cut. Ice compresses, antibiotics, and restricted activity were prescribed.

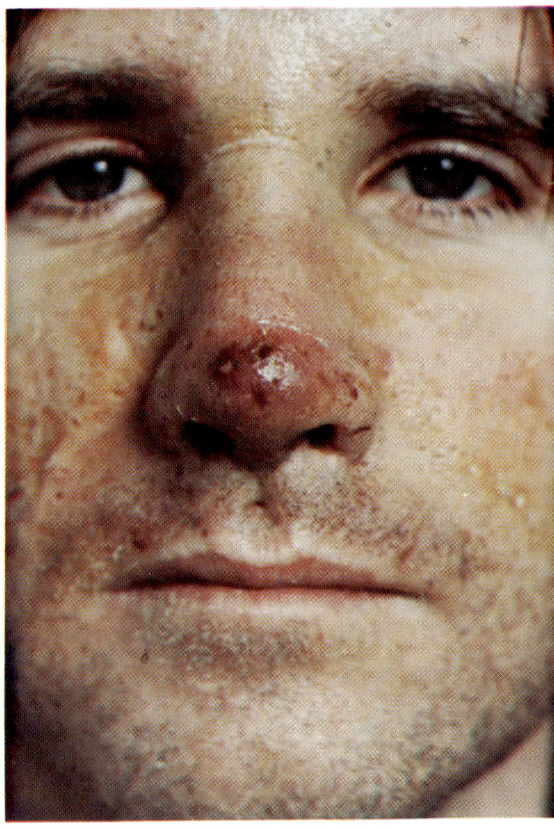

By the end of the first week, the tape was removed. The cyanosis and edema had subsided slightly.

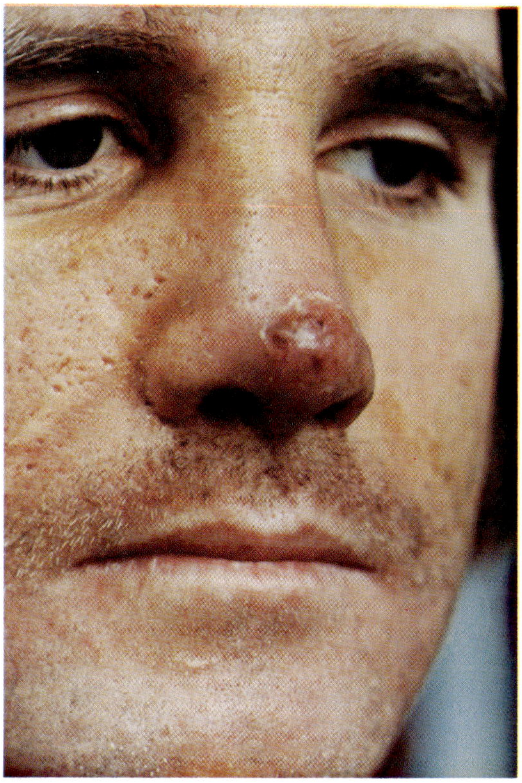

By the ninth postoperative day, there were favorable signs of resolution.

Twelve days after surgery the patient had almost complete resolution.

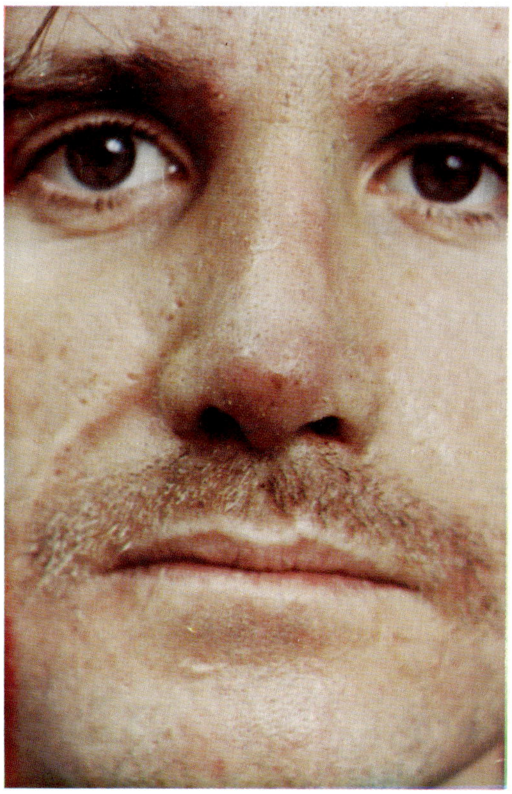

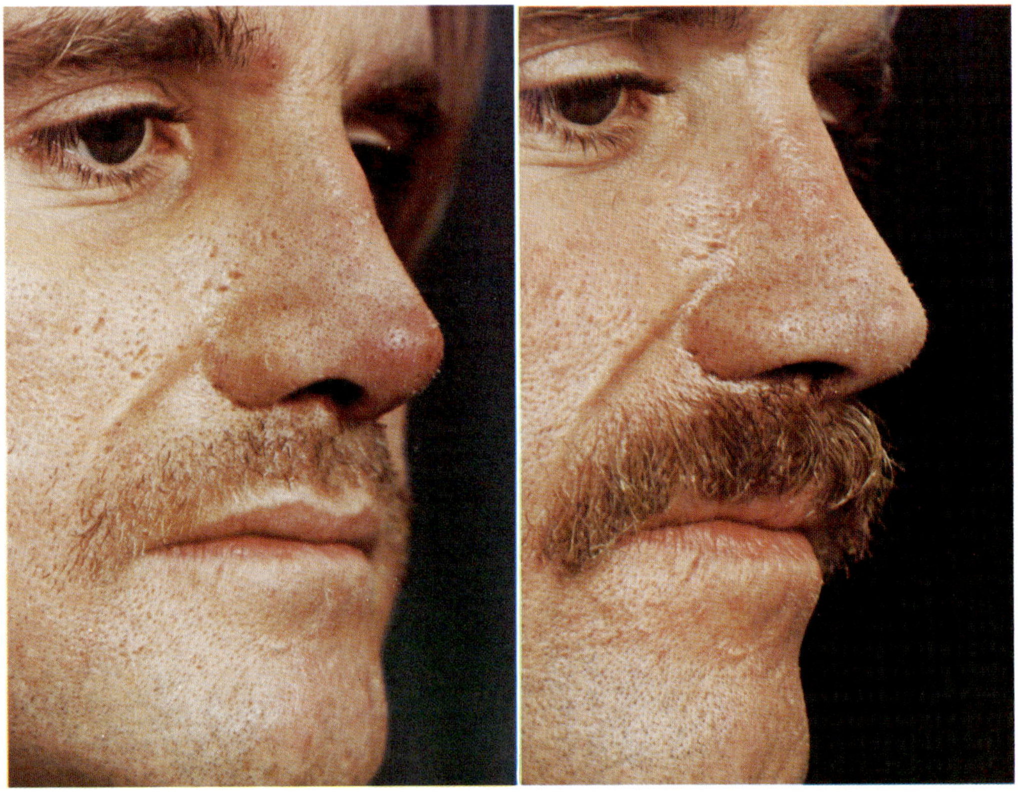

The patient is shown 12 days and 13 months after surgery.

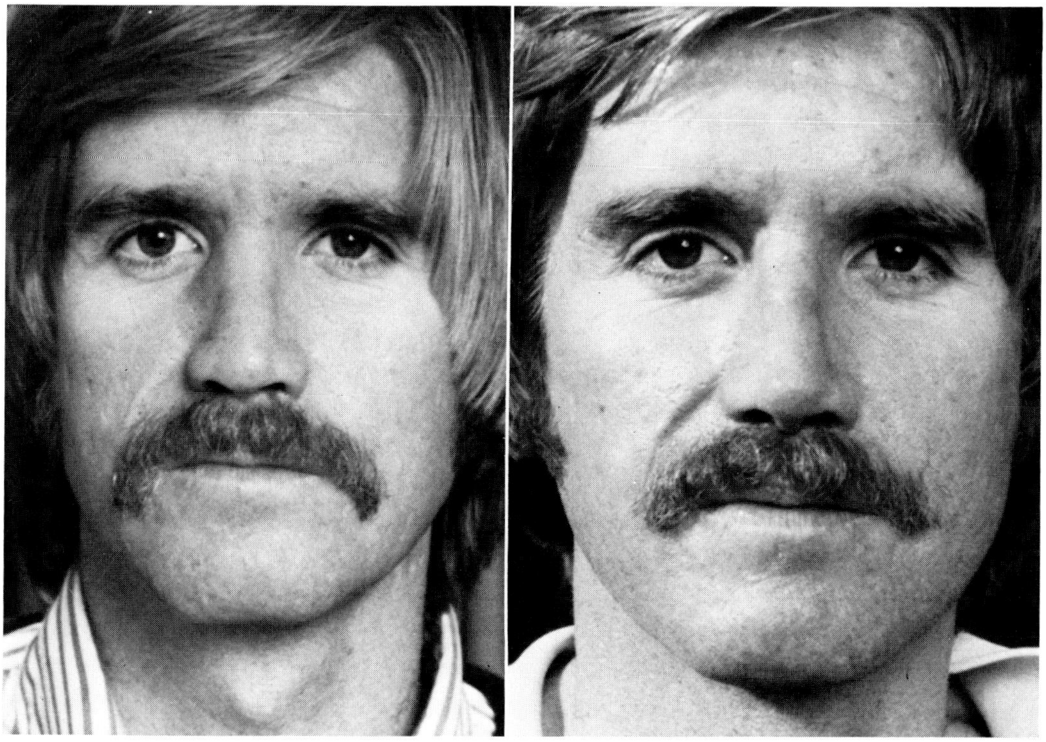

Fourteen months after surgery there is a narrower dorsum and greater tip definition. The relationships of the base have been improved by the slight cephalic rotation of the tip and the increase in tip projection from the graft.

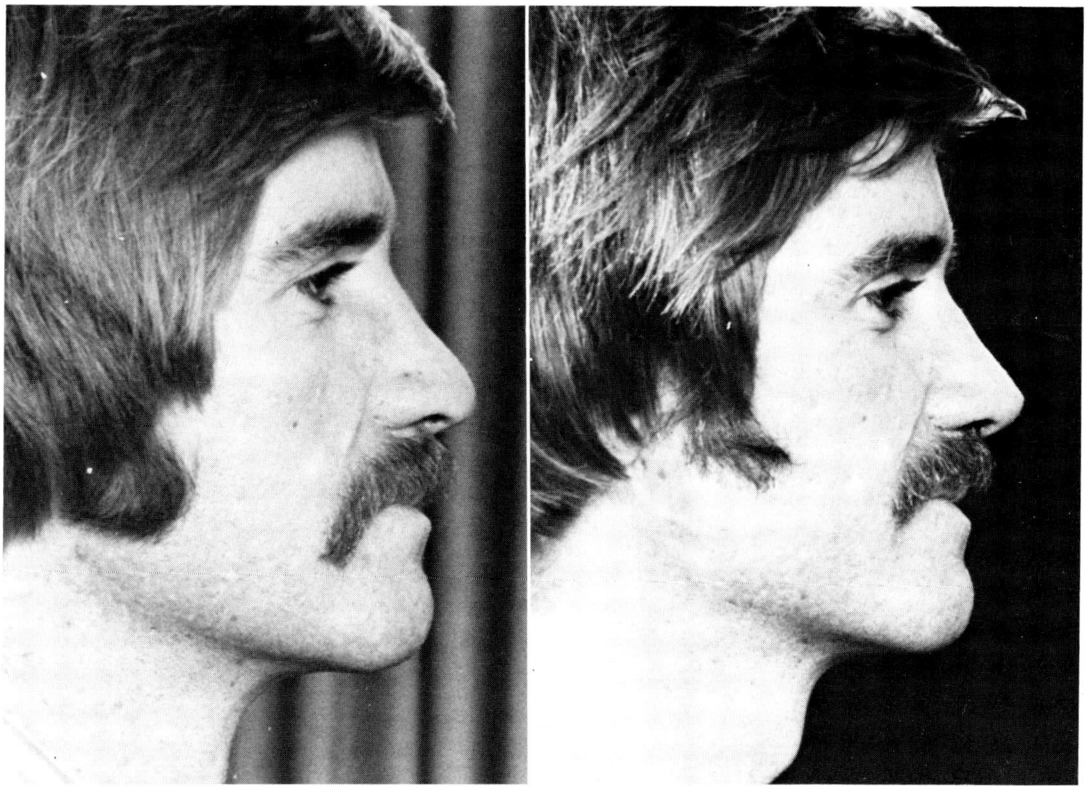

On right lateral view, the dorsum is straight, and the projection of the tip graft has eliminated the relative supratip fullness.

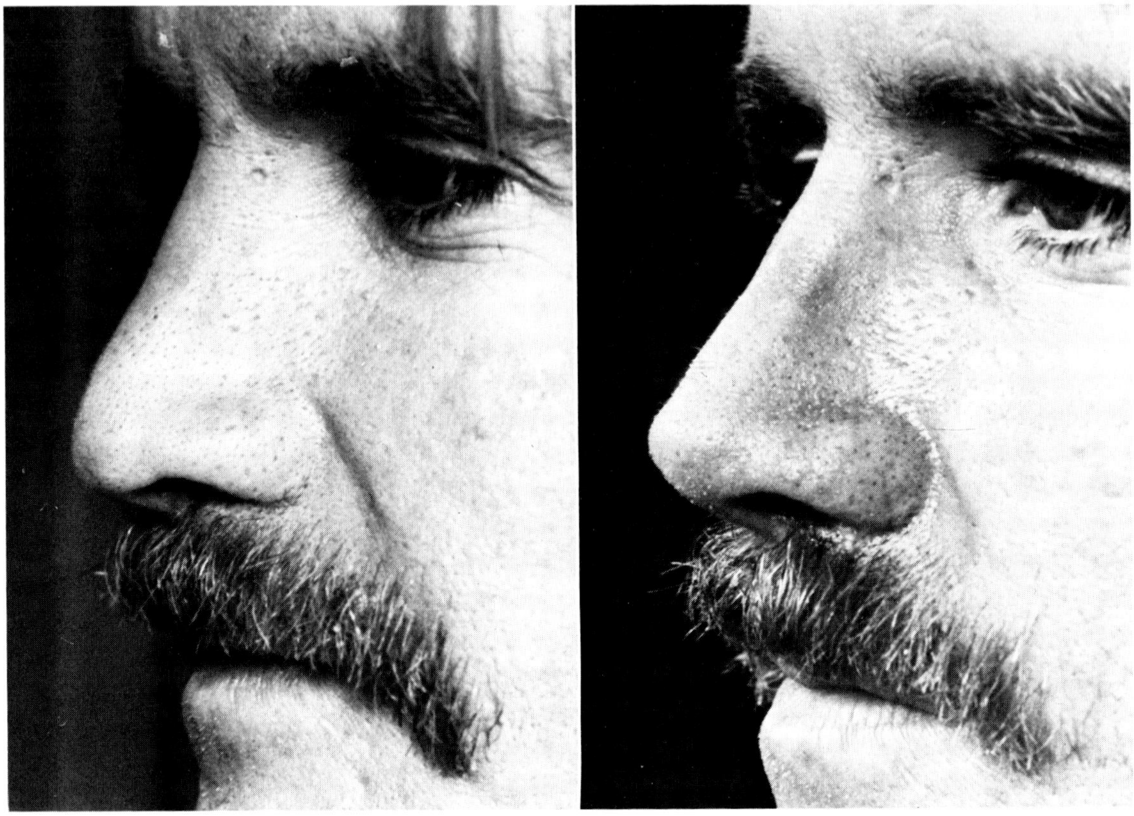

Postoperatively, the septal cartilage dorsal graft provides sufficient height and remains firmly implanted as a permanent part of the nasal pyramid. The structural effect of the tip graft adds refinement to the overall appearance of the nose.

DISCUSSION

In retrospect, this vascular compromise might have been avoided if unilateral rather than bilateral cartilage-splitting incisions had been made. These would have preserved one-half the blood supply to the tip. The tip was dissected from the dorsal tissues in order to allow proper tissue draping over the tip graft. However, one must realize that this dissection is a risk. My judgment to take this risk was influenced by the age of the patient and the apparent health of the tissues.

This case demonstrates the importance of vigilant postoperative observation of the secondary rhinoplasty patient. It further demonstrates that immediate treatment—release of the dressing, ice compresses, prophylactic antibiotics, and decreased patient activity—can prevent a serious complication.

Using only autogenous material

The use of alloplastic material in revisional rhinoplasty is a disservice to the patient and, too often, an embarrassment to the surgeon. The incidence of rejection, infection, or late extrusion is too high to recommend its use. There are donor areas that readily provide excellent autogenous material for a safe and permanent reconstruction.

The choice of material varies with the location of the defect. Listed in the order of preference, there are: septal cartilage, ear cartilage, and vomer or iliac bone for the dorsum; septal cartilage or ear cartilage for tip reconstruction; ethmoid for nasal wall deformities; and composite ear grafts for deformities of the vestibule. All of these grafts are autogenous, leave little or no deformity at the donor site, and provide permanent reconstruction.

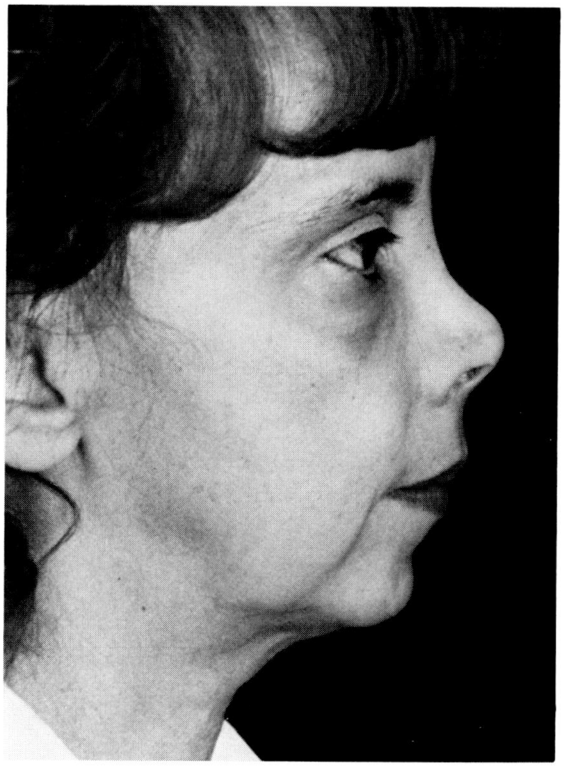

Case report

This woman is seen following five nasal surgeries. Her surgical history included postoperative infection and extrusion of a silicone prosthesis through the nasal tip. The tissues appeared too scarred and contracted to afford much hope for improvement. On internal examination, there was a septal perforation near the angle of the septum.

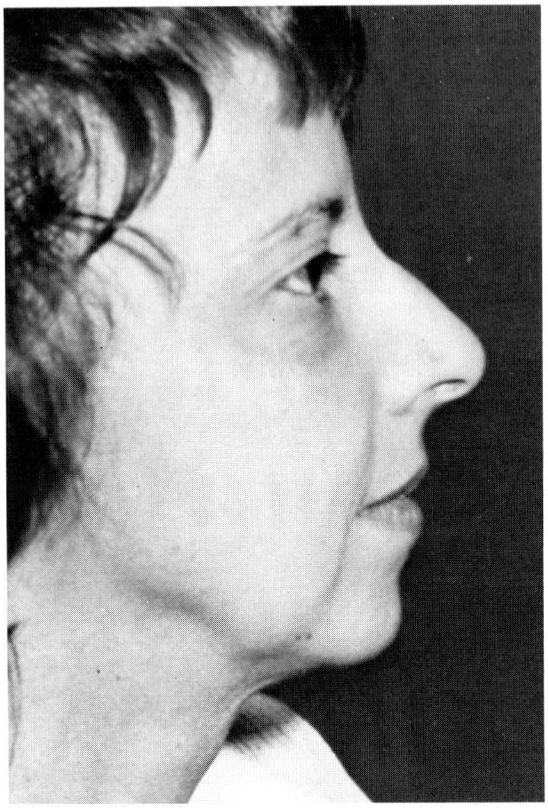

This preoperative photograph of the patient shows a slightly elevated dorsum. The relationships within the basal complex and appearance of the tissues are excellent. In retrospect, only a slight dorsal resection, lateral osteotomies, and tip refinement might have been sufficient for an excellent result.

Following the first surgical procedure, the patient displays the classic secondary rhinoplasty syndrome: low dorsum, high supratip, poor tip definition, open nasolabial angle, and flaring nostrils. At this point, appropriate treatment would have been to augment the dorsum with a septal cartilage graft and to obtain more tip definition with a septal cartilage tip graft.

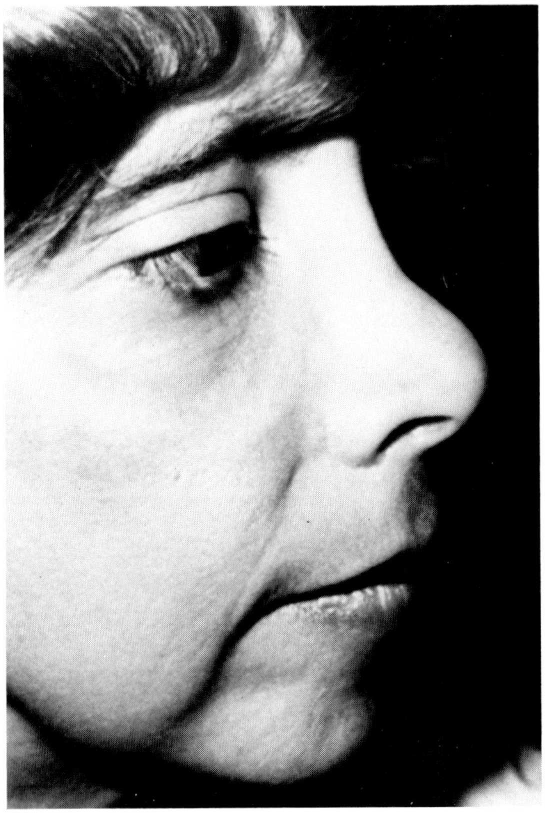

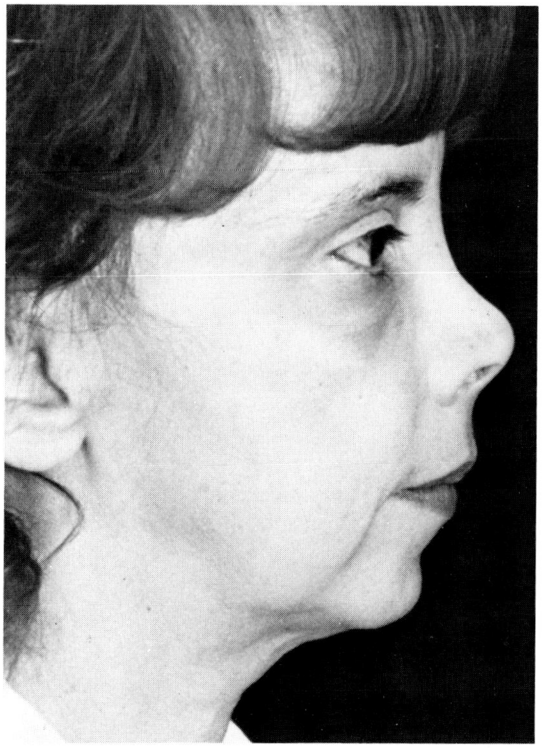

Following four more surgical procedures, all parts of the nose are severely reduced. All usable septal cartilage has been removed and a 1-cm perforation is present at the angle of the septum. The nasal tip appears to be turning away from the viewer.

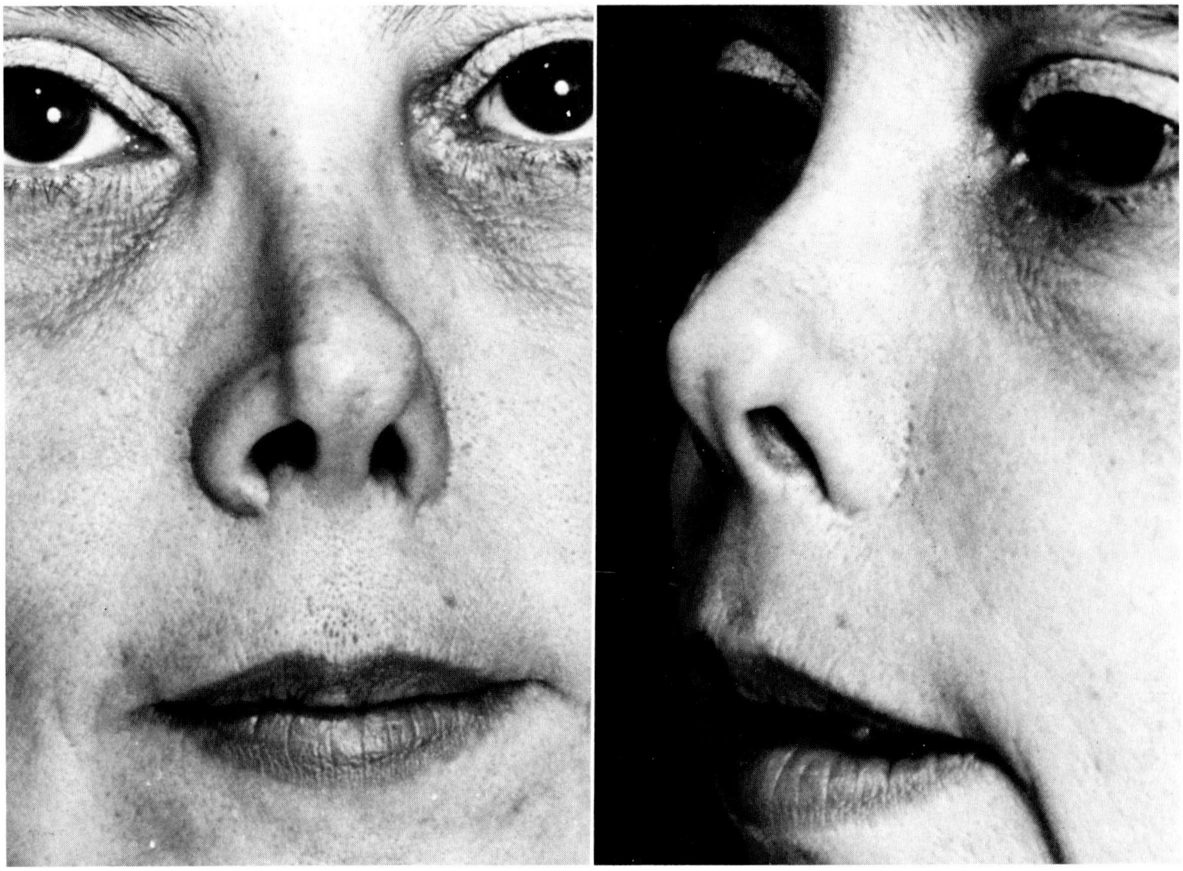

On close-up front view, there is a decided right-to-left twist to the nose, which is caused by the concavity on the left nasal wall and the projecting left dome of the lower lateral cartilage.

On left oblique view, the nasal tip appears to twist toward the viewer, bringing into view a depressed scar just above the columella.

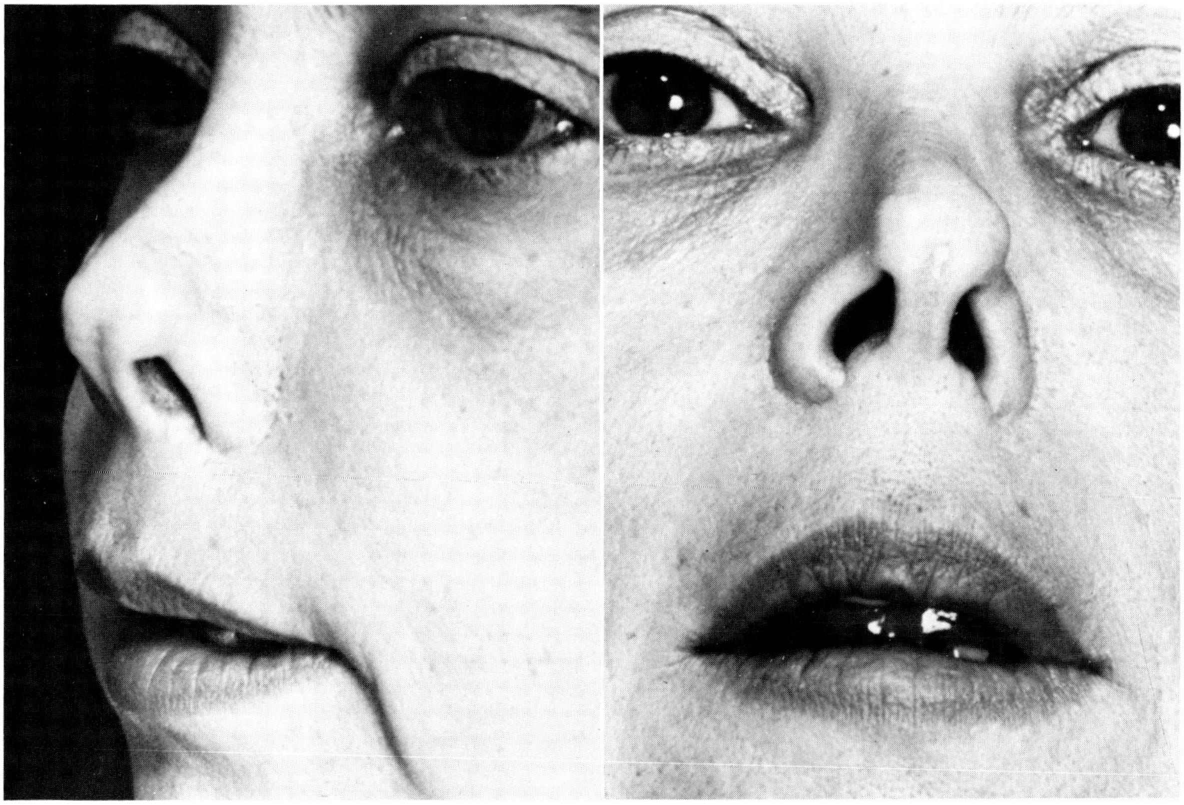

On close-up oblique view, the extreme reduction of the entire skeleton is evident. The nasolabial angle is unacceptably wide.

The basal view shows a depressed, well-healed scar at the center of the tip lobule. The nostrils are irregular, with bilateral notching that is greater on the left.

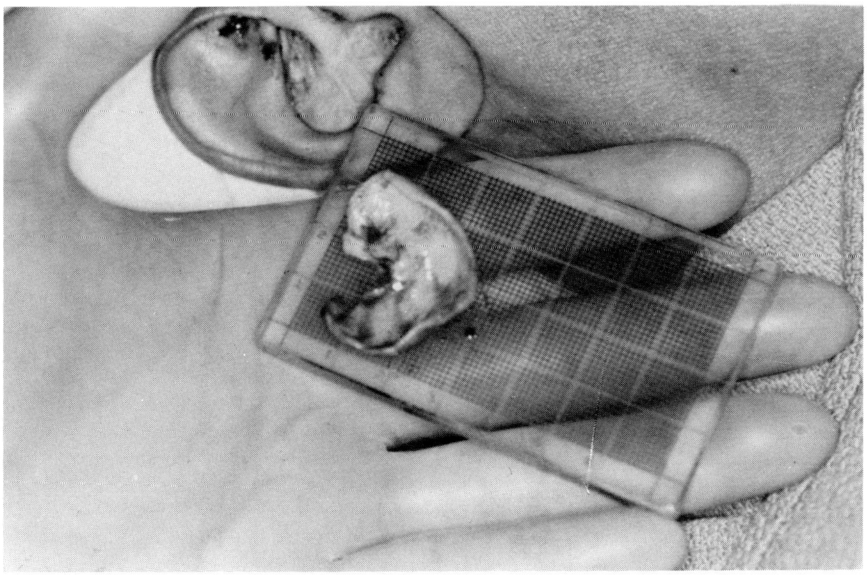

SURGICAL PROCEDURE

The specimen of conchal cartilage is shown lying on a 1-mm grid with the anterior, or concave, surface up.

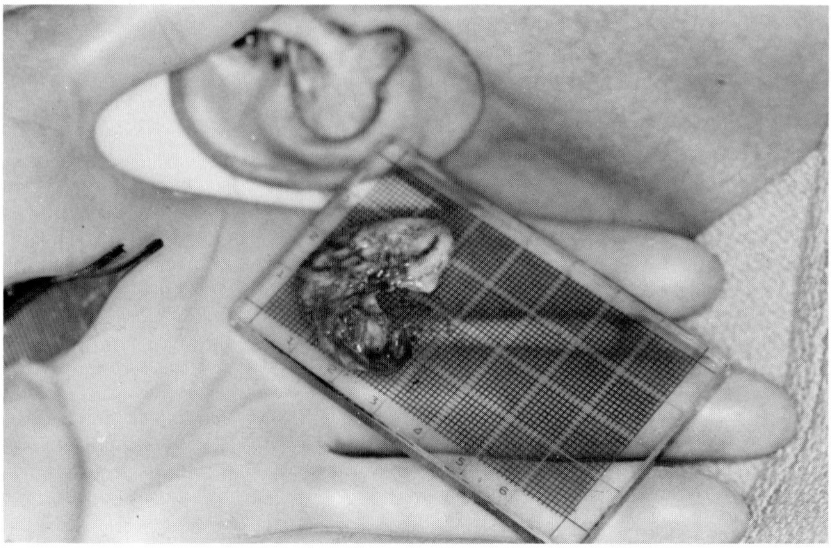

The posterior surface is shown with the attached perichondrium and soft tissues.

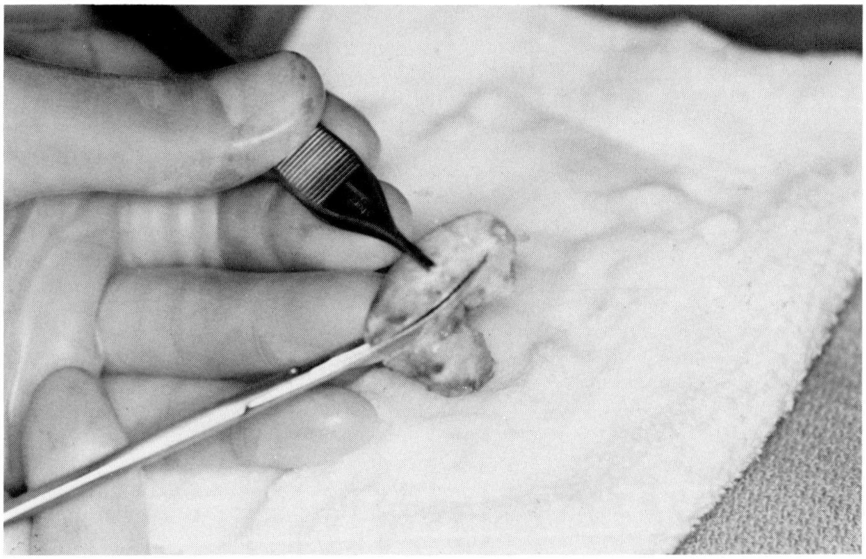

The cartilage is methodically cut to render the longest, most usable piece.

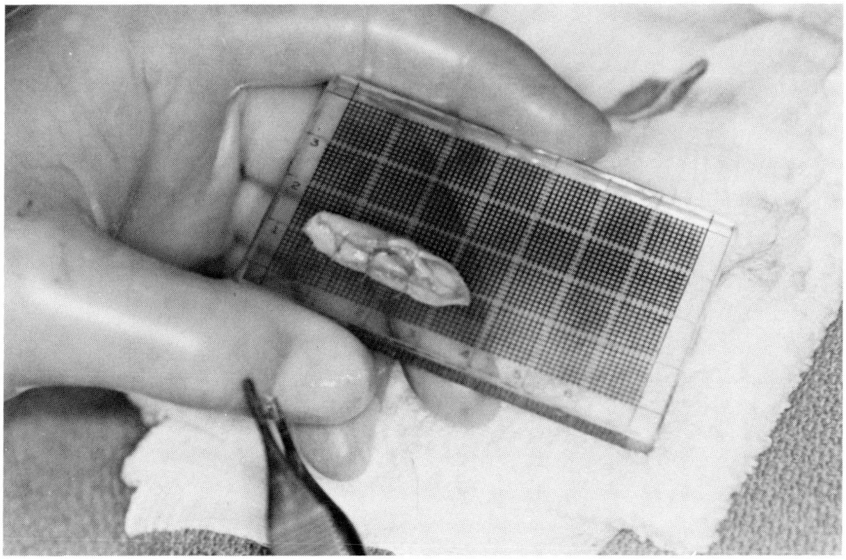

Following final contouring, the graft (ventral side up) is sutured over some cartilage fragments with 5-0 Dexon.

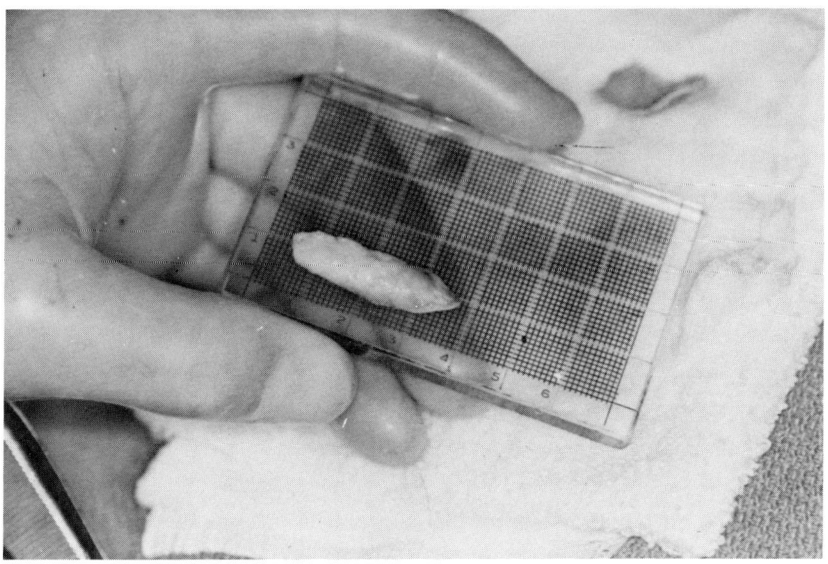

The conchal cartilage graft creates a remarkably smooth nasal dorsum.

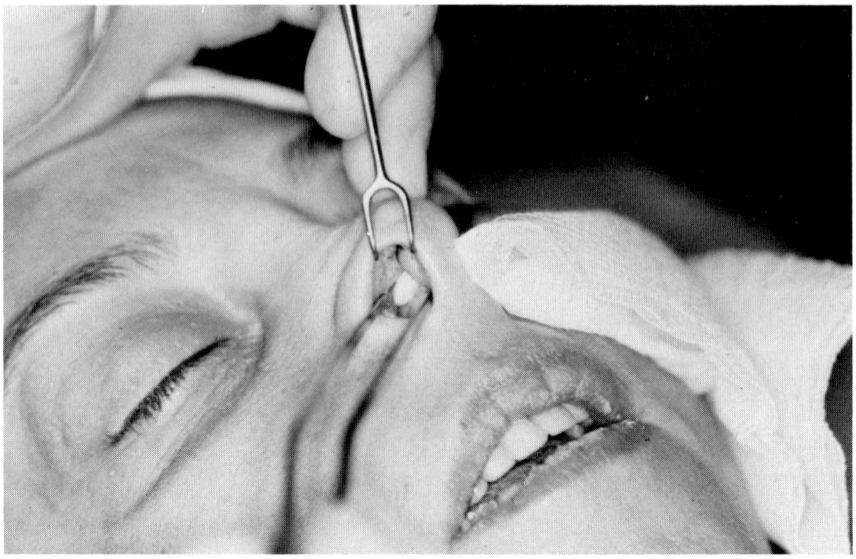

The septal fistula is shown from the right with a piece of gauze pulled through it.

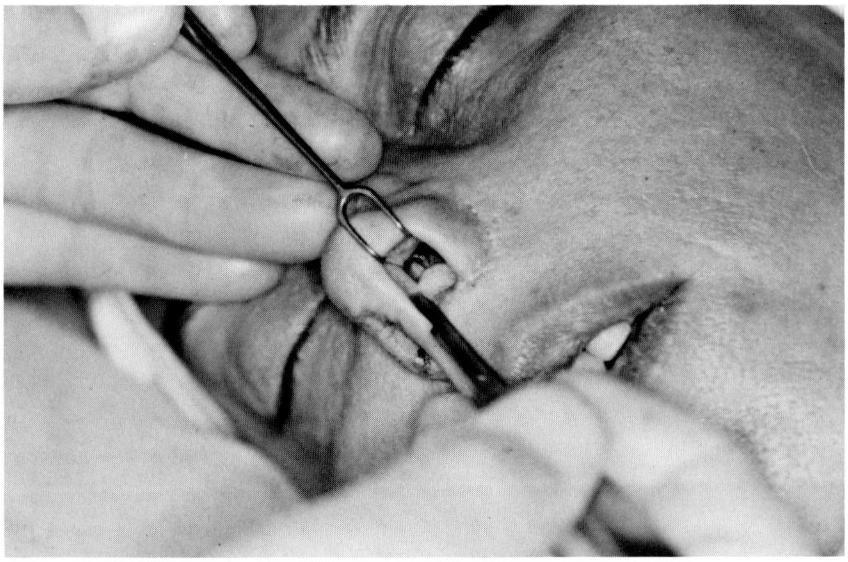

Shown from the left, packing in the right nasal airway is visible. Note the abundance of tissues at the posterior caudal septum—ideal for rotation into the defect.

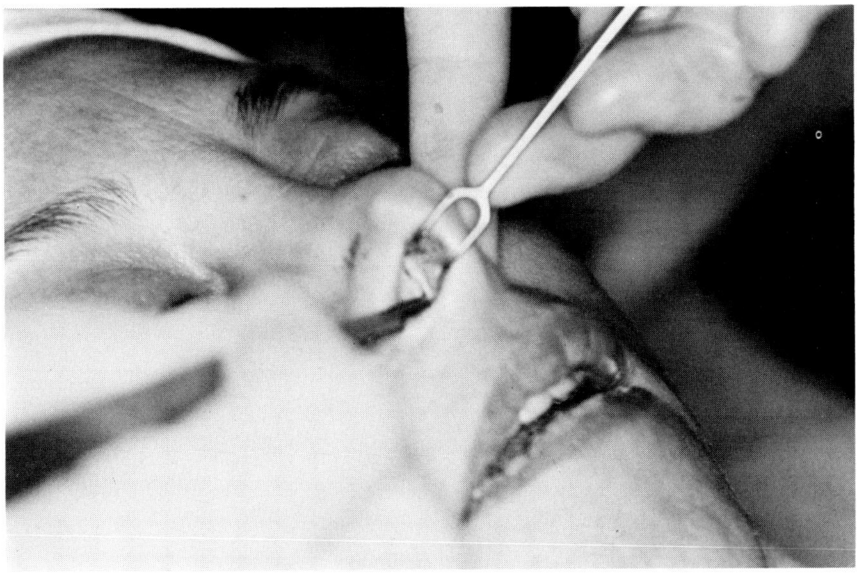

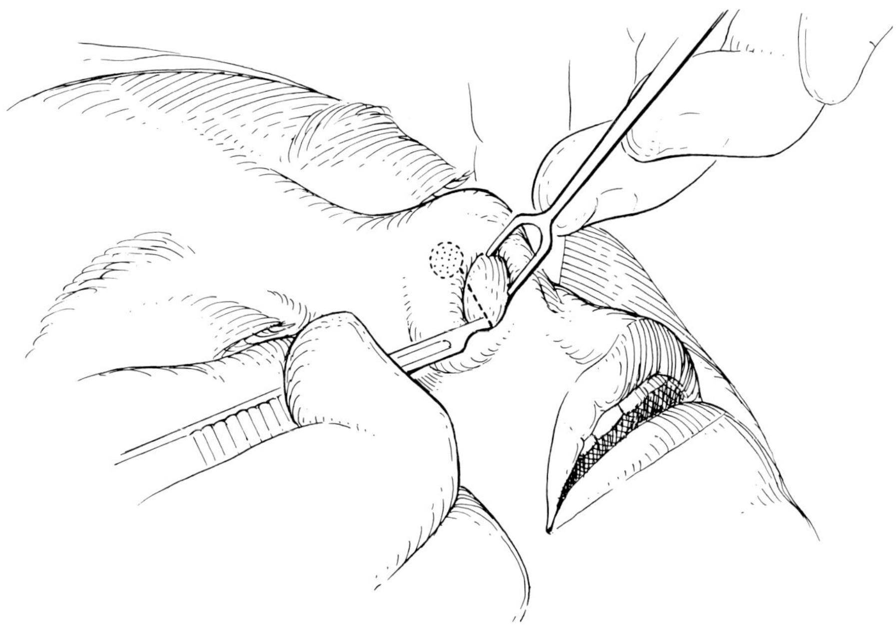

The initial incision is begun at the caudal arc of the perforation at about 5 o'clock, extending posteriorly to the nasal spine.

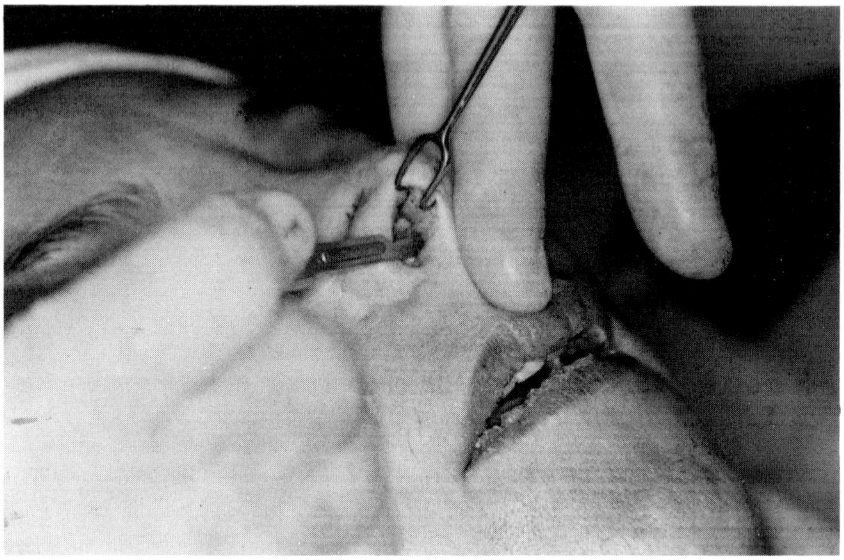

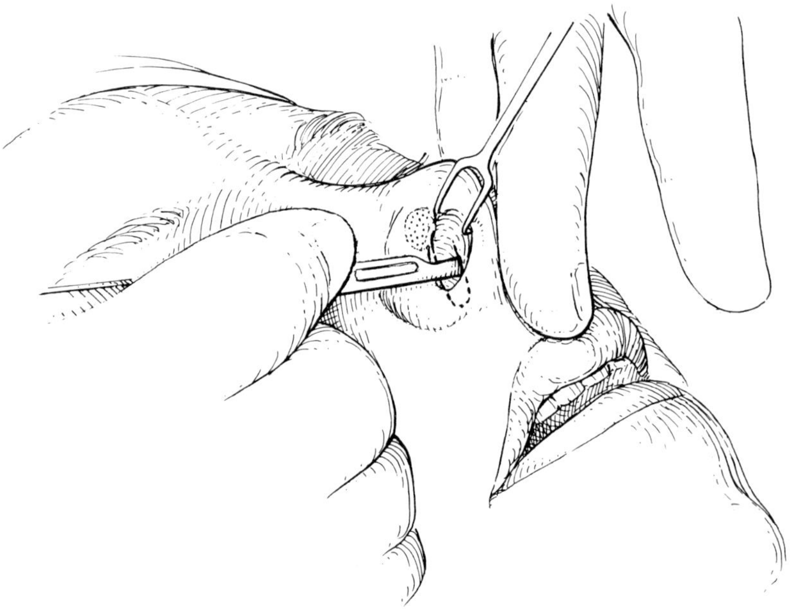

The posterior extent or distal edge of the flap is approximately 4 mm wide. The incision is returned toward the nasal tip, leaving a 4-mm bridge of tissue between the fistula and the caudal incision.

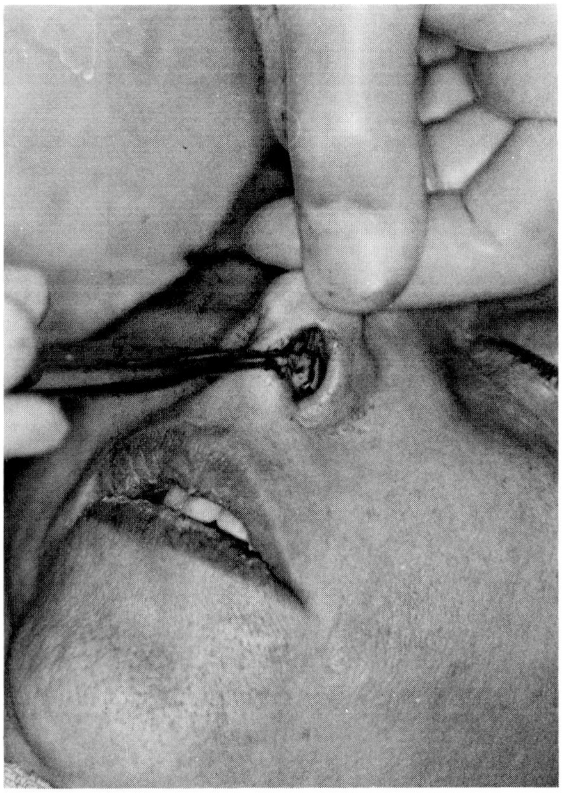

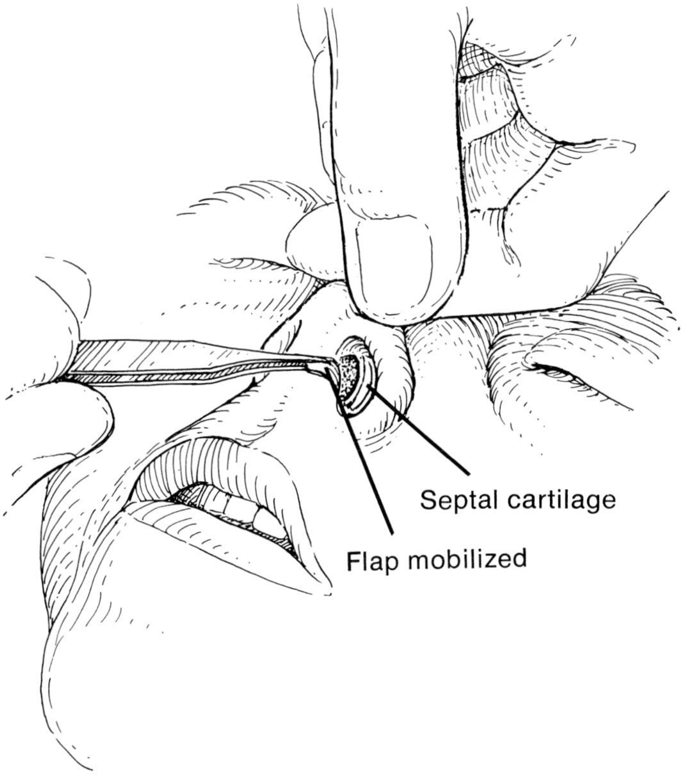

The flap, which is completely mobilized, is shown here with the posterior half ready to rotate into the trimmed fistula. The fistula appears white in the photograph because of the cotton in the opposite nostril.

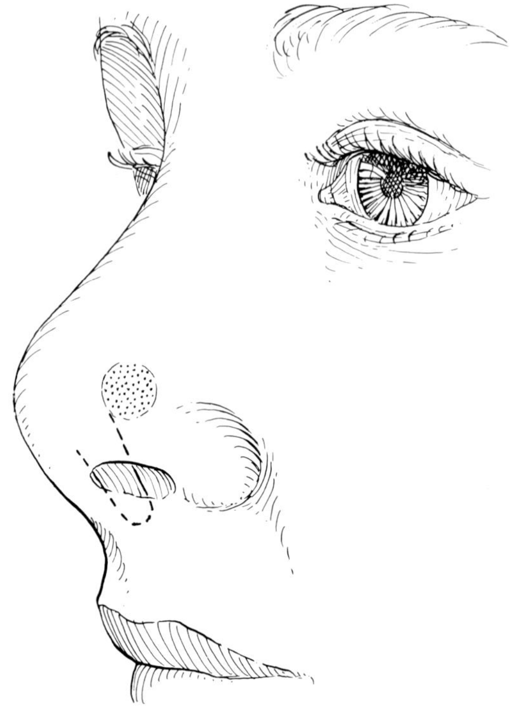

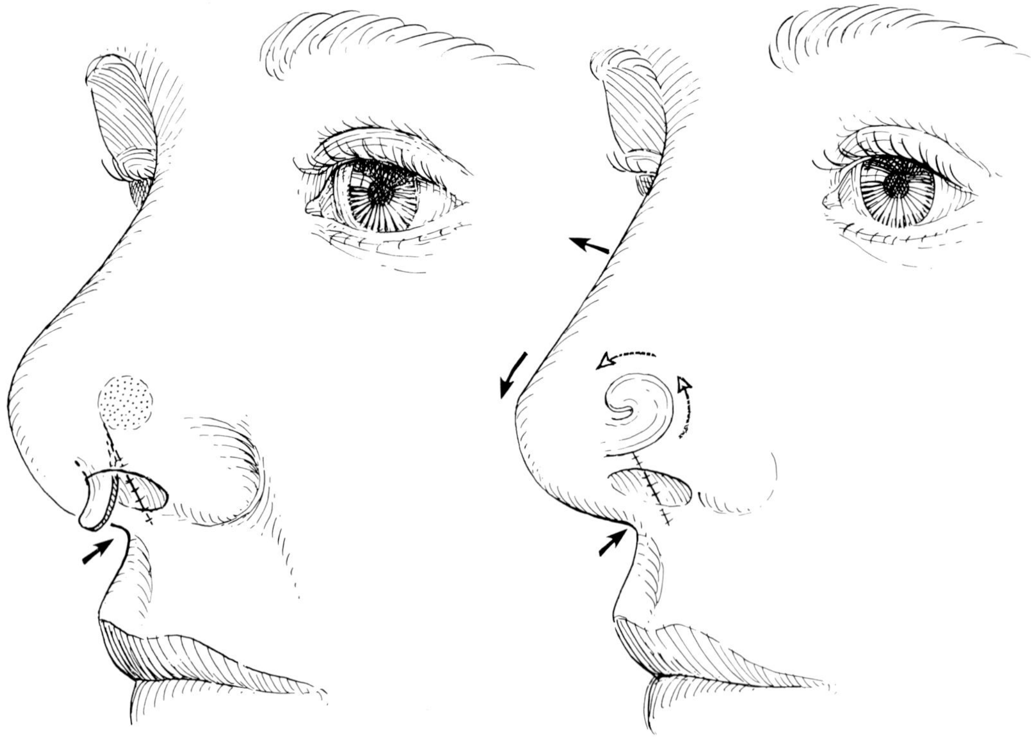

Following the mobilization of the graft, the wound is closed and the flap is rotated into the defect. The procedure is repeated on the opposite side.

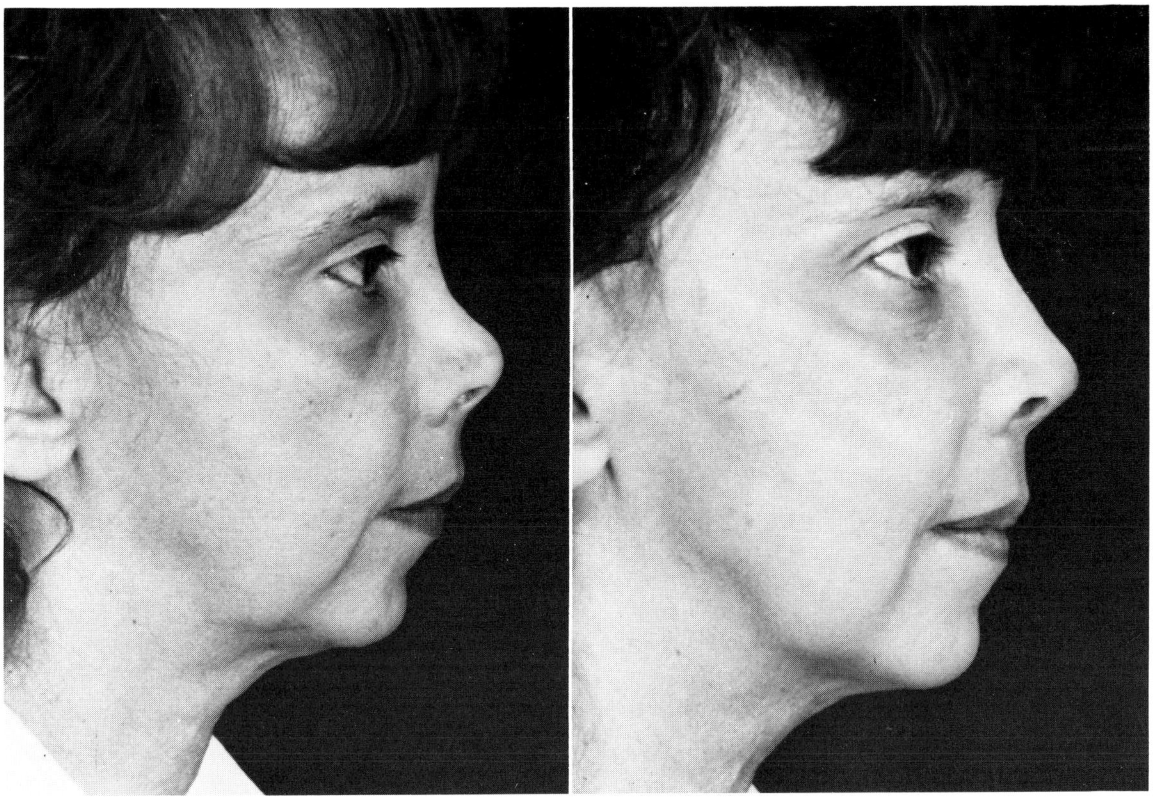

POSTOPERATIVE RESULTS

On postoperative lateral view, the decreased nasolabial angle and the somewhat retrusive subnasion are the result of reduction of the posterior, caudal membranous septum. This in conjunction with the dorsal graft has rotated the tip inferiorly, thereby adding length to the dorsal line.

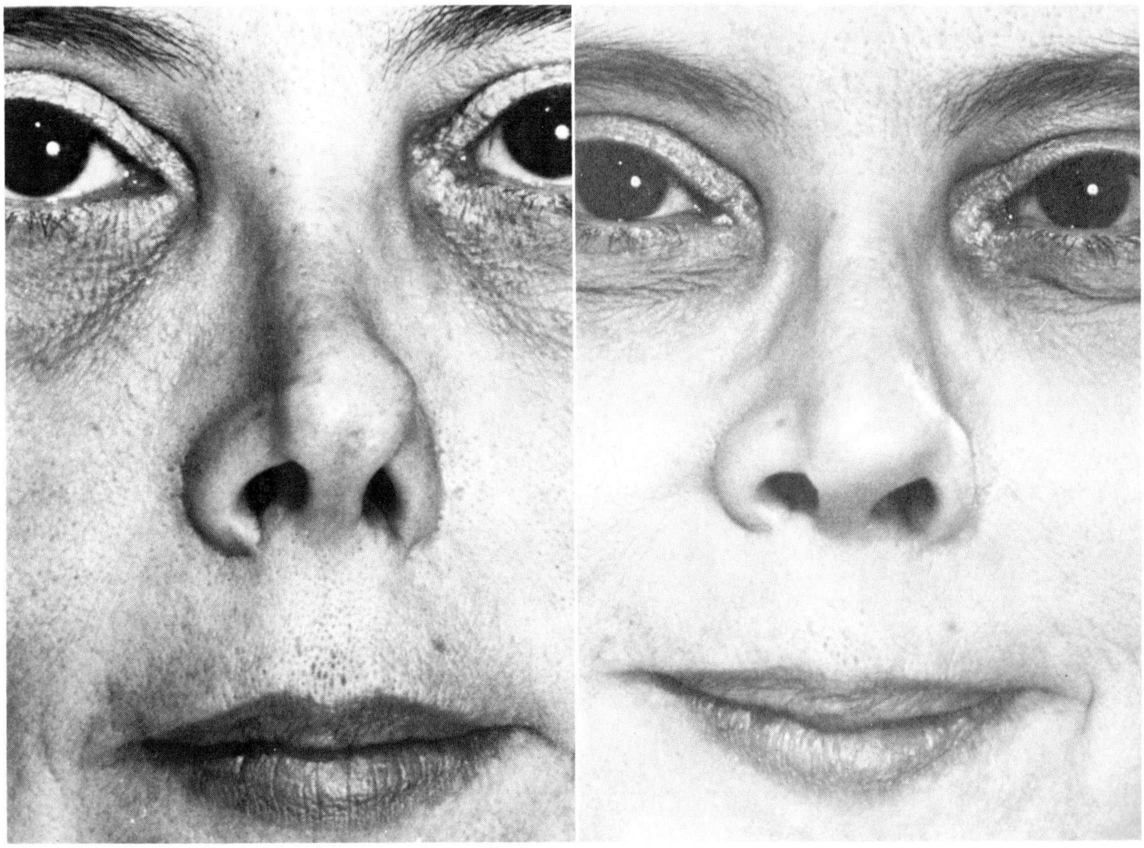

The nose is not entirely straight postoperatively, but the twisted appearance is corrected by the use of the dorsal graft and a small graft of crushed cartilage over the concavity on the left. Unfortunately, the thin tissues do not completely hide the cephalic end of the graft on the right side. The caudal rotation of the tip and a tip graft lessen the tip distortion and make the nostrils less visible.

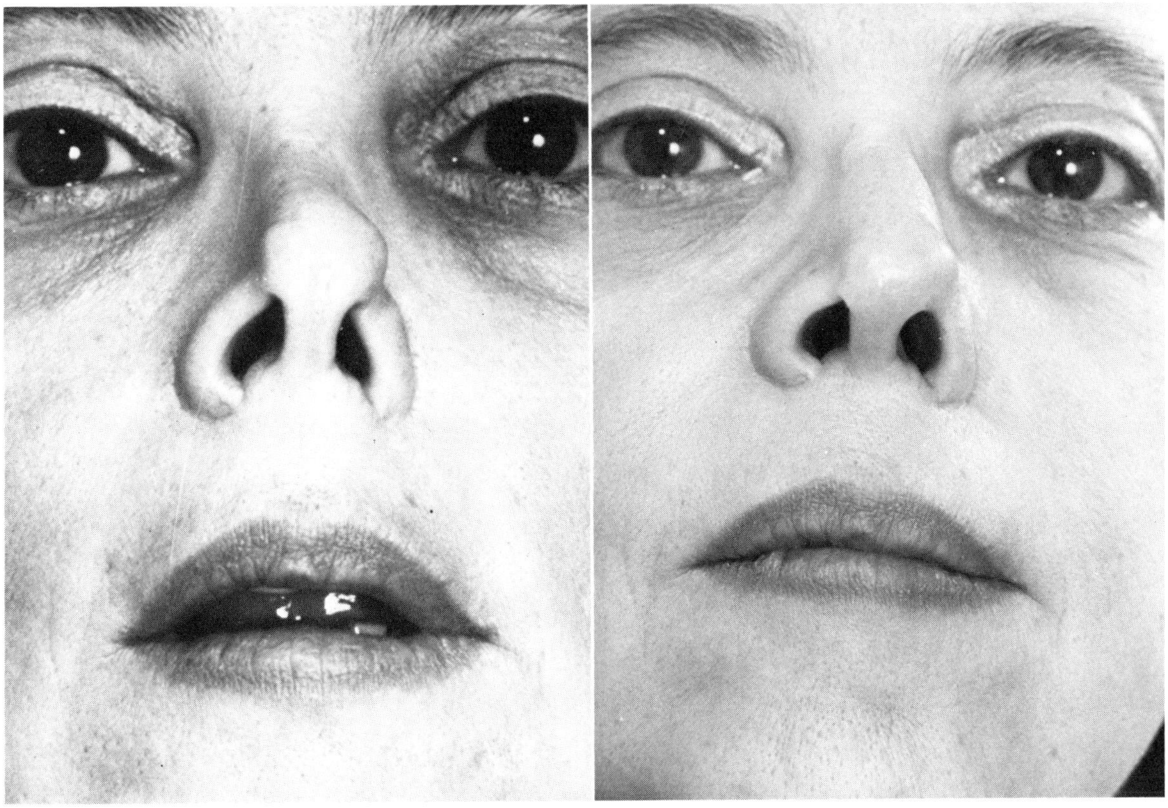

On basal view, the influence of a straight dorsal graft on the nasal contour is evident. The tip graft has minimized the residual cleft in the tip caused by the extrusion of the alloplastic implant.

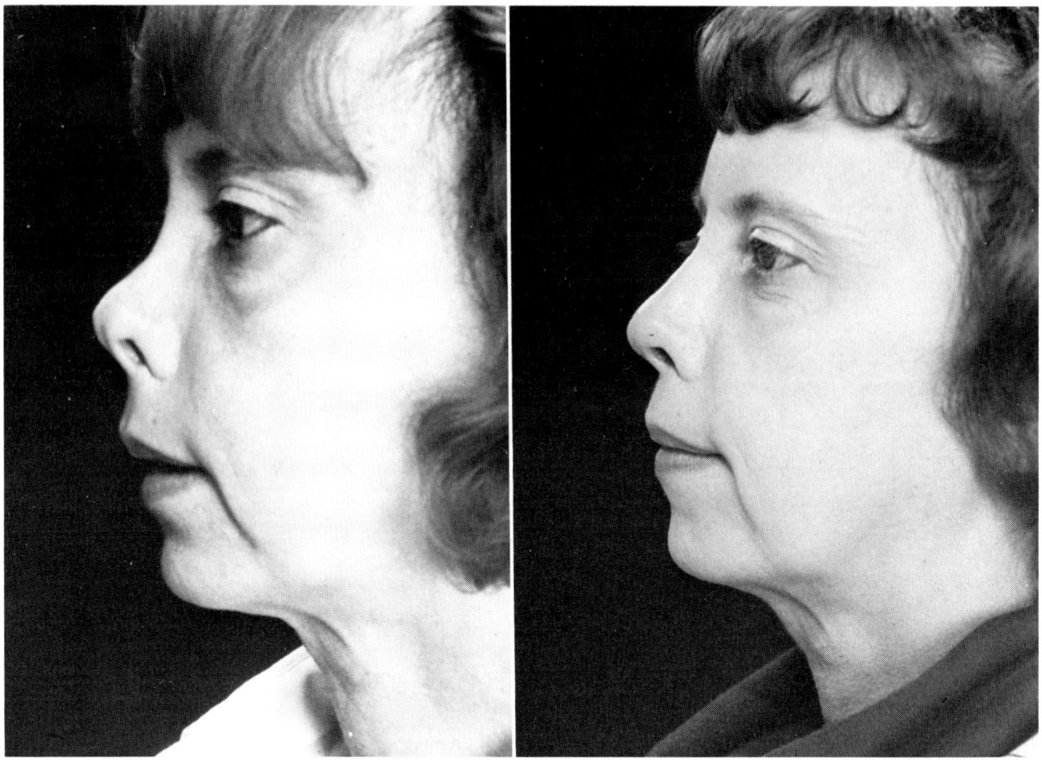

The use of a dorsal graft has succeeded in accomplishing a straight, nearly normal lateral profile.

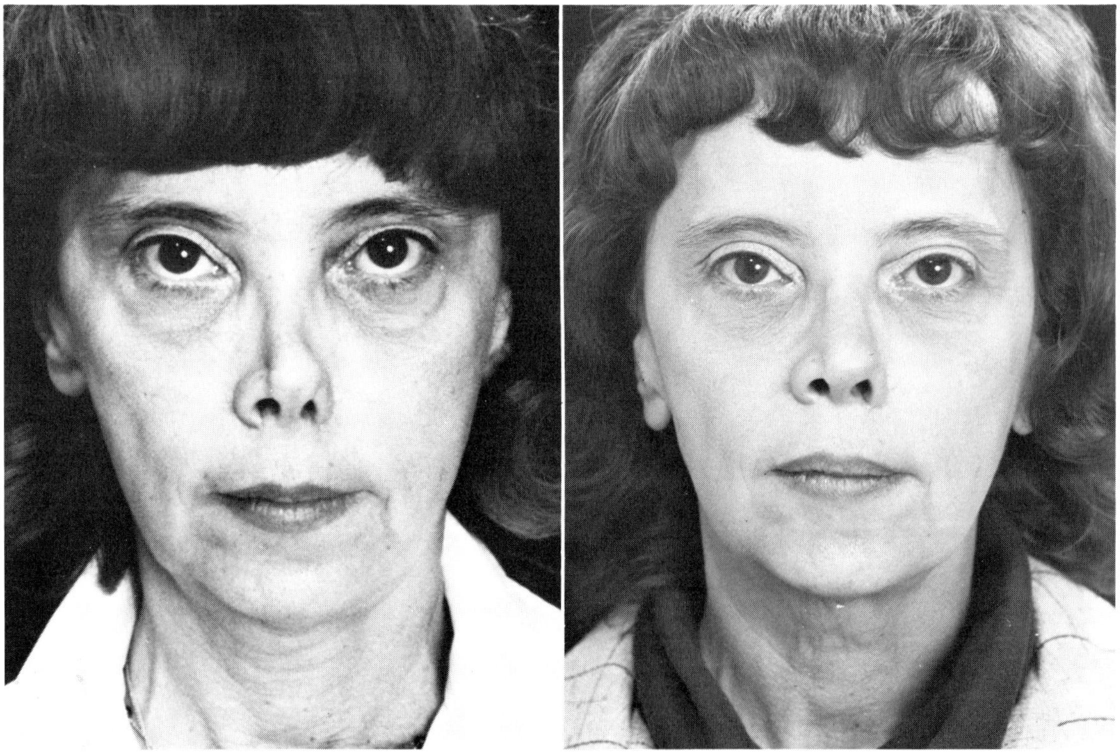

Elevating and widening the dorsum has made the nasal contour continuous with the orbital rims. Improving the confluence of nasal lines has made the nose a less distracting, more harmonious facial element.

DISCUSSION

The failure of alloplastic material, as in this patient, is the rule rather than the exception. Because the use of alloplastic materials has such a high failure rate in revisional rhinoplasty, I believe it is almost always contraindicated. In cases such as this, where three or more procedures have been performed, the compromised circulation and generally poor condition of the tissues simply will not support a synthetic implant for a long period of time.

A major concern for this patient was the preservation of vascularity. Therefore, tissue bridges were retained for tip circulation. For the same reason, the pocket for dorsal augmentation was made through a single incision on the right; the pocket for lateral augmentation was made through a small incision on the left. Dissection was kept to a minimum.

A WORD ABOUT LUCK

The kind of luck I am referring to falls about midway between science and superstition. Though its influence can be seen in all clinical practice, the role of luck in secondary rhinoplasty is especially noteworthy. For example, one might find quite unexpectedly *the* perfect piece of ethmoid bone with which to brace a collapsed ala. Or, as in the case just presented, enough tissues might be obtained from the posterior caudal septum for use as rotation flaps to cover the septal perforation. Under ordinary circumstances this would not seem very remarkable, but in a nose that has suffered five procedures and that was subsequently distorted by tissue deficit and scarring, nothing less than good fortune would provide this material for reconstructive use.

In rhinoplasty good luck usually is manifest in the appearance of rare opportunities. With experience and vigilance, one can recognize these opportunities; with good judgment and skill, one can transform them into exceptional results. The luck factor in revisional rhinoplasty should be recognized and appreciated but never depended on. It can be an advantage in the presence of sound judgment and technique but can never be a substitute for them.

CASE REPORT 1: CLASSICAL SECONDARY RHINOPLASTY

Identifiable postsurgical noses usually are similar because they are the consequences of similar procedural flaws. Routine overreduction of the dorsum, overreduction of the caudal septum, transection or overresection of the lateral crura, or suturing of the medial crura together produce a stereotypic nasal configuration that is not only characteristic of many rhinoplasties but also can sometimes be identified with specific surgeons.

These patients were operated on by different surgeons. Their similar noses exemplify the most frequently occurring combination of postsurgical traits seen in secondary rhinoplasty:

1. Low dorsum
2. High supratip
3. Blunted nasal tip, without definition
4. Open nasolabial angle
5. Flaring nostrils

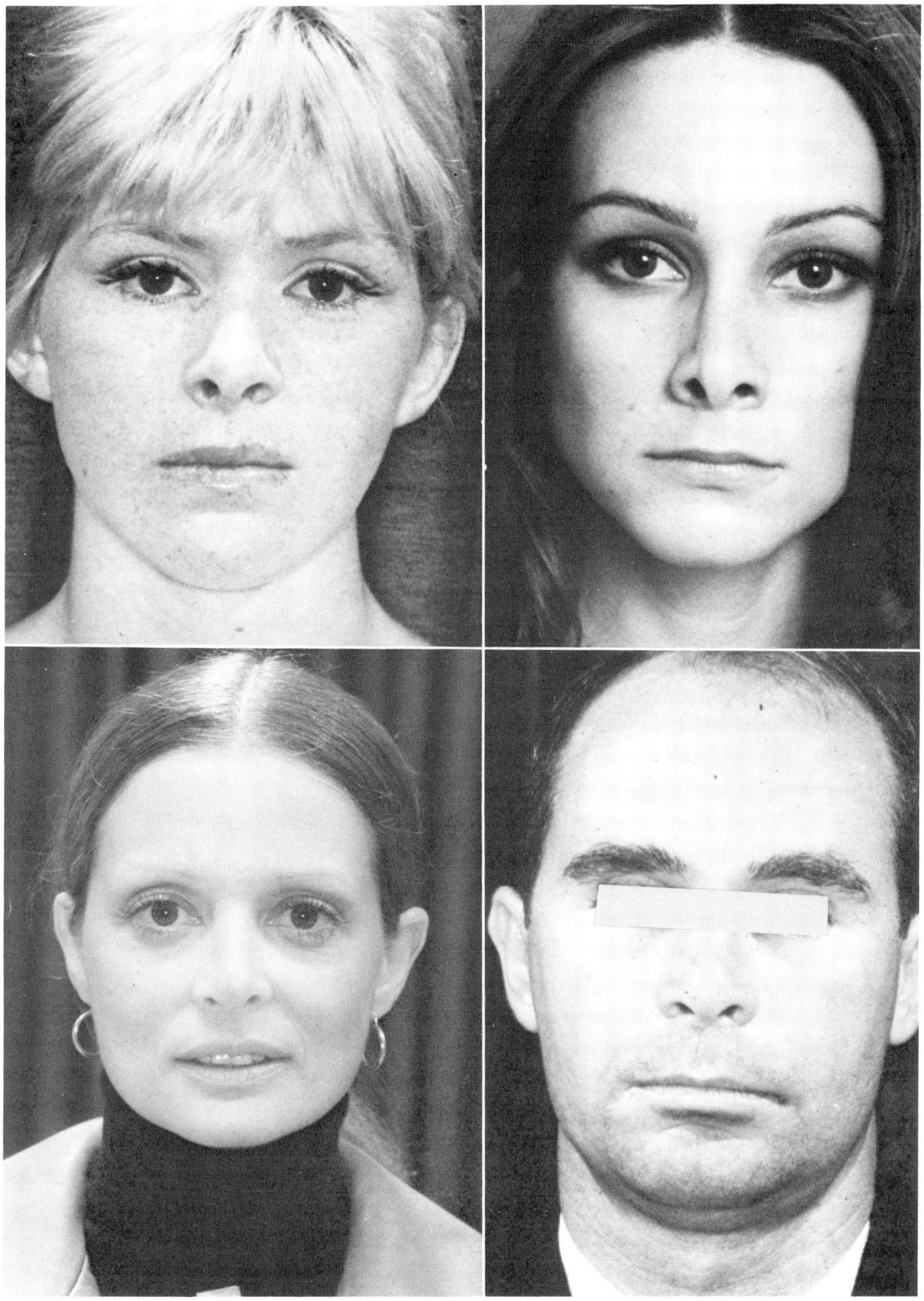

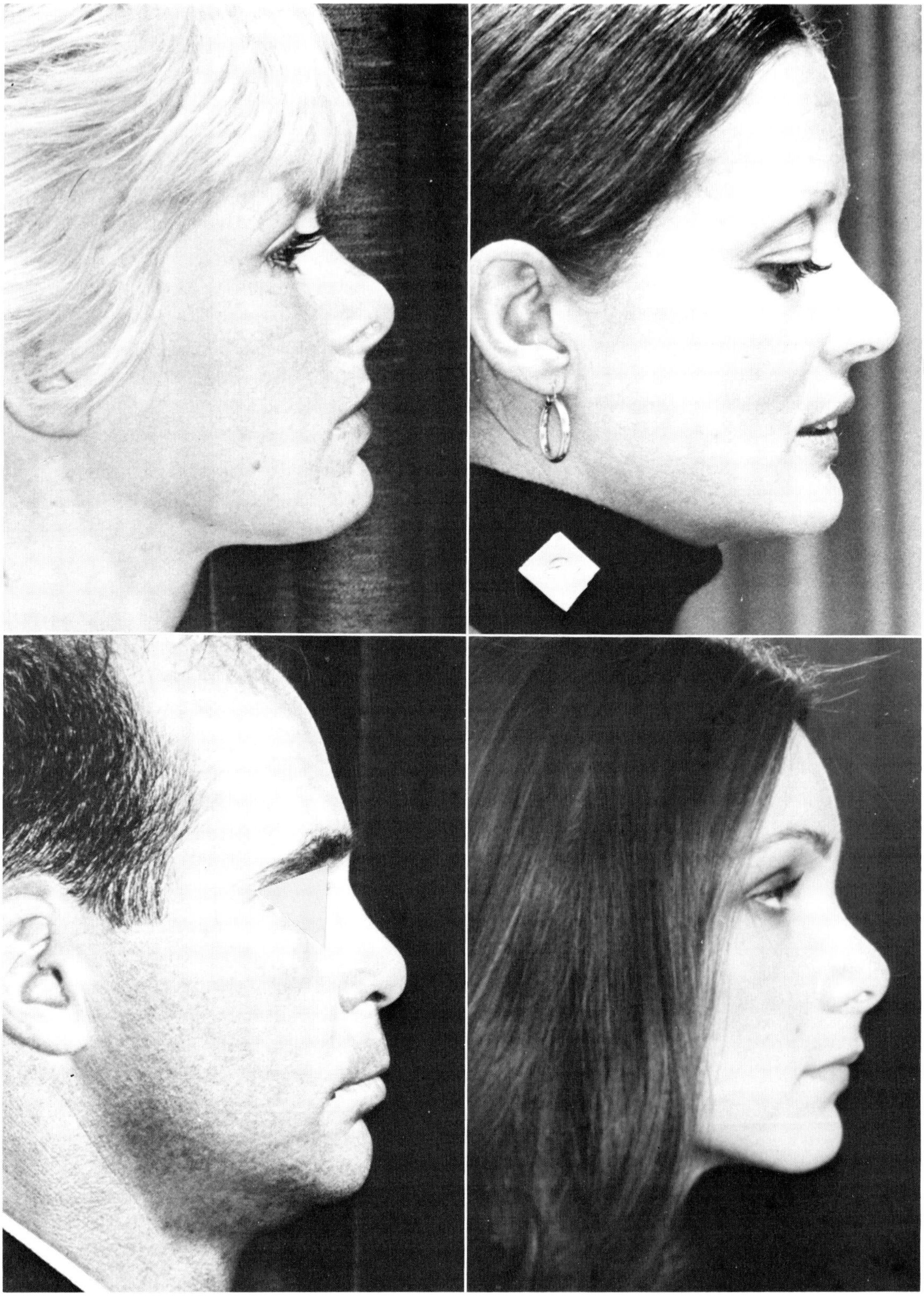

On lateral view, it is less apparent that the dorsum is low than the supratip area is high. Frequently patients are alarmed at the suggestion that the dorsum must be elevated, and their fears are sometimes reinforced by consultations with other surgeons who say that the supratip area should be reduced by resection of scar tissue.

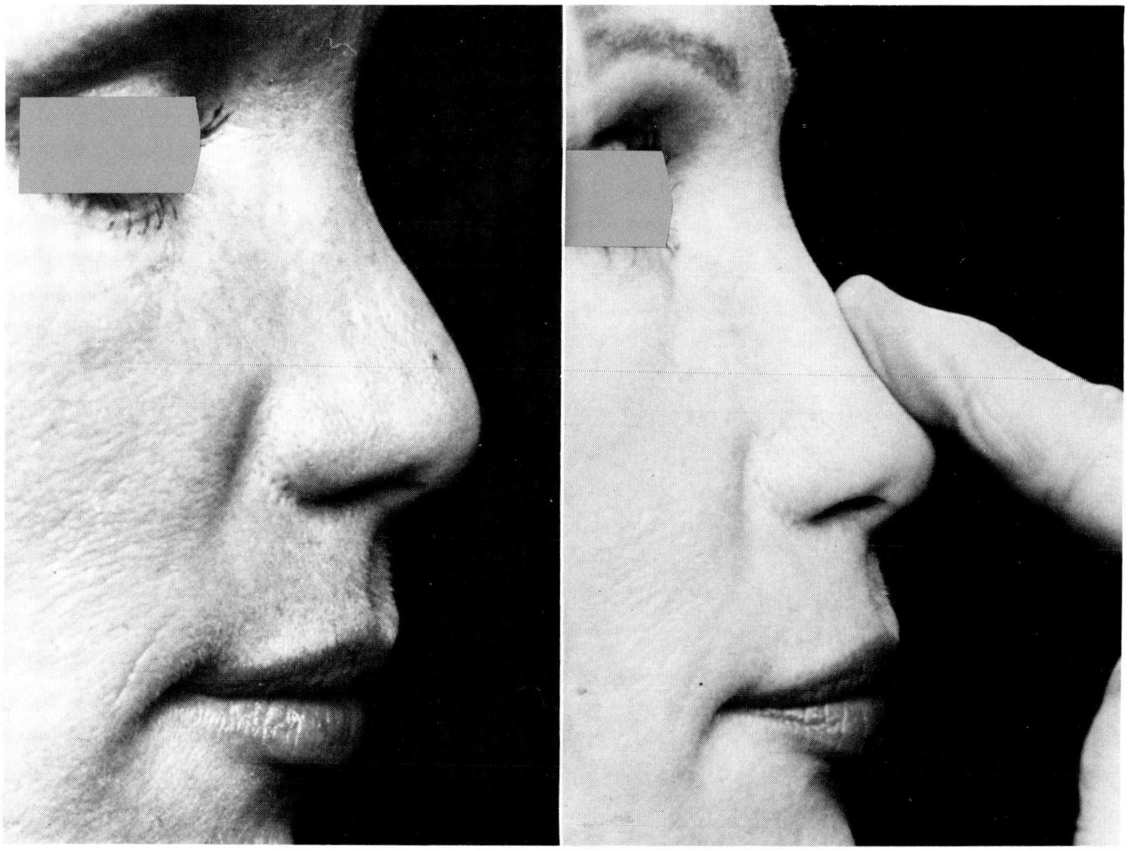

This patient has undergone five thinning procedures that have left vertical grooves along the middle third of the nose. The patient is shown with the tissues depressed to the level of the dorsal edge of the septum, thus demonstrating that this supratip fullness is caused by inadequate skeletal support—a problem that cannot be solved by repeated thinning.

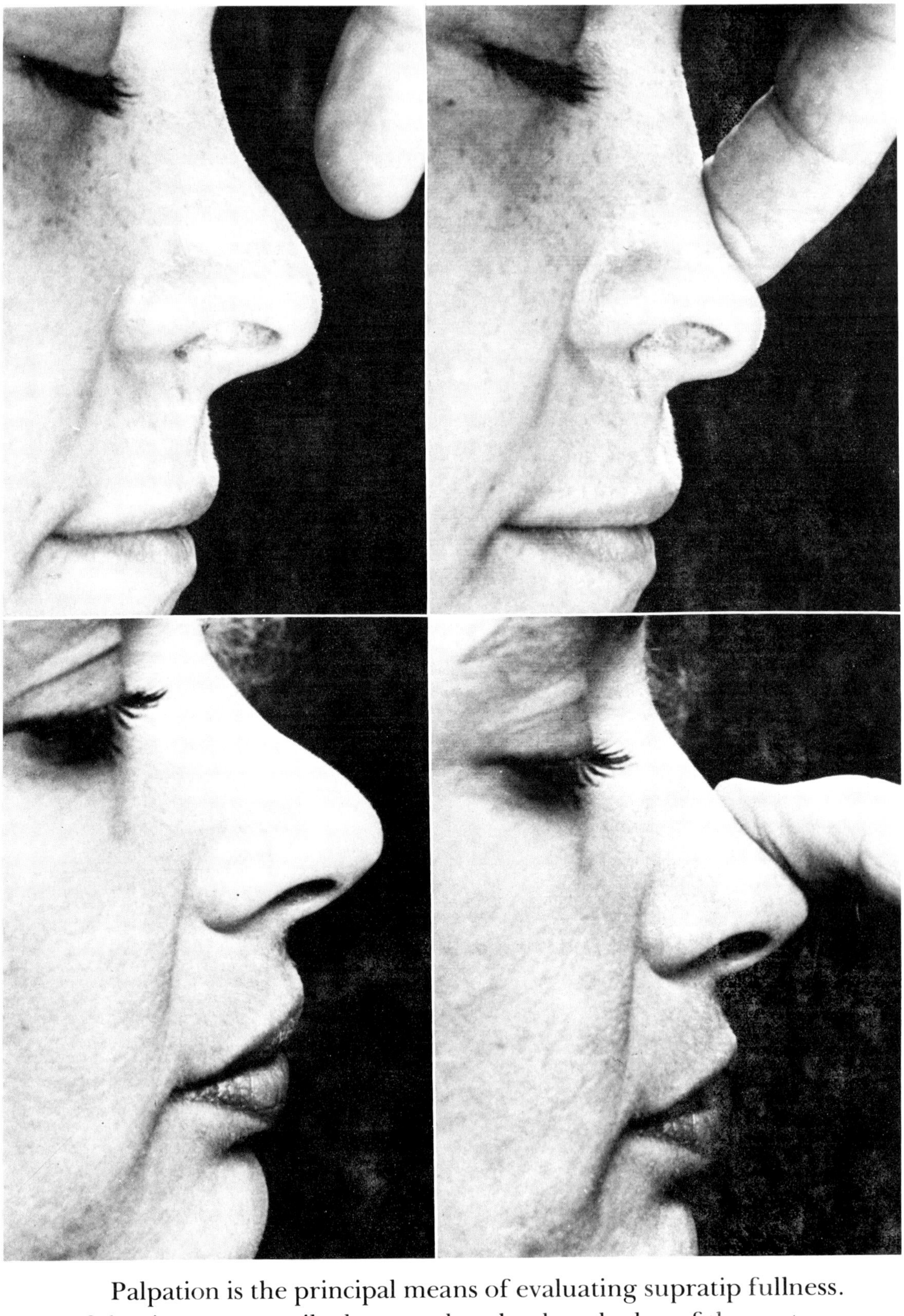

Palpation is the principal means of evaluating supratip fullness. If the tissues are easily depressed to the dorsal edge of the septum, thinning or scar resection is absolutely contraindicated.

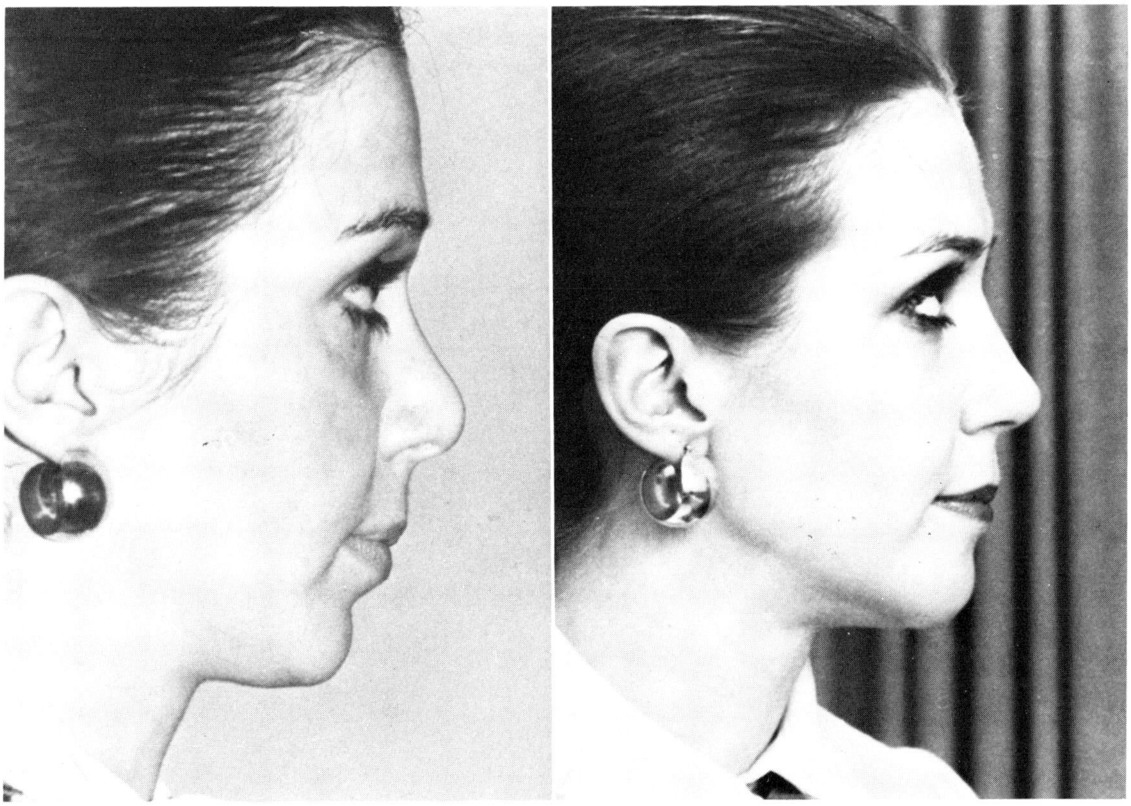

If the supratip tissues cannot be depressed, it does not necessarily indicate that they are supported by cartilaginous dorsum. Scar tissue may fill the void and palpate as firmly as cartilage.

On this patient, the supratip area was firm, yet at surgery (see Millard's *Symposium on Corrective Rhinoplasty)* the dorsum was found to be undercut 4 mm in the area of the supratip. The supratip fullness was corrected by dorsal augmentation and tip grafting. Additional cartilage was placed under the caudal edge of the graft in the immediate area of the supratip. No tissues were resected.

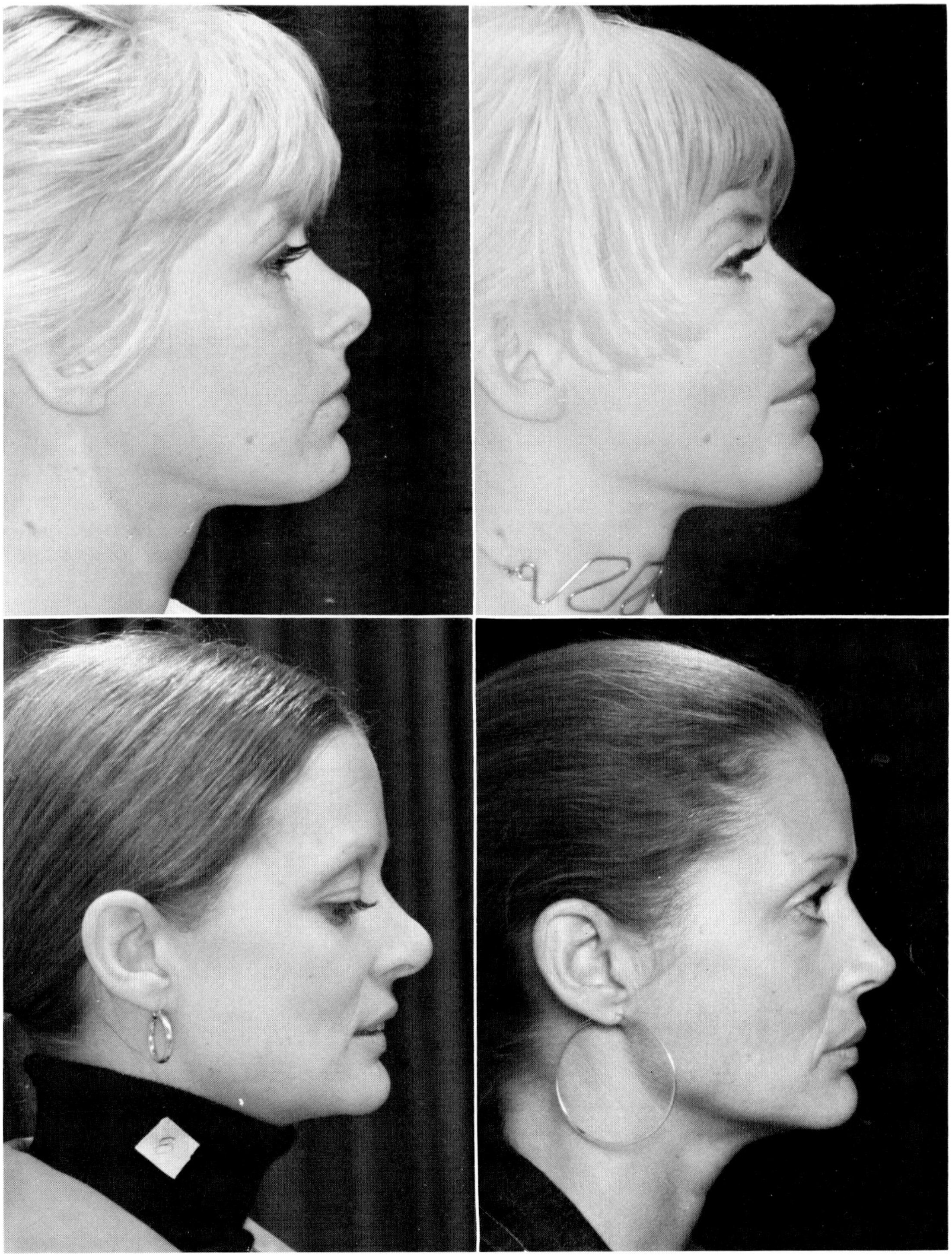

Although the noses of the following four patients are similar in concept postoperatively, they are anatomically more correct. Natural-appearing noses become well integrated into the facial gestalt and are no longer a distracting focal point.

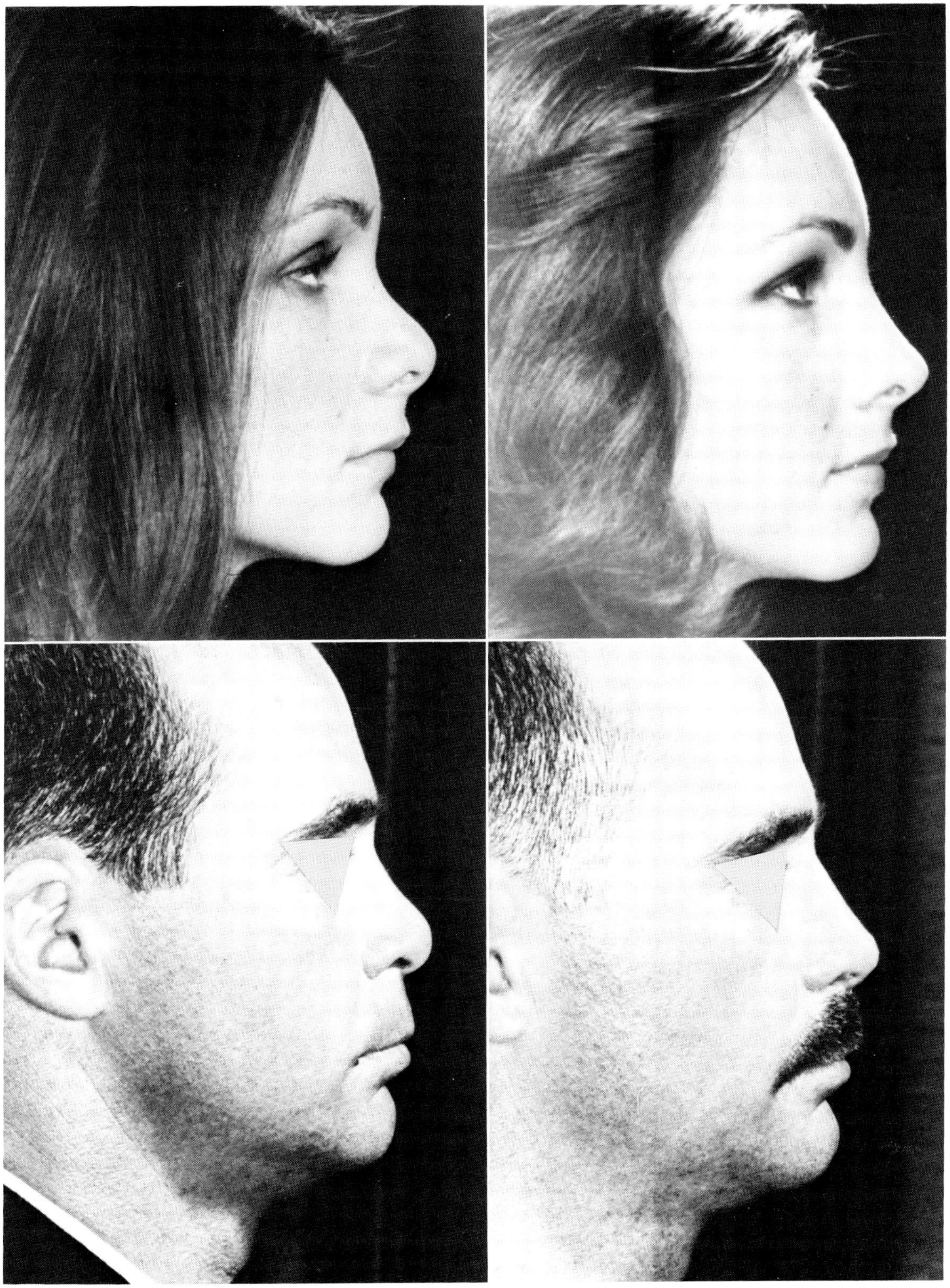

All four patients received dorsal grafts of septal cartilage, which began at the radix and extended into the area of the supratip. Tip definition was obtained by the use of a tip graft of septal cartilage.

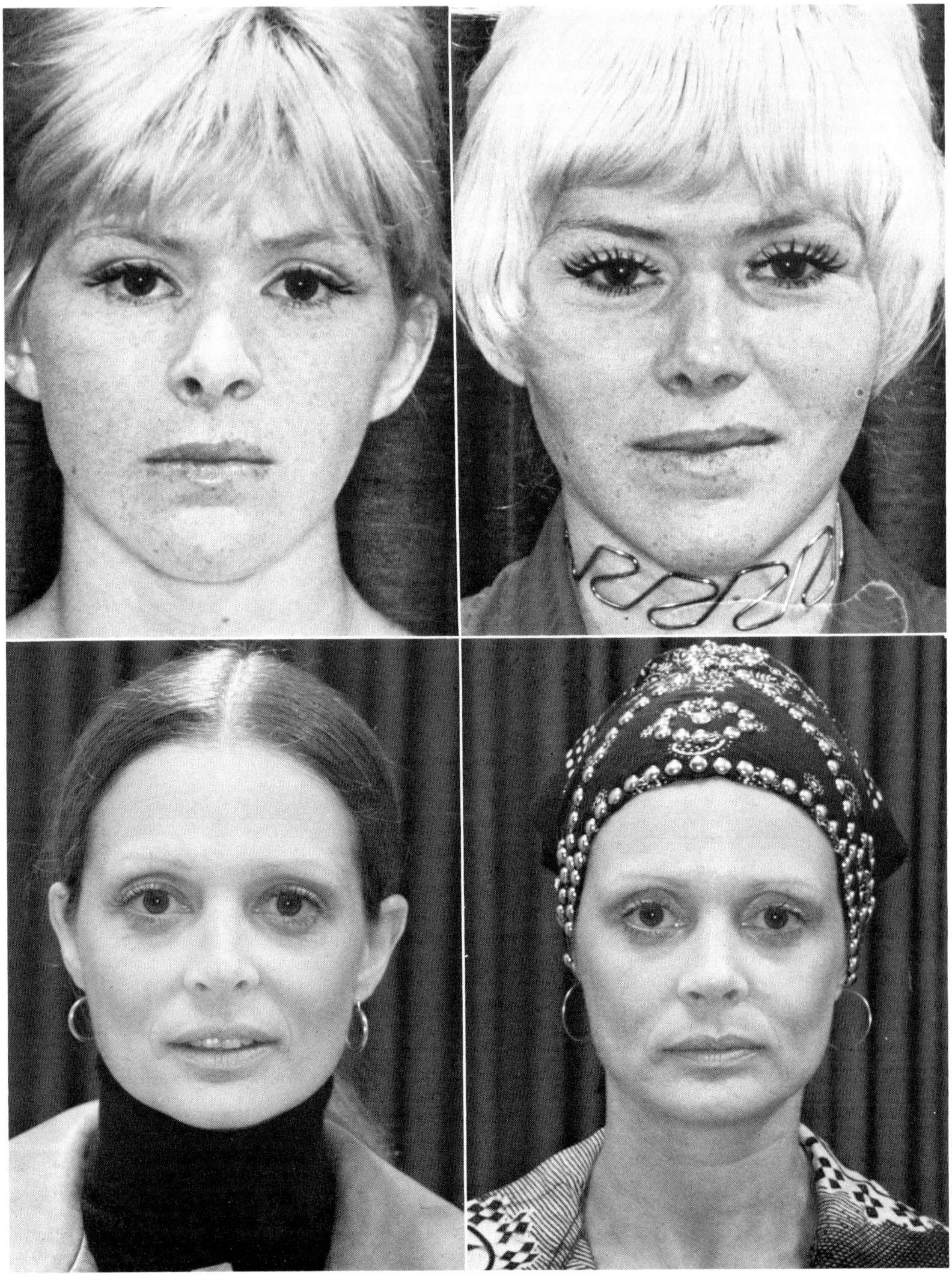

On postoperative front view, there is a restoration of nasofacial lines. Elevation of the dorsum has effected a favorable dimension to the midface. The position of the nostrils has been improved by the caudal rotation of the nasal tip and by the dorsal augmentation.

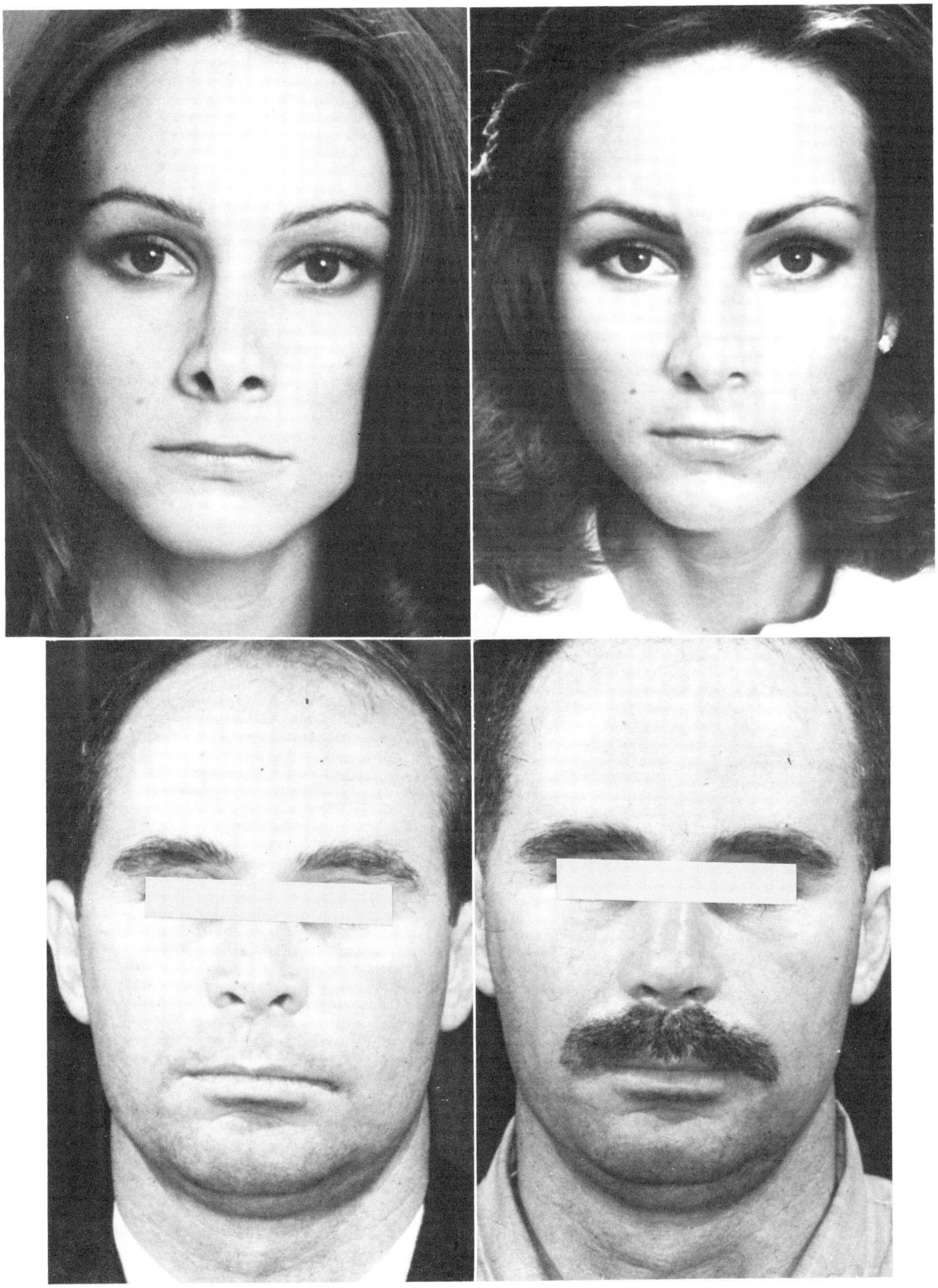

On oblique view, the correction of the classical postsurgical supratip deformity by augmentation of the dorsum and the tip is demonstrated.

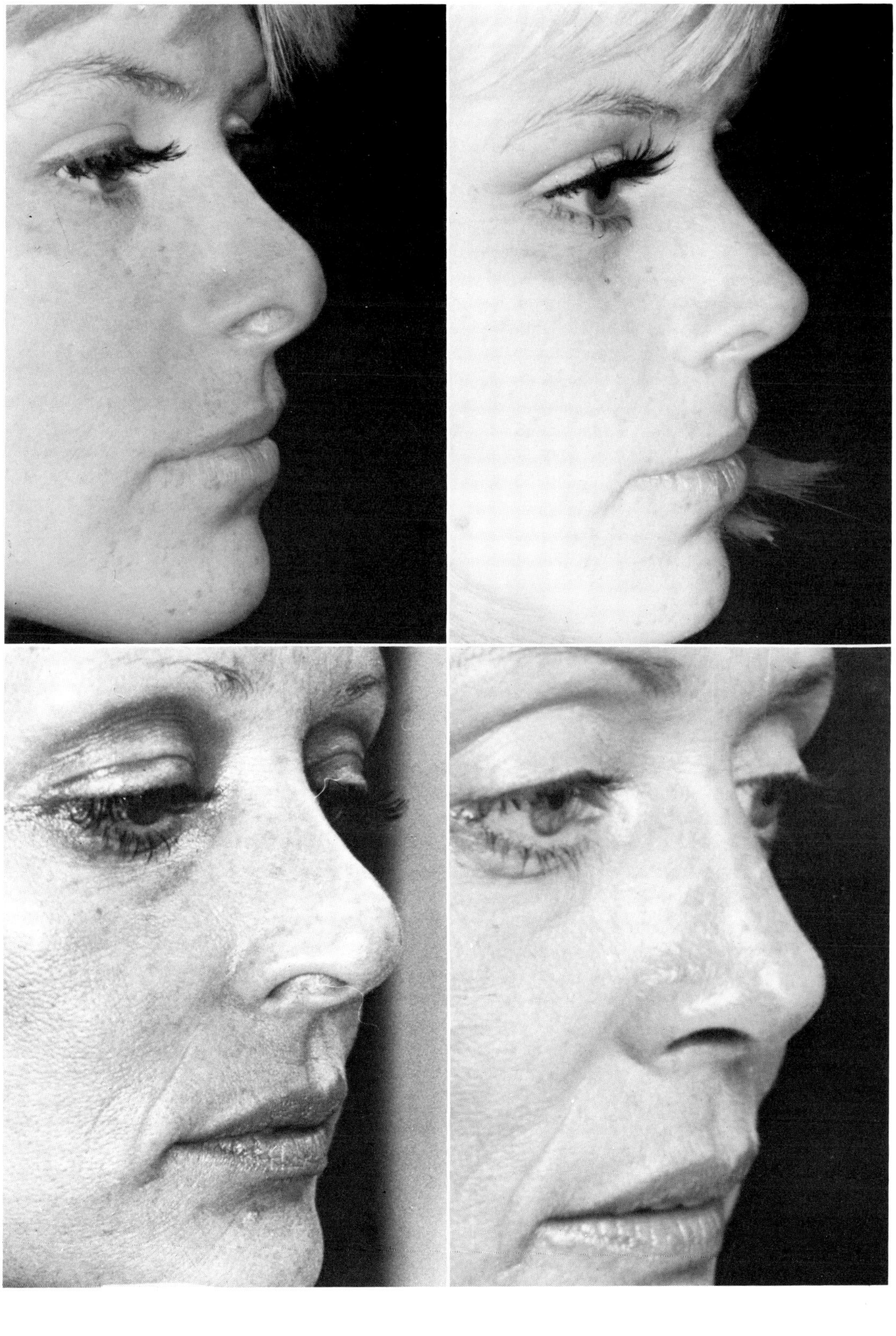

DISCUSSION

Because classical secondary rhinoplasty patients have similar nasal deficits, the surgical correction is necessarily similar. Except for minor variations in degree and placement, each of these patients received the same surgical treatment: dorsal augmentation, tip augmentation, reduction of the posterior caudal septum, and caudal rotation of the nasal tip.

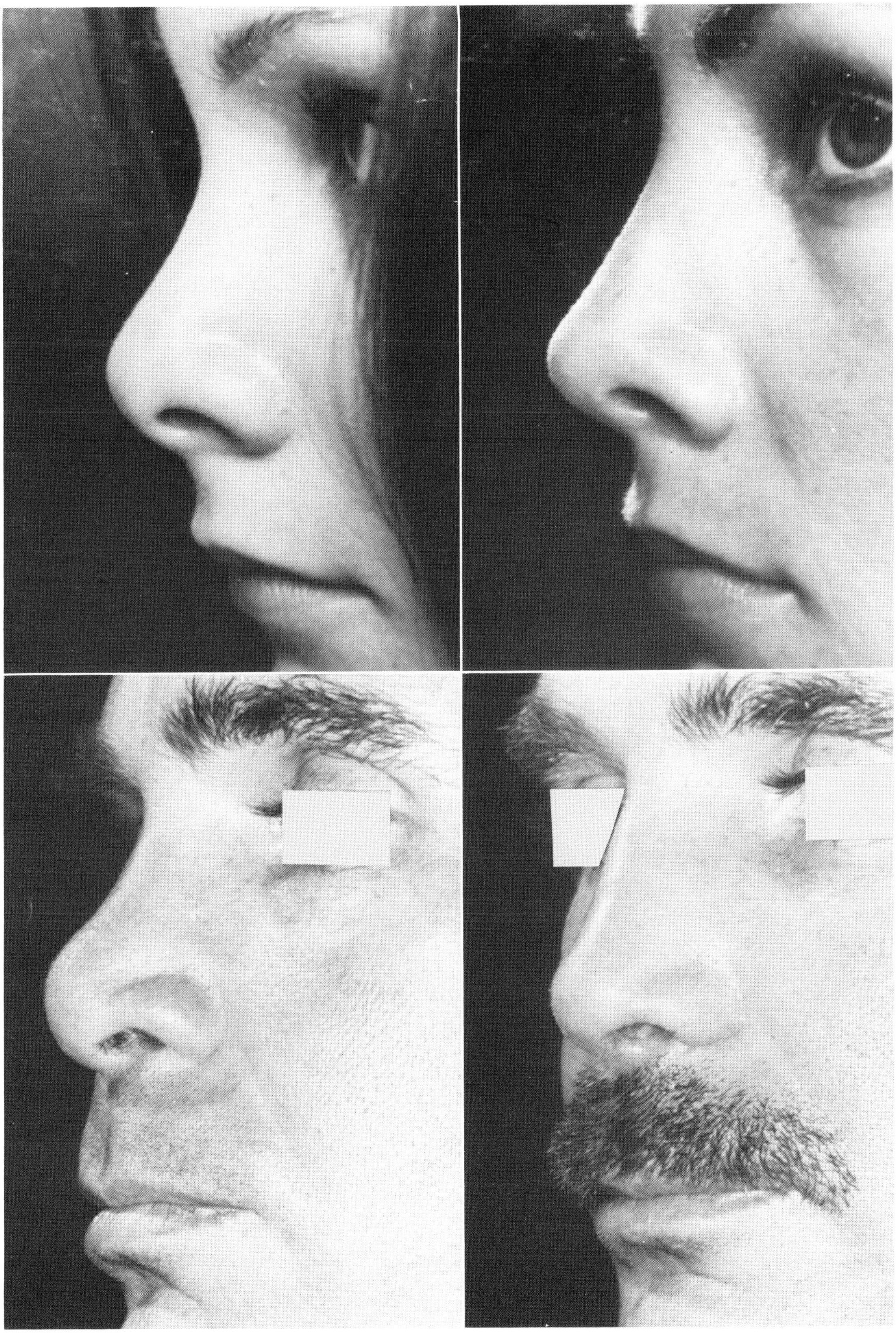

CASE REPORT 2: NASAL LENGTH

The length of the nose usually is measured from the radix to the base of the columella. However, the apparent length corresponds to the straight line of the dorsum that connects with the tip. If the nasal tip is rounded, eliminating the end point, or if the dorsum begins lower than the horizontal plane of the superior palpebral fold, the nose appears short.

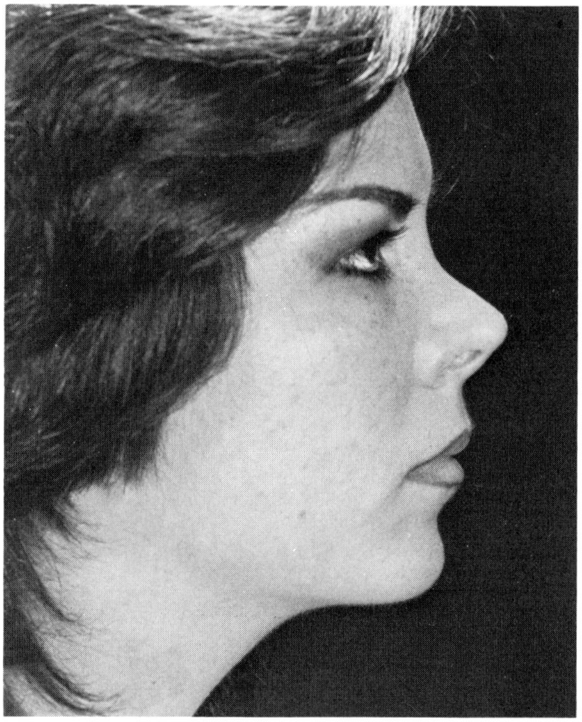

This 23-year-old student had a primary rhinoplasty 3 years before consultation. On lateral view, the dorsum begins too low—at about the level of the lower lid margin—and continues in a straight line to the overprojecting tip. The nasolabial angle is excessively wide, the columellar-alar relationship is poor, and the alar lobule is heavy and curls downward.

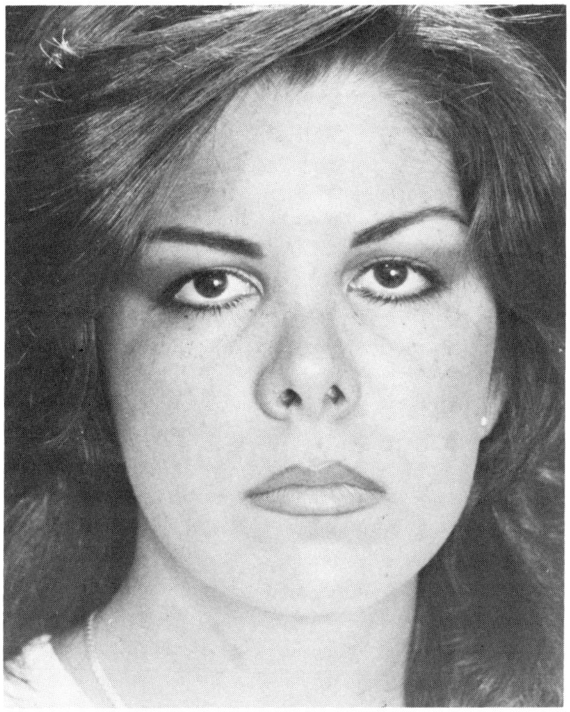

On front view, there is no continuity between the lateral nasal silhouette and the orbital rims. The appearance of the eyes has been adversely affected by the absence of suitable dorsal height. The nose appears extremely short on front view, and the nostrils are more visible than is desirable because of the wide nasolabial angle.

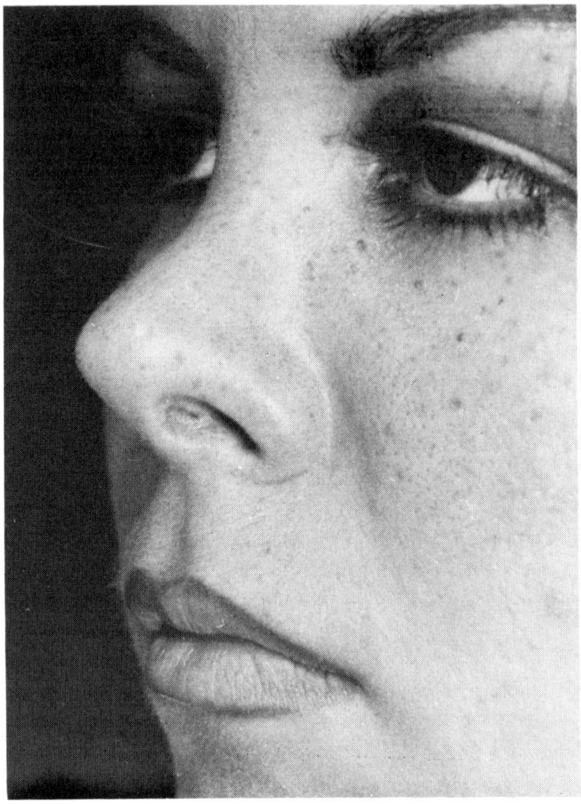

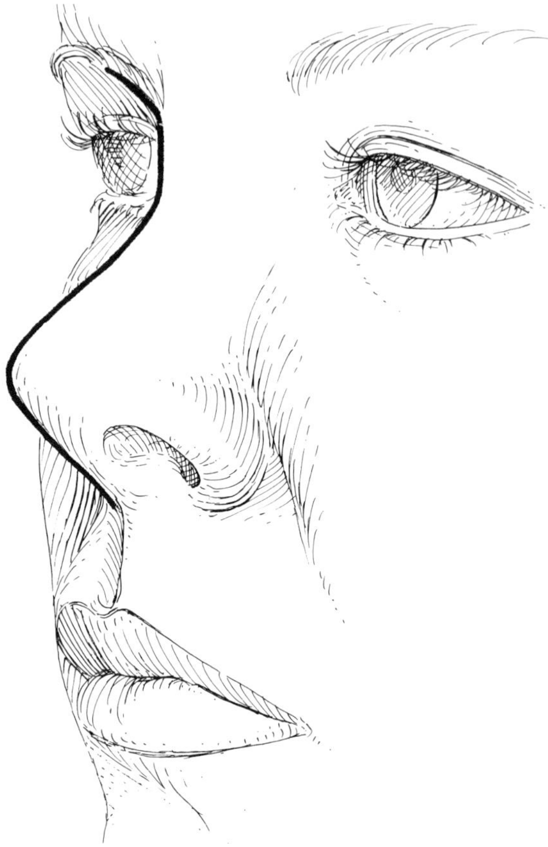

On left oblique view, there is an imbalance of parts. The base is overwhelming in contrast to the overreduced dorsum. There is a hint of supratip fullness, which warns of possible problems in reducing the projection of the tip. There is a crook in the ideal curve from the superciliary ridge to the nasal contour. The columella is too low for the alar rim, exposing vestibular skin and vibrissae.

SURGICAL PROCEDURE

Following limited skeletonization, the membranous septum was incised to the nasal spine. The spine was reduced with a bone-biting rongeur.

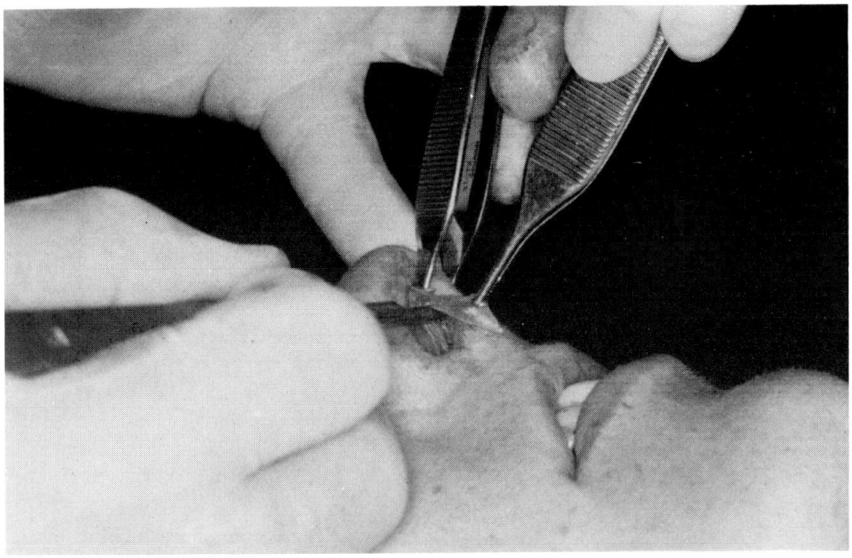

The posterior caudal septum was trimmed 4 mm posteriorly, gradually diminishing to 1 mm anteriorly.

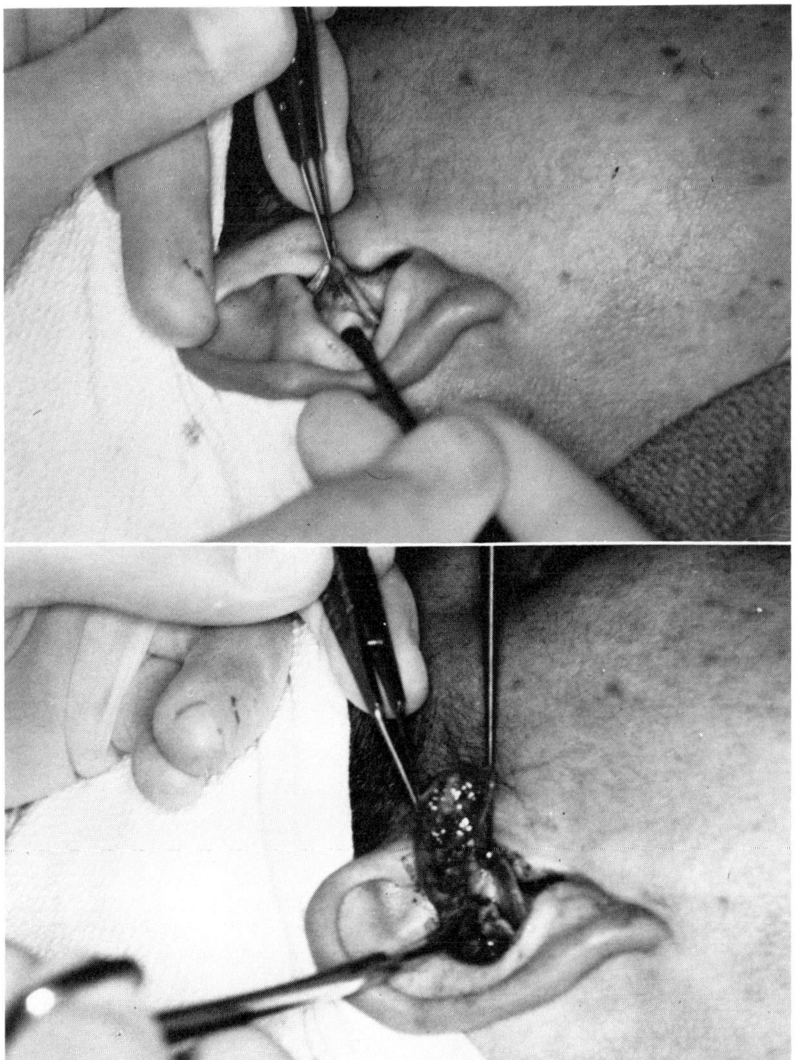

A conchal cartilage graft was obtained from the right ear.

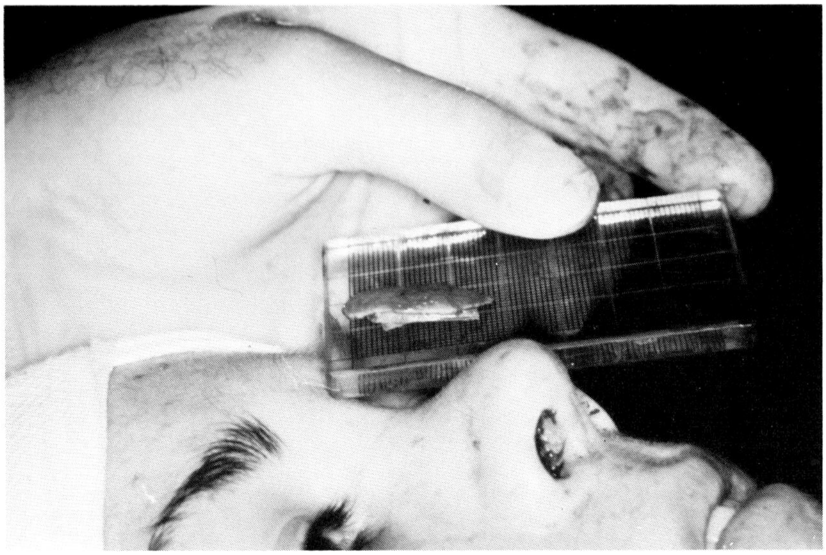

The conchal cartilage graft was made into a sandwich.

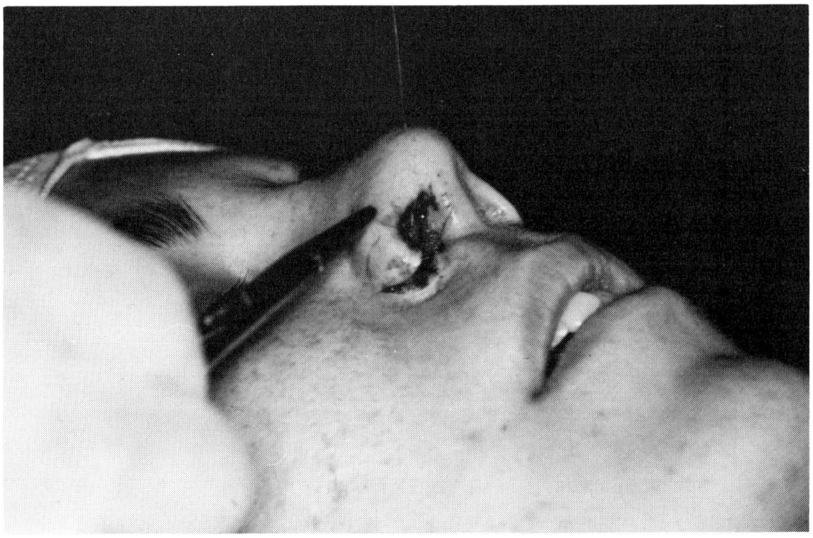

Bilateral alar wedge resections completed the procedure.

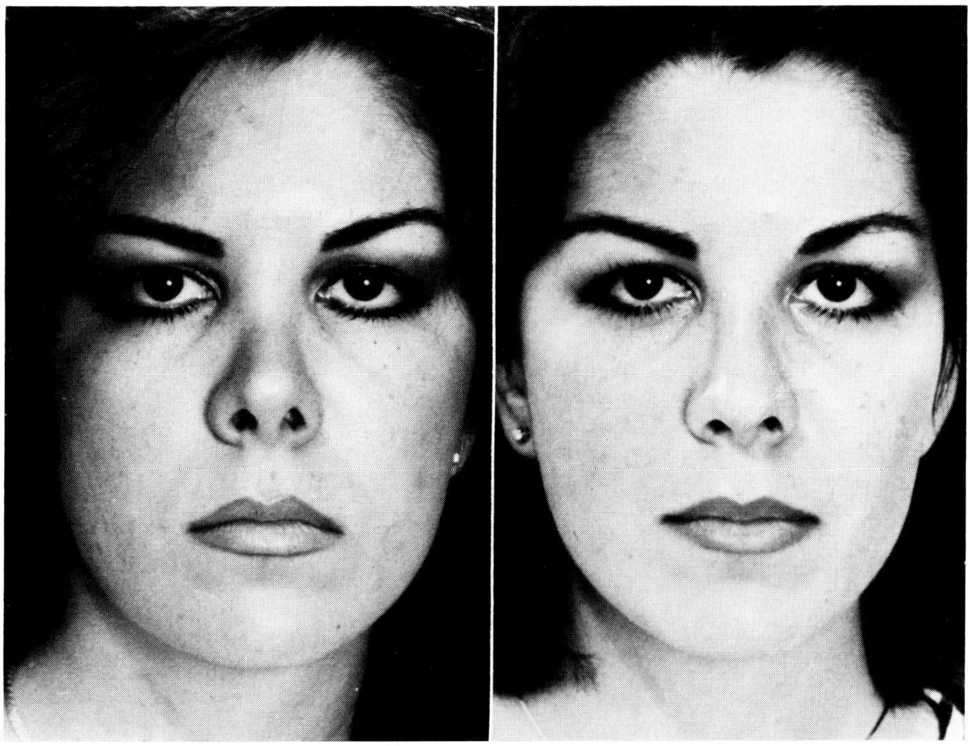

POSTOPERATIVE RESULTS

Postoperatively, there is a smooth, unbroken line connecting the superior orbital rim, radix, lateral nasal wall, and the nasal tip. Elevation of the dorsum and caudal rotation of the nasal base have decreased the show of nostrils and increased the apparent length of the nose.

On right lateral and left oblique views, the increase in length achieved by the large dorsal graft and surgical modification of the nasal base is demonstrated.

DISCUSSION

Ordinarily it is difficult to increase the length of a secondary patient's nose. However, if the combination of tissues is conducive to lengthening, as it was in this patient, dramatic changes can occur. With dorsal augmentation, the illusion of increased length occurred as the straight line of the dorsum was extended to the radix. Further length was obtained with the caudal rotation of the tip and the reduction of the tip projection. Because the tissues of her nasal tip were heavy, they would not respond to surgical reduction of the tip cartilages. Therefore, the reduction of tip projection had to come from a reduction in the parts of its supporting platform—the nasal spine and caudal septum. The slight retrusion of the subnasion was a compromise that was made for the reduction in tip projection. Alar wedge resection can reduce tip projection, but the technique seldom should be used for that purpose because of the necessarily small amount of lobule that can be resected without causing distortion.

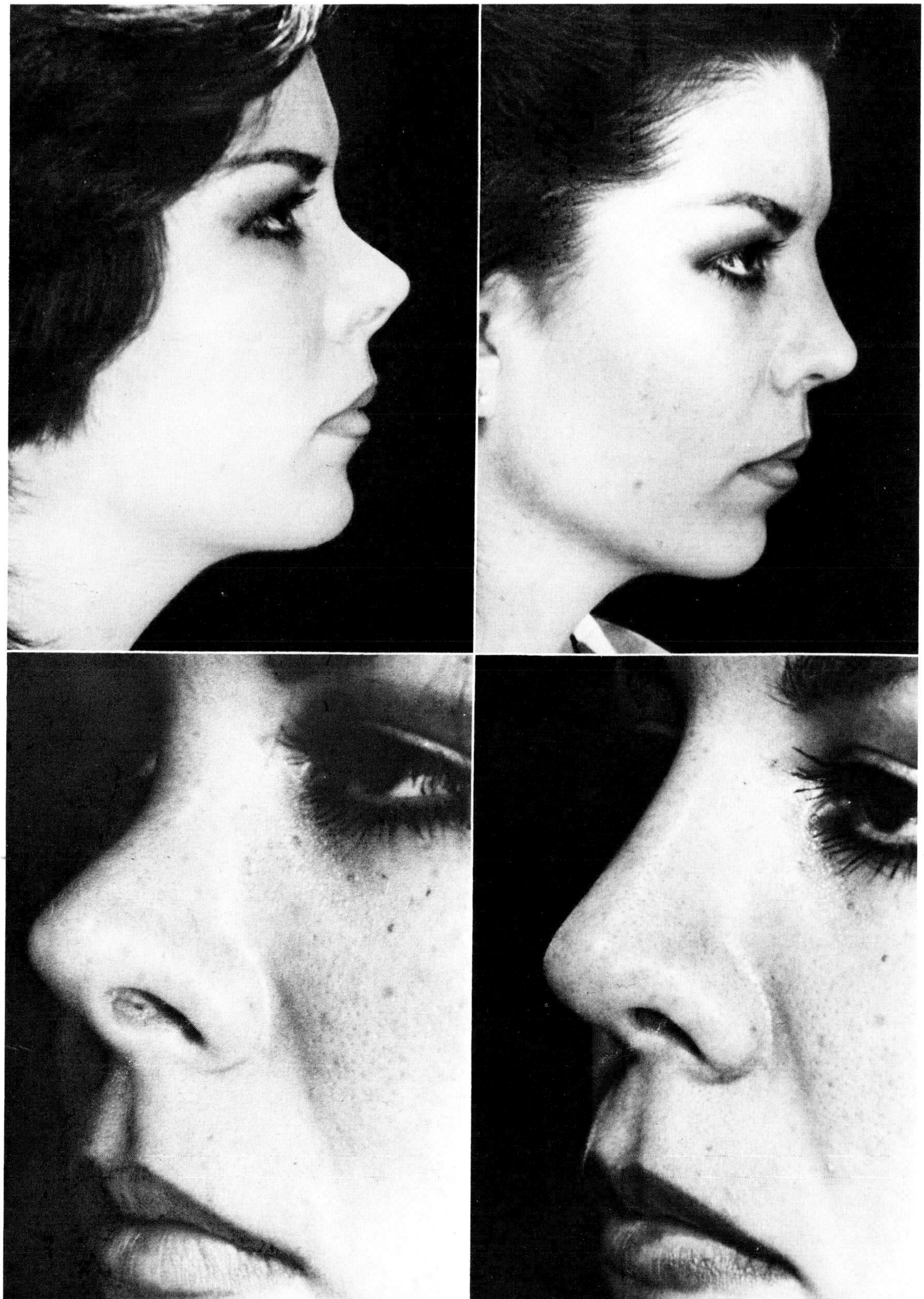

CASE REPORT 3: ETHMOID AND VOMER GRAFTS

Ethmoid or vomer is often the best material available for certain reconstructive needs. These bones have proved useful to support collapsed alae, provide structure for an impaired internal valve, or reconstruct a smooth contour for the lateral nasal walls.

The use of ethmoid or vomer for dorsal augmentation often is overlooked, but it does offer a feasible alternative to conchal cartilage in patients whose septal cartilage has been resected or who are uncomfortable with the idea of altering the structure of their ears.

Mucosal palpation with an applicator, following cocainization, will determine preoperatively whether or not the ethmoid or vomer appears to be adequate for the proposed use.

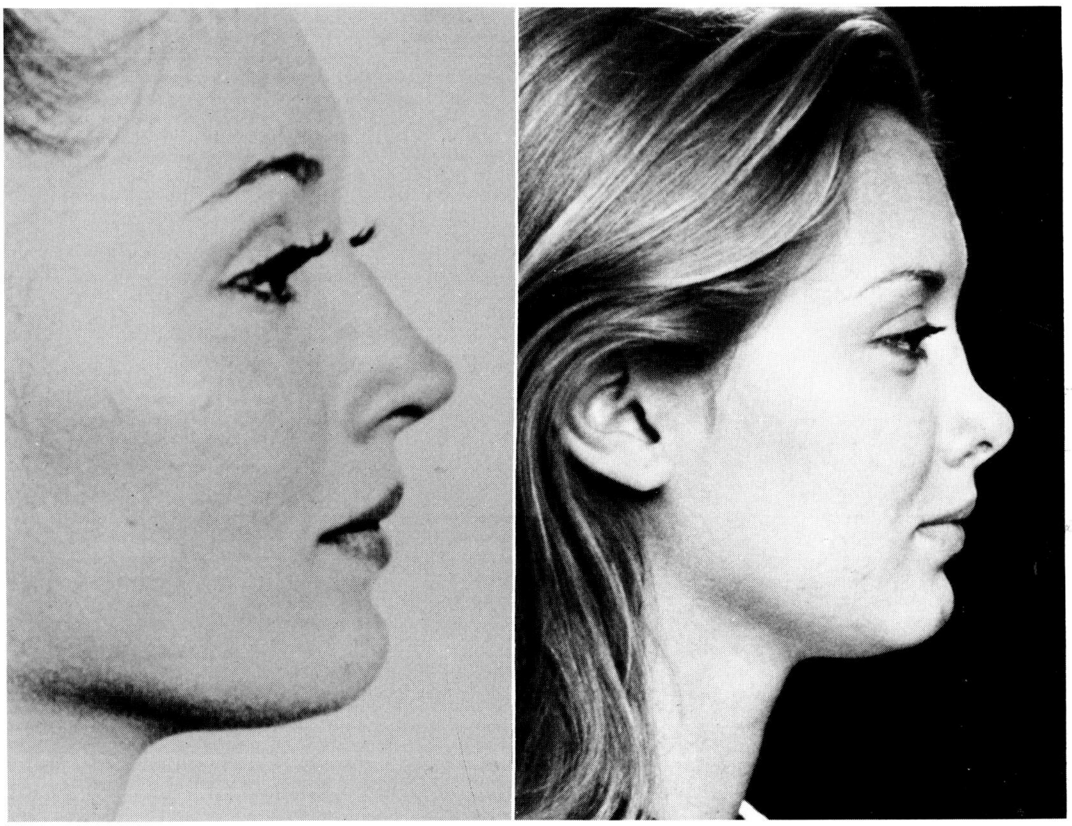

This fashion model originally requested that her slight dorsal irregularity be removed for professional reasons. Preoperatively, all of the relationships were excellent except for a very small dorsal hump. A conservative rasping of the dorsum without osteotomy or tip modification may have preserved the appearance of this exceptionally good nose.

A primary rhinoplasty resulted in a saddle deformity and a loss of tip projection. A major septoplasty removed virtually all of the septal cartilage except for narrow dorsal and caudal supports.

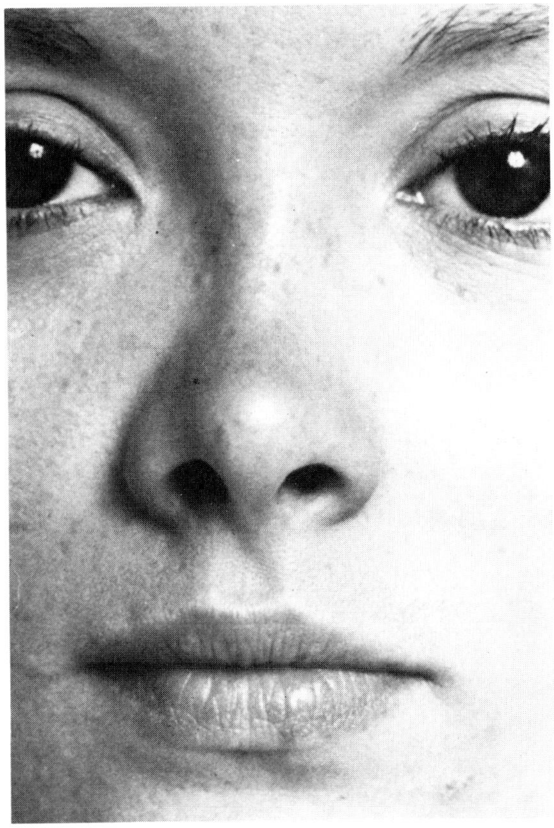

On front view, the overreduced and narrowed bony pyramid has an unfavorable effect on the appearance of the midface. The lines of the lateral nasal walls converge on a point at the supratip area. The single light reflex at the nasal tip indicates a small, rounded tip, resulting from overreduction of the lower lateral cartilages.

Summary of surgical procedure

1. Dissection of a small dorsal pocket through a right intercartilaginous incision
2. Resection of all available ethmoid and vomer
3. Placement of a dorsal graft of vomer, with bony fragments used as underfill
4. Dissection of two lateral nasal wall pockets through separate incisions
5. Placement of ethmoid grafts over lateral nasal walls, with underfill of ethmoid and vomer fragments to augment the width of the nasal pyramid

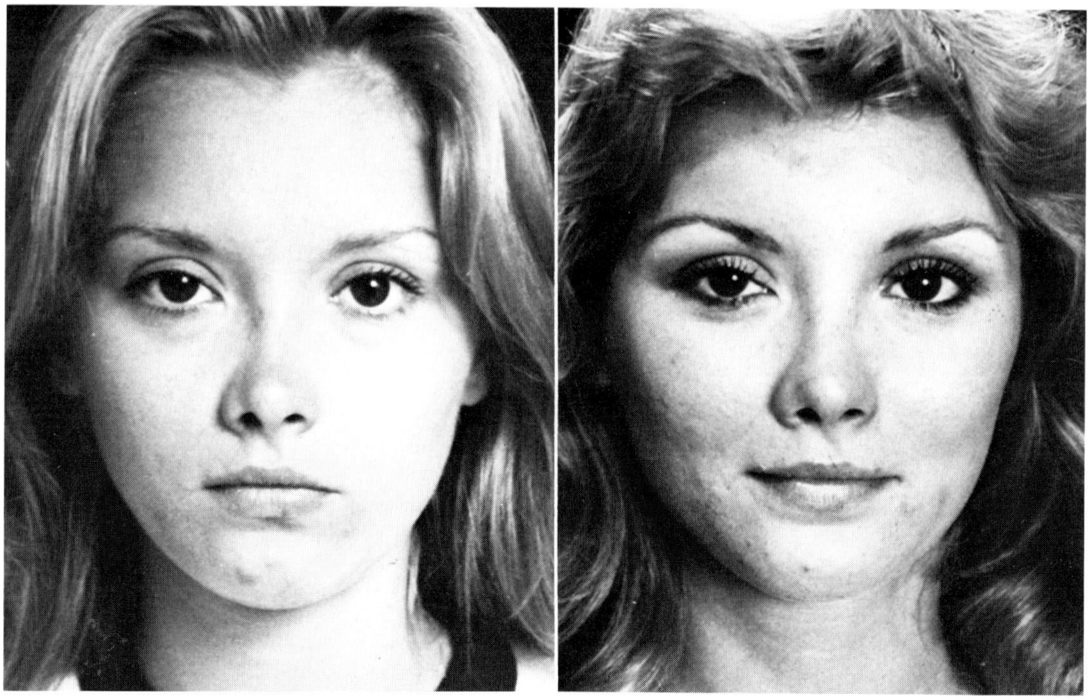

POSTOPERATIVE RESULTS

On front view, the reconstruction of the nasal pyramid has restored the normal confluence of nasofacial lines.

Postoperatively, the dorsum has been adequately elevated by the multiple bone grafts of ethmoid and vomer. The nasal tip is unchanged.

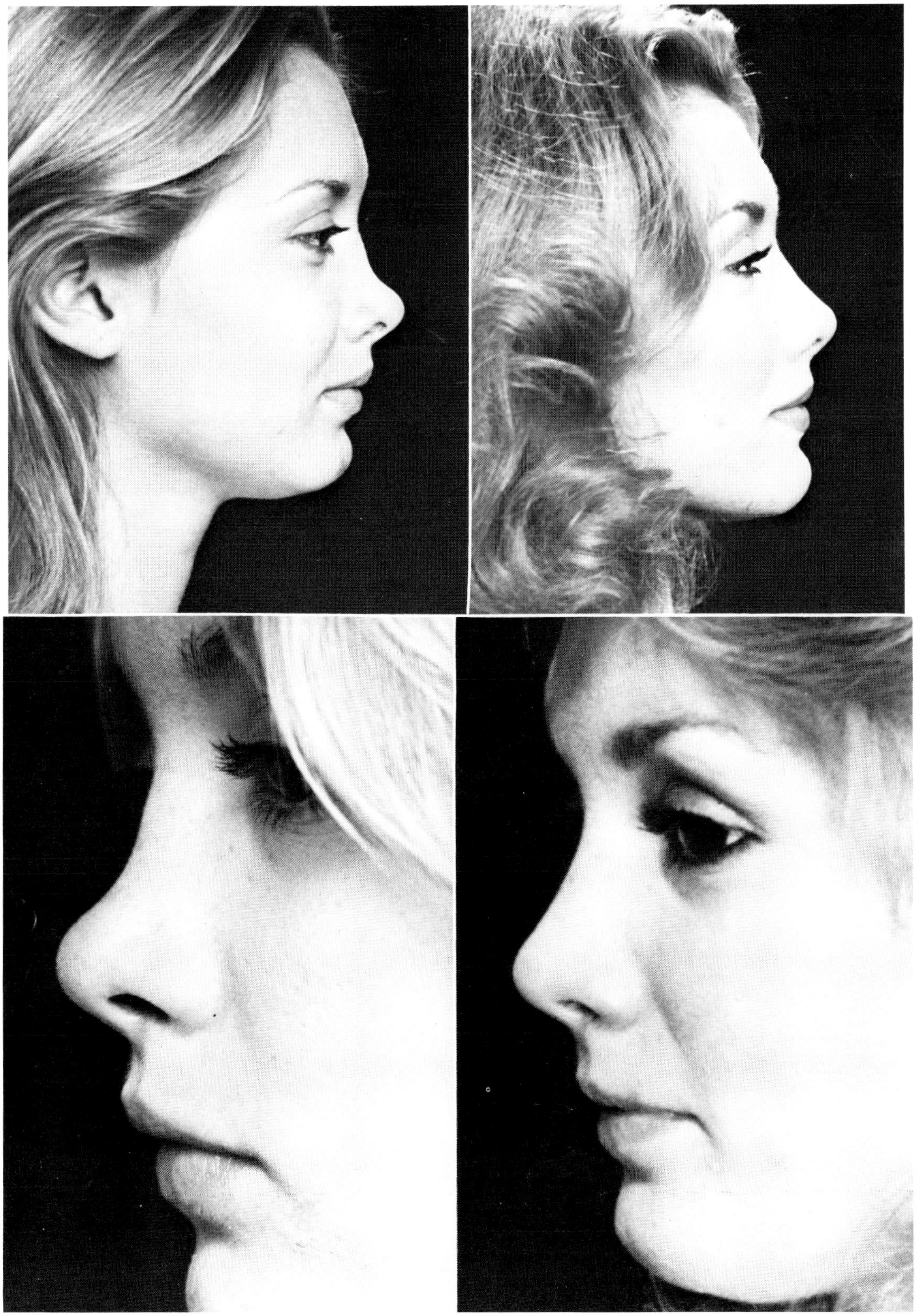

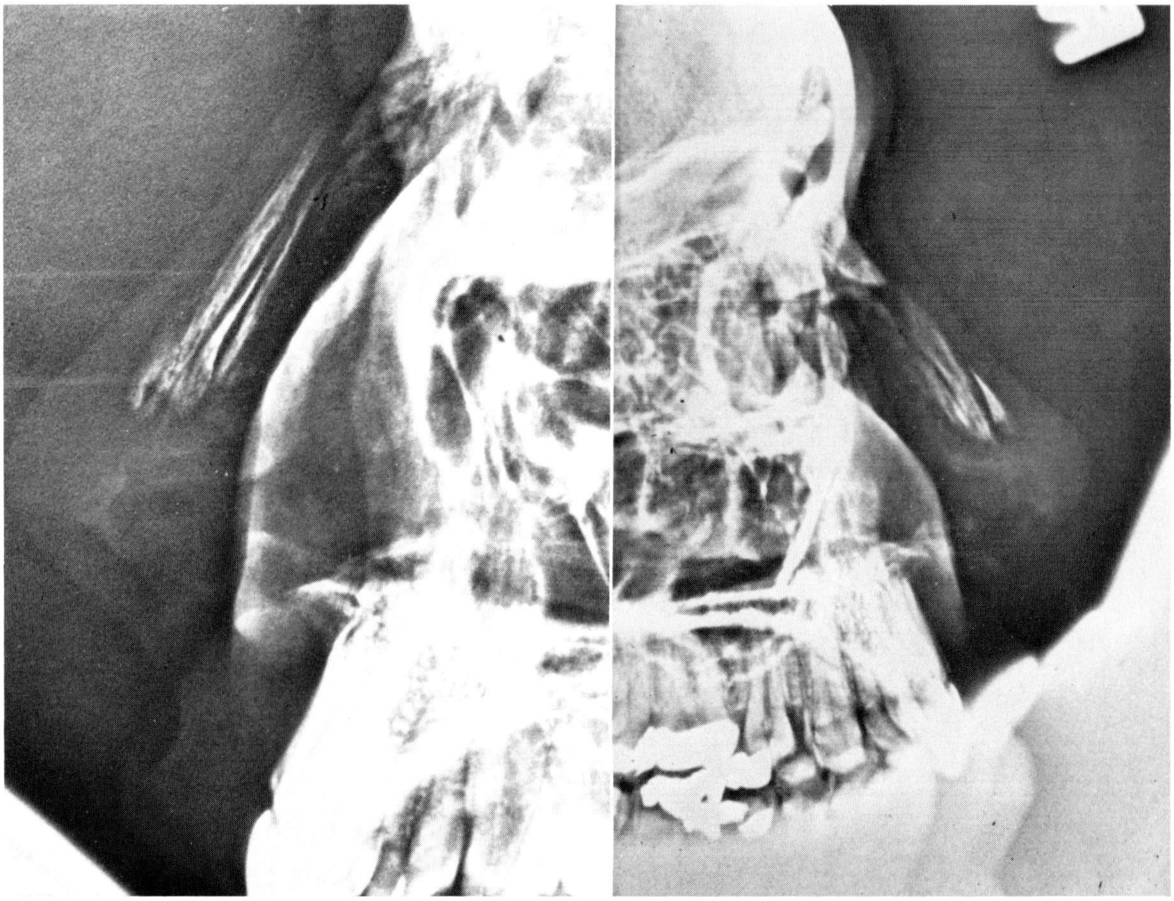

Xerograms were taken at 6 months. These right and left views show the three-tiered graft of vomer and ethmoid. There is faint evidence of the perpendicular plate that was used to re-create the lateral nasal walls on both sides.

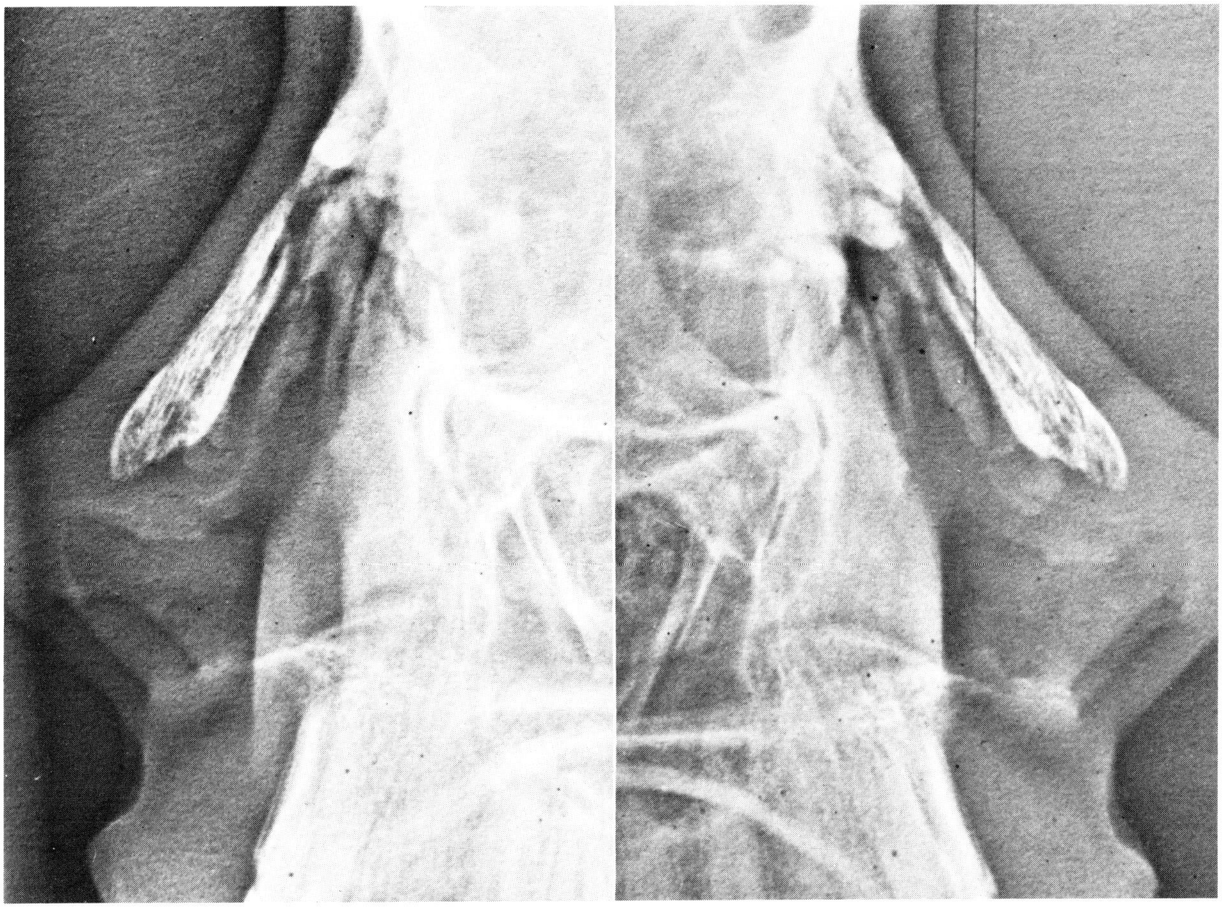

Xerograms taken of the same patient 3 years, 6 months after surgery show some interesting changes. There is consolidation of the dorsal grafts with trabeculation of bone between them. The graft size has not diminished as shown by x-ray film or by clinical comparison. Though the nose was a solid frame at 6 months, it was movable at the time of the second xerogram, which followed an accidental blow to the nose.

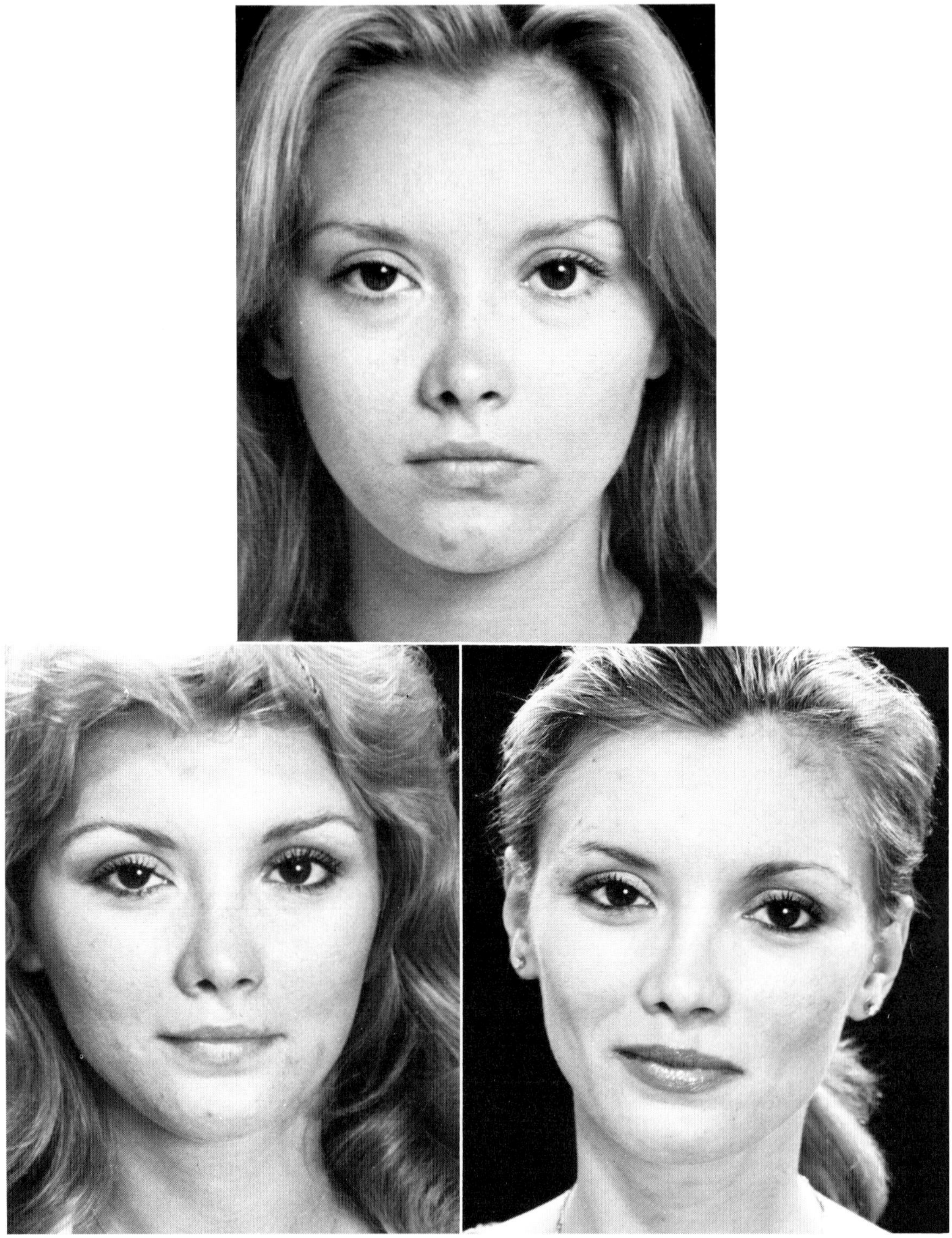

Comparative photographs of the patient at 6 months *(left)* and at 3½ years *(right)* after secondary correction indicate no appreciable change in nasal contour. The onlay grafts of ethmoid continue to provide support and width to the lateral nasal walls.

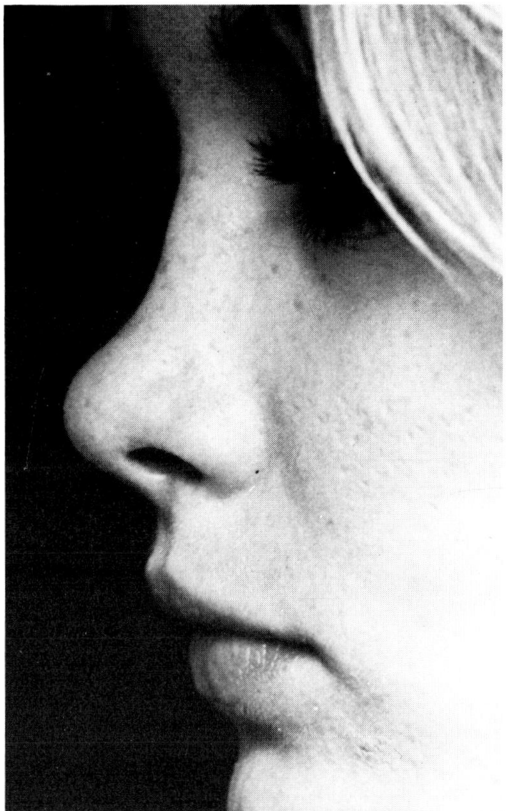

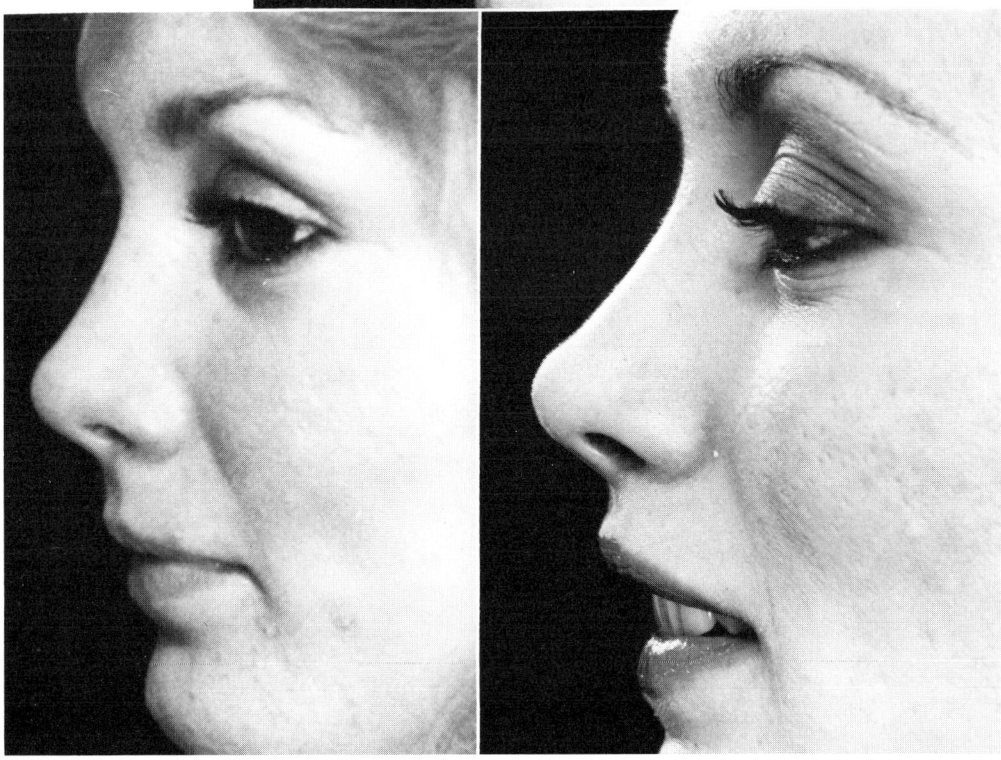

After 3½ years *(right),* there is a slight lowering of the supratip area, causing more differentiation of the tip from the dorsum. The dorsal height remains excellent, as does the smooth line from the superciliary ridge to the nasal tip.

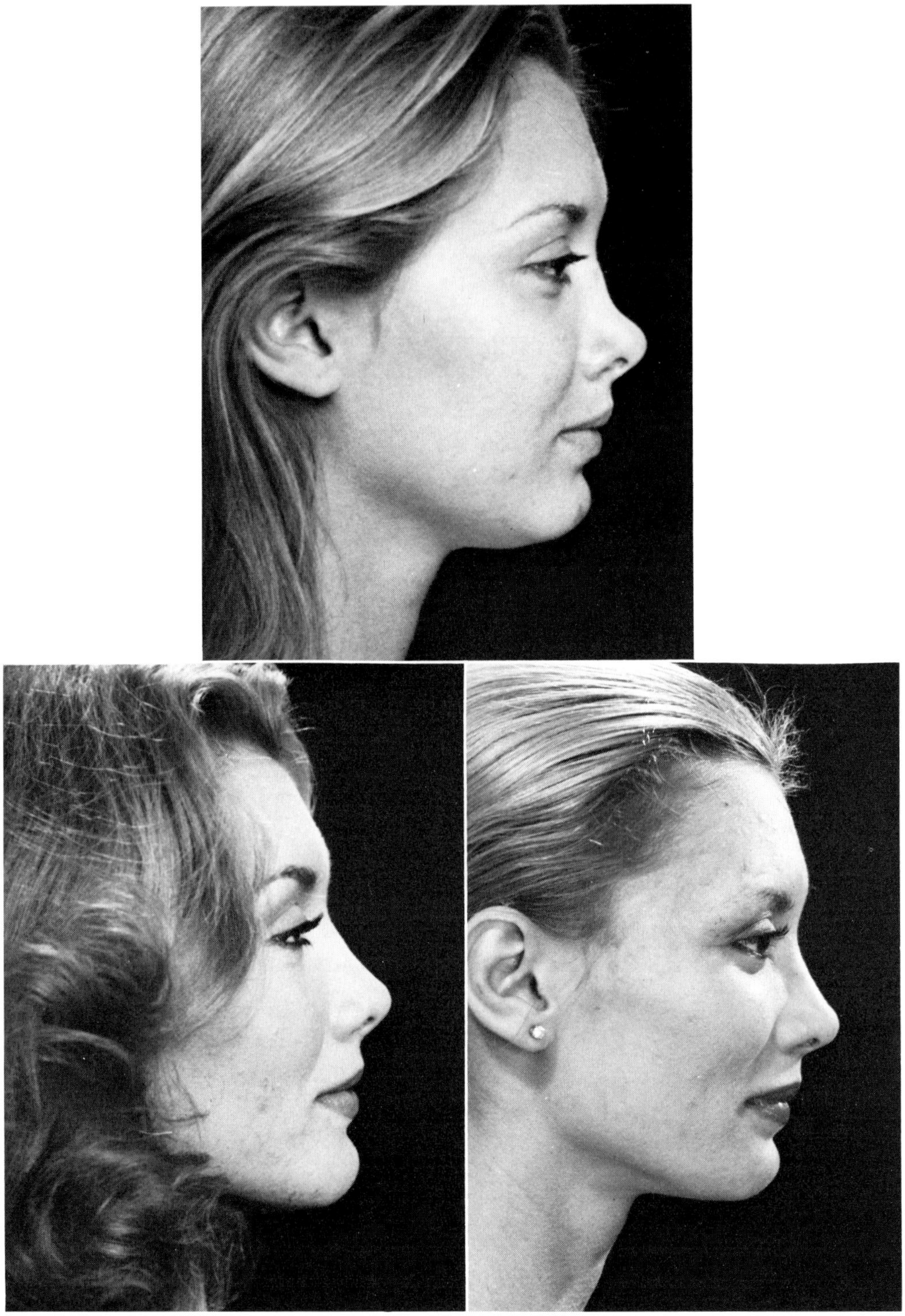

On right lateral view, the changes that have occurred over the 3-year period between secondary correction and final photograph are negligible. The vomer has furnished a dorsal graft that is aesthetically suitable and lasting.

DISCUSSION

Vomer is not recommended as a primary source of material for dorsal grafting. In fact, I consider this material to be a last resort because of the questionable effects of vomer resection on turbinate function. However, after 3½ years this patient's nasal airways are patent, and the turbinates appear normal. Moreover, this case illustrates the usefulness of vomer as a free graft and its perseverance over a significant length of time.

When one is attempting to harvest vomer, special precautions must be taken to preserve the integrity of the mucoperichondrial flap. The dissection should proceed from a tunnel below the vomerian groove to the septal cartilage. If the dissection is attempted from cartilage to bone, tearing of the mucosa and an improper plane of dissection are likely occurrences.

It is also advisable to fill the septal void with any leftover cartilage or bone to provide some rigidity to the septum. Crushed pieces of bone, remnants of lower lateral cartilage, small bits of caudal septum—any such leftovers—can be flattened with a cartilage crusher and then used as septal filling.

CASE REPORT 4: SEPTAL CARTILAGE GRAFT

Septal cartilage is the most practical, versatile, and predictable material available for nasal reconstruction. Usually it can be harvested in adequate amounts and is amenable to carving, crushing, layering, and other manipulations to produce a variety of sizes and shapes. Unlike costal cartilage, septal cartilage does not have a tendency to curl.

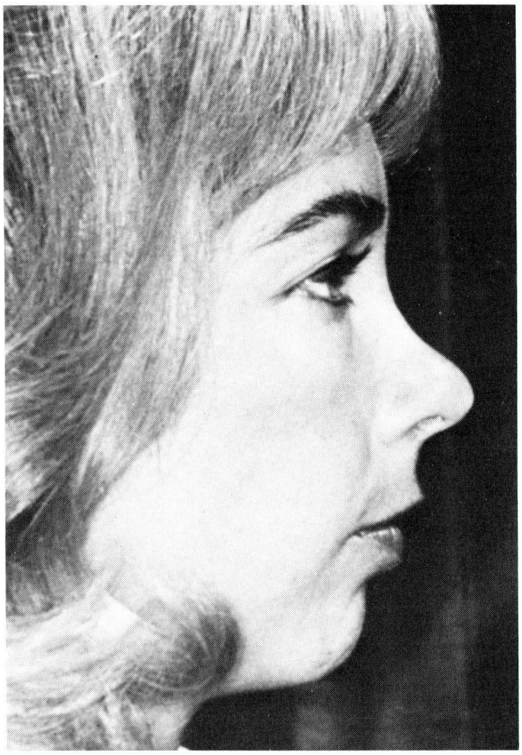

This patient had a primary rhinoplasty 8 years before consultation. On lateral view, there is a very low dorsum, a slightly high supratip, a poorly defined nasal tip, and an open nasolabial angle. The chin is slightly retrusive.

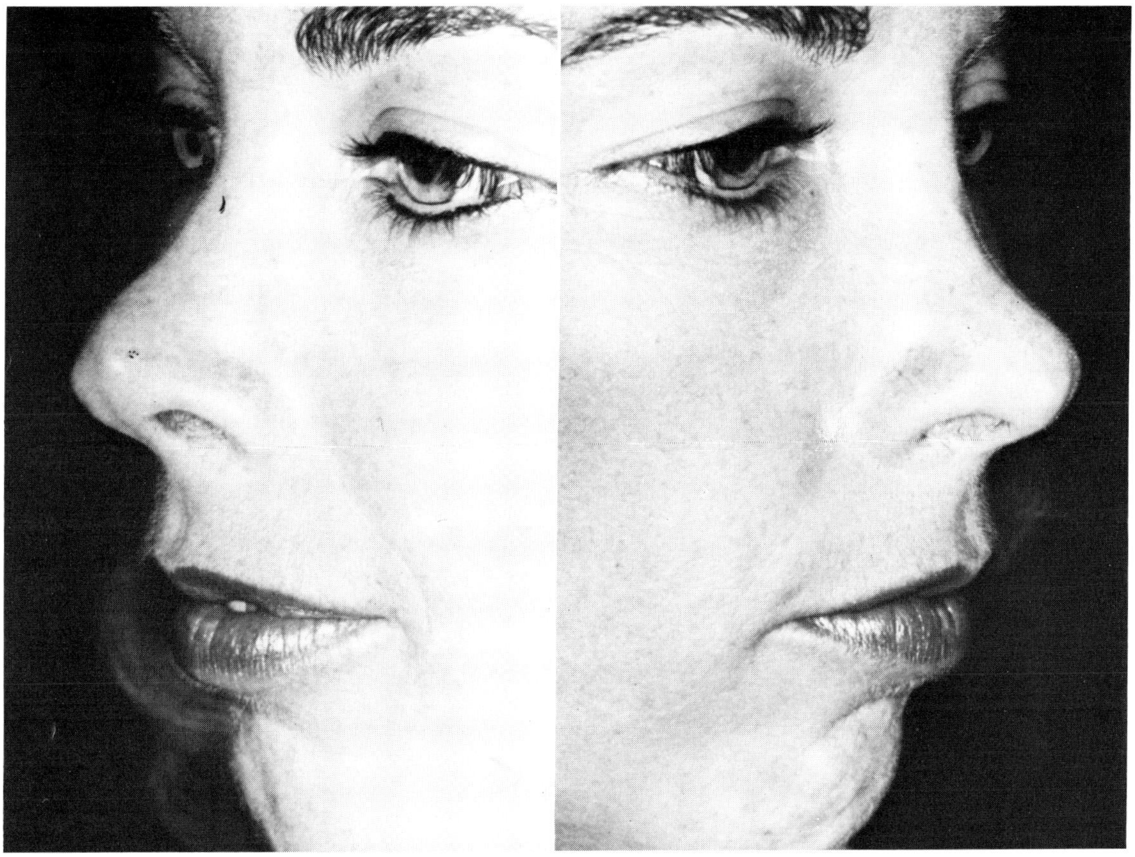

On left oblique view, irregular tip projections are visible, and the tip appears to be twisting toward the viewer. On right oblique view, the tip appears to be twisting away from the viewer.

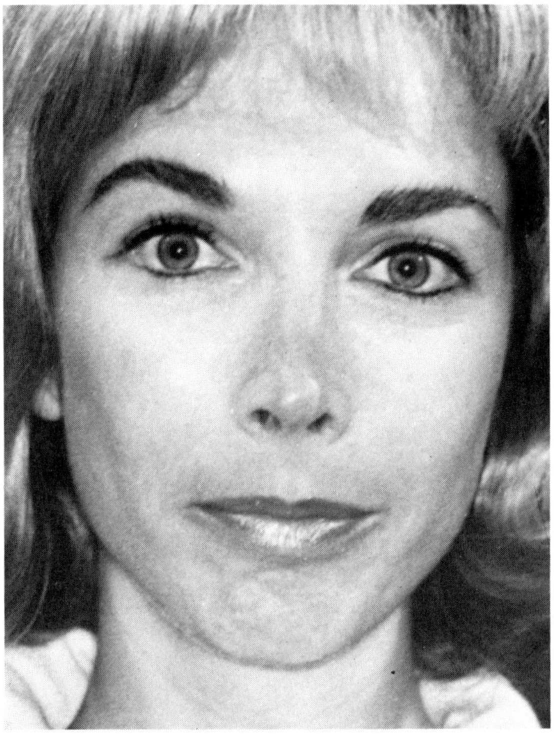

On front view, the lateral nasal lines are uneven, reflecting the flat and irregular nasal dorsum. The low dorsum creates a characteristic vacant appearance to the midface. The domes of the lower lateral cartilages are prominent and asymmetrical.

A

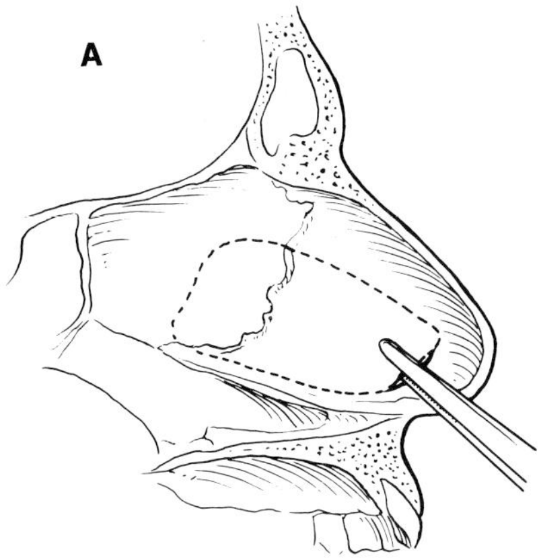

B

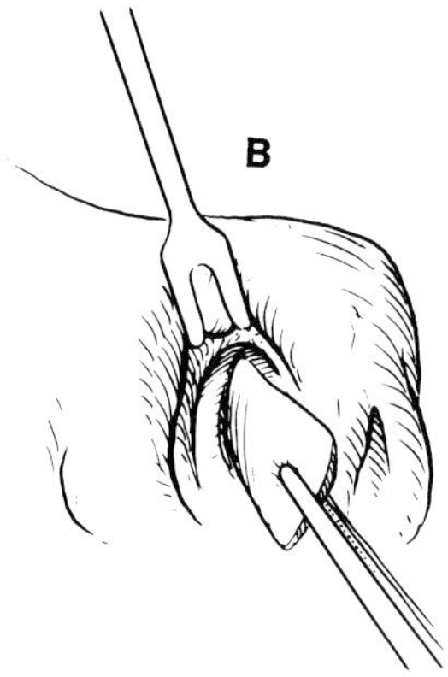

D

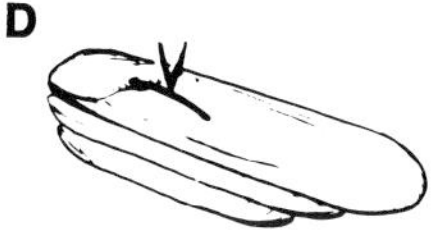

C

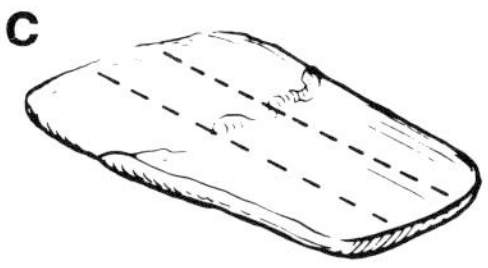

E

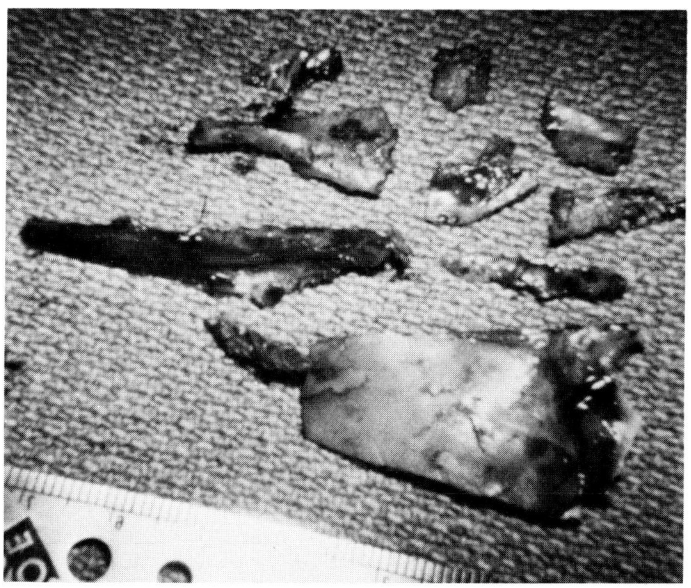

F

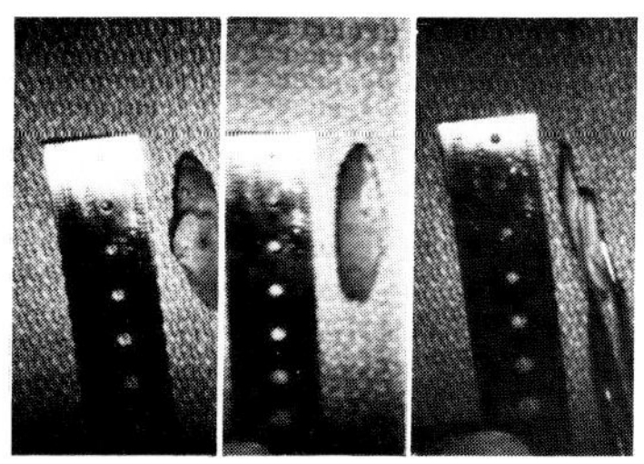

SURGICAL PROCEDURE

Septal material was obtained as shown in *A* and *B*. The actual specimen is shown in *E*. *C* and *D* illustrate the preparation of the graft from the largest piece of cartilage and perpendicular plate. The photographs in *F* are the three views of the prepared graft. Note the broad and smooth dorsal surface of the graft and the thick central part that coincides with the deformity.

Summary of surgical procedure

1. Limited skeletonization
2. Major submucous resection for the graft material
3. Exploration of the tip, with resection of cartilaginous projections
4. Preparation and insertion of a three-tiered dorsal graft
5. Insertion of a graft
6. Mentoplasty

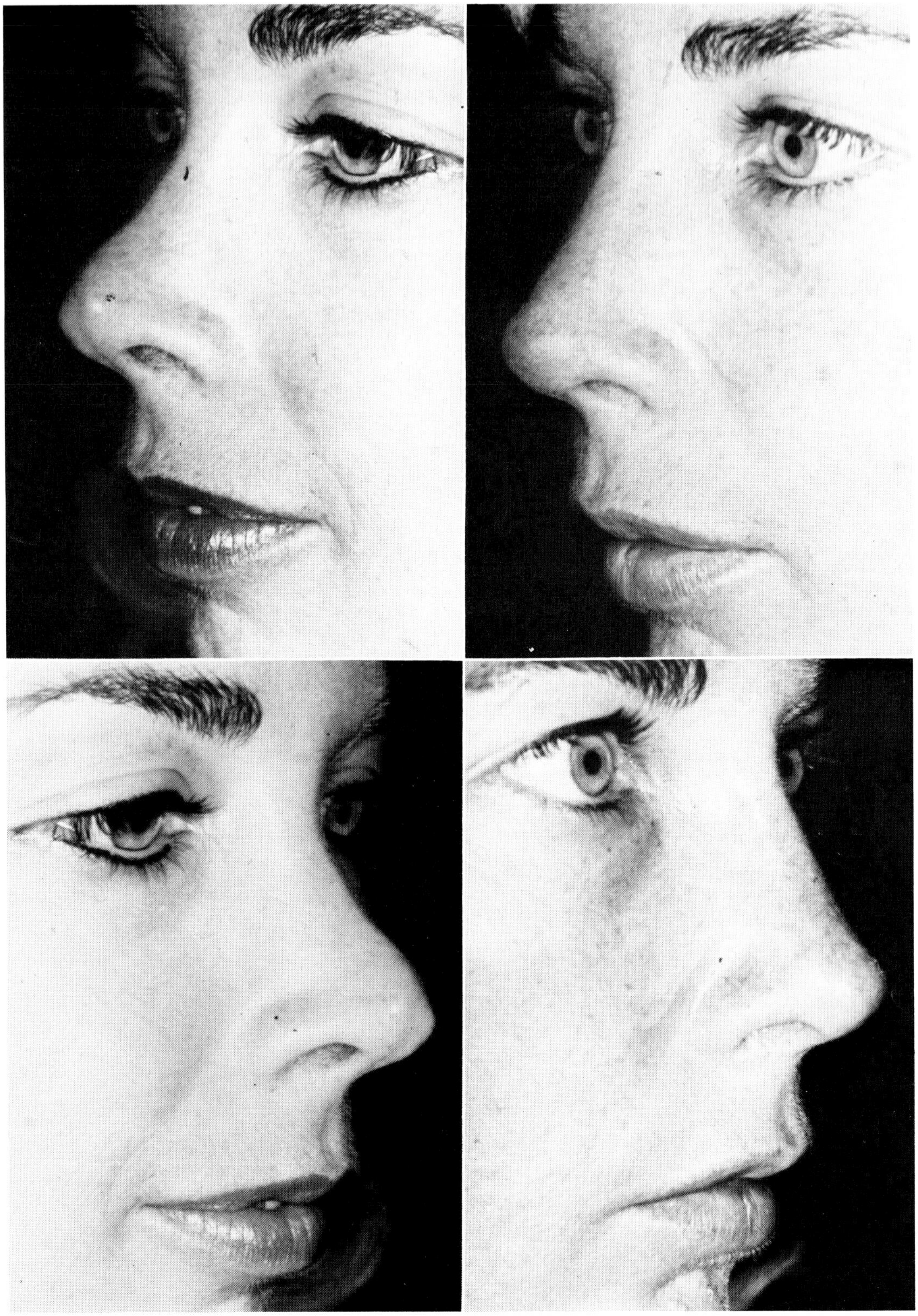

POSTOPERATIVE RESULTS

Postoperatively, the two oblique views are almost symmetrical with the tip in a central position. The septal graft has provided a smooth, broad, straight dorsum.

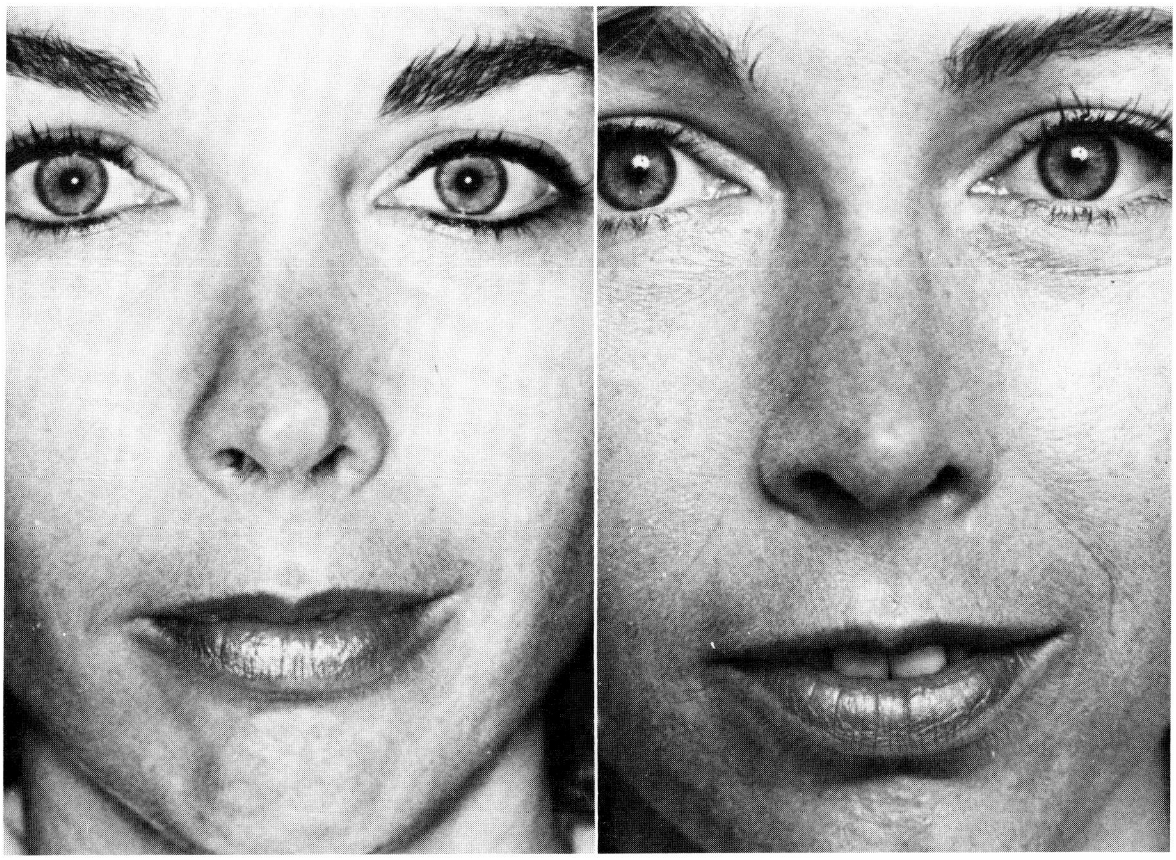

After 4 years, the dorsal graft remains virtually unchanged. The central light reflex from the nasal tip indicates a narrower tip than is ideal; this is the result of a necessary compromise to obtain symmetry and controlled projection.

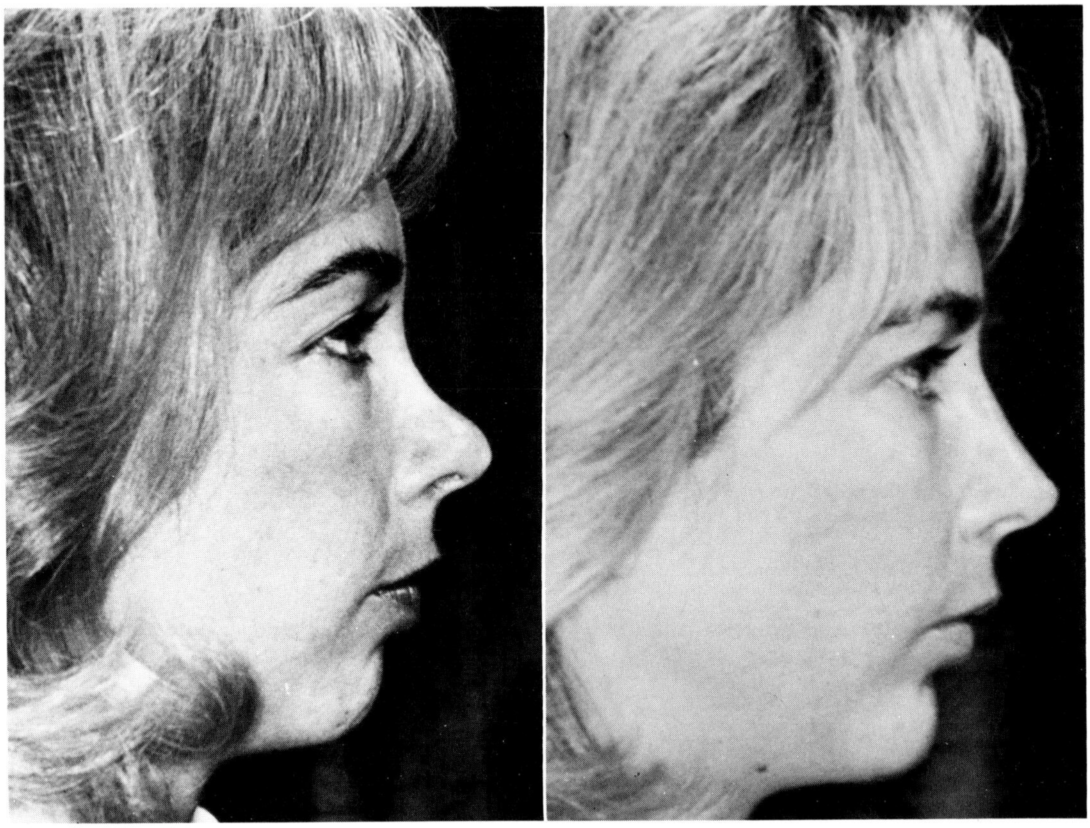

On lateral view, the postoperative nasal contour is fine and natural appearing. A mentoplasty has made a significant improvement in the facial balance.

DISCUSSION

This case was successful because of the abundance and quality of the available septal cartilage. Luck provided a large, straight substantial piece of cartilage with which to re-create a smooth, straight dorsum. The dorsum can be sufficiently elevated by filling in or layering pieces of cartilage under a good "contour graft," while maintaining a smooth surface regardless of the number or shape of the pieces used as filler.

Although this patient's nasal asymmetry was corrected primarily by the dorsal reconstruction, tip reconstruction was also necessary to rectify the distortion of the tip cartilages. Since the lower lateral cartilages were found to be unserviceable, the asymmetrical "knuckles" were resected, and a tip graft of septal cartilage was used to provide support and contour for the tip.

CASE REPORT 5: A MEDLEY

The combination of a straight dorsum and a short bony pyramid made this case especially hazardous for the original surgeon. The results following standard primary and secondary rhinoplasties are almost predictable, based on an understanding of the inherent problems with this type of nose. Examination of the photographs of the original nose was helpful in planning the complex tertiary reconstruction, which utilized grafts of septal cartilage, ethmoid, and vomer.

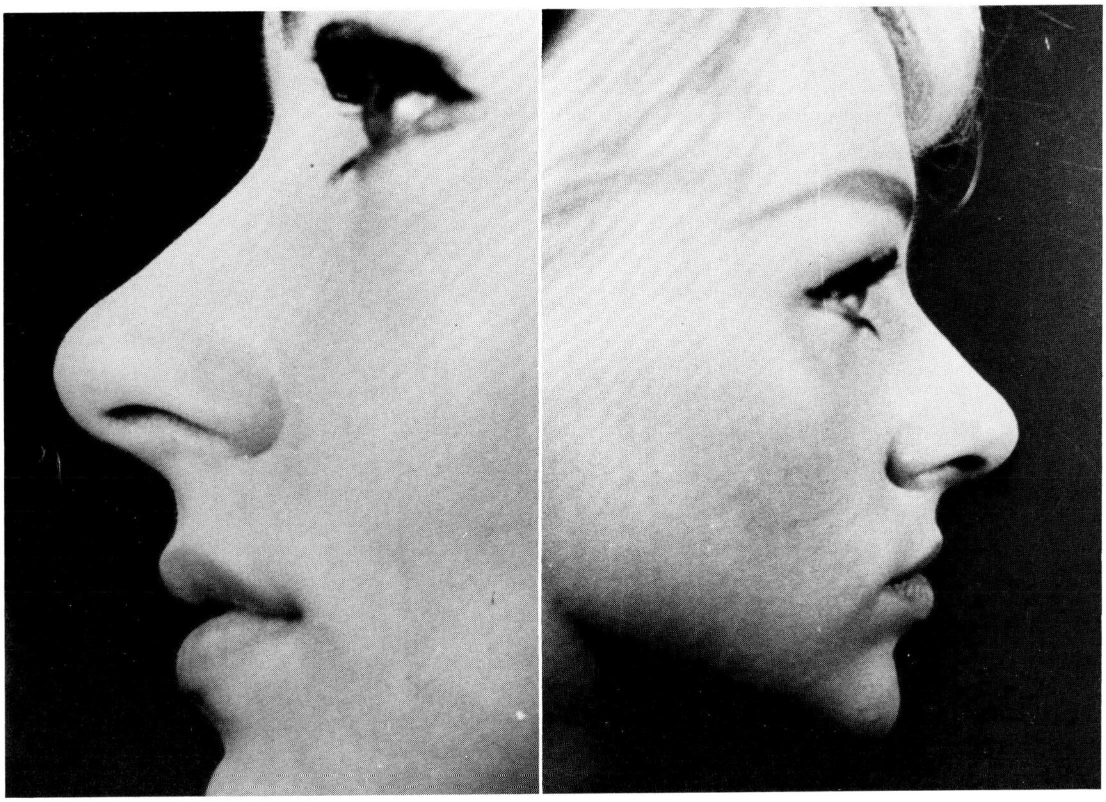

The preoperative right and left lateral views are nearly symmetrical. The radix is low, and the dorsum is straight. The nasal tip is poorly differentiated. The relationship of columella to ala is good, and the nasolabial angle is excellent.

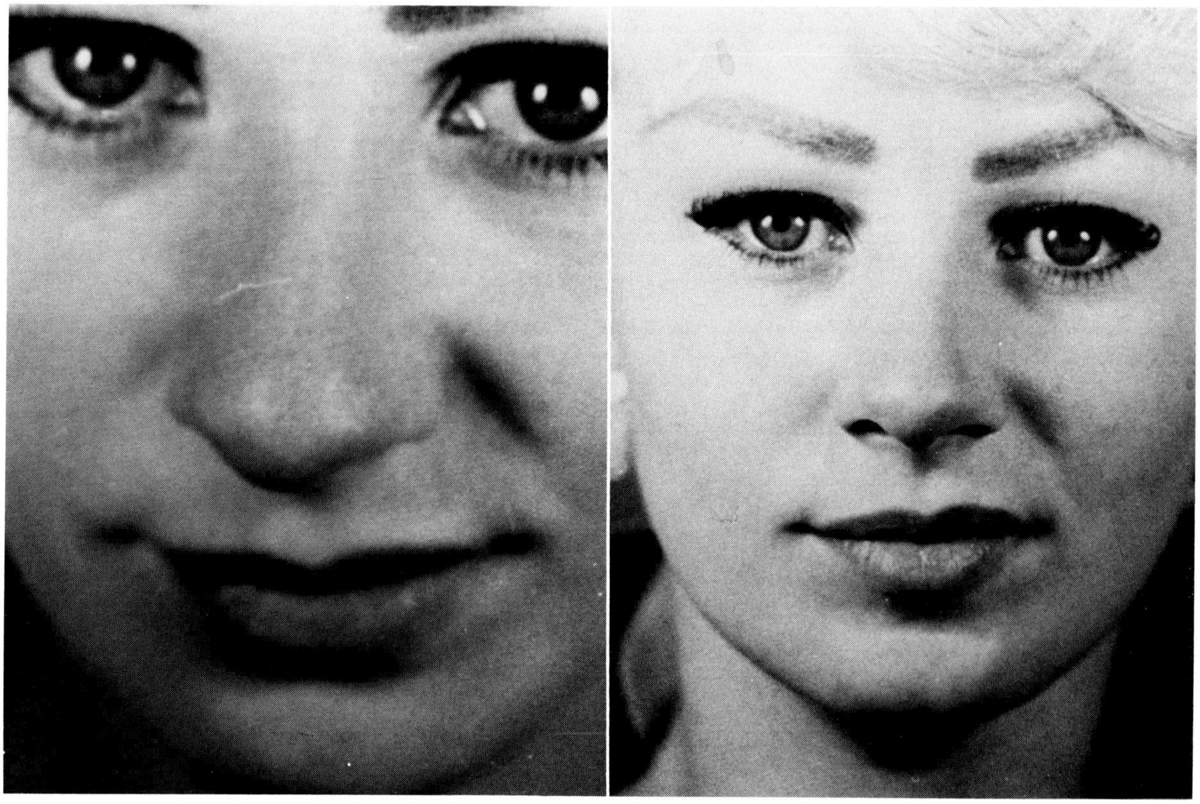

The upper part of the nose is narrow in proportion to the base—a warning that osteotomy would be detrimental. With the head tilted slightly, the hint of a concavity on the right side suggests a short nasal bone. The tip is excellent, though slightly wide. The basal contour demonstrates a perfect gull-in-flight configuration.

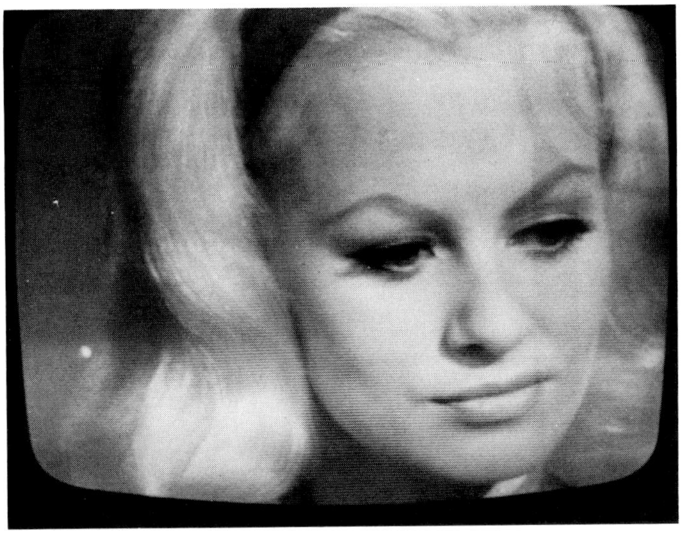

A photograph taken of the patient as she appeared on television clearly shows the borders of the bony pyramid. The central concavity is emphasized by a cross light.

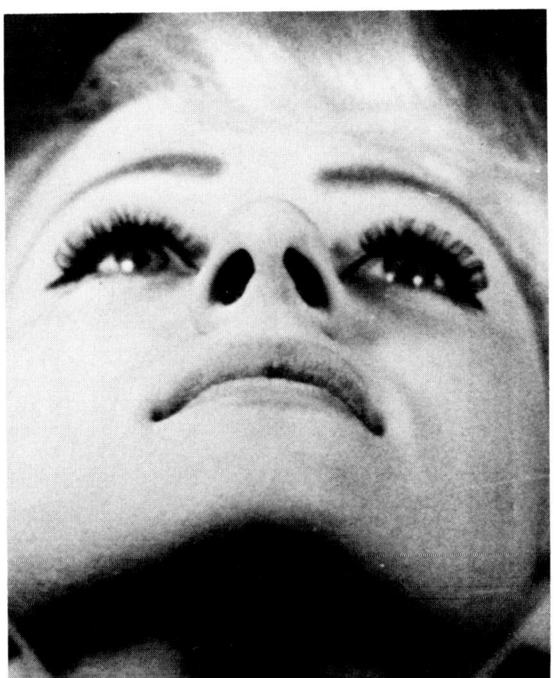

The basal view is close to ideal. The nostrils incline toward the apex of a triangular base.

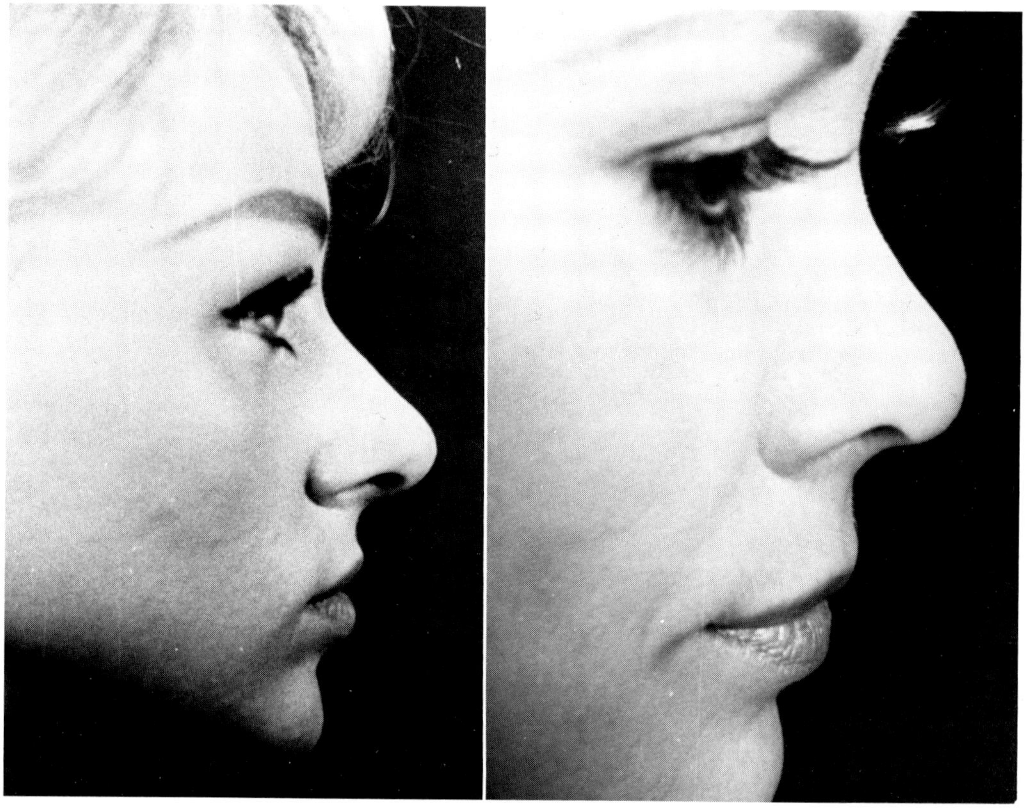

The preoperative nose is compared with the appearance of the nose following two rhinoplasties, illustrating overreduction of the nasal dorsum, tip, and caudal septum.

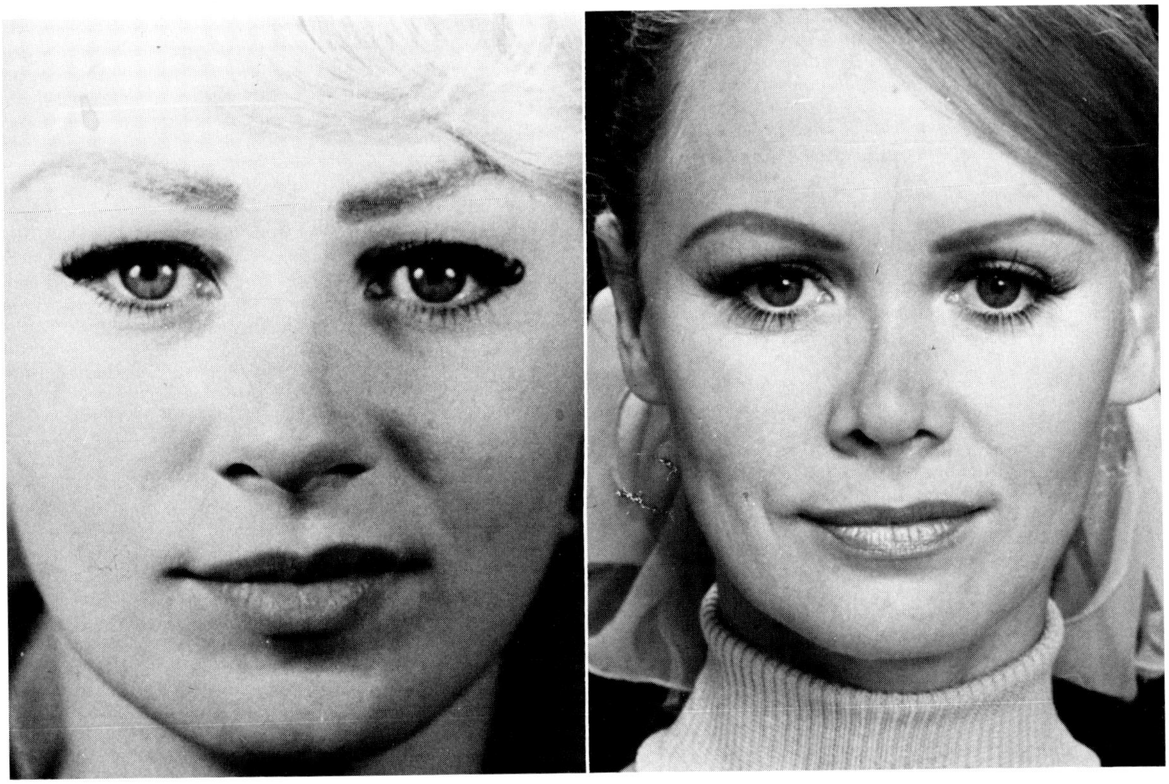

On postoperative front view, the consequence of osteotomies is apparent. The short nasal bones no longer support the lateral nasal walls, which have collapsed toward the septum. There is discontinuity of the line from radix to tip, which accentuates the imbalance of the upper and lower vaults.

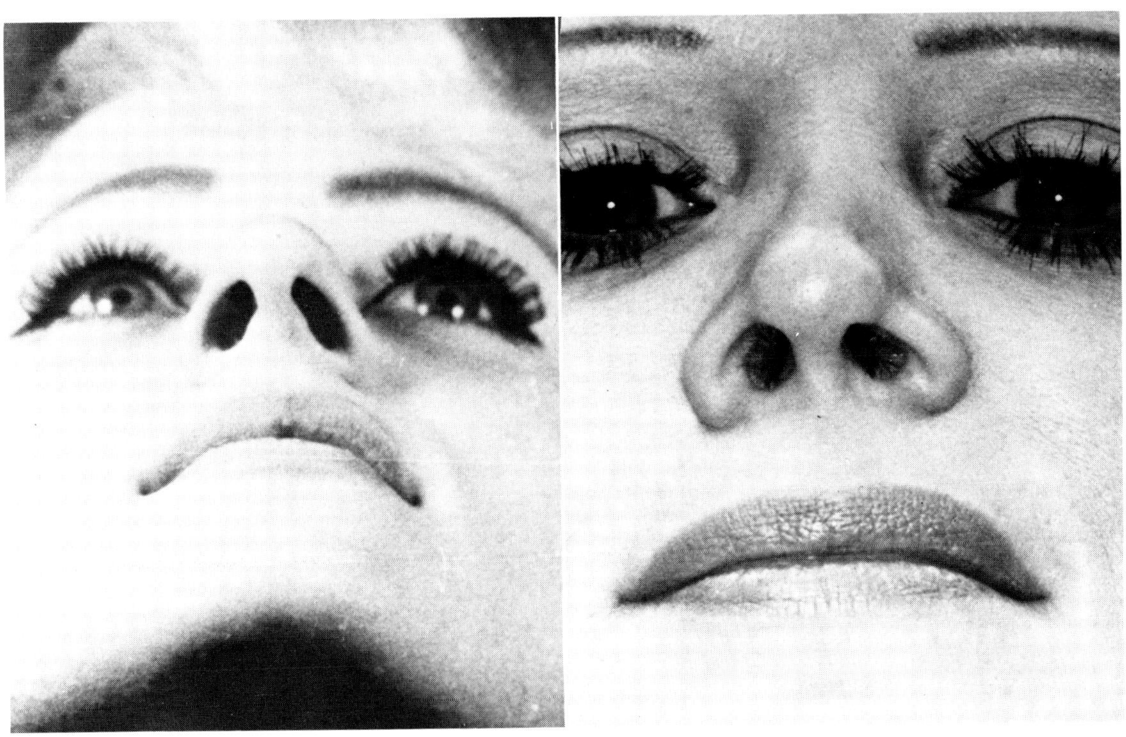

The nostrils flare postoperatively, resulting from a loss of dorsal support and tip projection. The basal perimeter appears to be flattened.

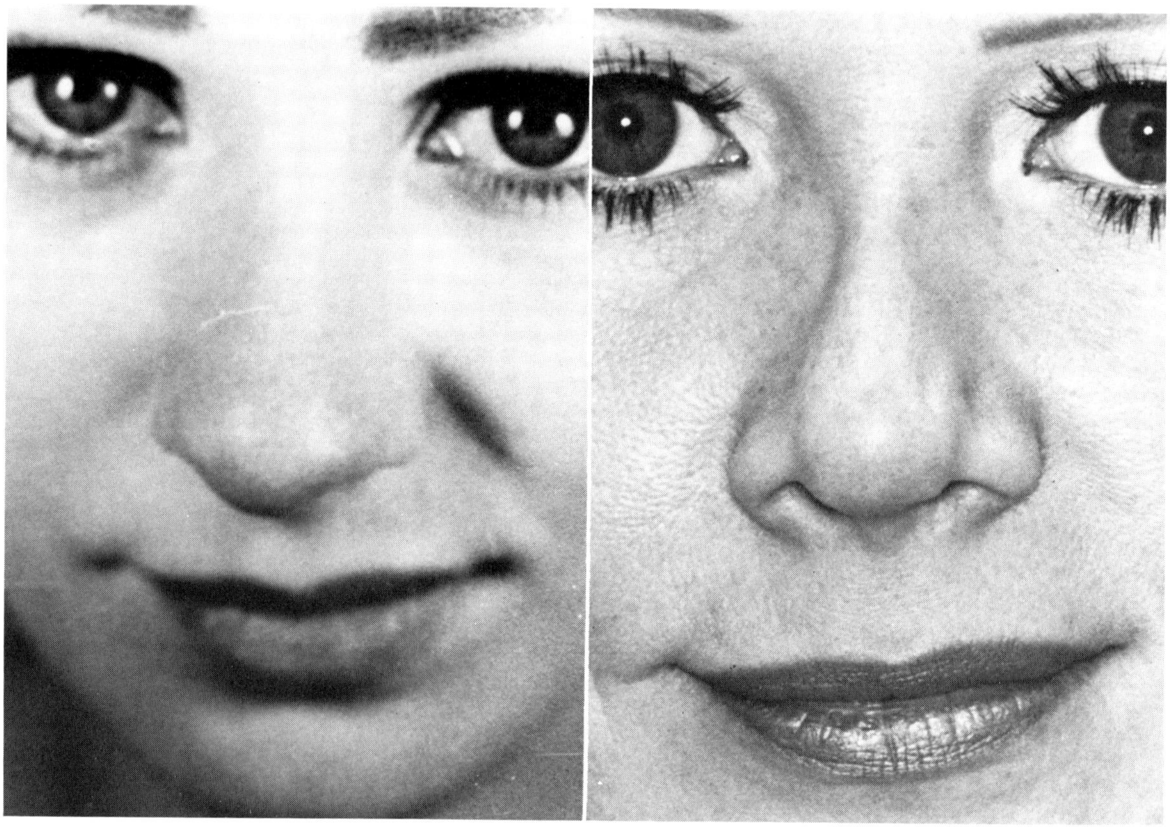

A close-up view illustrates the effects of an attempt to reduce the tip mass to match the overreduced dorsum. The vertical grooves are a permanent deformity that can be improved but never removed.

The aims for reconstruction were to reverse the aesthetic effects of overreduction and to regain good nasal function.

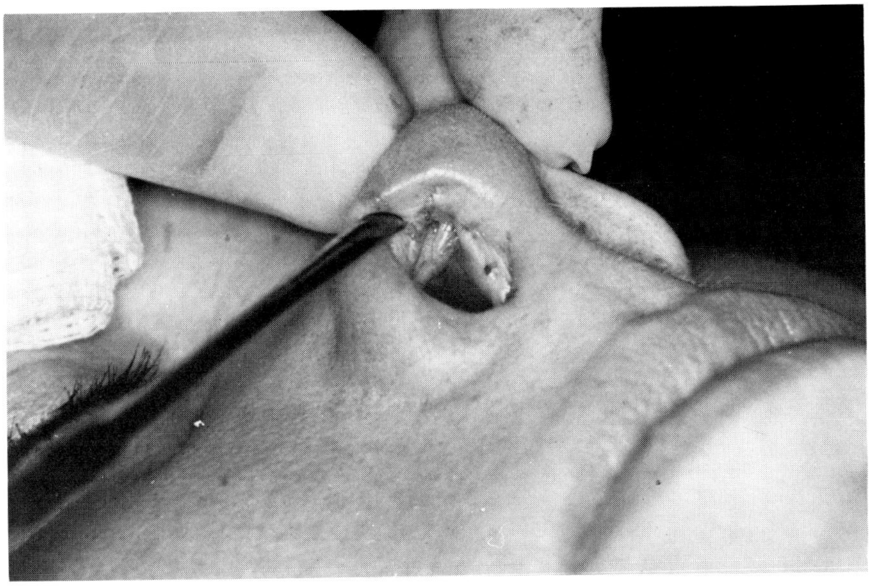

SURGICAL PROCEDURE

A grade I atresia can be seen in the vestibule as the nostril is retracted laterally.

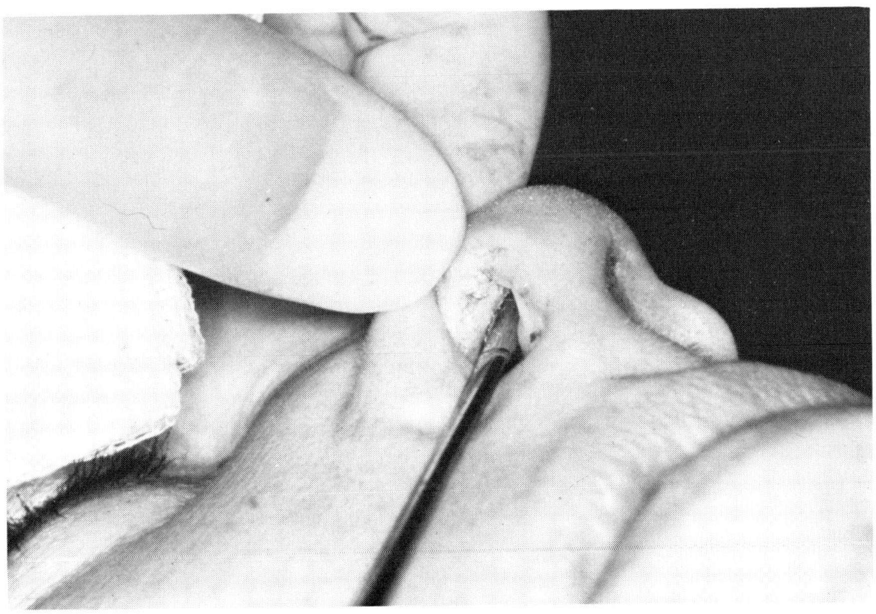

An instrument is placed in a blind pouch that is present behind the web.

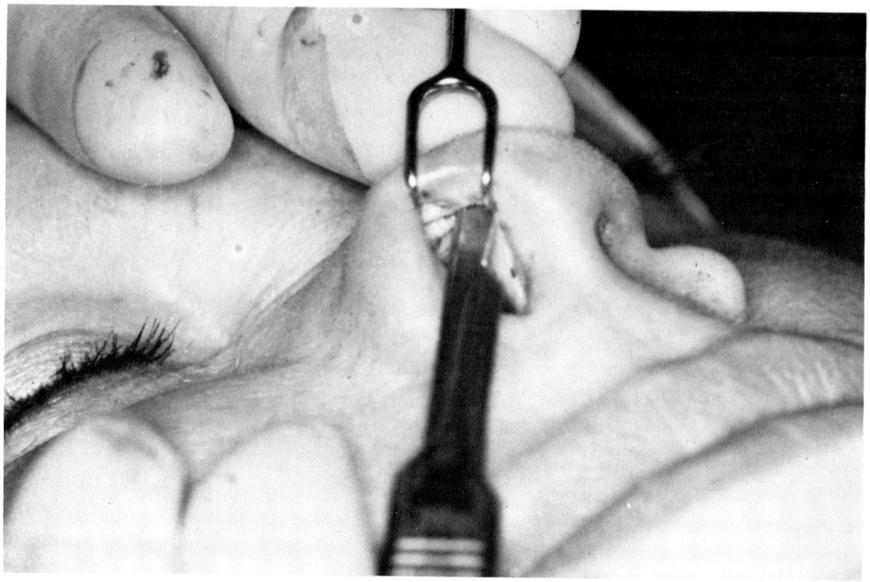

The opening incision is a gull-wing incision that ends just below the angle of the septum.

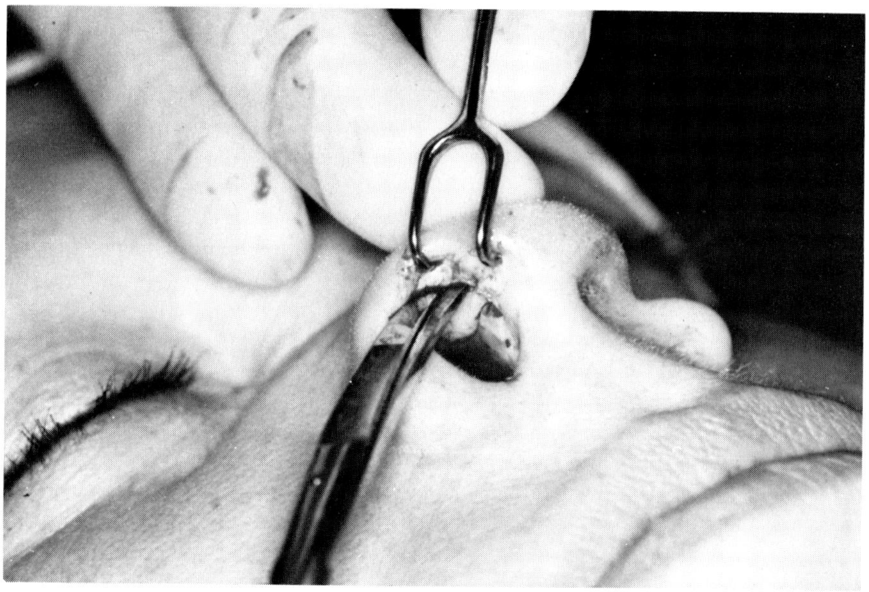

Dissection of the soft tissues proceeds in a subdermal plane.

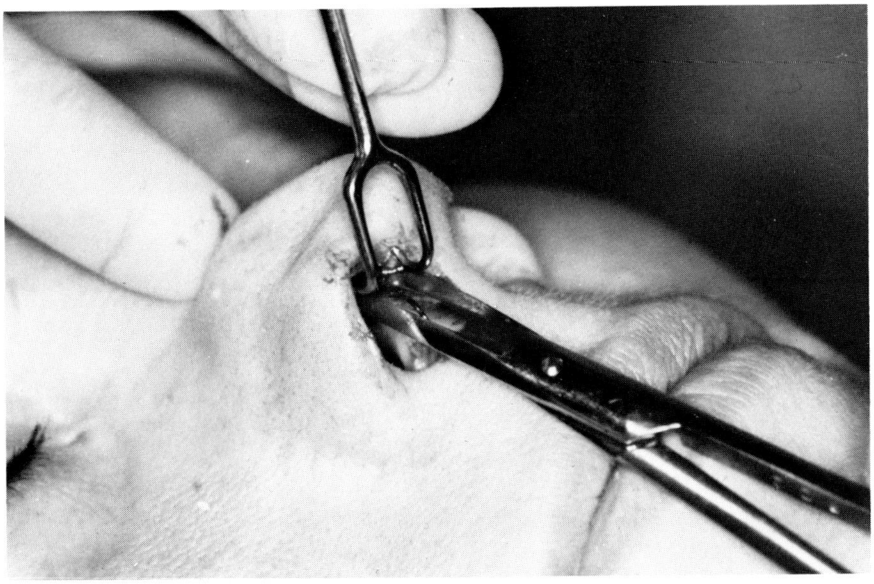

The dissection is carried to the caudal border of the bony vault, which in this patient is almost at the radix.

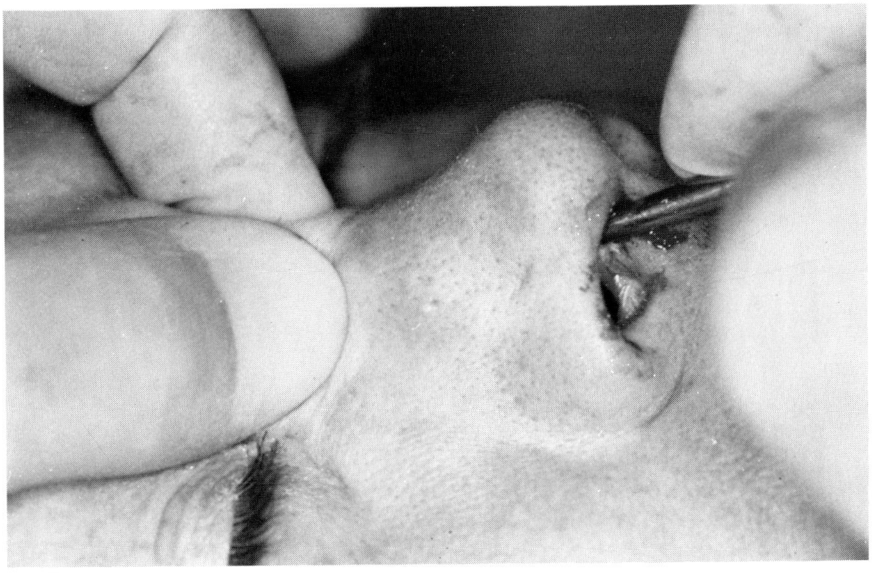

A Joseph periosteal elevator is placed at the bony edge and, with a rocking motion, slipped under the periosteum. It then proceeds to the radix, where it is swept toward the midline.

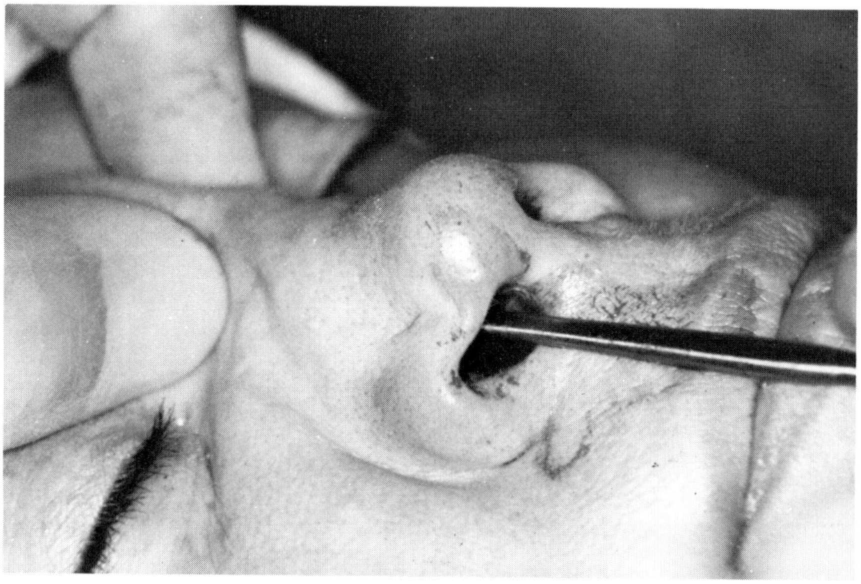

The skeletonization is completed with a right-angle (hockey stick) knife with the handle held below the level of the dorsum to preserve all the soft tissues. The knife is carried around the angle of the septum.

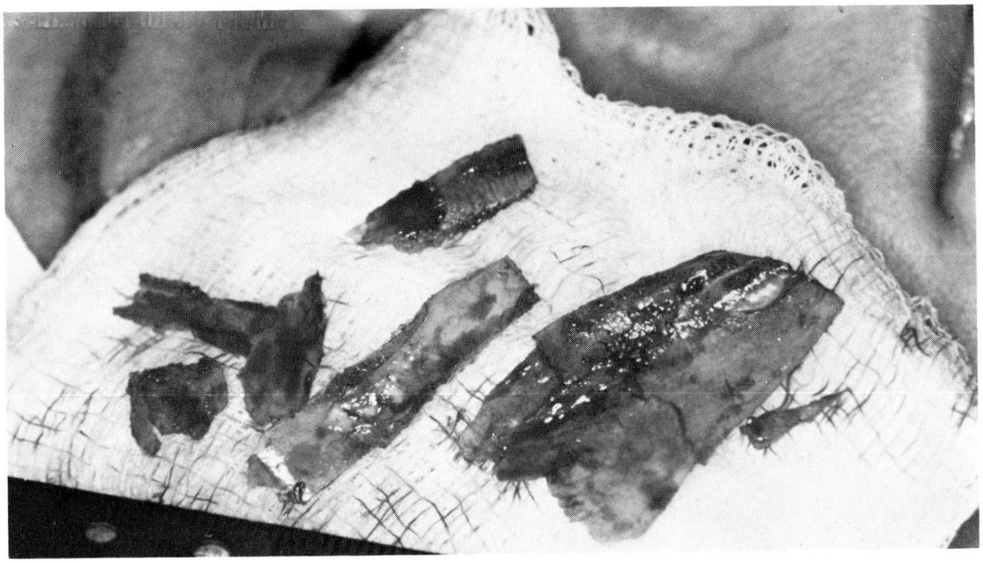

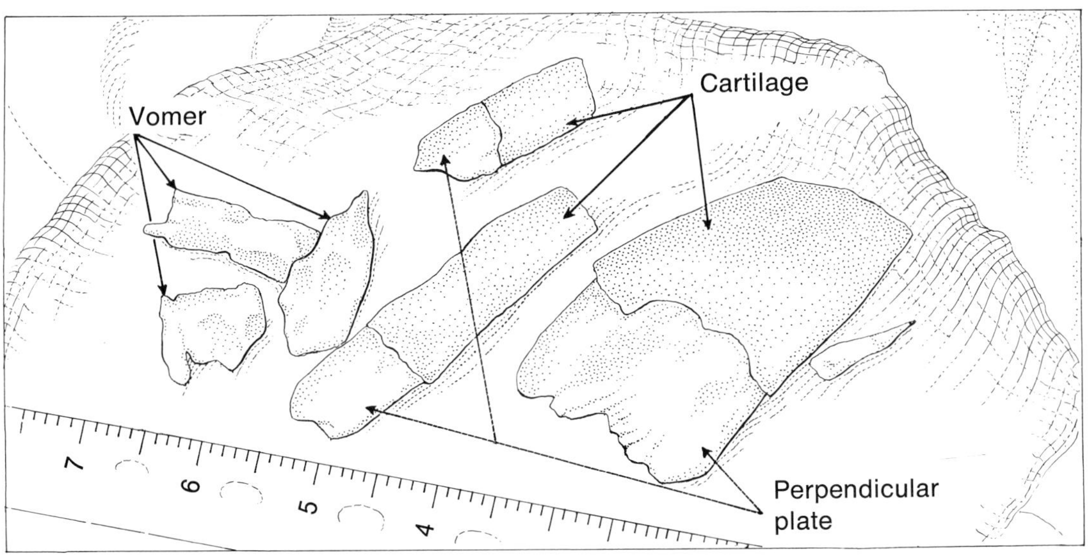

Following resection of septal cartilage and parts of the ethmoid and vomer, all parts are evaluated for their prospective roles in the reconstruction.

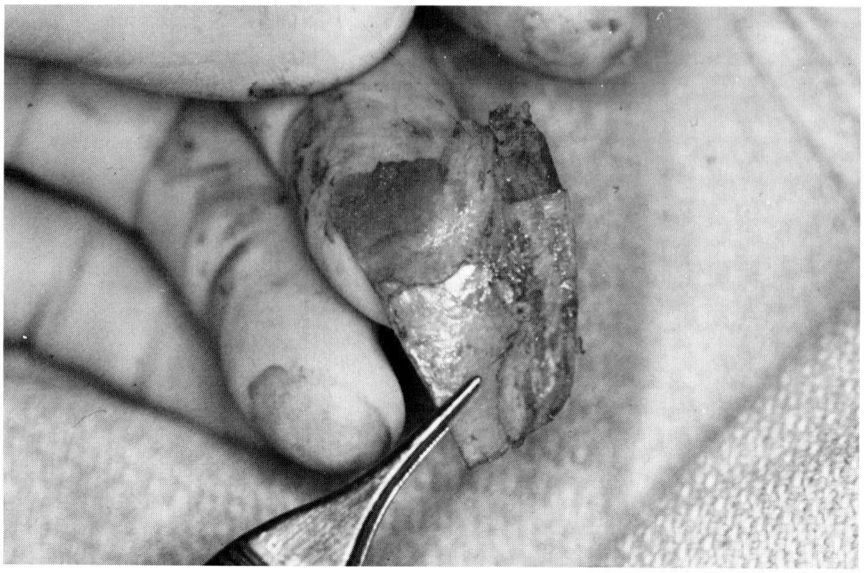

The largest piece was dissected from the vomerian groove. Old fracture lines outline an ideal tip graft.

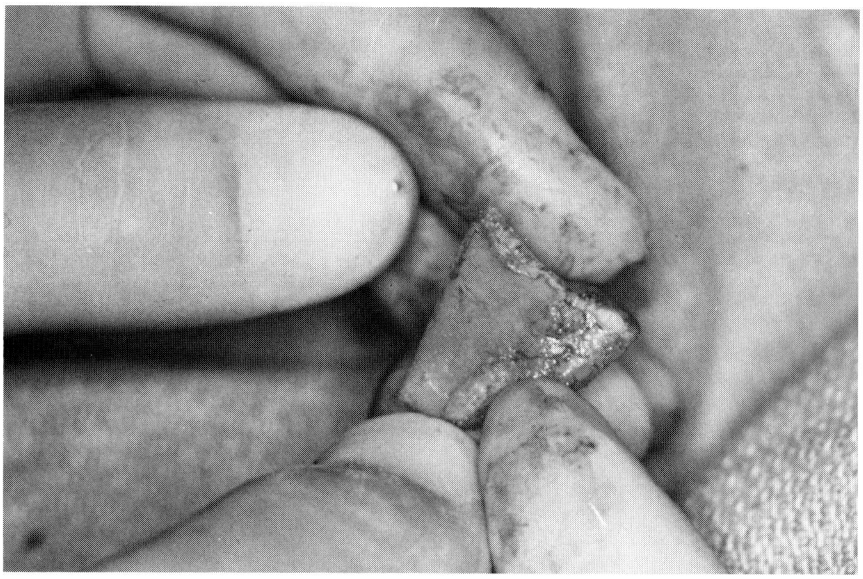

The projecting end of the tip graft is made from the thick cartilage at the osteochondral articulation.

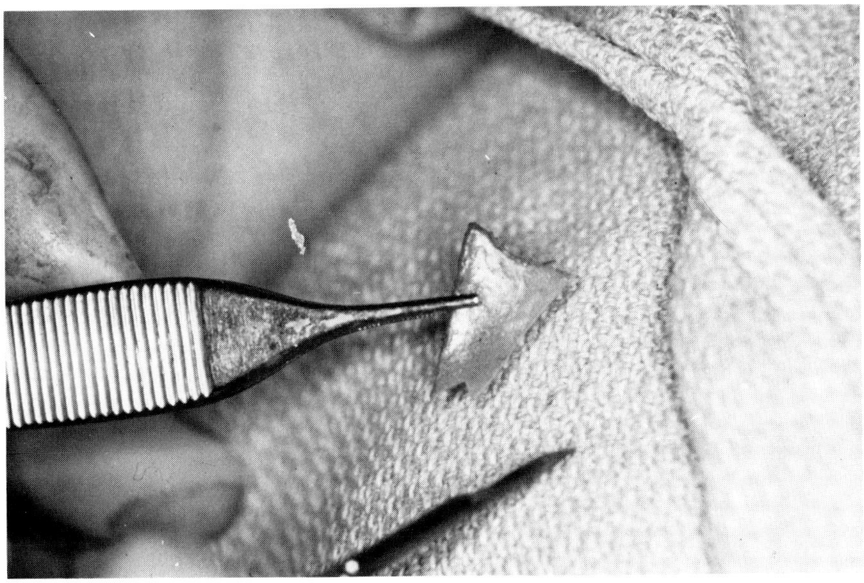

A preliminary graft is rendered, tested in place, then finished just before final placement.

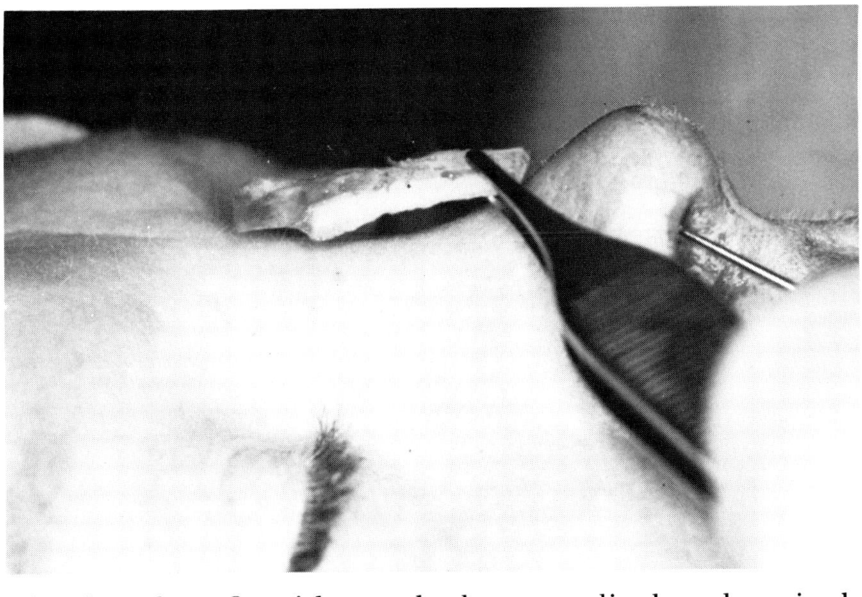

The dorsal graft, with attached perpendicular plate, is shown before insertion. The sides have been beveled with a No. 15 blade.

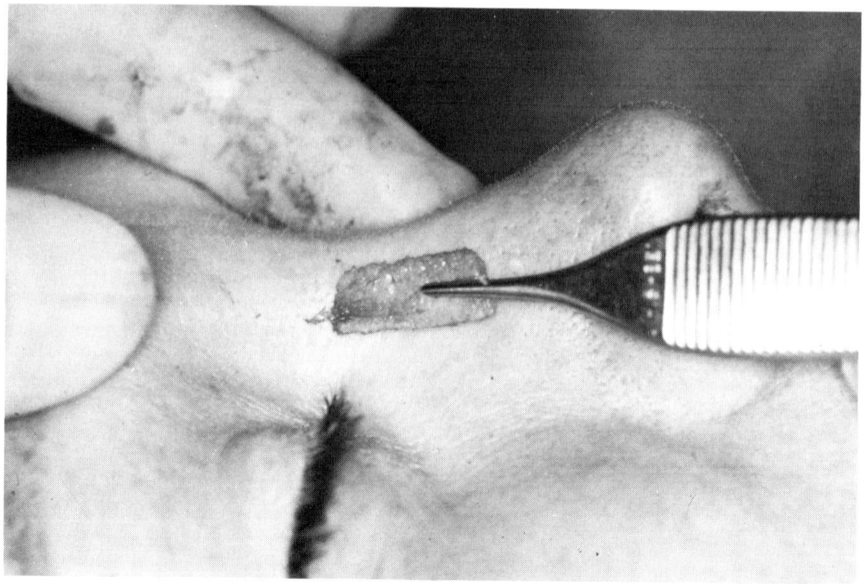

The right lateral bony vault is augmented by a rectangular cartilage graft, placed in a separate pocket.

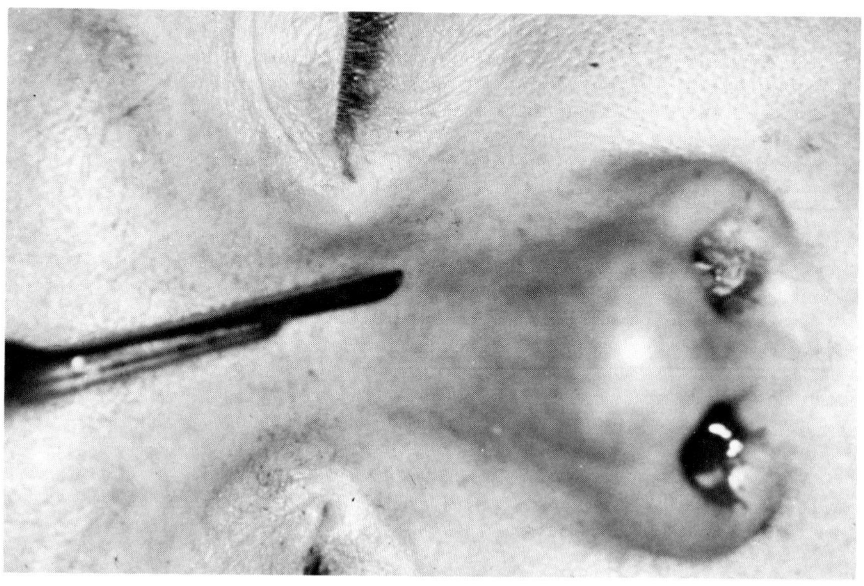

Following the right lateral graft, the nasal wall is in good alignment with the radix and nasal base. However, a concavity remains on the left side at the point of the scalpel.

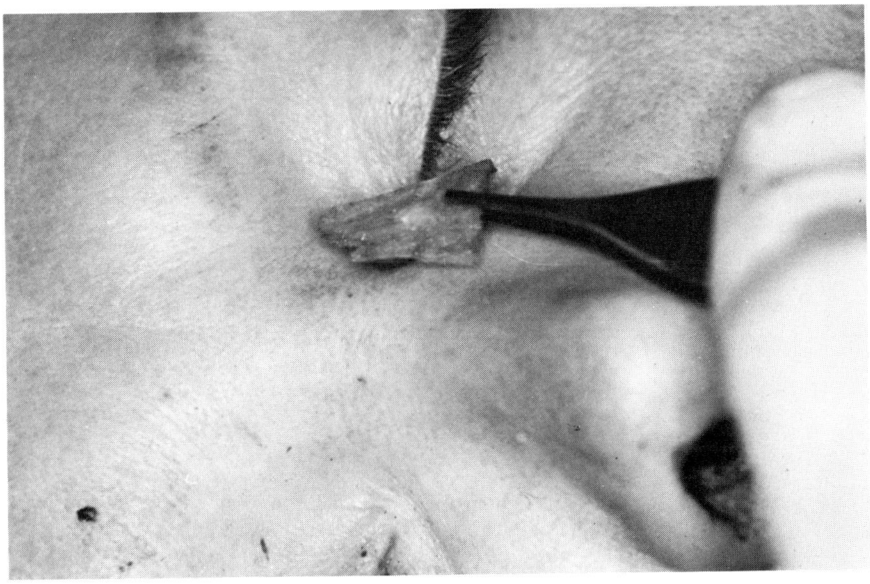

A piece of vomer is used to fill out the left side. It too is placed in a separate pocket.

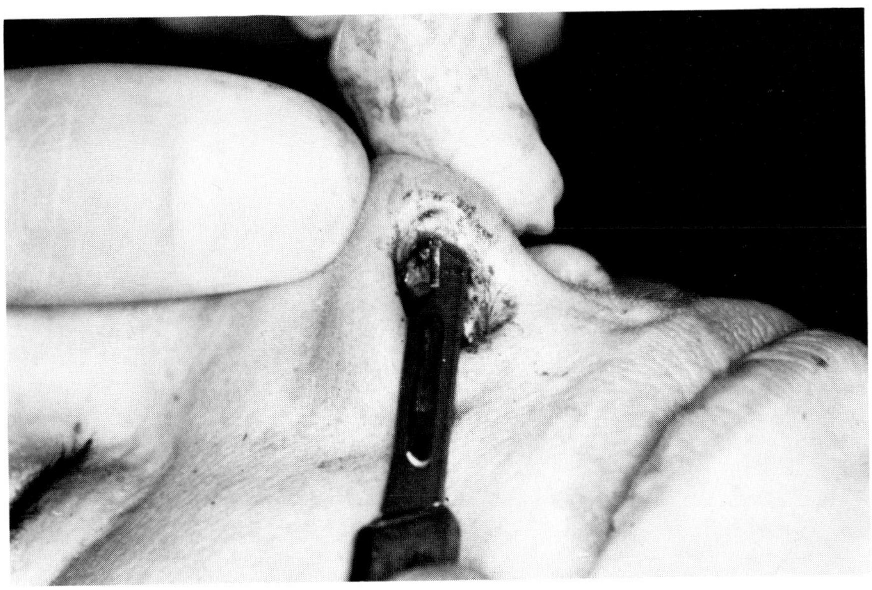

The opening incision for the tip graft is caudal to the terminal point of the initial gull-wing incision.

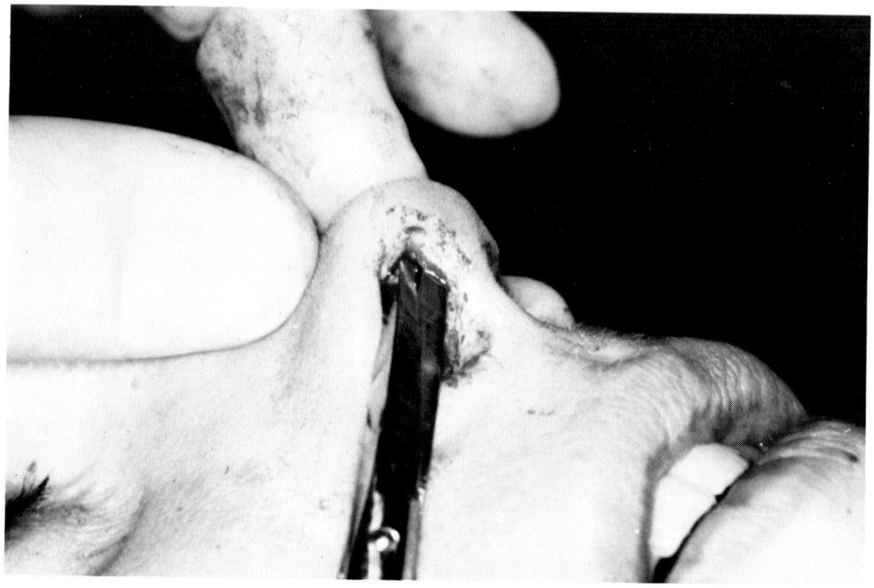

The pocket is dissected with a 35-degree cephalic tilt.

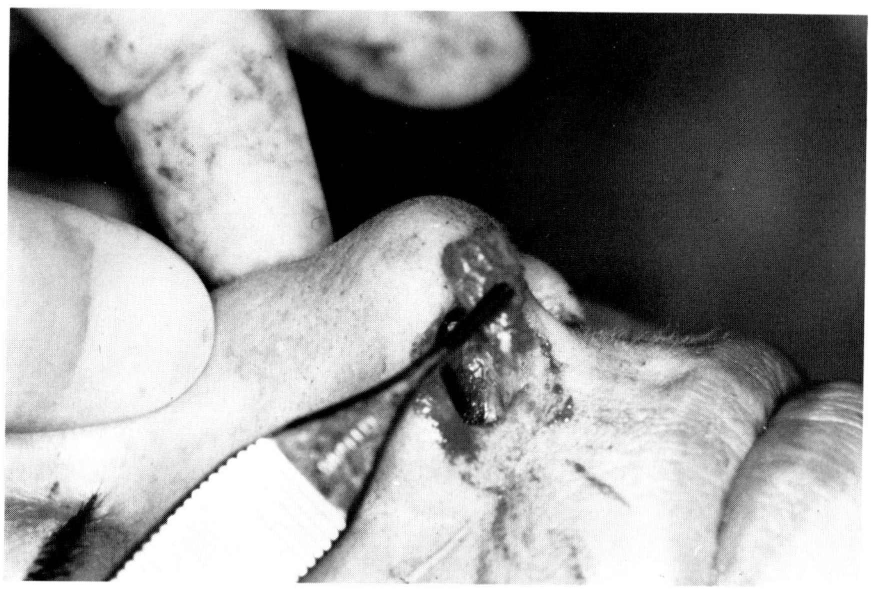

The final contour of the tip graft is shown before its insertion.

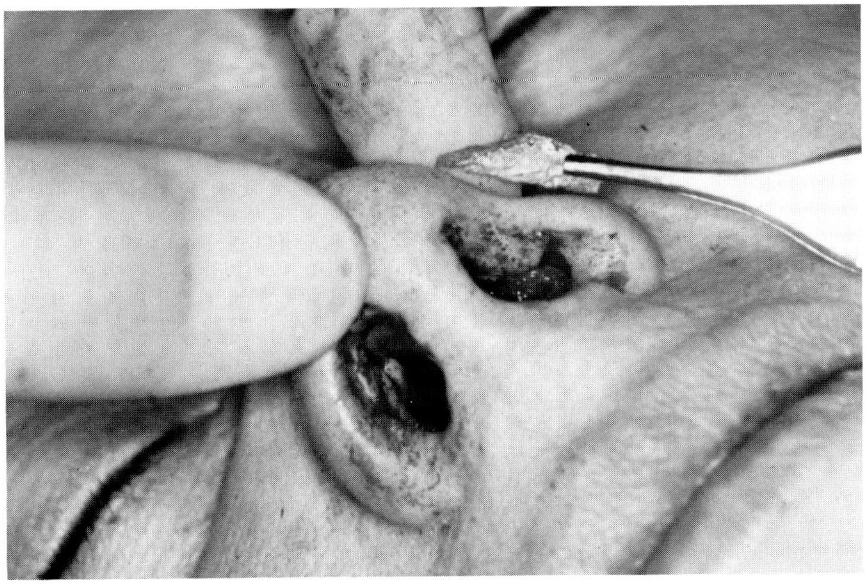

To correct the collapse of the left ala, a 6-mm incision is made low on the nasal wall perpendicular to the rim. A piece of perpendicular plate has been prepared for insertion into a pocket made in a subdermal plane.

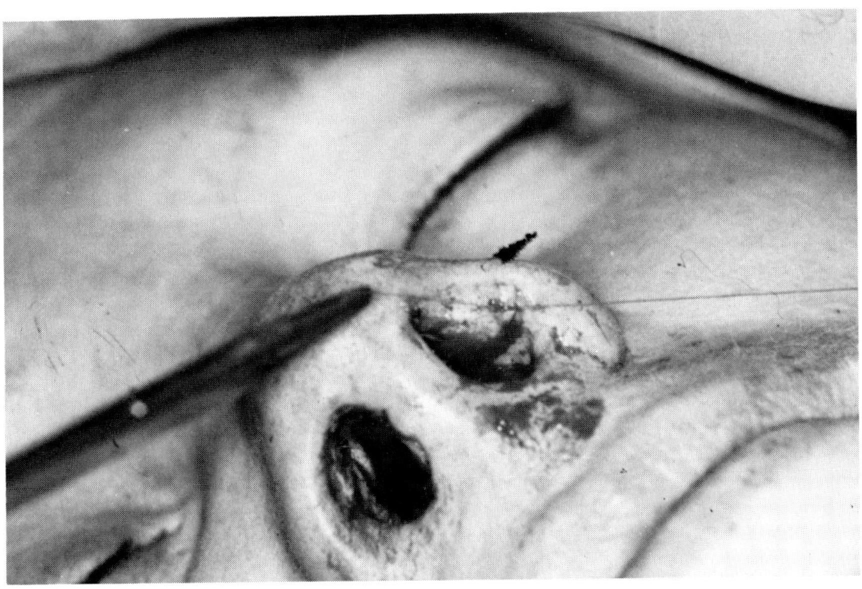

After placement of the graft, the wound is closed with interrupted 5-0 plain catgut.

Summary of surgical procedure

1. Limited skeletonization
2. Submucous resection for graft material
3. Dorsal graft of septal cartilage with attached perpendicular plate
4. Right lateral graft of septal cartilage placed in separate pocket
5. Left lateral graft of vomer placed in separate pocket
6. Tip graft of septal cartilage
7. Graft of perpendicular plate of the ethmoid placed in the left alar rim

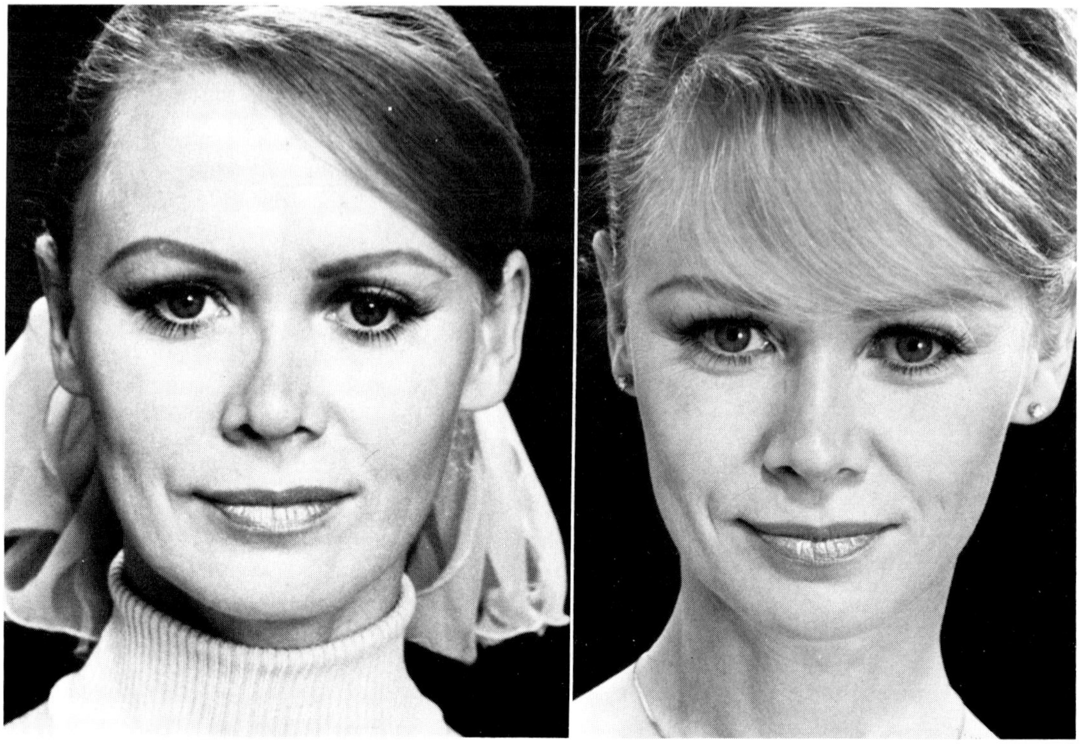

POSTOPERATIVE RESULTS

Three years following tertiary rhinoplasty, a smooth contour of the lateral nasal walls can be seen. Reconstruction of the entire bony pyramid has resulted in a wider dorsum that flows in continuity from radix to tip. The vertical ridges around the tip persist, though augmentation has provided some improvement.

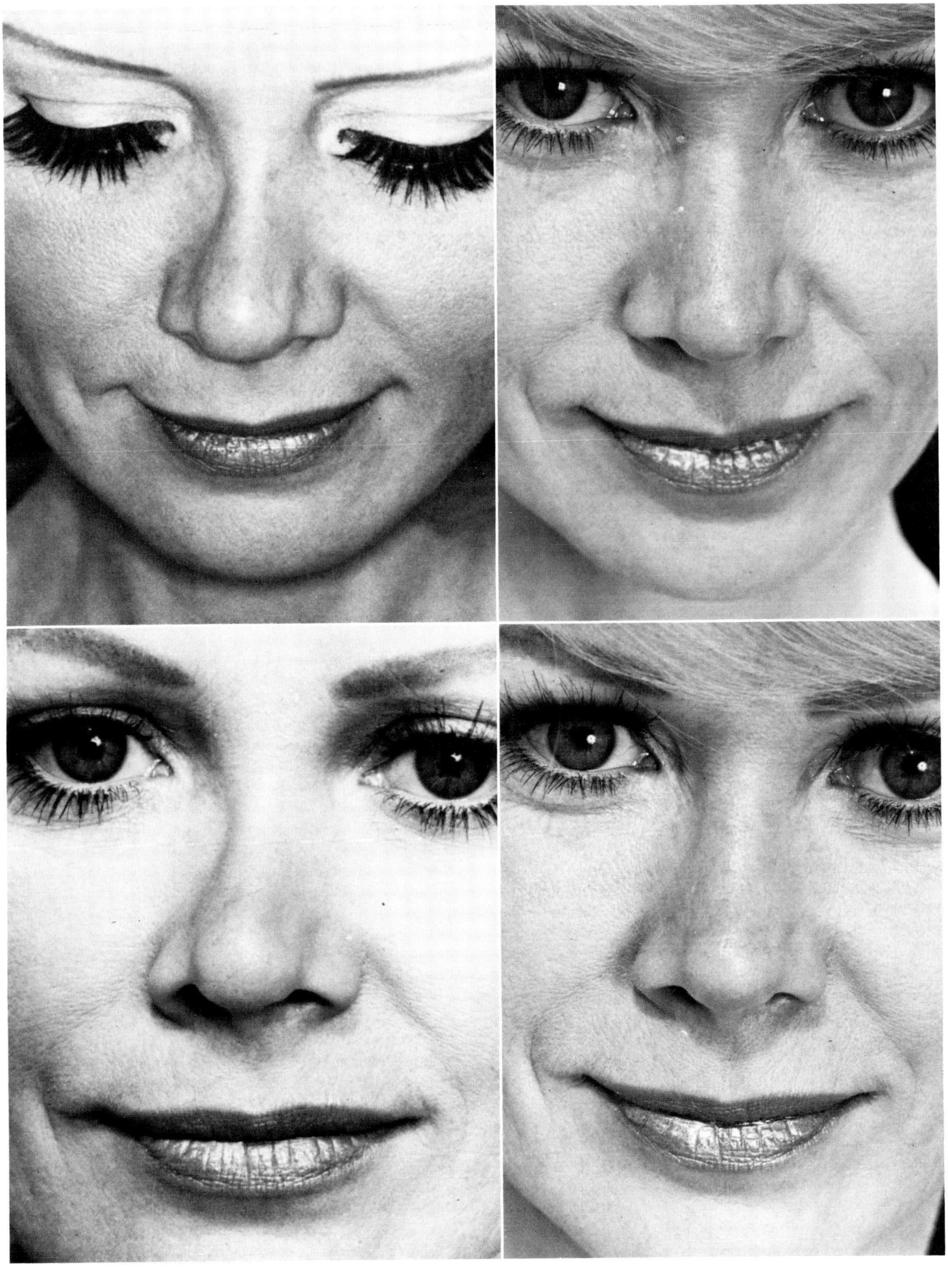

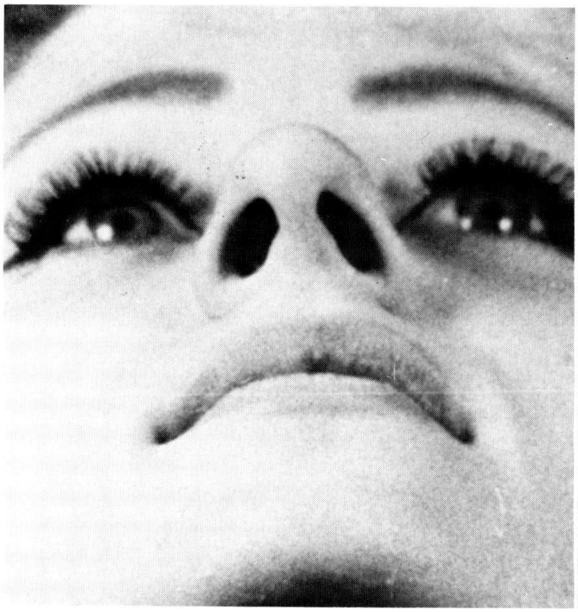

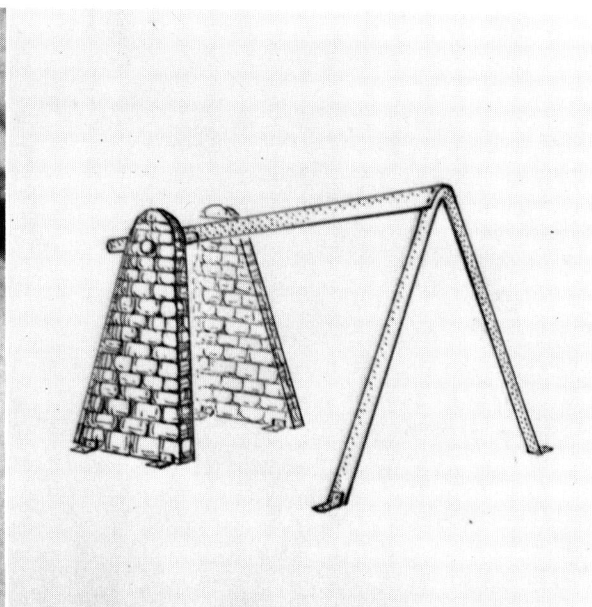

The preoperative basal view is triangular, with elliptical nares and a projecting tip. It is represented schematically as being supported by a cantilevered rod from a stationary base (bony pyramid).

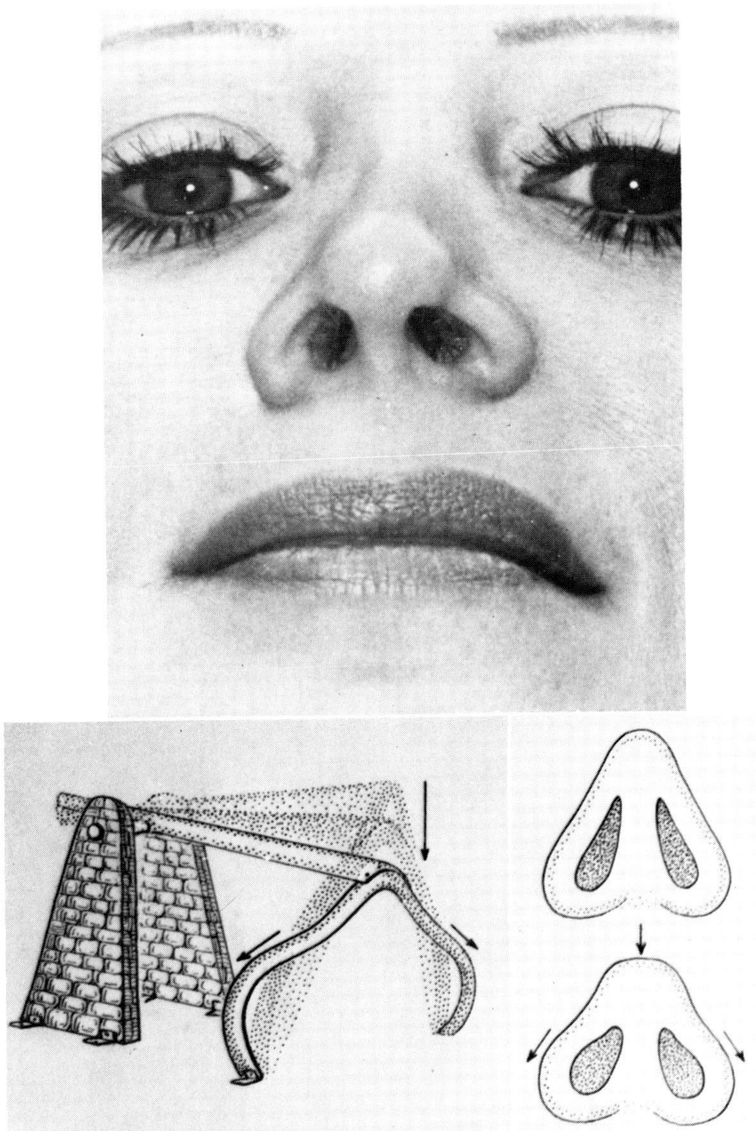

Following two surgeries, the lowered dorsum has caused the basal perimeter to flatten. The nostrils have changed from a vertical to an almost horizontal plane. There is a notch in the left ala. The internal valve areas are narrowed to small slits. The relationship of dorsum to basal contour is shown schematically.

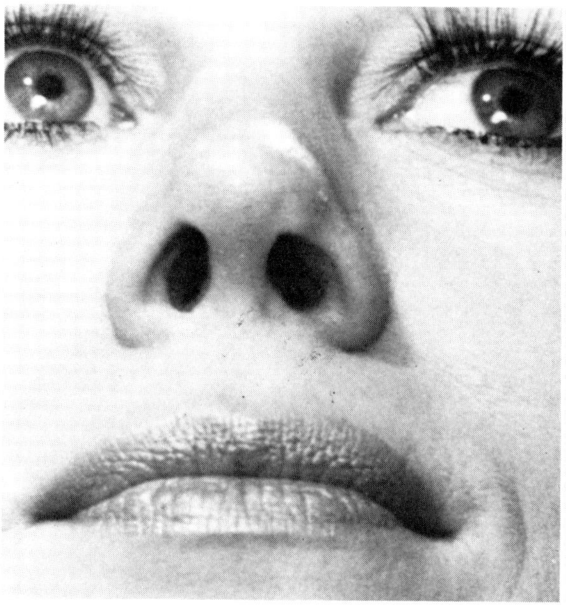

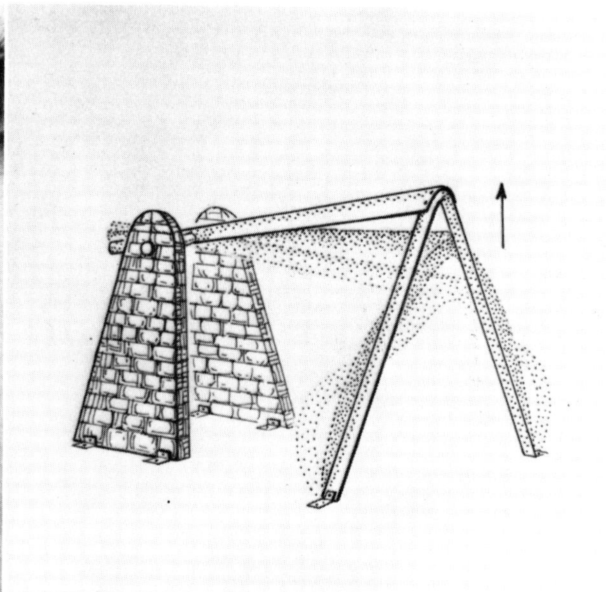

Following reconstruction of the nasal skeleton, there is a reversal of the effect of the dorsal reduction on the basal perimeter. The nares are restored to a vertical plane, and the internal valve has almost doubled in size. There can be no doubt concerning the improved function in this area. The tip projection is close to the original height. The notch in the left ala has been corrected by the ethmoid bone graft.

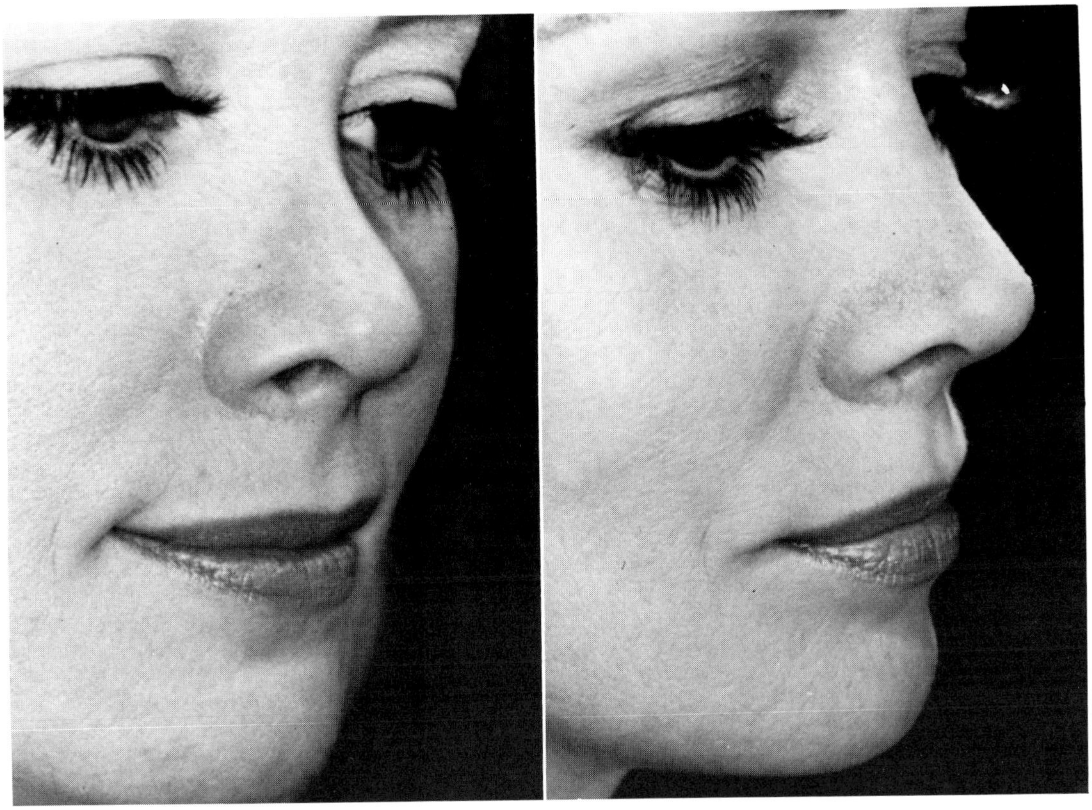

On right oblique view, the substantial augmentation of the entire nasal pyramid is evident. The tip graft has refined the tip as well as extended it above the dorsal line.

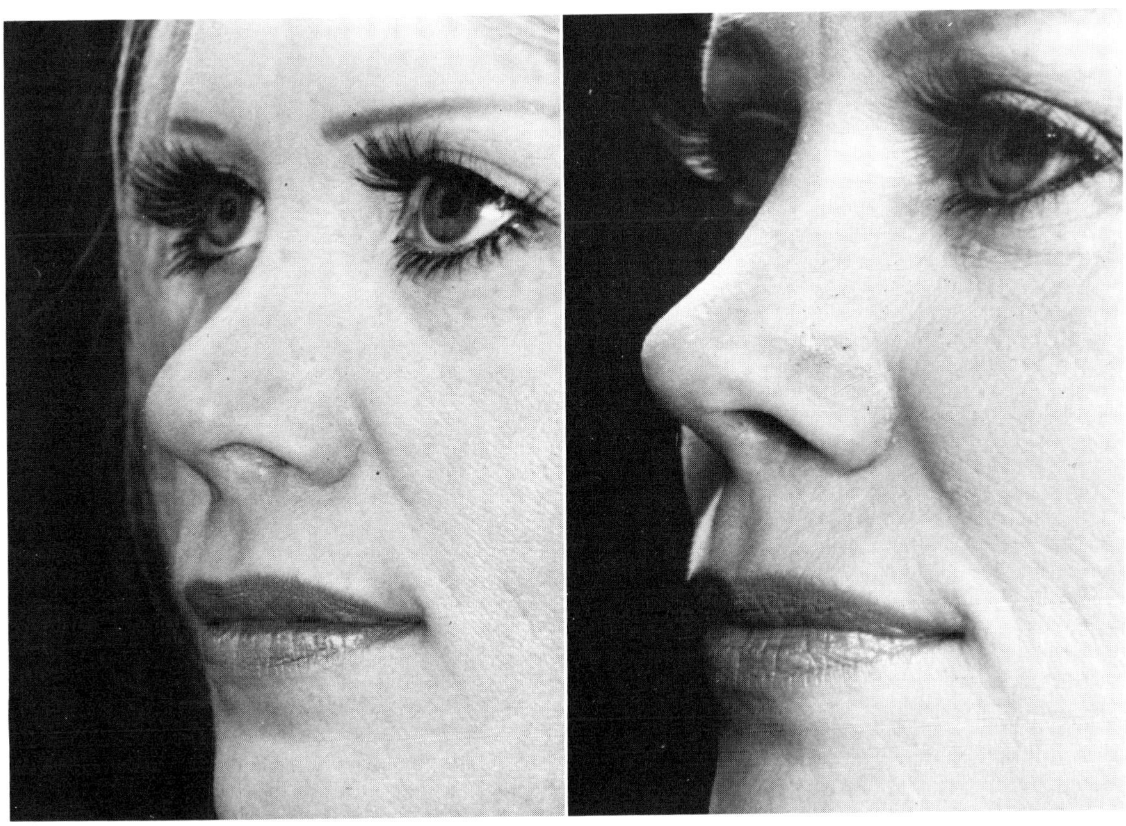

On left oblique view, the piece of ethmoid bone that was placed in the left ala has provided support to the nostril with virtually no distortion.

CASE REPORT 6: ANALYSIS OF A FAILURE

The mental and technical exercises of secondary rhinoplasty have been an invaluable part of my education in nasal surgery. The postsurgical nose poses immediate problems but also offers one a special opportunity to evaluate the nose retrospectively, to investigate the causes of an unsuccessful surgery, and in the process of investigation, to glean insights that will benefit one's own patients in the future. When an unsatisfactory result is evaluated, part of the exercise is to ask "What caused this result?" Another part is to ask "How would *I* have done this nose?" In the following case report an analysis is offered from the perspective of these questions.

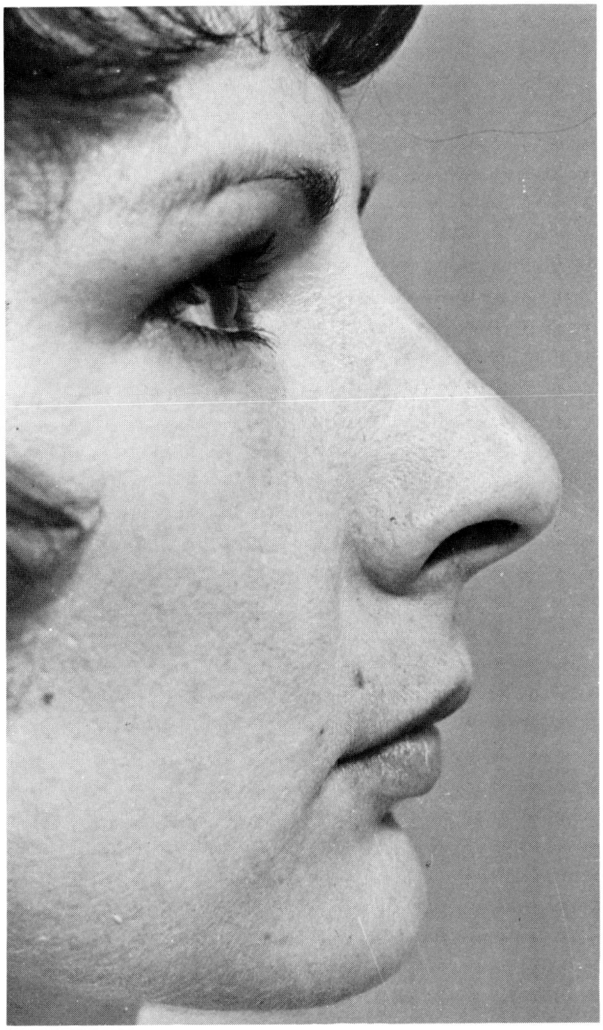

The patient is shown before two nasal surgeries. The first procedure was done primarily for airway dysfunction. The surgeon performed a major septoplasty and rasped the dorsum, which produced some irregularity along the lateral nasal walls. Subsequently, she consulted another surgeon, who performed a "standard rhinoplasty."

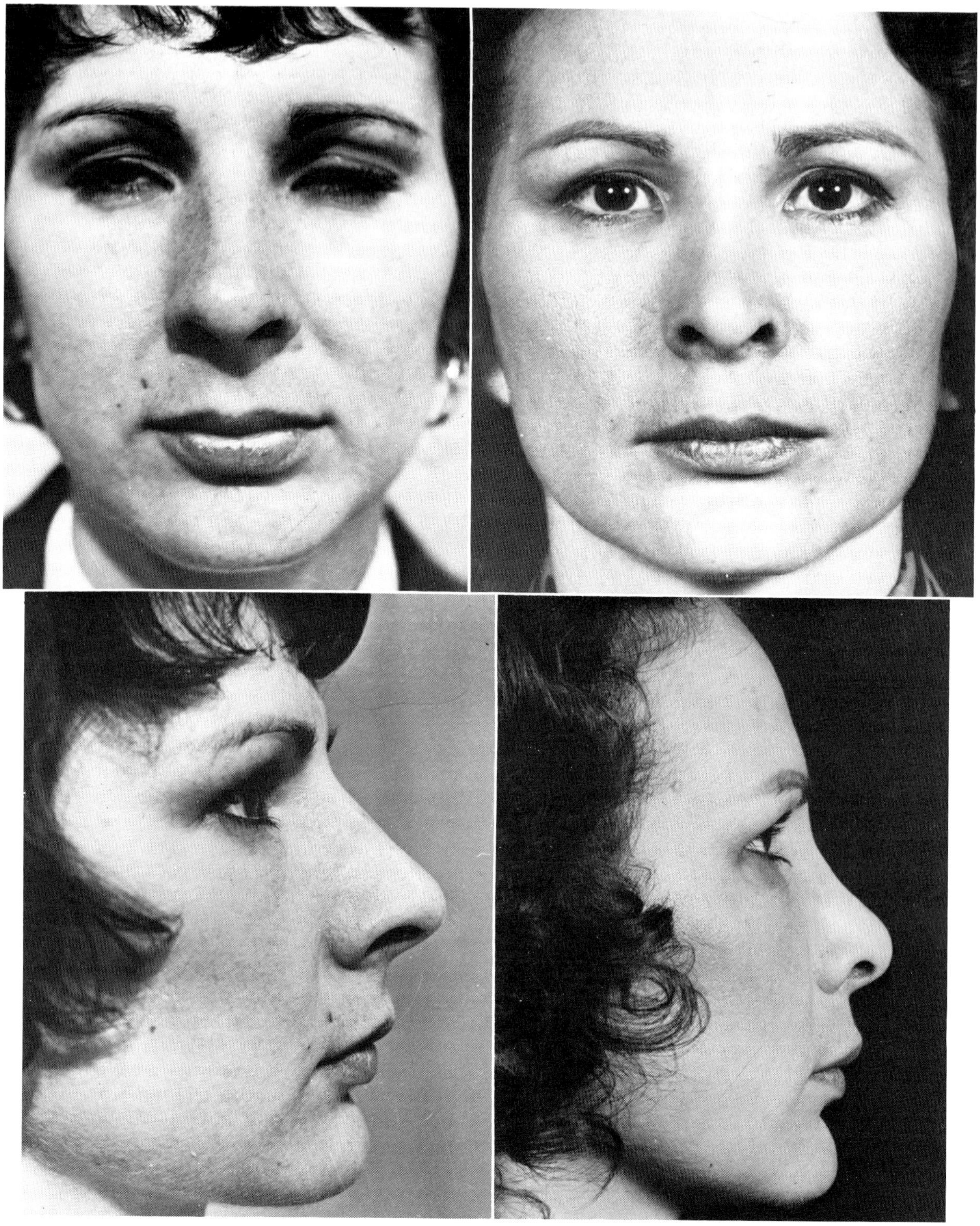

Postoperative photographs give evidence of general overreduction of nasal parts: low dorsum, rounded tip, retrusive subnasion, and small, rounded nostrils.

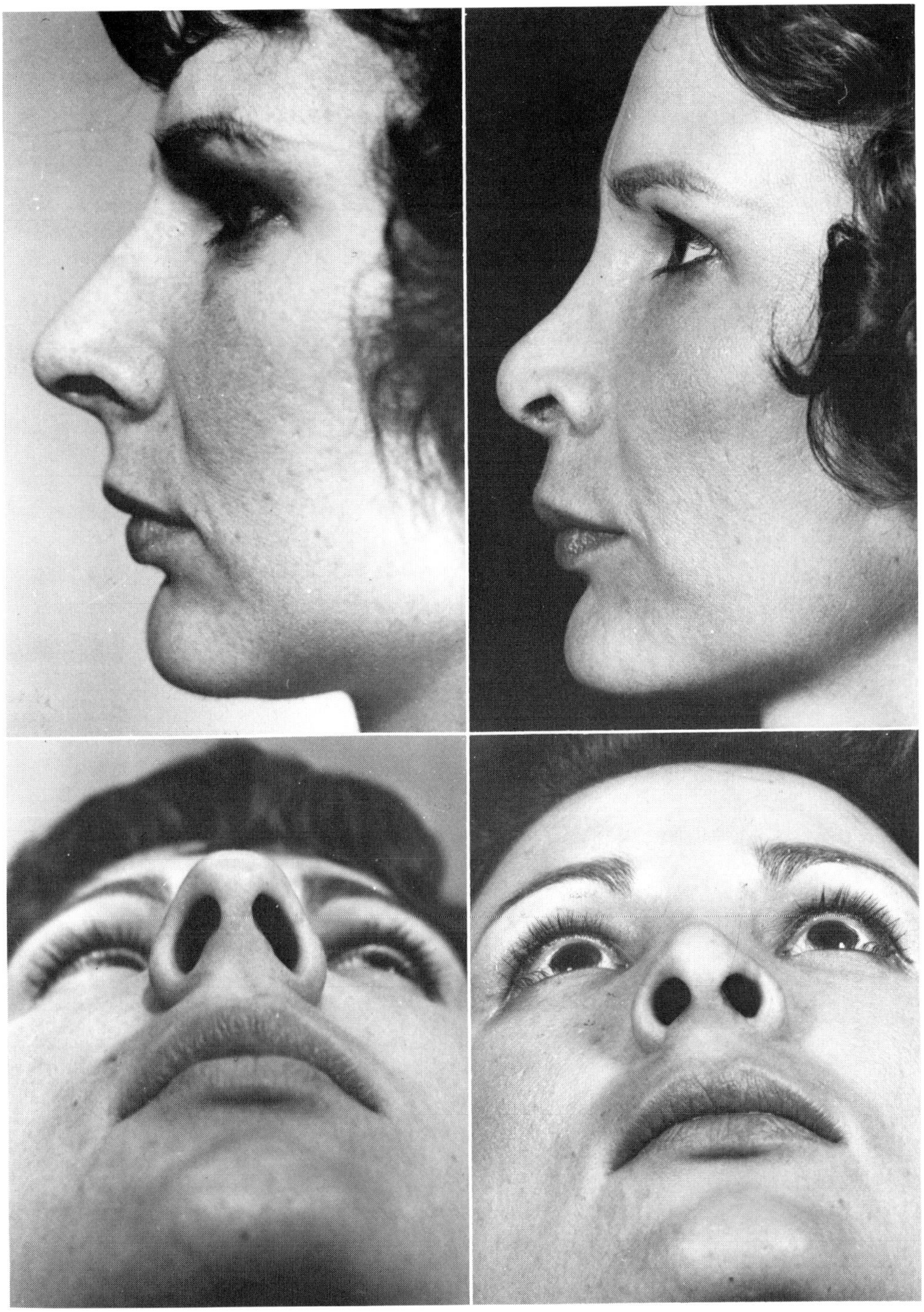

To answer the question—What caused this result?—it is helpful to study the operative record, step by step. Direct quotes from the operative note are followed by my own observations and comments.

First step: Skeletonization

Preoperative diagnosis: Deformity of the nose due to trauma
Postoperative diagnosis: Same
Operation: Rhinoplasty
Procedure: After the packing was removed, an incision was made between the upper and lower lateral nasal cartilages. The skin over the entire nose was freed up . . . transfixion carried to the nasal spine.

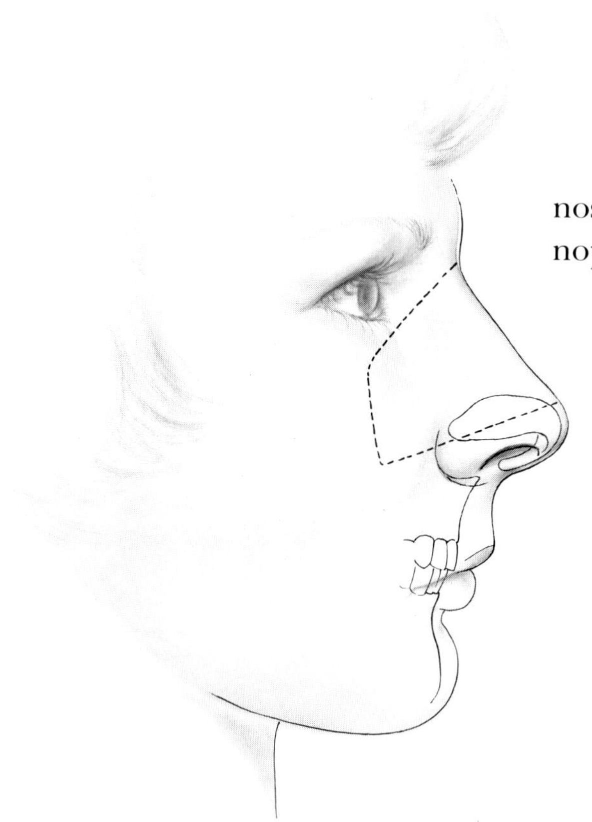

The surgeon widely skeletonized the nose, a step generally accepted for rhinoplastic procedures.

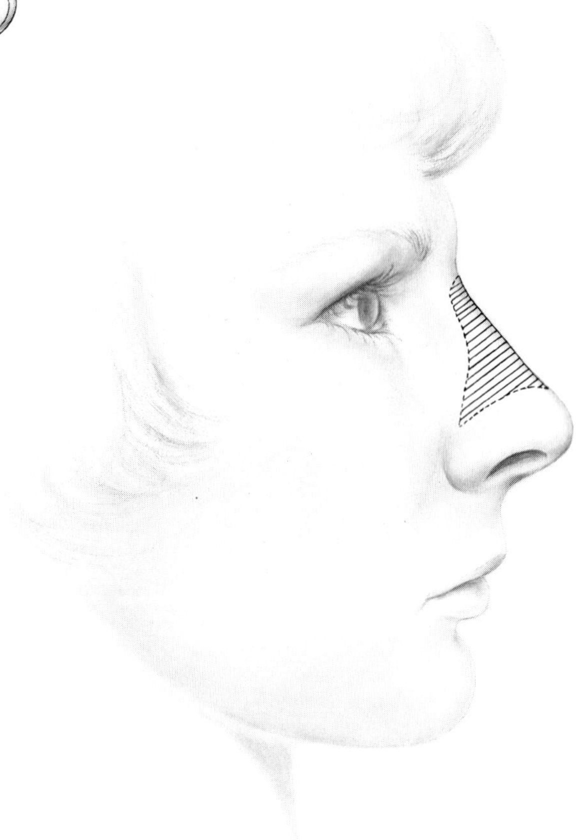

With a nose requiring only slight changes, the skeletonization should have been just enough to gain access to the nasal parts needing modification. No transfixion of the membranous septum was necessary because the nasolabial angle was excellent. The alae and columella were in good relation to each other, and the full subnasion set off an attractive mouth and upper lip.

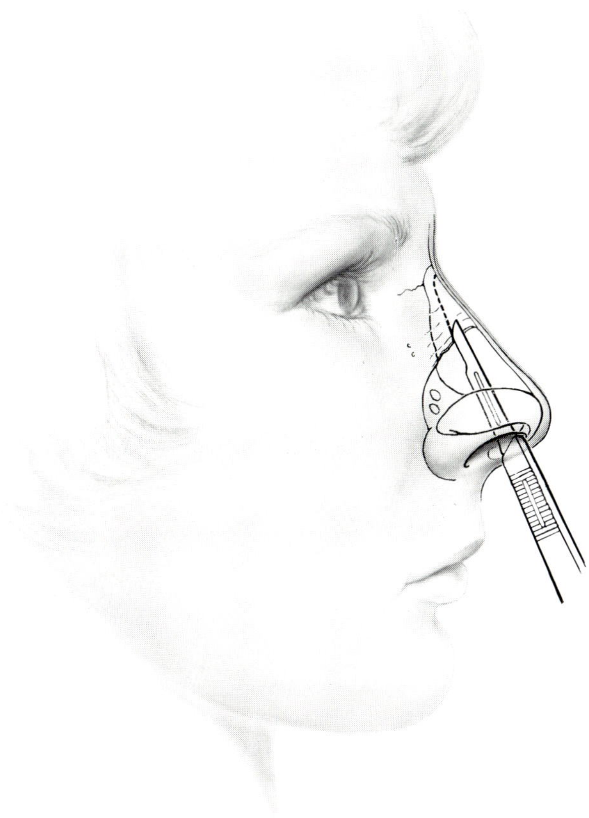

Second step: Hump removal

A scalpel was used to groove the area of incision for the removal of the hump. A Joseph saw was then used to saw through the hump on the right side first and then the left side. A large straight scissor was used to cut through the septal cartilage and then the hump was removed with a double-action rongeur or a straight hemostat.

The reduction of this dorsum should not have exceeded 2 mm. The Joseph saw is poorly suited to perform this critical task, which can be done easily and predictably with the use of a rasp.

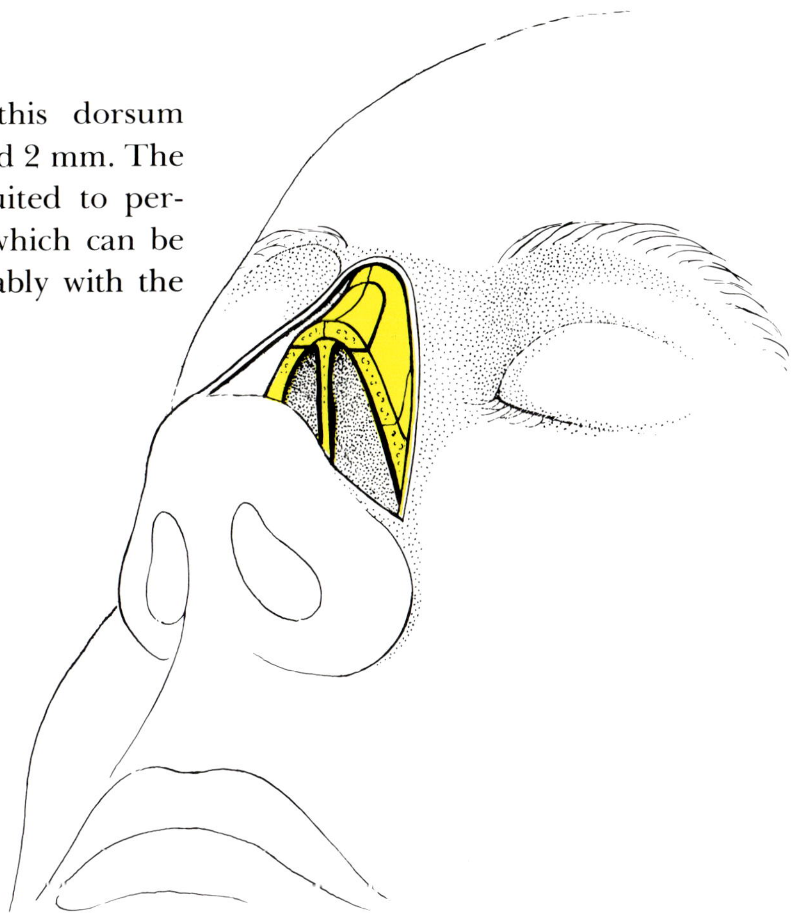

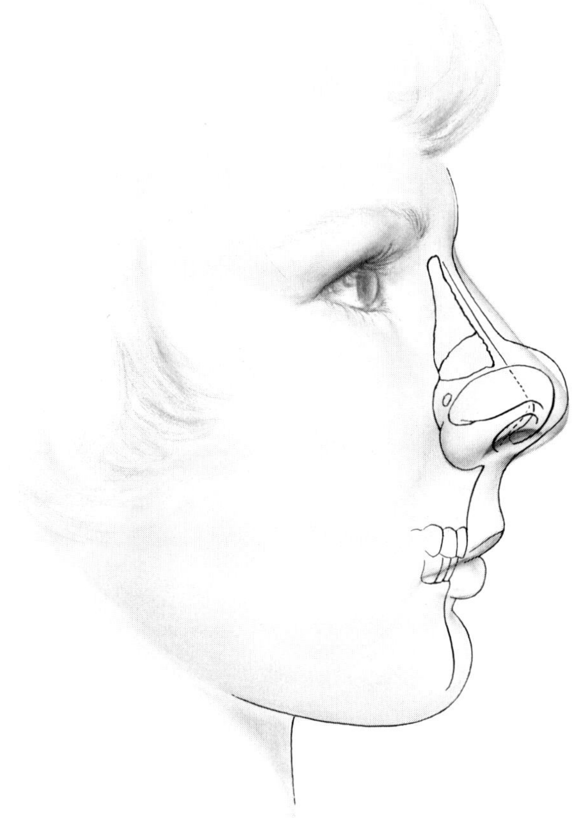

Third step: Tip reduction

It was decided that the height of the tip needed to be lessened as well as the width, so the dome of the cartilage was excised with a scalpel to change the same.

The need to reduce the projection of the tip was predicated on overreduction of the dorsum. After the dorsum was resected, the strong nasal tip became proportionately overprojecting. At this point, replacement of the resected dorsal segment may have saved the day by making reduction of the tip unnecessary.

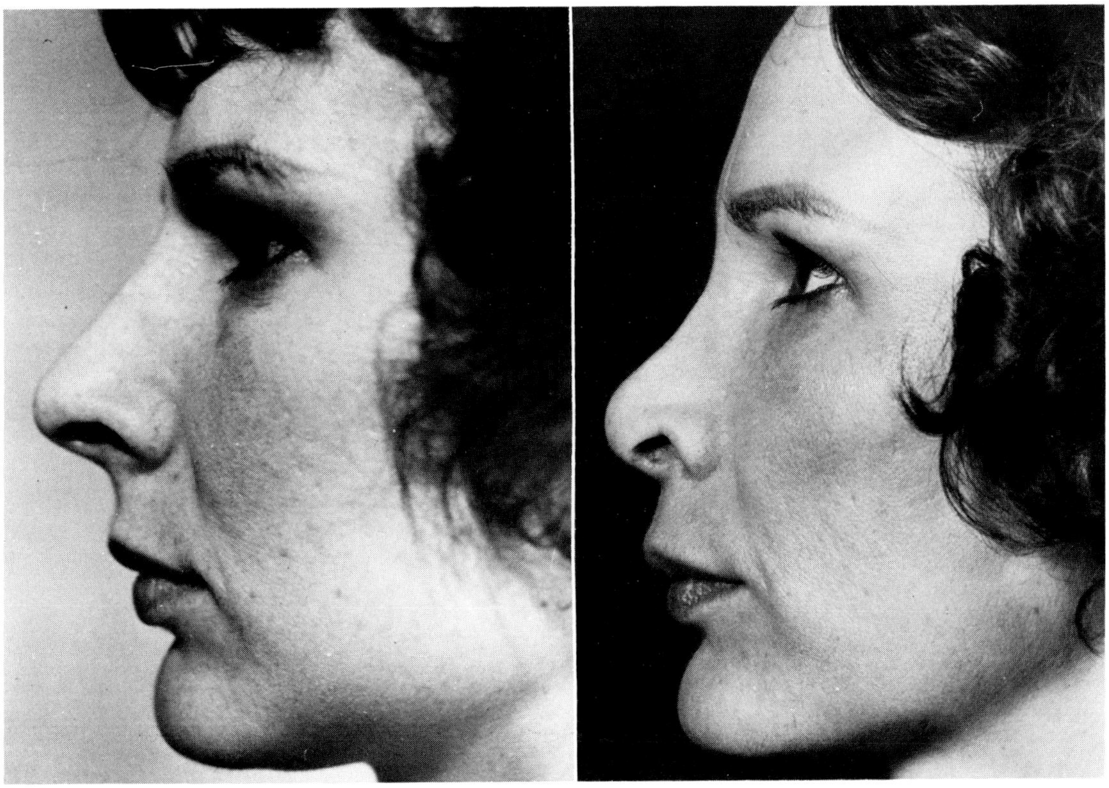

Fourth step: Resection of caudal septum and nasal spine

There is no mention in the operative note concerning the resection of the caudal septum and nasal spine. However, there is no doubt that a generous resection of both caudal septum and nasal spine was done at surgery. Preoperatively, the nasolabial angle was soft and open. Postoperatively, the area of the subnasion is sharp, accentuating the upper lip, which was made too long and retrusive. Consequently, the appearance of the mouth has been severely altered. Resection of the nasal spine must be thought out carefully and performed with deliberate conservatism to avoid the look this patient demonstrates.

Fifth step: Alar wedge resection

On this particular patient, it was necessary to lessen the diameter of the nostril by excising a wedge resection at the base and suturing it with a buried No. 38 wire suture followed by 6-0 nylon. A nasal splint and dressing were then applied. The patient went back to her room in good condition.

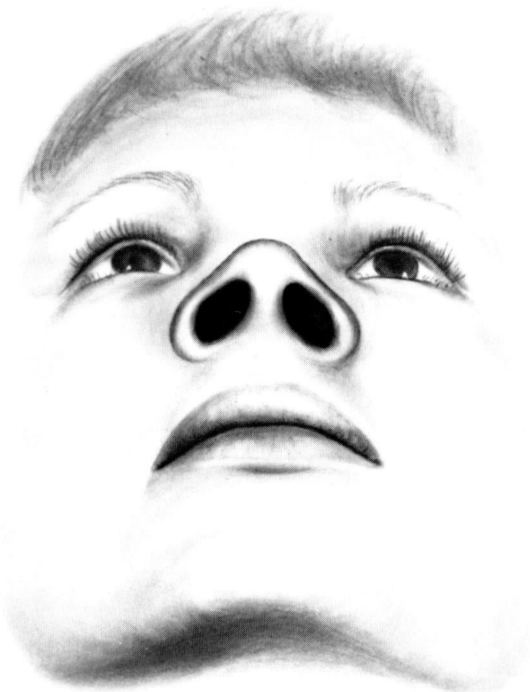

This is an artist's drawing of what the surgeon probably saw as he made the decision to narrow the nasal base by wedge resection. The base of the nose was broad and the nares were flaring. To bring the base into proportion, it must have seemed logical to narrow the nostrils. Had he understood the influence of dorsal height on the nasal base, he might have reversed the flare by elevating the dorsum.

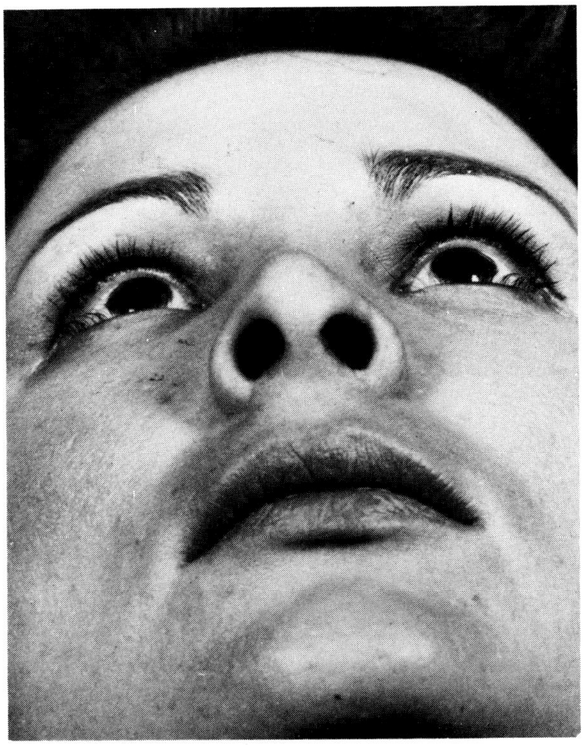

Following reduction, the alar base has been narrowed at the expense of normal nostril contour.

This case illustrates the effect of dorsal height on the basal perimeter. When the dorsum is lowered, the tip height is reduced, the base broadens, and the nostrils flare.

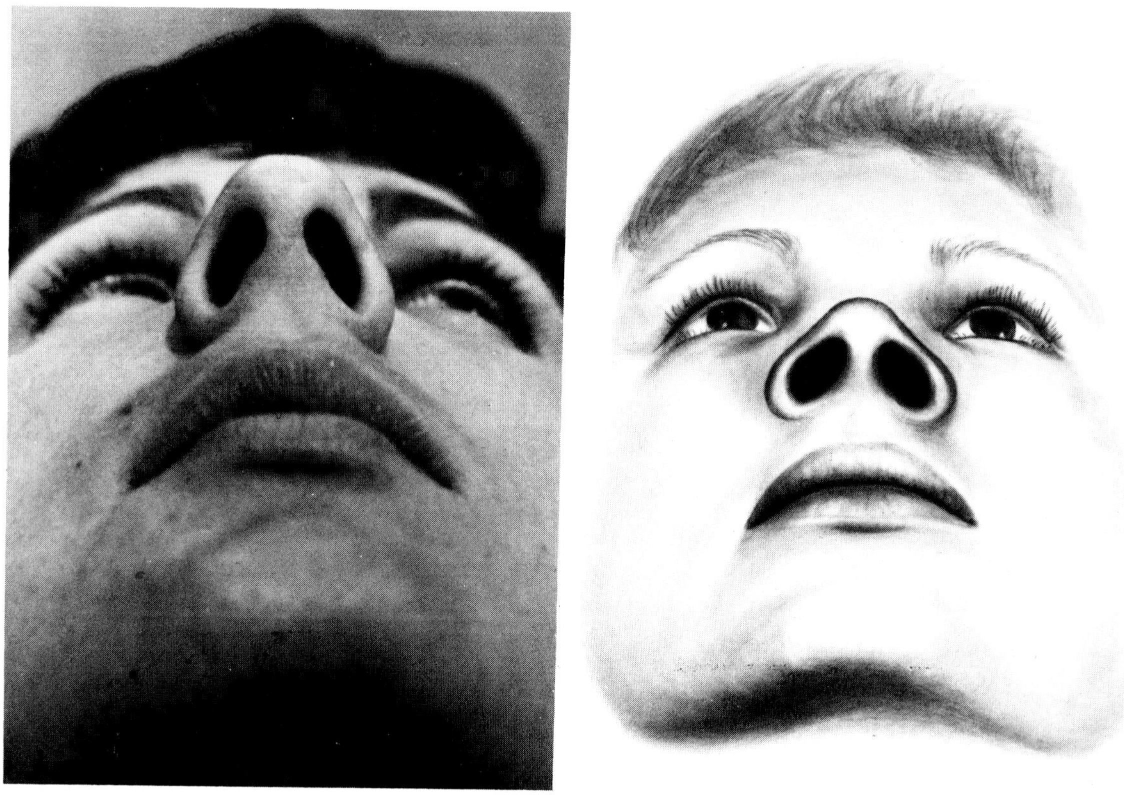

The patient is shown preoperatively and then following reduction of the dorsum. With the loss of dorsal support, the flattening of the nasal base is predictable.

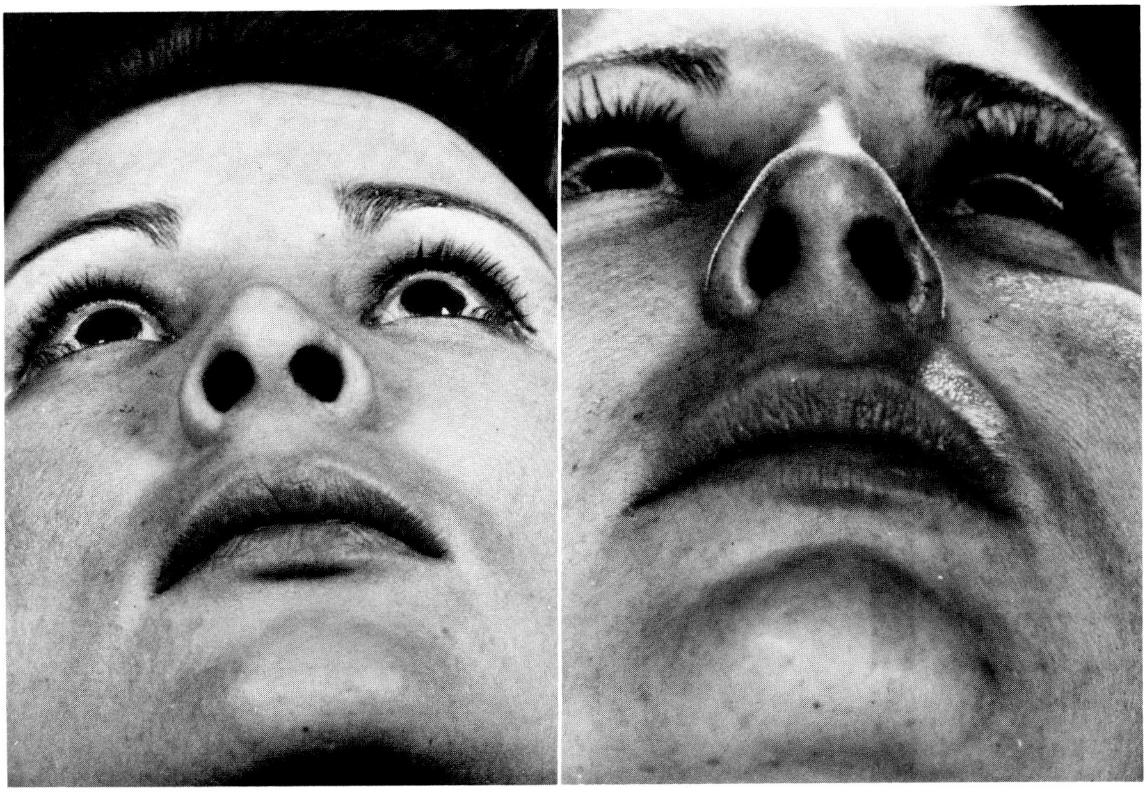

The patient is shown before and following dorsal augmentation and tip grafting. The nostrils have changed from round to elliptical, improving both their appearance and function.

Tertiary reconstruction

The plan for tertiary reconstruction was for augmentation of the dorsum, nasal tip, and maxilla.

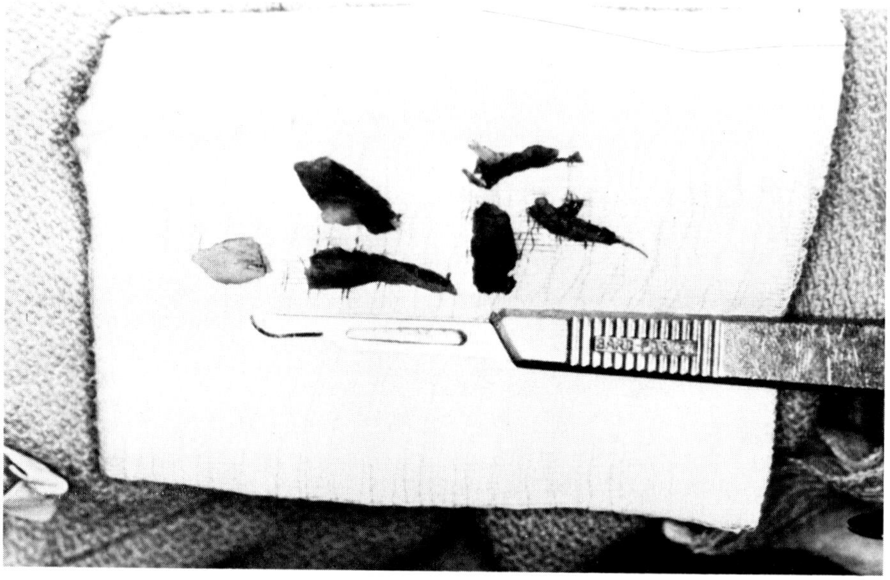

Since most of the septal cartilage had been resected, the available graft material was primarily vomer and ethmoid bone.

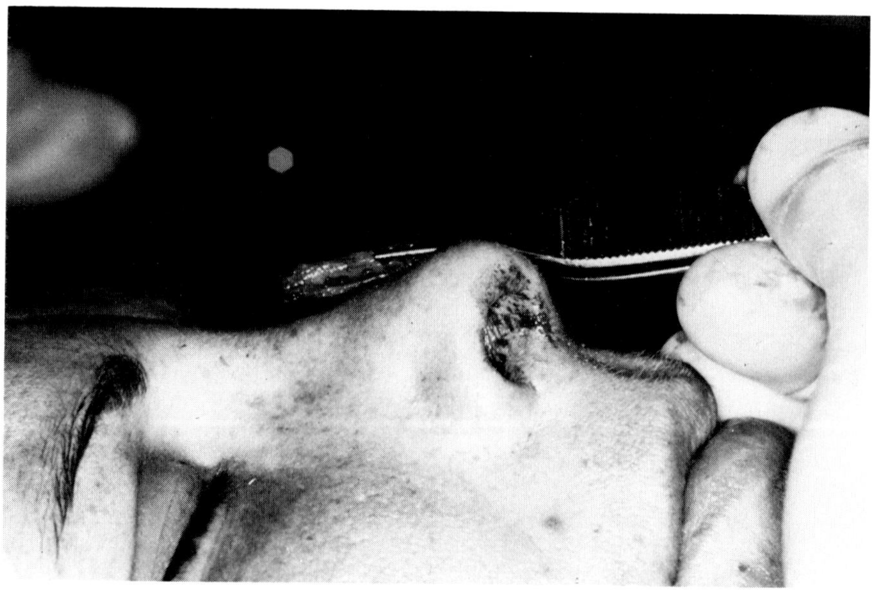

The dorsal graft of vomer bone was carefully contoured to recreate a smooth dorsal line. Because the pocket was small, there was no need for fixation. Further elevation by insertion of fragments of ethmoid under the caudal end of the graft brought the dorsal line to its proper height.

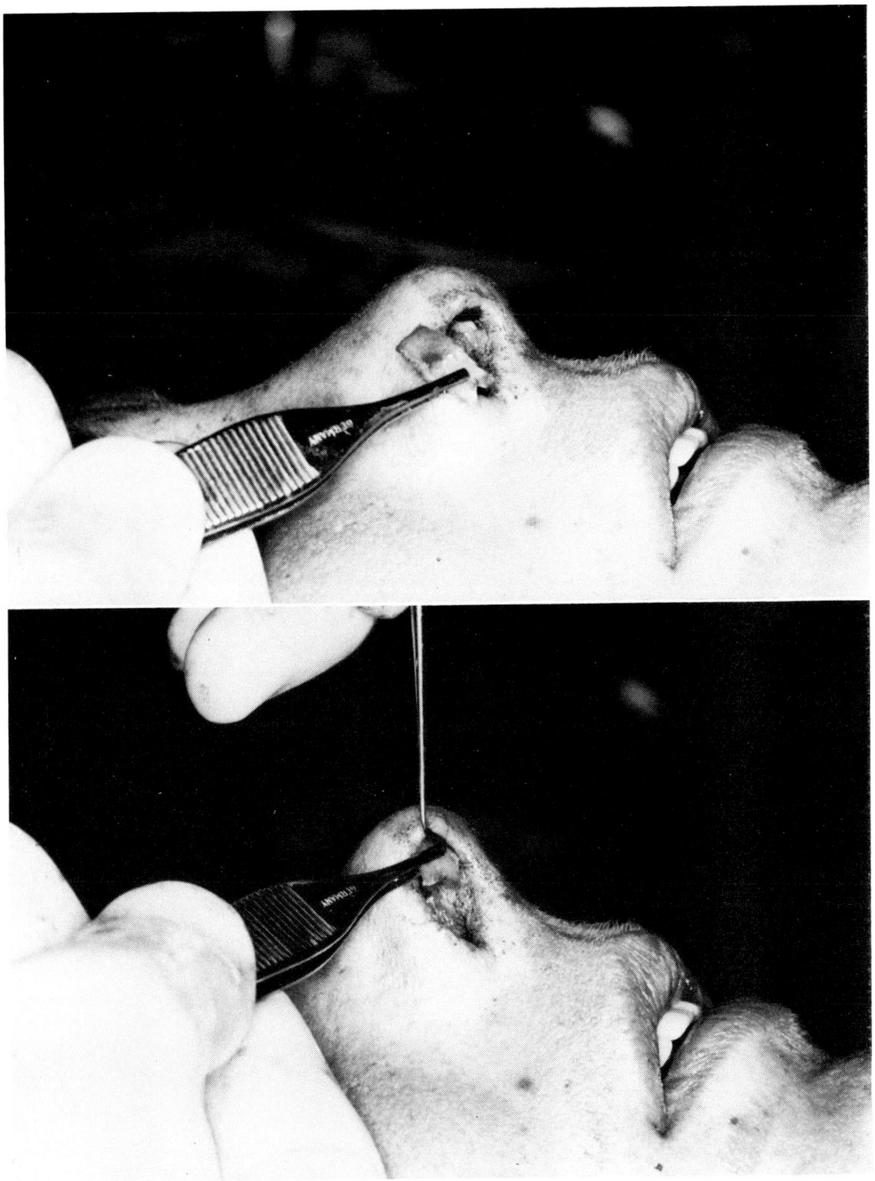

The only usable material for a tip graft was a small piece of residual cartilage attached to a small piece of ethmoid.

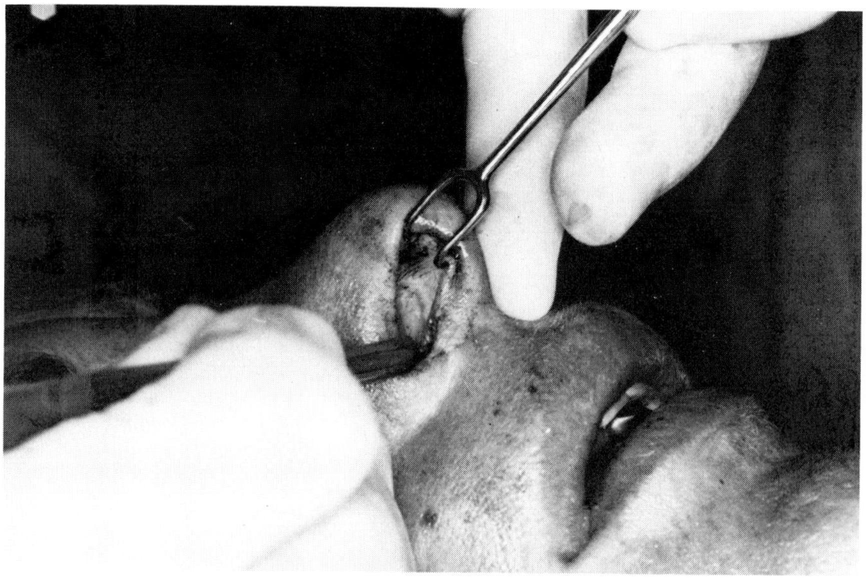

An incision along the nasal floor was carried to the maxilla, where the tissues were elevated lateral to the nasal spine. A silicone prosthesis (with holes) was inserted.

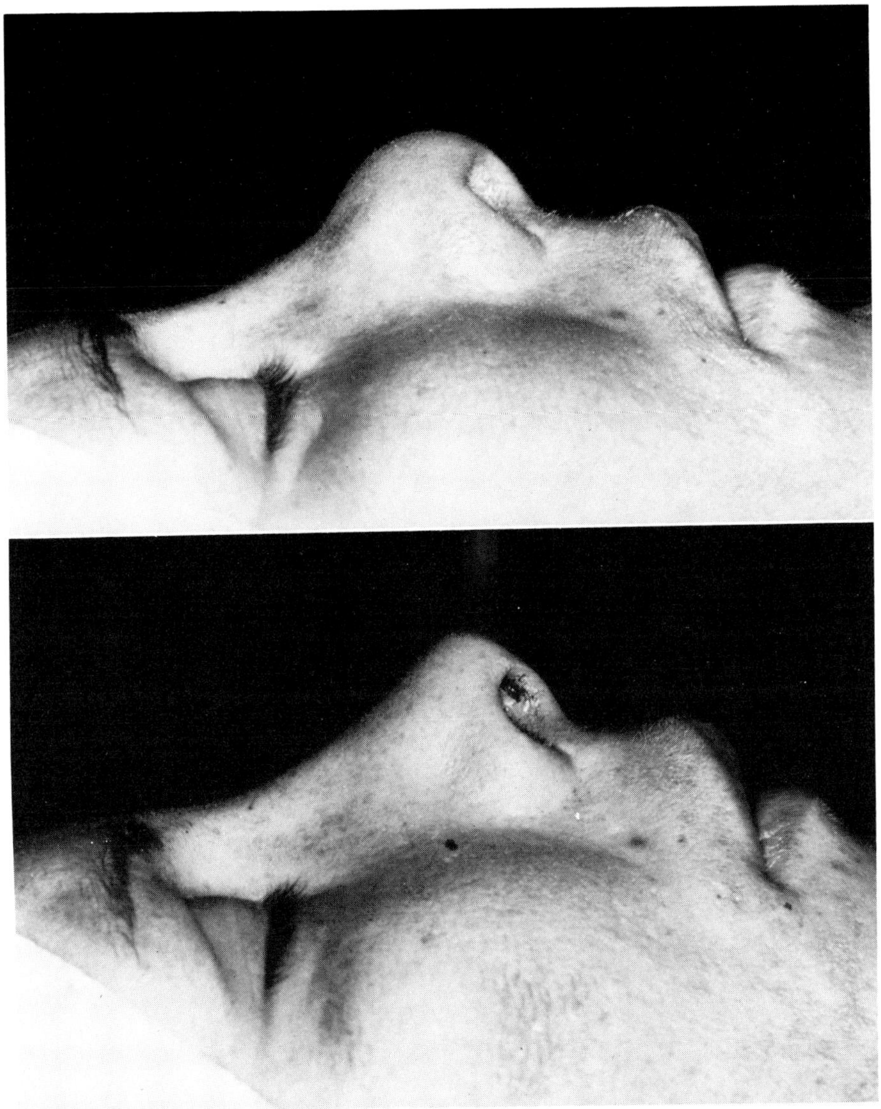

These photographs compare the patient at the beginning and completion of the procedure.

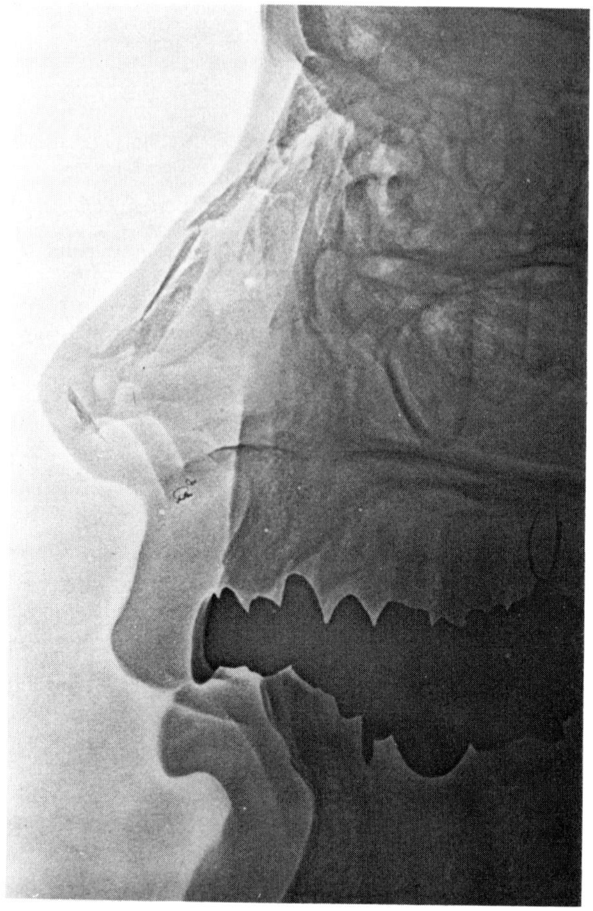

A xerogram taken 2 years following surgery shows all the vomer and ethmoid bone grafts placed in the dorsum. The dorsal line has been maintained. Some loss of tip projection has occurred, although the ethmoid bone graft can be seen in the tip.

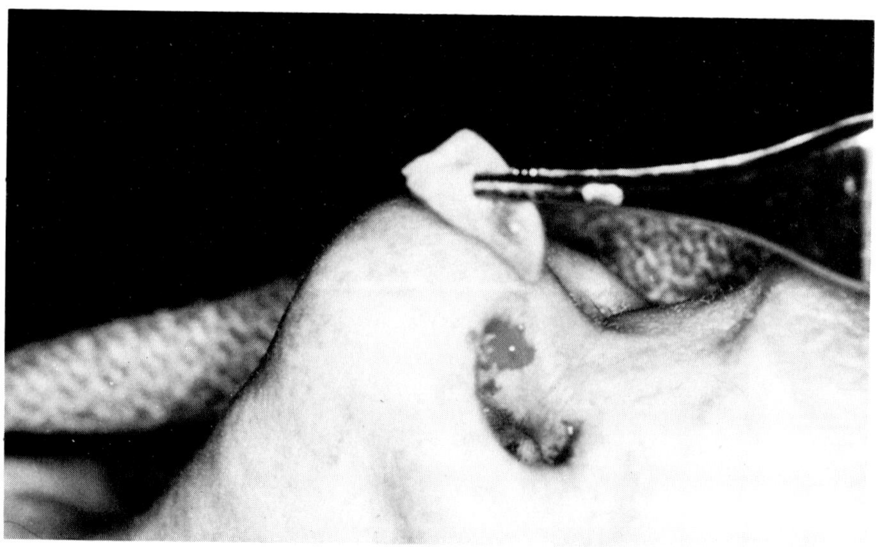

Because of the decrease in tip projection 2 years after tertiary reconstruction, an ear cartilage graft was placed anterior to the first tip graft.

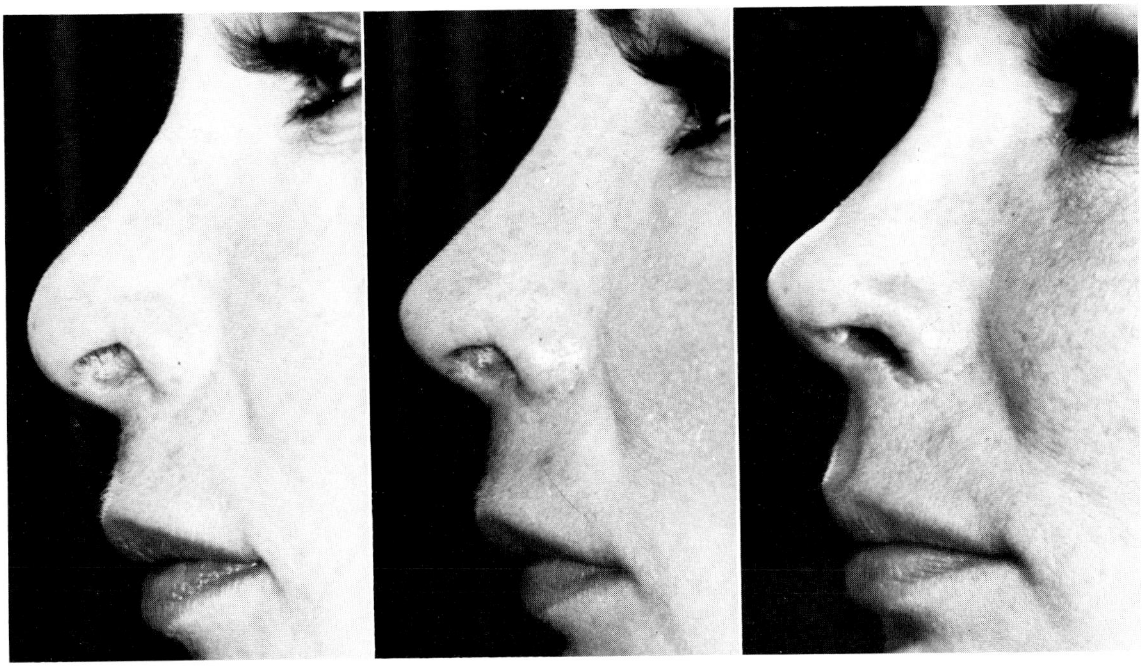

Left lateral views show the patient preoperatively; 2 years following tertiary reconstruction, in which the relationship of the nostril to the columella needs improvement; and following a conservative resection of alar lobule and a conchal cartilage tip graft.

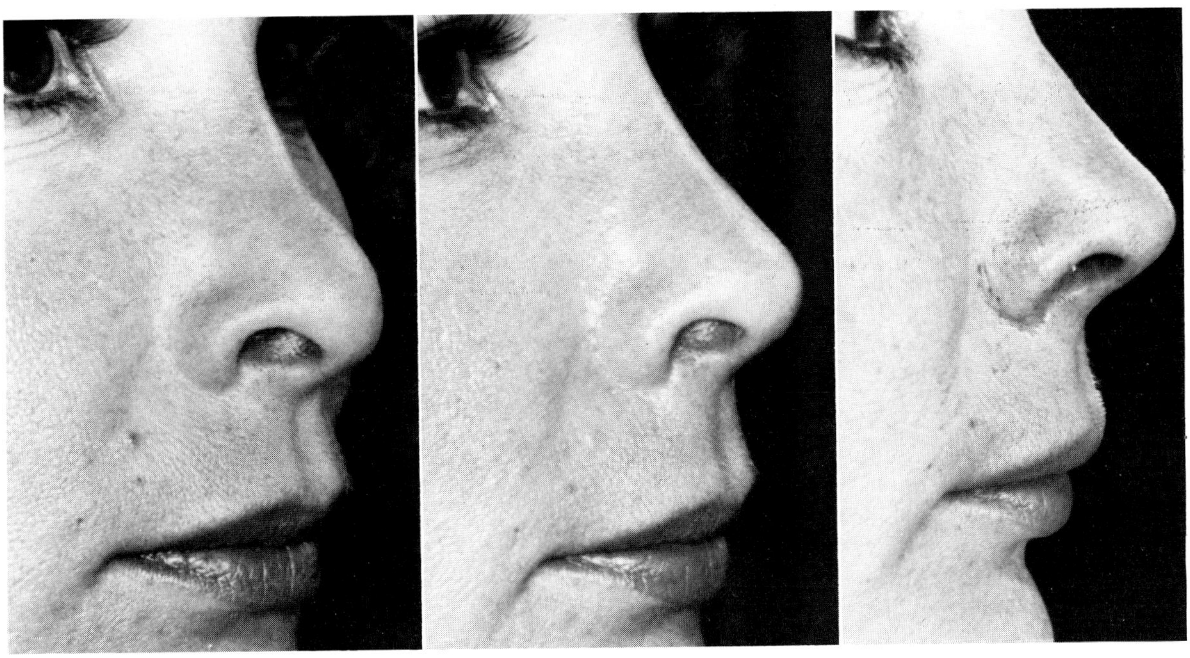

Right lateral views show the patient preoperatively, 2 years following tertiary reconstruction, and following reduction of the alar lobule and conchal cartilage tip graft, but with no incision of the nasal sill on either side. Note that 2 years after the tertiary reconstruction there is a slight decrease in the projection of the tip because of either slippage of the graft or absorption of the bony portion.

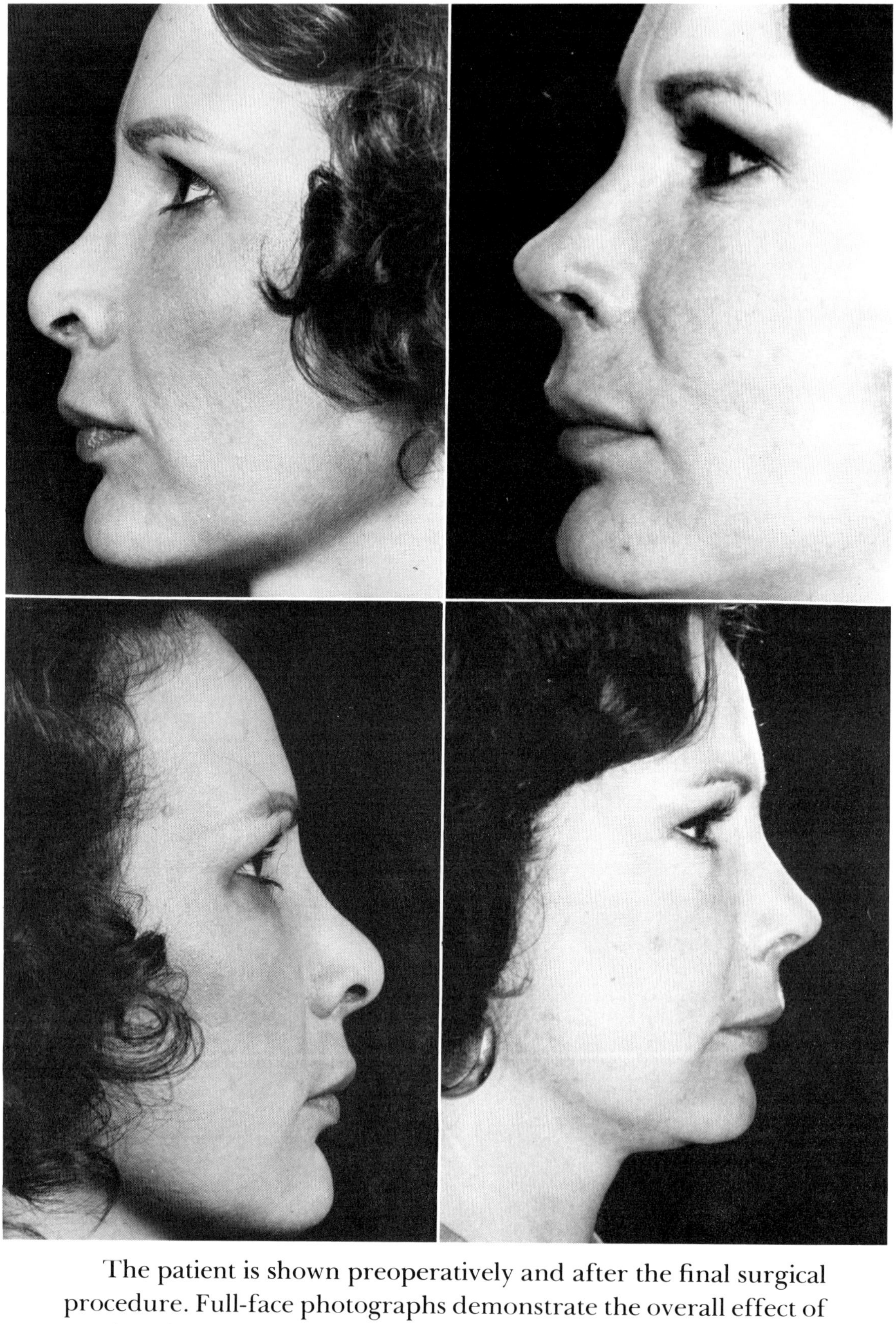

The patient is shown preoperatively and after the final surgical procedure. Full-face photographs demonstrate the overall effect of nasal and maxillary augmentation on the facial relationships.

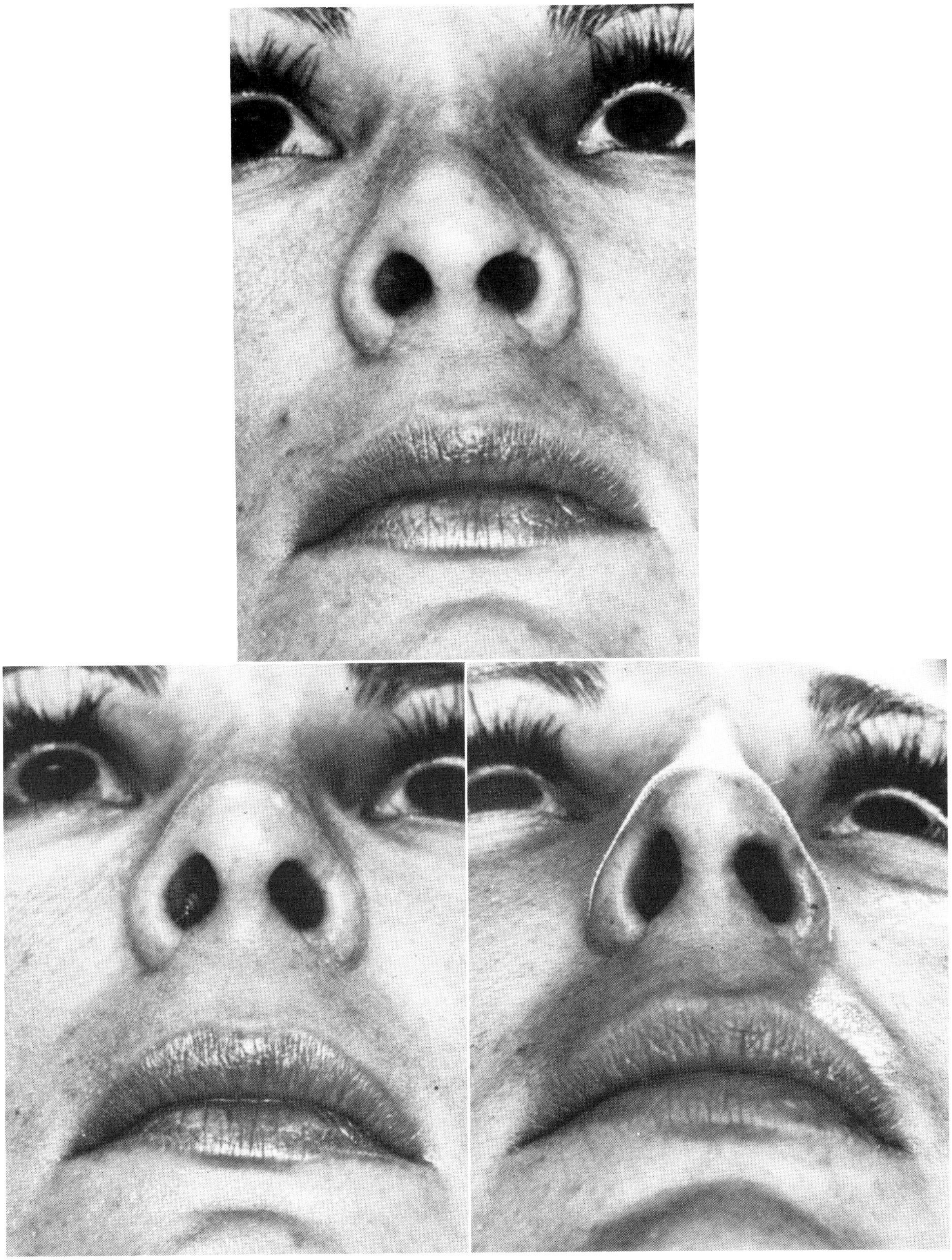

Basal views show the patient preoperatively; 2 years following tertiary reconstruction, with some resorption of the tip graft; and following conchal cartilage graft to tip and alar lobule "thinning." Note the progressive elongation of the nostrils.

Discussion

My response to the question "How would I have done this nose?" is "Conservatively." This patient had a strong, straight nose that required only some refinement. The primary aesthetic fault of the nose was a lack of differentiation of parts. My surgical plan would have been as follows:

1. Limited skeletonization, with no transfixion of membranous septum
2. Reduction of 1 to 2 mm of the bony dorsum with a rasp
3. Reduction of the cartilaginous dorsum 1 to 2 mm
4. Cephalic trim of the lower lateral cartilages, no modification of the domes
5. Lateral osteotomies
6. No resection of mucosa or cartilage from the caudal borders of the upper lateral cartilages

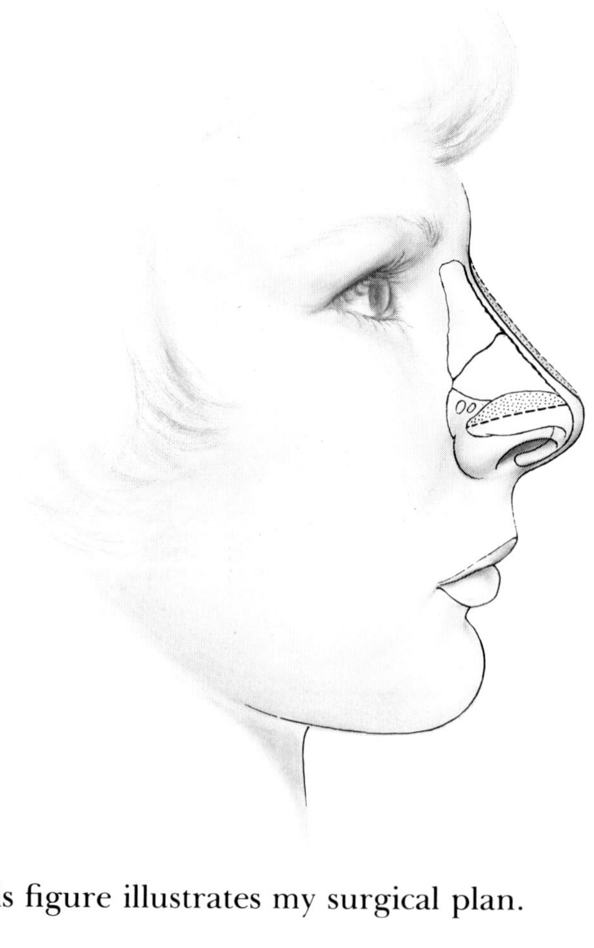

This figure illustrates my surgical plan.

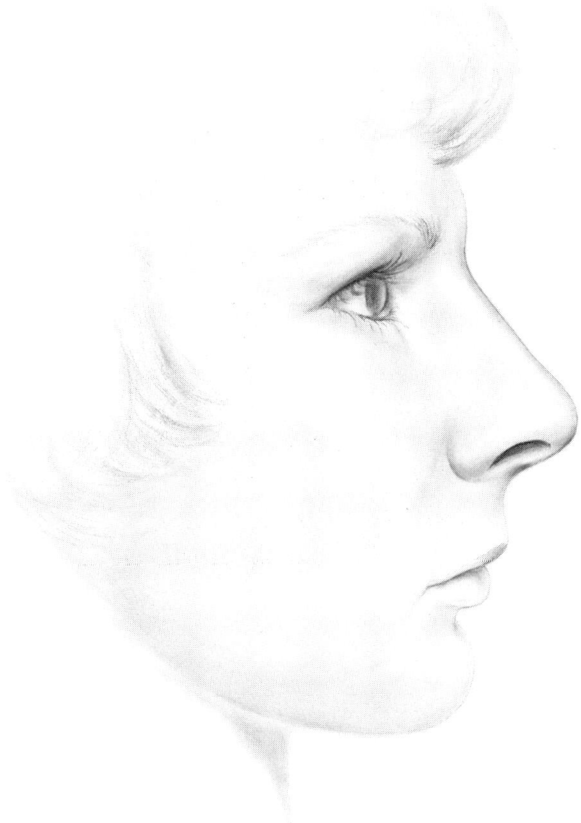

A preoperative drawing of the patient is shown on the left.

The drawing on the right illustrates the anticipated result.

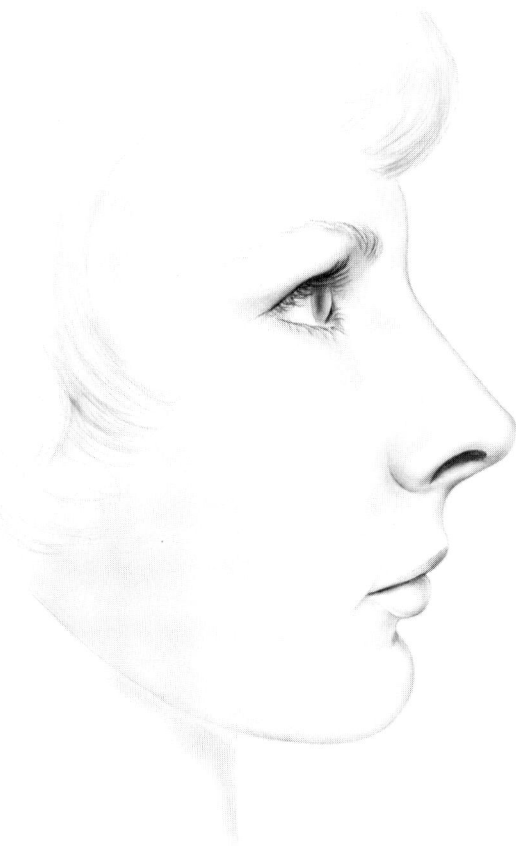

It is true that hindsight makes the right course of action seem obvious and makes what seemed obvious at the time, a question. But it is possible to foresee unfavorable results if hazards, such as the straight dorsum, are recognized. Certainly I have been humbled by less difficult cases than this. They were constructive defeats.

Although the game "duplicate bridge" cannot be applied to rhinoplasty, a hypothetical surgical plan can be tested by evaluating surgical results on similar noses. I have selected three patients whose nasal configurations are similar to the patient in the previous case report. The surgery performed on all of these patients closely paralleled the surgical plan proposed for the patient just described.

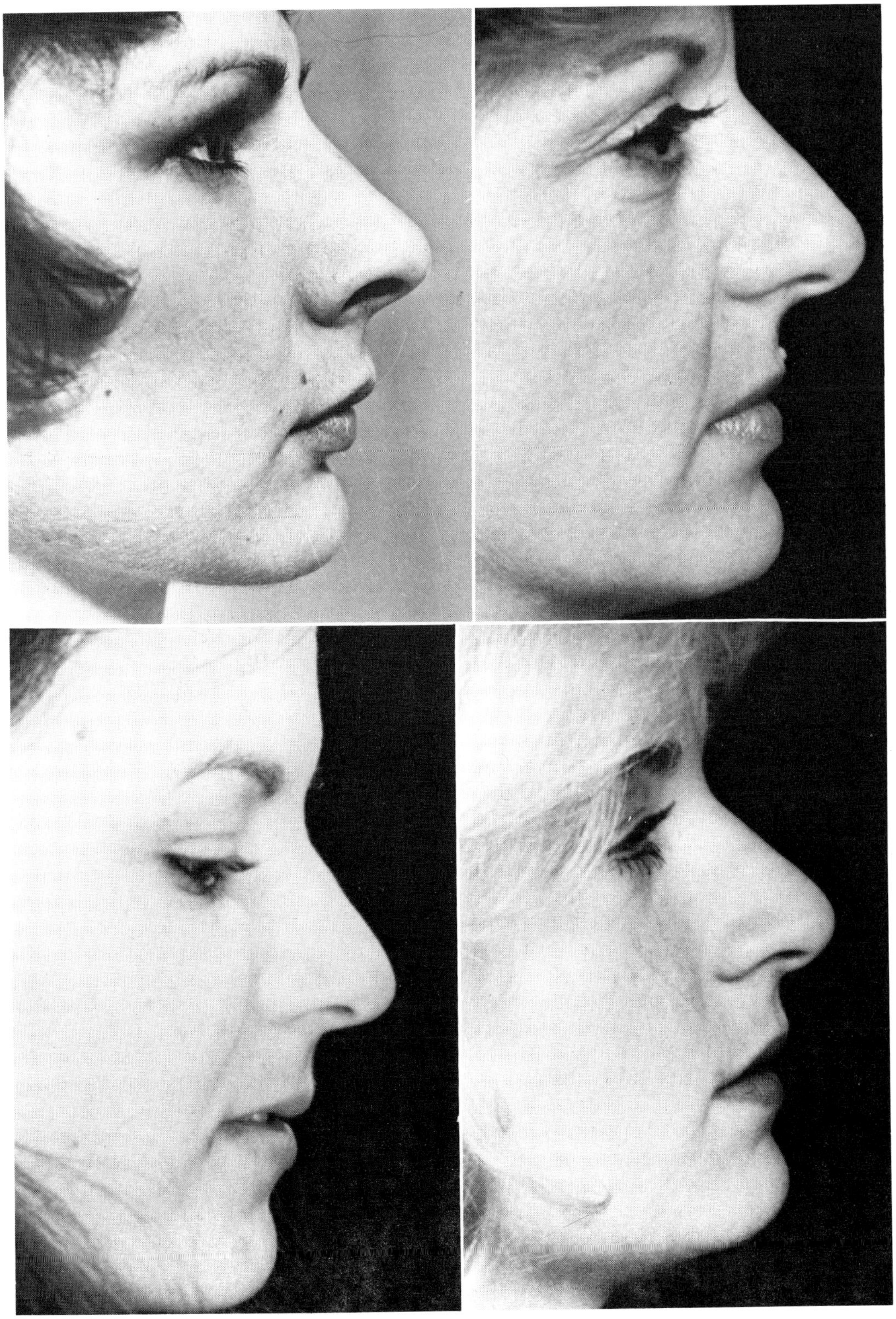

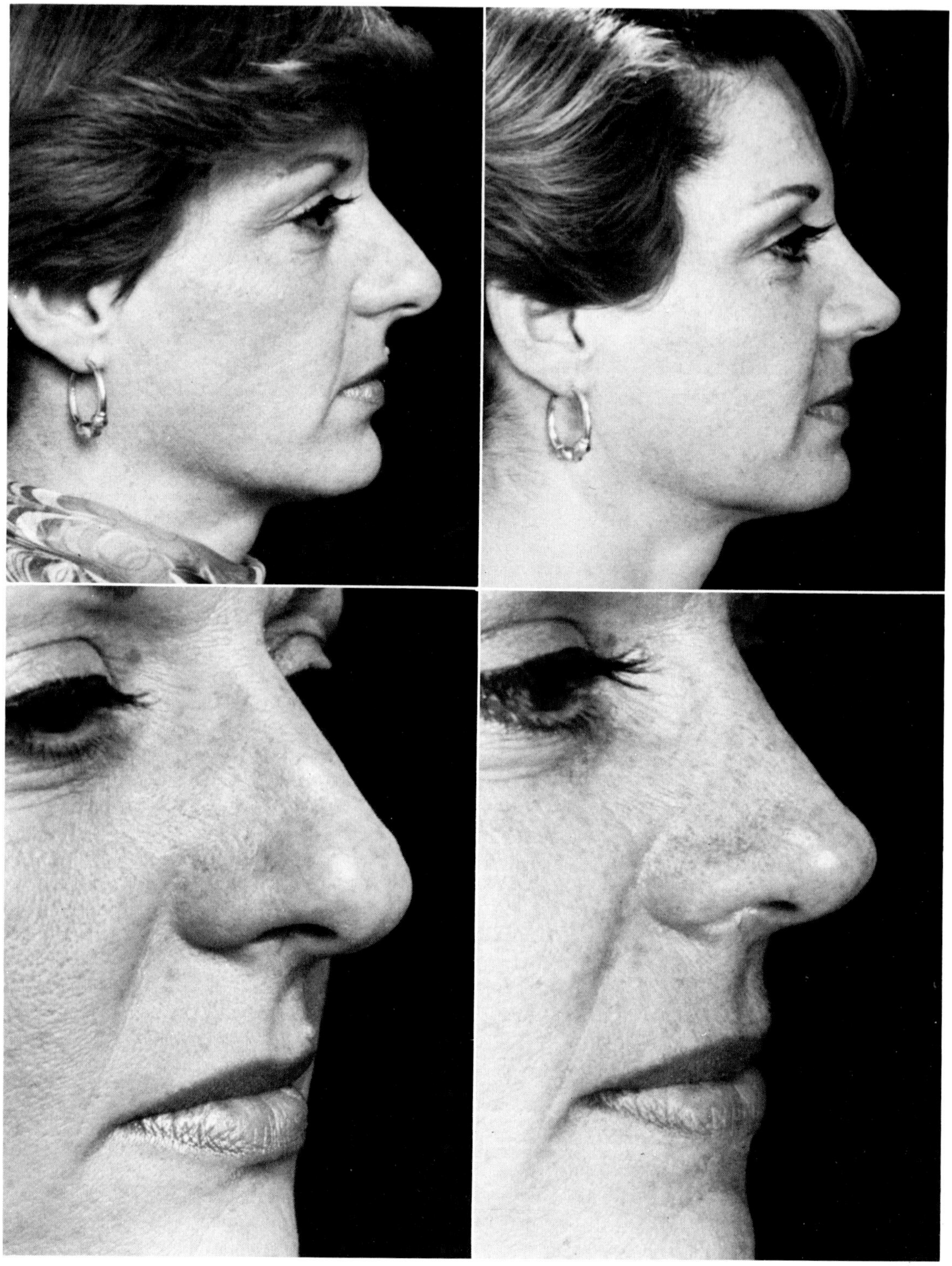

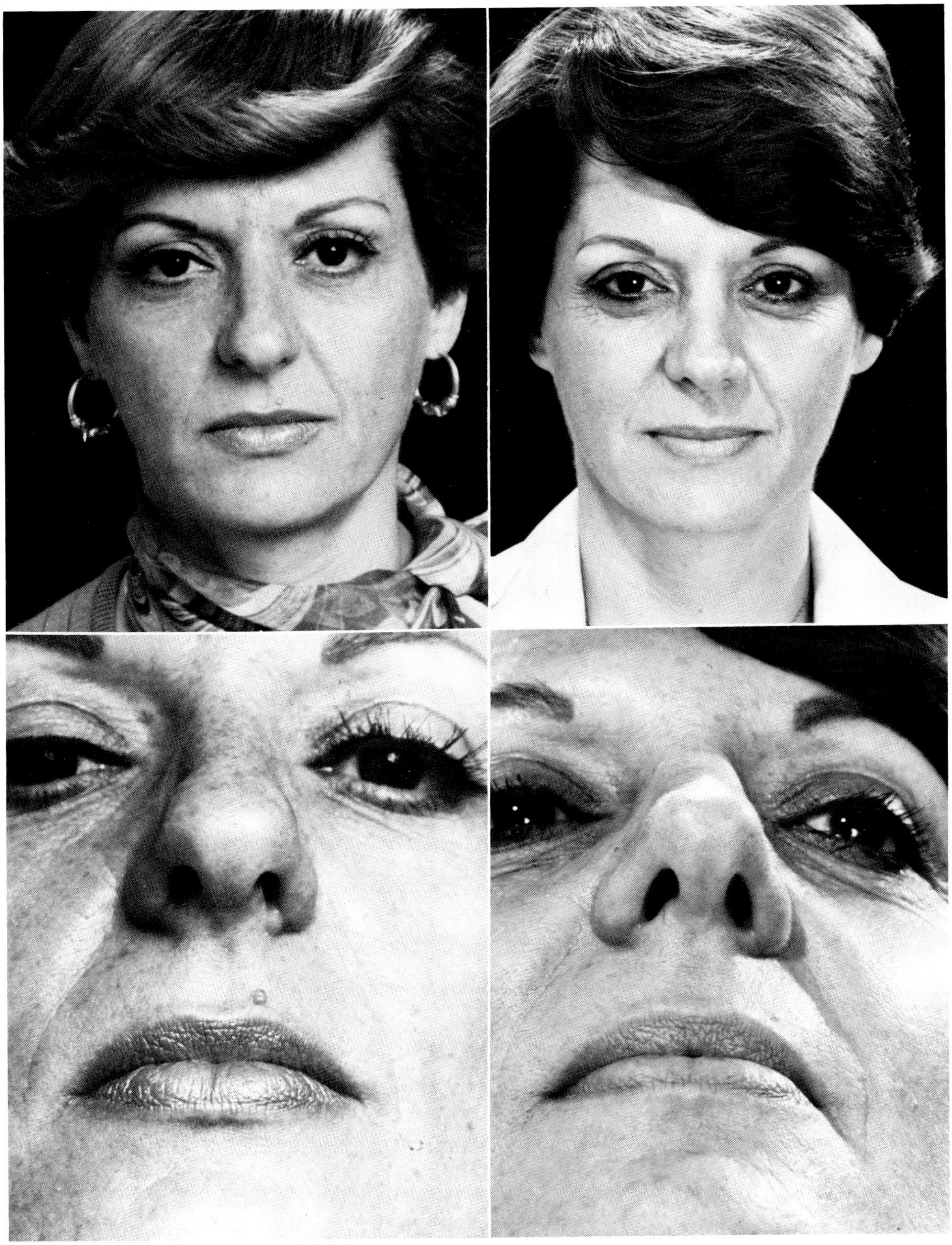

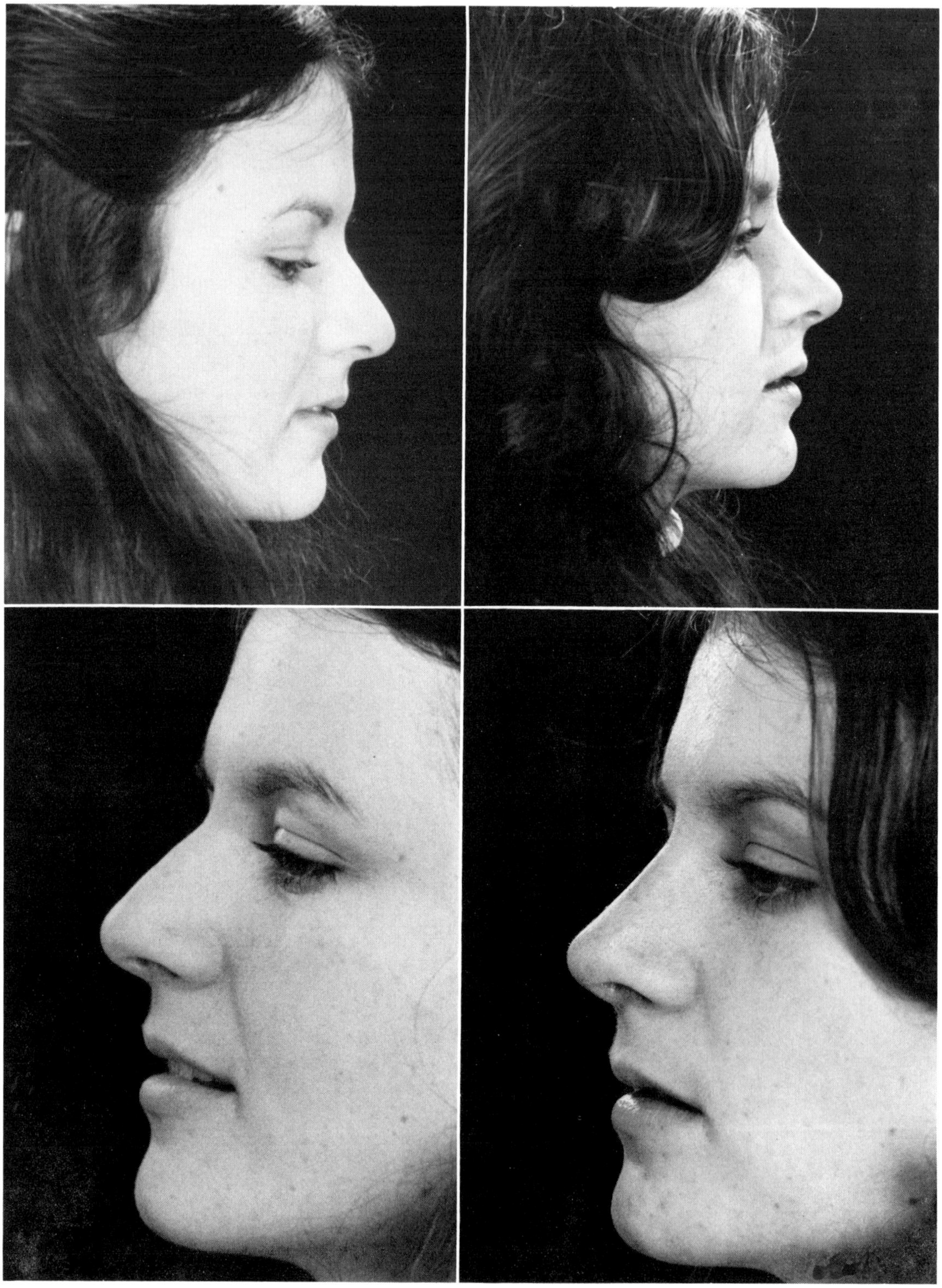

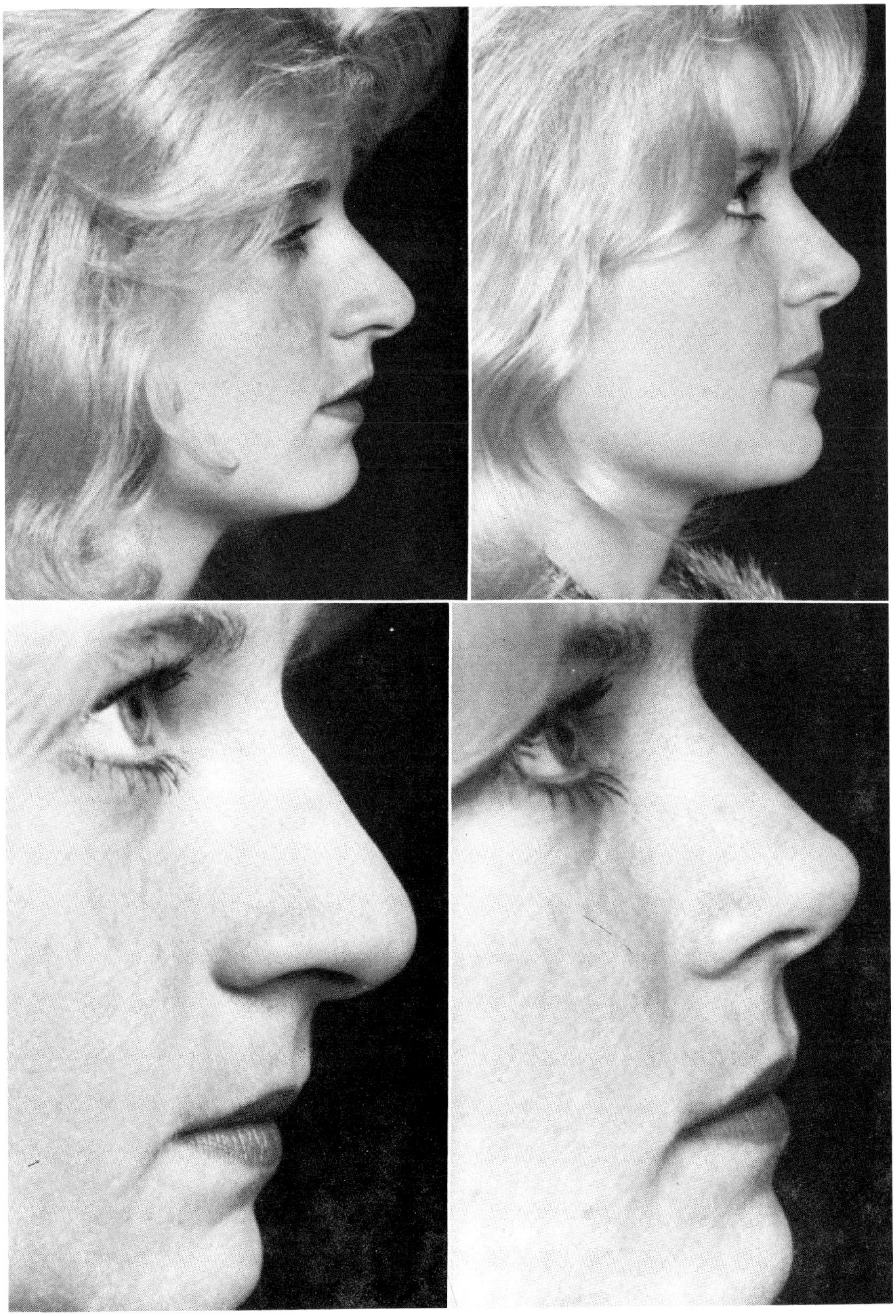

Bibliography

Benton, C. D.: Chemical cauterization of the inferior nasal turbinates, Eye Ear Nose Throat Mon. **45:**90, 1966.

Brent, B.: Personal communication, 1977.

Bridger, G. P.: Physiology of the nasal valve, Arch. Otolaryngol. **92:**543, 1970.

Brobeck, J. R., editor: Best and Taylor's physiologic basis of medical practice, ed. 9, Baltimore, 1973, The Williams & Wilkins Co.

Brown, J. B., and McDowell, F.: Plastic surgery of the nose, St. Louis, 1951, The C. V. Mosby Co.

Butler, J.: The work of breathing through the nose, Clin. Sci. Mol. Med. **19:**55, 1960.

Clark, G. M.: Analysis of nasal support, Arch. Otolaryngol. **92:**118, 1970.

Cohen, S.: Complications following rhinoplasty, Plast. Reconstr. Surg. **18:**213, 1956.

Cole, P.: Nasal turbinate function, Can. J. Otolaryngol. **2:**259, 1973.

Converse, J. M.: Reconstructive plastic surgery, Philadelphia, 1964, W. B. Saunders Co., pp. 694-828.

Cook, T. A.: Statistical analysis of the alterations of blood gases produced by nasal packing, Laryngoscope **83:**1802, 1973.

Cottle, M. H.: The structure and function of the nasal vestibule, Arch. Otolaryngol. **62:** 173, 1955.

Cottle, M. H.: Nasal breathing pressures and cardiopulmonary illness, Eye Ear Nose Throat Mon. **51:**331, 1972.

Denecke, H. J., and Meyer, R.: Plastic surgery of the head and neck; corrective rhinoplasty, New York, 1967, Springer-Verlag New York, Inc.

DeWeese, D. D., and Saunders, W. H.: Textbook of otolaryngology, ed. 5, St. Louis, 1977, The C. V. Mosby Co., pp. 187-266.

Ersner, M. S.: Rhinoplastic procedures to establish normal physiologic nasal function, Pa. Med. J. **51:**749, 1948.

Falces, E., and Gorney, M.: Use of ear cartilage grafts for nasal tip reconstruction, Plast. Reconstr. Surg. **50:**147, 1972.

Fomon, S., and Bell, J.: Rhinoplasty new concepts evaluation and application, Springfield, Ill., 1970, Charles C Thomas, Publisher.

Fomon, S., and others: Physiological principles in rhinoplasty, Arch. Otolaryngol. **53:** 256, 1951.

Fry, H. J.: Judicious turbinectomy for nasal obstruction, Aust. N.Z. J. Surg. **42:**291, 1973.

Goldwyn, R. M., and others: The unfavorable result in plastic surgery, Boston, 1972, Little, Brown & Co.

Grabb, W. C., and Smith, J. N., editors: Plastic surgery; a concise guide to clinical practice, ed. 3, Boston, Little, Brown & Co. (to be published).

Hinderer, K. H.: Diagnosis of anatomic obstructions of the airways, Arch. Otolaryngol. **78:**660, 1963.

Hinderer, K. H.: Fundamentals of anatomy and surgery of the nose, Birmingham, Ala., 1971, Aesculapius Publishing Co.

Holloway, R. M.: Nasal airway physiology, J. Fla. Med. Assoc. **58:**42, 1971.

Joseph, J.: Nasenplastic und sonstige gesichtsplastic, Leipzig, 1931, C. Kabitsch.

Kazanjian, V., and Converse, J. M.: Surgical treatment of facial injuries, ed. 3, Baltimore, 1974, The Williams & Wilkins Co., pp. 729-948.

Littell, J. J.: Partial decortication of the inferior turbinate body, Trans. Indian Acad. Ophthalmol. Otolaryngol. **45:**57, 1962.

Little, S. W.: Management of enlarged turbinates, Va. Med. Mon. **90:**484, 1963.

Maliniac, J. W.: Prevention and treatment of sequelae in corrective rhinoplasty, Am. J. Surg. **50:**84, 1940.

Masters, F. W., and Lewis, J. R.: Symposium on aesthetic surgery of the face, eyelid, and breast, St. Louis, 1973, The C. V. Mosby Co.

Masters, F. W., and Lewis, J. R.: Symposium on aesthetic surgery of the nose, ears, and chin, St. Louis, 1974, The C. V. Mosby Co.

Millard, R. D., Jr.: External excisions in rhinoplasty, Br. J. Plast. Surg. **12:**340, 1960.

Millard, R. D., Jr.: Adjuncts in augmentation mentoplasty and corrective rhinoplasty, Plast. Reconstr. Surg. **36:**48, 1965.

Millard, R. D., Jr.: Alar margin sculpturing, Plast. Reconstr. Surg. **40:**337, 1967.

Millard, R. D., Jr.: Secondary corrective rhinoplasty, Plast. Reconstr. Surg. **44:**545, 1969.

Millard, R. D., Jr.: Symposium on corrective rhinoplasty, vol. 13, St. Louis, 1976, The C. V. Mosby Co.

Murray, A. B.: The appearance of the turbinates and nasal allergy in children, Ann. Allergy **30:**245, 1972.

O'Connor, G. B., and McGregor, M. W.: Secondary rhinoplasties, Plast. Reconstr. Surg. **15:**404, 1955.

Ogura, J. H.: Physiologic relationships of the upper and lower airways, Ann. Otol. Rhinol. Laryngol. **79:**495, 1970.

Paparella, M. M., and Shumrick, D. A.: Otolaryngology, vol. 1, Basic sciences and related disciplines, Philadelphia, 1973, W. B. Saunders Co., pp. 329-346.

Peer, L. A.: The fate of autogenous septal cartilage after transplantation in human tissues, Arch. Otolaryngol. **36:**696, 1941.

Peer, L. A.: The neglected septal cartilage graft, Arch. Otolaryngol. **42:**384, 1945.

Pollet, J.: Utilisation des exérèses osteo-cartilagineuses au cours de la rhinoseptoplastie, Ann. Chir. Plast. **17:**91, 1972.

Proctor, D. F.: The nose; a defense against the atmospheric environment, Inhal. Post **1:** 59, 1970.

Proetz, A. W.: Respiratory air currents and their clinical aspects, J. Laryngol. Otol. **67:**1, 1953.

Rao, S.: Nasal airflow with body in various positions, J. Appl. Physiol. **28:**162, 1970.

Rees, T. D., and Wood-Smith, D.: Secondary rhinoplasty, Plast. Reconstr. Surg. **46:**332, 1970.

Rees, T. D., and Wood-Smith, D.: Cosmetic facial surgery, Philadelphia, 1973, W. B. Saunders Co.

Rogers, B. O.: The importance of delay in timing secondary and tertiary corrections of post-rhinoplastic deformities. In Transactions of the Fourth International Congress of Plastic and Reconstructive Surgeons, Amsterdam, 1967, Excerpta Medica.

Safian, J.: Corrective rhinoplastic surgery, New York, 1935, Paul B. Hoeber, Inc.

Schaeffer, J. P.: The nose and olfactory organ, New York, 1920, McGraw-Hill Book Co., pp. 55-56.

Seltzer, A. P.: Inferior turbinate surgery; a new technique, J. Natl. Med. Assoc. **64:**476, 1972.

Shapiro, S. L.: Concerning nasal reflexes, Eye Ear Nose Throat Mon. **49:**332, 1970.

Sheen, J. H.: Secondary rhinoplasty. In Grabb, W. C., and Smith, J. N., editors: Plastic surgery; a concise guide to clinical practice, ed. 3, Boston, Little, Brown & Co. (to be published).

Sheen, J. H.: Absorption of small bone graft in nasal tip (letter to editor), Plast. Reconstr. Surg. **56:**332, 1975.

Sheen, J. H.: Achieving more nasal tip projection by the use of a small autogenous bone or cartilage graft, Plast. and Reconstr. Surg. **56:**35, 1975.

Sheen, J. H.: Limited turbinectomy; an adjunct to rhinoplasty, presented at the American Society of Plastic and Reconstructive Surgeons meeting, Toronto, 1975 (unpublished).

Sheen, J. H.: Secondary rhinoplasty, Plast. Reconstr. Surg. **56:**135, 1975.

Sheen, J. H.: The small dorsal hump. In Transactions of the Sixth International Congress of Plastic and Reconstructive Surgeons, Paris, 1975, Masson Publishing USA, Inc., pp. 479-482.

Sheen, J. H.: Finesse in rhinoplasty. In Millard, D. R., Jr., editor: Symposium on corrective rhinoplasty, St. Louis, 1976, The C. V. Mosby Co.

Sheen, J. H.: Secondary rhinoplasty. In Millard, D. R., Jr., editor: Symposium on corrective rhinoplasty, St. Louis, 1976, The C. V. Mosby Co.

Sheen, J. H.: A new look at supratip deformity, presented at the American Society of Aesthetic Plastic Surgeons meeting, San Francisco, 1978 (unpublished).

Stark, R. B.: Plastic surgery, New York, 1962, Harper & Row, Publishers, Inc.

Taylor, G.: Assessing degree of nasal patency by measuring peak expiratory flow rate through the nose, J. Allergy Clin. Immunol. **52:**193, 1973.

Taylor, G.: The nose as a model for the study of respiratory tract allergy disease, Ann. N.Y. Acad. Sci. **221:**117, 1974.

Tresley, I. J.: Personal communication, 1964.

Von Mangoldt, F.: Reconstruction of saddlenose by cartilage overlay, Dtsch. Gesell. F. Chir. **29:**460, 1900. (Reprinted in Plast. Reconstr. Surg. **46:**498, 1970.)

Watkins, A. B.: Middle turbinate headache, Med. J. Aust. **1:**382, 1970.

Webster, R.: Personal communication, 1972.

Index

Index